Case Studies in Public Health

Case Studies in Public Health

Theodore H. Tulchinsky, MD MPH
Emeritus, Braun School of Public Health, Hebrew University,
Jerusalem, Israel
Head of School of Health Professions, Ashkelon Academic College,
Ashkelon, Israel

With: M. Joan Bickford, BSc MSN
Former Chief Public Health Nurse, Province of Manitoba, Canada

Foreword by: Walter A. Orenstein, MD DSc (Honorary)
Professor of Medicine, Pediatrics, Global Health, and Epidemiology,
Associate Director, Emory Vaccine Center, Emory University,
Atlanta, GA, United States

Recommended Citation
Tulchinsky TH. Case Studies in Public Health. Elsevier Press etc 2017

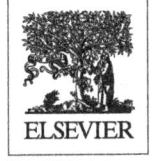
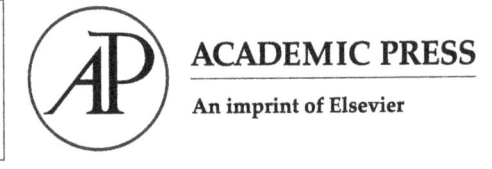

ACADEMIC PRESS
An imprint of Elsevier

Academic Press is an imprint of Elsevier
125 London Wall, London EC2Y 5AS, United Kingdom
525 B Street, Suite 1800, San Diego, CA 92101-4495, United States
50 Hampshire Street, 5th Floor, Cambridge, MA 02139, United States
The Boulevard, Langford Lane, Kidlington, Oxford OX5 1GB, United Kingdom

British Library Cataloguing-in-Publication Data
A catalogue record for this book is available from the British Library

Library of Congress Cataloging-in-Publication Data
A catalog record for this book is available from the Library of Congress

ISBN: 978-0-12-804571-8

For Information on all Academic Press publications
visit our website at https://www.elsevier.com/books-and-journals

Working together
to grow libraries in
developing countries

www.elsevier.com • www.bookaid.org

Publisher: Mica Haley
Acquisition Editor: Erin Hill-Parks and Kattie Washington
Editorial Project Manager: Tracy Tufaga
Production Project Manager: Priya Kumaraguruparan
Cover Designer: Matthew Limbert

Typeset by MPS Limited, Chennai, India

Cover image, with permission from: Consistency between US dietary fat intake and serum total cholesterol concentrations: the National Health and Nutrition Examination Surveys, by N D Ernst, C T Sempos, R R Briefel and M B Clark in *Am J Clin Nutr* (1997;66 (4 Suppl):965S−972S), American Society for Nutrition *The American Society for Nutrition, Inc., does not endorse any commercial enterprise.*

I wish to dedicate this book to the loves of my life: My wife Joan (54 years married), our children (Daniel, Joel, and Karen) and grandchildren (Guy, Noah, Amir, Ariella, Jonathan, Or, and Tommy) whose ages range from 23 to three years. Their love and support sustain me.

Contents

About the Author   xiii
Foreword   xvii
Preface   xxi
Acknowledgments   xxv

1. James Lind and Scurvy

Background   2
Current Relevance   4
Ethical Issues   6
Economic Issues   9
Conclusion   10
Recommendations   11
Student Review Questions   12
Recommended Readings   12

2. Edward Jenner, Vaccination and Eradication of Smallpox

Background   17
Current Relevance   22
Ethical Issues   23
Economic Issues   24
Conclusion   25
Recommendations   27
Student Review Questions   28
Recommended Readings   29

3. From Panum to Eradication of Measles

Background   36
Current Relevance   39
Ethical Issues   47
Economic Issues   48
Conclusion   49
Recommendations   51
Student Review Questions   51
Recommended Readings   52

4. **Semmelweiss, Credé, Lister, and Nightingale: Pioneers in Controlling Hospital Infections**

    Background   58
    Current Relevance   64
    Ethical Issues   67
    Economic Issues   70
    Conclusion   71
    Recommendations   71
    Student Review Questions   72
    Recommended Readings   73

5. **John Snow, Cholera, the Broad Street Pump; Waterborne Diseases Then and Now**

    Background   79
    Current Relevance   84
    Ethical Issues   88
    Economic Issues   91
    Conclusion   93
    Recommendations   94
    Student Review Questions   95
    Recommended Readings   95

6. **Pasteur on Microbes and Infectious Diseases**

    Background   102
    Current Relevance   109
    Ethical Issues   111
    Economic Issues   112
    Conclusion   113
    Recommendations   113
    Student Review Questions   114
    Recommended Readings   114

7. **Robert Koch and Paul Ehrlich: Criteria of Causation of Disease and Chemotherapy as "Magic Bullets"**

    Background   119
    Current Relevance   122
    Ethical Issues   124
    Economic Issues   125
    Conclusion   125
    Recommendations   127
    Student Review Questions   127
    Recommended Readings   128

8. Bismarck and the Long Road to Universal
   Health Coverage

Background	133
Current Relevance	163
Ethical Issues	164
Economic Issues	166
Conclusion	168
Recommendations	171
Student Review Questions	172
Recommended Readings	172

9. Joseph Goldberger, Pellagra, and Nutritional
   Epidemiology

Background	182
Current Relevance	190
Ethical Issues	191
Economic Issues	192
Conclusion	192
Recommendations	195
Student Review Questions	196
Recommended Readings	196

10. Endemic Goiter and Elimination of Iodine Deficiency
    Disorders

Background	202
Current Relevance	205
Ethical Issues	214
Economic Issues	216
Conclusion	216
Recommendations	218
Student Review Questions	218
Recommended Readings	219

11. Elmer McCollum and Edward Mellanby:
    Vitamin D and Cod Liver Oil for Prevention
    of Rickets and Osteoporosis

Background	229
Current Relevance	232
Ethical Issues	237
Economic Issues	240
Conclusion	241
Recommendations	243
Student Review Questions	244
Recommended Readings	245

12. **Norman Gregg and Congenital Rubella Syndrome**

Background	258
Current Relevance	261
Ethical Issues	265
Economic Issues	266
Conclusion	268
Recommendations	270
Student Review Questions	271
Recommended Readings	271

13. **Ethical Issues in Public Health**

Background	279
Current Relevance	296
Ethical Issues	306
Conclusion	308
Recommendations	309
Student Review Questions	310
Recommended Readings	311

14. **Framingham and North Karelia: Studies that Changed the Cardiovascular Disease Pandemic**

Background	318
Current Relevance	333
Ethical Issues	341
Economic Issues	343
Conclusion	345
Recommendations	348
Student Review Questions	349
Recommended Readings	350

15. **Milton Roemer, Hospital Bed Supply and Economics of Health**

Background	358
Ethical Issues	374
Economic Issues	375
Conclusion	376
Recommendations	377
Student Review Questions	378
Recommended Readings	378

16. **John Enders, Jonas Salk, Albert Sabin and Eradication of Poliomyelitis**

Background	385
Current Relevance	392

Ethical Issues 396
Economic Issues 398
Conclusion 399
Recommendations 400
Student Review Questions 401
Recommended Readings 402

17. Preventing Vitamin K Deficiency Bleeding in Newborns

Background 408
Current Relevance 411
Ethical Issues 413
Economic Issues 414
Conclusion 414
Recommendations 415
Student Review Questions 416
Recommended Readings 416

18. Eliminating Beta Thalassemia Major and Other Congenital Blood Disorders

Background 424
Current Relevance 428
Ethical Issues 432
Economic Issues 433
Conclusion 434
Recommendations 435
Student Review Questions 436
Recommended Readings 436

19. Maurice Hilleman: Creator of Vaccines That Changed the World

Background 444
Current Relevance 449
Ethical Issues 454
Economic Issues 457
Conclusion 461
Recommendations 464
Student Review Questions 465
Recommended Readings 465

20. Robert Guthrie and Nicholas Wald: Screening and Preventing Birth Defects

Background 473
Current Relevance 500

Ethical Issues	503
Economic Issues	505
Genomics/Genetics	507
Conclusion	508
Recommendations	510
Recommended Readings	511

21. Marc Lalonde, the Health Field Concept and Health Promotion

Background	524
Current Relevance	529
Ethical Issues	532
Economic Issues	533
Conclusion	535
Recommendations	536
Student Review Questions	537
Recommended Readings	537

22. Warren, Marshall, *Helicobacter Pylori*, Peptic Ulcers and Gastric Cancer

Background	545
Current Relevance	550
Ethical Issues	551
Economic Issues	552
Conclusion	553
Recommendations	554
Student Review Questions	555
Recommended Readings	555

Index	561

About the Author

I was born and raised in Brantford, Ontario, Canada as the youngest in a Jewish family including two sisters and one brother. Married to Joan Tulchinsky, my beloved wife of 54 years, we now live in Ashkelon, Israel with a magnificent view of the Mediterranean Sea. We have three children and seven grandchildren.

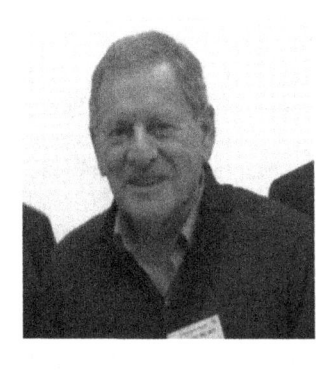

Following graduation from the University of Toronto, Faculty of Medicine in 1961, and internship in Montreal, Quebec, I went to Saskatchewan to support the province's pioneering provincial medical care insurance program bitterly opposed in the medical community by the "Doctor's Strike", resolved in compromise after 21 days. The Saskatchewan approach to public universal health insurance became the basis for Canada's much revered national health insurance Medicare program. Following practice as a primary care physician (general practice) in a Saskatoon Community Clinic and training in internal medicine at University of Saskatchewan Hospital I studied public health at Yale University graduated with a MPH in 1968. Subsequently, I became Director of a union-sponsored community clinic in Ontario.

My public health career of over 50 years began in Canada as a family physician and organizer of community clinics. Later, I served as Deputy Minister of Health and Social Development in Manitoba, responsible for a department with over 5,000 employees including social welfare and occupational health services and the mental hospitals and provincial prison.

At that time, many new innovations were occurring in Manitoba and throughout Canada. This included provincially-insured services such as home care, community mental health, nursing homes, and financial assistance with orthotics and drugs for nonhospitalized individuals. These programs based on results of provincial research of population health needs, led to alternatives to acute-care hospital-based services such as nursing homes and organized population-based community service programs.

Immigrating to Israel in 1976, I joined the Ministry of Health as head of the Public Health Service, then Coordinator of Health in the West Bank and Gaza (1980–94) up to the transfer of health responsibility to the Palestinian Authority. Key issues were safe community water supply, including implementation of mandatory chlorination and sanitation, expanding the immunization program to eradicate polio, measles, tetanus and other vaccine preventable diseases, Rift Valley Fever, occupational health and nutrition, maternal and child health, hospital specialty development, medical and other staff training programs, growth studies of children, and micronutrient fortification of flour later mandated by the Palestinian Authority.

As lead author, an internationally focused public health textbook was published in three editions from 2000 to 2014,[1] used widely in Israel, Europe, and North America by teachers, practitioners and students in academic programs. *The New Public Health* has been translated into many languages: Russian, Albanian, Bulgarian, Georgian, Moldovan, Macedonian, Mongolian, Romanian, Uzbek and Turkish Uzbek.

I taught at the Braun School of Public Health International MPH program as an external teacher continuously since 1982 until retirement with Emeritus status in 2016. The academic environment was stimulating and the interchange with students from around the world included publishing articles on global health issues with graduates in Africa and India, as well as colleagues in Israel, the West Bank, and Gaza.

I have authored more than 110 articles in peer-reviewed journals and many book chapters on a wide range of public health topics including infectious disease policies such as immunization (e.g., polio, measles, tetanus), nutrition policies, maternal and child health, blood disorders (vitamin K and thalassemia), mesothelioma, geriatric care, community health workers, public health ethics, development of academic public health education, and global health.

In the 1990s, I served as a consultant to the World Bank and later to the Open Society Institute with onsite visits to establish many schools of public health across Russia as well as in Central Europe (Macedonia, Moldova, Albania, Bulgaria and Georgia), and in Central Asia (Kazakhstan, Uzbekistan, and Mongolia).

From 2004 to 2008, I was a member of the Executive Board of the Association of Schools of Public Health in the European Region (ASPHER). I served on the Ethics and Undergraduate Education Working Groups. In 2010 I was awarded the ASPHER's *Andreas Stampar Medal* "for excellence in promoting public health education in Europe". I also continued to work with the Israel Ministry of Health on nutrition issues.

Since 2010, I have been the Deputy Editor of *Public Health Reviews* and also developer and Head of the School of Health Professions including a BA program in public health at Ashkelon Academic College, the first undergraduate public health education program in Israel. In 2016, I was coordinator/moderator of Salzburg Workshops on behalf of the Austrian-American

1. TH Tulchinsky, EA Varavikova, *The New Public Health*, Third Edition. San Diego: Academic Press/Elsevier, 2014

Foundation and ASPHER on the topics "Migrant and Minority Health" and "New Issues in Public Health Education."

Case Studies in Public Health published by Academic/Elsevier Press in 2018 is the outcome of a long career in public health practice, teaching, and publication. I hope it will contribute to student and public appreciation of how population health advanced so much in the past two and a half century, and what it can achieve in the coming decades of the 21st century.

Theodore H. Tulchinsky, MD MPH

Foreword

Tremendous gains in our overall health and duration of life have been made over the past two centuries. For example, the National Institute on Aging estimates among eight industrialized countries that the average life expectancy during the 1840s was <50 years.[1] In contrast, the life expectancy was >80 years by the 2000s. Since 1900, the average lifespan in the United States has lengthened by more than 30 years; 25 years of this gain are attributable to advances in public health.[2]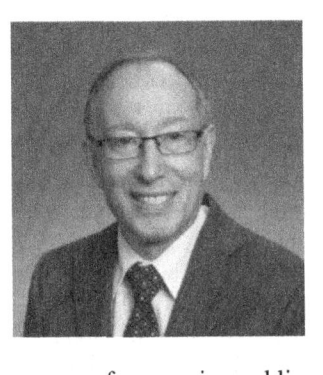

Much of the credit deserved for these advances comes from major public health breakthroughs including discoveries related to sanitation, water and food safety, the adverse effects of nutritional deficiencies and ways to prevent them, the role of infectious diseases and ways to prevent and treat them, determination of causes of chronic diseases and supporting diagnosis, treatment and prevention, and much more. There has been an epidemiologic transition with a shift from infectious and parasitic diseases to chronic diseases as the leading causes of death—even in developing countries—and the many advances in science and practical methods of prevention have made public health vital for the future of global health.

While one is often tempted to focus just on the "hard science," the results of scientific observations and/or experiments, scientific breakthroughs often take a long time until they become common knowledge and accepted by the public health and medical professions, and the public at large. What it has taken are champions who have insights, who perform the science, put the information together to convince others, deal with skeptics, and push, push, and push until the world accepts the findings and, more importantly, acts on those findings.

---

1. National Institute on Aging. Global health and aging: living longer. Available at: https://www.nia.nih.gov/research/publication/global-health-and-aging/living-longer (accessed 18.05.17).
2. Centers for Disease Control and Prevention. Ten great public health achievements—United States, 1900–1999. MMWR Morb Mort Wkly Rev. 1999;48(12):241–243. Available at: https://www.cdc.gov/mmwr/preview/mmwrhtml/00056796.htm (accessed 19.05.17).

Case Studies in Public Health by Ted Tulchinsky contains a superlative collection of stories of many of the key people who have changed our lives for the better, and in so doing, the book provides lessons on approaches to what can be done in the future to improve the quality of our lives and life expectancy. The stories range from the pivotal discovery of vaccines by Edward Jenner, the first epidemiologic study of nutritional deficiencies and how to correct them by James Lind in 1756, the sentinel epidemiologic study by John Snow determining the role of contaminated water in the Broad St Pump causing cholera epidemics, other pioneers besides Jenner in vaccine development and much more.

There is a strong focus on modern public health matters, including the importance of nutritional deficiencies and socioeconomic status as significant underlying factors in population health. Both the social sciences and the hard sciences, and their interrelationships, are factors in achieving better health through immunization and living circumstances, especially in developing countries.

As a vaccinologist, I have always been intrigued by the story of Jenner, who recognized that milk maids with cowpox lesions were protected against smallpox. It is remarkable how this pioneering physician, took pus from a lesion of the milkmaid, Sarah Nelmes, and inoculated a boy, James Phipps, whom he later challenged with smallpox virus and showed that he was protected. Jenner had to finance publication of his superb report on his findings. His work formed the basis of modern vaccinology albeit at the time based on empirical observations and now based on many factors including a much better understanding of immunology, infectious etiologies, pathogenesis, genetics, and sociology of vaccine acceptance. From this beginning in 1796, the world health community managed to eradicate the horrific scourge of smallpox by 1980, showing the way to eliminate many other infectious diseases including poliomyelitis, measles, and others.

Tulchinsky devotes multiple chapters to vaccine pioneers, including Louis Pasteur, the developer of rabies vaccine and considered by many as the founder of modern day immunology, Jonas Salk and Albert Sabin, developers of polio vaccines, and Maurice Hilleman, the outstanding 20th century developer of many of the vaccines in use globally today including those against measles, mumps, rubella, varicella, hepatitis A and B, and others.

The list of chapters reads like a "Who's Who" in public health starting with the discovery of scurvy around 1756 by Lind going all the way to the discovery of *Helicobacter pylori* and its role in cancer in the 1980s by Warren and Marshall. Tulchinsky does not focus on "every key contributor" to our public health. That would be impossible. But his stories are illustrative of what goes into making a major impact. The text gives the reader the opportunity to learn from history to make new and deeply significant history in mitigating the health burden of diseases during the rest of the 21st century, and beyond.

The book is outstanding because its author has himself made major contributions to public health and understands from personal experience what the obstacles are which need to be overcome to make an impact. He is currently Emeritus with the Braun School of Public Health and Community Medicine of Hebrew University-Hadassah and Head of the School of Health Professions at Ashkelon Academic College. Dr. Tulchinsky is the lead author of a textbook of public health now in its third edition. He has been Deputy Editor of *Public Health Reviews* since 2010 and has worked in numerous areas of public health in Canada, Israel, the West Bank, and Gaza, countries of the former Soviet Union and the Balkans. His fields of professional activity range from health planning, vaccination policy, primary health care, nutrition, water chlorination, occupational health, and more.

His background and experience provide a great basis for framing the contributions of major public health pioneers, which in turn will hopefully motivate even greater achievements for the future of population and individual health globally. I predict that this book should be great for students to educate them in what it takes to make major contributions to our health. Hopefully it will inspire students to aspire to achievements and to become our next generation of public health heroes.

Walter A. Orenstein, MD, DSc (Honorary)
Professor of Medicine, Pediatrics, Global Health, and Epidemiology,
Associate Director, Emory Vaccine Center, Emory University, Atlanta, GA, United States

Preface

The Classic Epidemiologic Triangle and its Wider Context

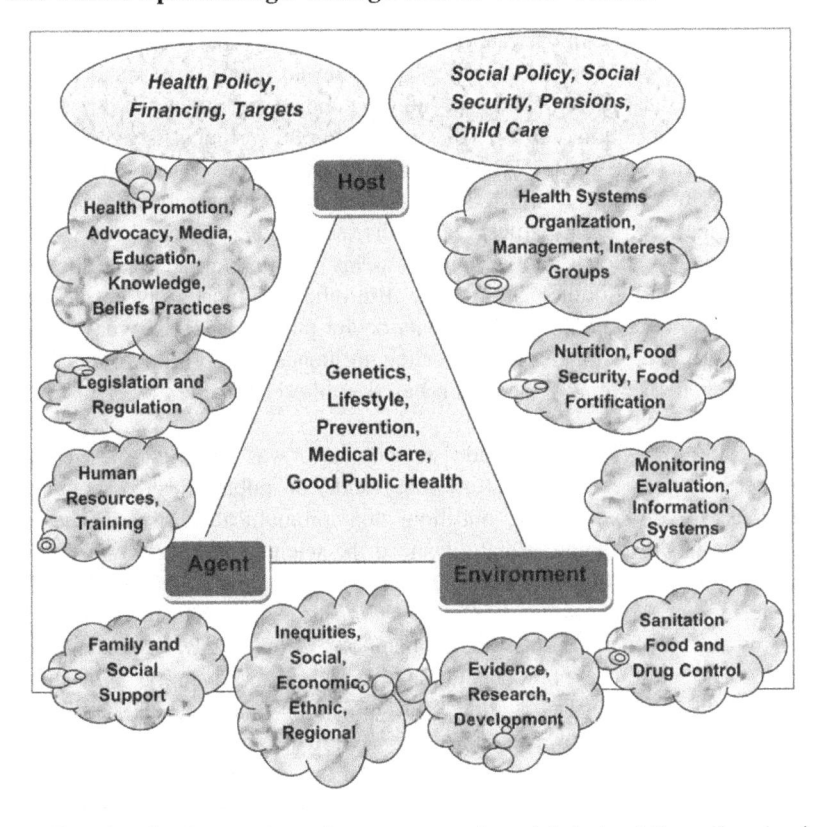

The triangle shown above is a conceptual model derived from the classic infectious disease triangle of epidemiology (Host-Agent-Environment) with the modifications of Lalonde[1] adding genetics and medical care including public health and health promotion. As seen in this figure, disease causation is complex with many surrounding personal, familial, and societal factors that impinge on population health. Over the years, public health has evolved conceptually from the classic model of disease-recognizing contextual

---

1. Lalonde, M. *A New Perspective on the Health of Canadians*. Ottawa: Government of Canada, 1974.

factors that impinge on health including education, employment, poverty, societal protection programs, organization of health care, and others. The figure represents the immediate factors as well as the many contributory societal influences on population health and wellbeing.

The case study approach chosen for this book is meant to provide examples of the development of breakthrough ideas of public health, and the struggles for their acceptance, that over time changed the world for the better forever. Hopefully these stories will show students and readers how the role of individuals created game-changing events which happened and how their issues remain with us today.

The case studies demonstrate how public health workers of today should appreciate the contributions of those described and how we all stand on the shoulders of these precursors, and other game changers, as in Sir Isaac Newton's elegant quotation: "If I have seen a little further it is by standing on the shoulders of giants." These people did not discover new continents, nor conquer other nations, nor write great literature or music, but they started processes that won great battles against diseases, and so changed the world. Some are widely known and recognized as history-making personas, such as Louis Pasteur and Florence Nightingale. But others included may not be recognizable by name among professionals or the public, or often even among public health professionals. And yet their influence was profound and their contribution helped make population-based public health the powerful force for good that it became.

Choosing the cases to include in this book was not easy. I tried to select people who worked in different fields of public health, including infectious diseases, sanitation, nutrition, non-communicable diseases, health policy, and health promotion that advanced the science and practice of public health, changing the life expectancy and wellbeing of populations globally.

The idea of *Case Studies in Public Health* arose in 2000, in discussions with my wife Joan and with international MPH students while teaching at the Braun School of Public Health at the Hebrew University, Jerusalem, Israel, along with preparation of *The New Public Health* (NPH) textbook. The initial work was, however, put aside to prepare second (2009) and third (2014) editions of *The New Public Health*. In the earlier stage, during 2005, I had the assistance of many wonderful, capable young international MPH students and summer interns at the Braun School of Public Health.

In 2015, a proposal for a book on Case Studies submitted to Elsevier was sent to external academic reviewers and accepted after receiving favorable comments with helpful suggestions. So the project restarted in 2015 and being published in 2018 being a little later than hoped due to unavoidable factors.

Despite the great advances that arose from these outstanding pioneers, in many of the cases the issues they dealt with are still present in the world, so that revisiting them can help students and community leaders to understand—and face dealing with—present and future health issues.

We live in a world of ever-increasing globalization, migration, demographic, epidemiologic, and technological changes with many unresolved health issues and new challenges appearing frequently. Yet, the potential for improving population health has been demonstrated beyond doubt, including in low-income countries by successes such as those achieved in the United Nations initiated Millennium Development Goals. International cooperation has proven to be effective in reducing the burden of many diseases and elimination of some such as smallpox, and soon poliomyelitis, with others to follow such as measles, rubella, and even "neglected tropical diseases" such as river blindness (onchocerciasis) and leprosy.

Although society has made noteworthy gains in longevity, we cannot be complacent to the need for constant pursuit of science of factors and interventions for old challenges such as tuberculosis and malaria, along with new and changing disease patterns. The search for new methods and strategies is vital to improve population health. This includes universal health access programs with a clear understanding of their organization for effective use of resources.

This book is intended to be of interest not only to students in academic public health programs, but also to others in the health field, such as analysts, policy-makers, economists, lawyers, and others. Public health should be a subject taught in undergraduate and graduate schools for other professionals whose work relates to health and who will participate in the ongoing evolution of public health and the search for appropriate universal care access, standards and policies, and for addressing the challenges of inequality.

I hope readers will appreciate and internalize the struggles and achievements of risk-taking pioneers who developed dramatically successful approaches to improve population health. This will help students to understand the struggles and potential contribution of individuals and foster a sense of personal commitment to be involved in the search for ways to improve the health of the world's population, whether in local communities, nationally or internationally.

Theodore H. Tulchinsky, MD MPH[1,2]
[1]Ashkelon Academic College, Ashkelon, Israel,
[2]Emeritus, Braun School of Public Health, Hebrew University, Jerusalem, Israel

Acknowledgments

This book was conceived in 2005, but set aside for 10 years with demands associated with preparing the second (2005) and third (2014) editions of *The New Public Health*.

Case Studies could not have been accomplished without the steadfast support, dedication, high-quality ideas and editing of Joan Bickford of Winnipeg, Manitoba, retired Chief Public Nurse, Manitoba Health, a colleague since the 1970s.

I want to thank my wife Joan for raising ideas for the development of these cases and Professor Walter Orenstein of Emory University for kindly agreeing to prepare a Foreword to this book.

Many students and interns at the Braun School of Public Health have worked on this book since 2005. Among these are Shiri Ourian, Yael Wolfe Sagy, Alex Brown, and Ann Blake. My thanks to Dr EA Varavikova for co-authorship of *The New Public Health*, over the period 1992 to 2014.

Many colleagues in Canada, Israel, and other countries have been invaluable confidants in developing a range of ideas over my career.

Editing assistance from Lore Leighton (Paris), Lisa Ploeg (Portugal), and Amanda Shriwise (WHO) was enormously helpful in the later stages of preparation.

My appreciation also goes to Elsevier staff who kept the process moving including Kattie Washington, Erin Hill Parks, Tracy Tufaga, Julia Haynes, Sandhya Narayanan, and especially to the technical staff headed by Priya Kumaraguruparan in Chennai, India.

I also wish to express special appreciation to the courtesies of sources and organizations which provided access to information and/or photos displayed in each chapter. These included: the Centers for Disease Control and Prevention; World Health Organization; the Wellcome Foundation; the US National Institutes of Health; the National Library of Medicine; the Framingham Heart Study; the Smithsonian Institution; the American Society for Nutrition; the American Heart Association; the Edward Jenner Museum, the John Snow Society; the James Lind Library; Dr. Androulla Eleftheriou of the International Thalassaemia Federation (ITF), Nicosia, Cyprus; the College of Physicians of Philadelphia History of Vaccines; the US National Library of Medicine; the Danish Royal Society; Merck Company; the United Nations Multimedia, the James Lind Library; World Health Organization Infographics;

the Reference Laboratory for Haemoglobinopathies, Ministry of Health, Nikosia, Cyprus; the Cooley's Anemia Foundation; the Florence Nightingale Museum; the Wellcome Trust Science Museum; the University of California Los Angeles (UCLA) Jonathan and Karin Fielding School of Public Health; the Semmelweiss Society International, the Universities of Vienna and Pest; the University of Sydney Archives; the Harvard University Francis A Countway Library of Medicine, Department of Rare Books and Special Collections; the Hauck Center for the Sabin Archives, University of Cincinnati Libraries; the Jonas Salk Polio Vaccine Collection, University of Pittsburgh Library System, University of Pittsburgh; the Saint Louis University Libraries, Saint Louis, MO; the London School of Economics Image Library; Marxists Internet Archive; the Science Museum UK; the Pasteur Institute Paris; President Franklin Delano Roosevelt Presidential Museum, President Lyndon Baines Johnson Presidential Library; the White House Museum; PKUTest; Wikimedia; the March of Dimes; and other organizations which provided access to the photos displayed in each chapter.

Special thanks belong to the families and individuals who kindly gave permission to publish photos of their family members cited in this book including Lorraine Hilleman, Patricia Guthrie, Joan Douglas, Robin Warren and Barry Marshal, and Marc Lalonde.

Appreciation is also extended to Ashkelon Academic College for a grant to assist in editing this book and to organizations which provided access to the photos displayed in each chapter.

With kind regards and thanks to all, I take personal responsibility for this project to summarize selected game-changing ideas and struggles of pioneers in health. I hope to have given them the admiration and respect they deserve, along with their institutions, colleagues, friends, and families, made spectacular contributions to conquer diseases and save the lives of countless millions of people from much suffering and premature death. They advanced population health globally, and yet there is still so much more that needs to be done.

Ted Tulchinsky
27 February 2018

Chapter 1

James Lind and Scurvy

ABSTRACT

Scurvy is a disease that results from lack of fresh fruit and vegetables, now known to be caused by vitamin C (ascorbic acid) deficiency, causing symptoms of fatigue, lethargy, limb pains, swollen and bleeding gums, joint pain, shortness of breath on exertion, skin bruising, and, if untreated, death. Identified as a disease in the 16th century and widely attributed to infection, it was common among seamen with disastrous loss of life on long voyages. In 1747, James Lind, a young naval surgeon, conducted a clinical trial of comparing nutritional treatment of sailors with scurvy, which showed the cure to be citrus fruit, and reported on his finding to the Royal Society. The Royal Navy later made consumption of lemon juice mandatory to preserve the health of sailors and to allow ships to stay at sea longer. Lind's study is considered a first in epidemiology as a case-control study opening the field of nutritional epidemiology with vital public health implications that continue today. Scurvy gradually passed from public health consciousness but vitamin C has recently attracted attention as a common micronutrient deficiency globally with dietary intake of fruit and vegetables daily, and vitamin C fortification of basic foods as public health nutritional intervention.

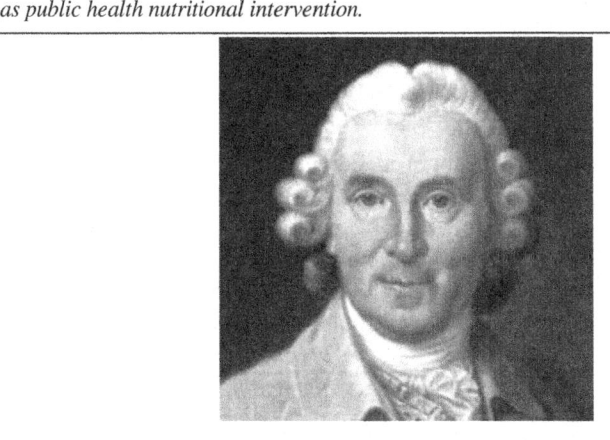

James Lind (1716–1794) a 30-year-old surgeon's mate on HMS Salisbury in 1746 conducted the first documented randomized controlled clinical-epidemiologic trial using various nutritional regimens for sailors sick with scurvy, and reported: *"They all in general had putrid gums, skin spots and lassitude, with weakness of their knees. Two others had each two oranges and one lemon given them every day. These they ate with greediness, at different times, upon an empty stomach. The consequence was, that the most sudden and visible good effects were perceived from the use of oranges and lemons; one of those who had taken them, being at the end of 6 days fit for duty."* Source: James Lind—Quotes. Available at: http://www.sciencemuseum.org.uk/broughttolife/people/jameslind.

Case Studies in Public Health. DOI: http://dx.doi.org/10.1016/B978-0-12-804571-8.00018-4
1

BACKGROUND

Studies in nutritional sciences began in the early 18th and 19th centuries with identification of the basic food elements - carbohydrates, protein and fats. Revolutionary developments that enabled identification of the elements led to the development of methods of testing with chemical analysis, quantitative analysis and new scientific approaches to nutrition. Development of studies in chemistry and physiology advanced the field, which today is still dynamic and productive of information vital to public health.

The practice of nutrient supplementation of foods dates back to the year 400 BCE when the Persian physician Melanpus suggested adding iron filings to wine to increase soldiers' "potency." In 1831, the French physician Boussingault urged adding iodine to salt to prevent goiter. In 1912, Casimir Funk identified "vital amines" as essential trace elements for human health. With the development of nutritional sciences from the early part of the 20th century, knowledge grew rapidly of the vital role of vitamins and minerals, now called essential micronutrients, and they became part of the public health arena.

Scurvy was a common illness and cause of death for ship crews on long sea voyages during the 17th and 18th centuries. Although no scientific knowledge of the cause of scurvy existed, in 1617, John Woodall, a surgeon and author of *Surgeon's Mate*, described the disease. He listed lemon juice as the cure, which was subsequently adopted by the East India Company, which started providing lemon juice for its sailors. The famed round-the-world voyage of a Royal Navy fleet of eight ships led by Commodore George Anson in 1740−44 lost a majority (145 men survived out of a total of nearly two thousand, most dying of scurvy), of the sailors who died from the "great sea plague" as scurvy was then called.

James Lind (1716−1794) was born in Edinburgh in 1716, the son of an Edinburgh merchant with family medical connections. In 1731 he was apprenticed to an Edinburgh surgeon supplemented by studies at Edinburgh University Medical School. He joined the Royal Navy in 1738 as a surgeon's mate and in 1740 was posted to the 50-gun vessel HMS Salisbury. His major works included *"Treatise of the Scurvy"* published in Edinburgh in 1753, *"An Essay on the Most Effectual Means of Preserving the Health of Seamen."* (1762), and *"An Essay on Diseases Incidental to Europeans in Hot Climates"* (1771).

On a ten-week voyage in 1746 scurvy struck 80 out of 350 sailors on the Salisbury. Lind then at age 30, with little academic education, undertook an investigation of the problem by randomly assigning 12 sailors sick with scurvy to different dietary regimens. Each group of two received a different diet of frequently recommended regimens for a two week period while Lind monitored progress of the clinical picture. One group was given oranges and lemons, others seawater, cider, vinegar, or various medications thought to be effective against scurvy. This study is recognized as the first recorded experimental randomized controlled clinical trial, which became a hallmark of general and nutritional epidemiology.

The sailors in Lind's study who received lemon and other citrus fruits showed dramatic clinical improvement within several days, in such a way that one was able to help care for the other group of sailors in the trial who did not improve. Lind reported in his book *Treatise of the Scurvy* that in a short time this group was fit for duty. Lind further concluded that "*experience indeed sufficiently shows that green or fresh vegetables with ripe fruit were the best remedies for it (scurvy), so they prove the most effectual preservatives against it,*" and "*oranges are the most effectual preservatives against the distemper.*" Lind also promoted hygienic improvements in ventilation, regular bathing, changes of clothing and bedding for sailors to reduce infectious diseases including typhus.

Lind found difficulty convincing naval authorities of the importance of these findings. Captain James Cook (1728−1779), one of the greatest sea explorers of all time, took great efforts to maintain the health of his seamen on his circumnavigation voyages with ventilation and mandatory hygiene and antiscorbutic foods. During his second voyage, a companion ship, whose captain paid less attention to diet and hygiene of the sailors, experienced many cases of scurvy, while Cook's crew members were free of scurvy. Cook documented the benefits in health of sailors on his ship as compared to the companion ship which ignored these requirements in his official logbook of the voyage.

Further efforts by experts on scurvy, such as Gilbert Blane (1749−1834) and Thomas Trotter (1760−1832), and the documented experience of seasoned sailors such as Captain Cook on the efficacy of dietary discipline in preserving the health of his crews on long sea voyages, helped convince the British Admiralty. In 1796, the Admiralty mandated daily issuing lemon juice to all sailors at sea to prevent scurvy. Application of the new dietary regulations eliminated scurvy from the Royal Navy, allowing voyages to go beyond the previous 6−8 week limit of sea time without replenishment of supplies of fresh vegetables, shore leave, or both. A naval expert of the time noted that this effectively doubled the fighting strength of the Royal Navy at sea during the Napoleonic wars of 1797−1814, in a common saying of the time that Lind, as much as Nelson, broke the power of Napoleon. In 1867, the British Parliament mandated provision of a daily lime ration to sailors in all ships of both the Royal Navy and the Merchant Navy to prevent scurvy. This resulted in the use of the term "limey" for British sailors and British people generally in America.

Lind's study was the first clinical-epidemiologic study, and is considered the first randomized control trial (RCT). It was also the first documentation of effective intervention in a nutritional-occupational disease. Identification of an active nutritional factor led to cure and prevention of a well known clinical disease of major public heath importance. Lind anticipated the discovery of vitamins by 150 years, describing "*various qualities, of which all*" *vegetables possess one or more in various degrees, and do from thence accordingly become more or less antiscorbutic."*

Vitamin C was isolated from lemon juice in 1932 by Hungarian and British scientists. The Nobel Prize for Physiology or Medicine was awarded to Albert Szent-Györgyi for his studies of the biological functions of L-ascorbic acid (vitamin C). In 1937 the Nobel Prize for Chemistry was awarded to two scientists. Norman Haworth received the Prize for his investigations on carbohydrates and vitamin C and "for determining the structure of ascorbic acid" Paul Karrer received the Prize "for his investigations on carotenoids, flavins and vitamins A and B2". Further studies of the nutritional and public health importance of vitamin C are ongoing. Examples of these are studies on how to enhance the nutritional value of ascorbic acid in agricultural crops, for prevention of heart disease, stroke, and cancer.

CURRENT RELEVANCE

Nutritional sciences in the 19th century focused mainly on calories, carbohydrates, protein, and fats. Early in the 20th century, the identification of other essential or "vital amines", later shortened to vitamins, became part of the field of study. Lind's demonstration that specific foods that could cure and prevent a serious disease of sailors on long voyages proved to be a prescient change in nutritional science, and pioneered the development of the vital research methods of the clinical trial.

Today, micronutrient deficiencies (MNDs) of vitamins and minerals that are necessary for health, especially for pregnant women, children and adults, are considered to affect some 2 billion persons globally. Vitamins are organic compounds that are essential in small amounts for specific functions and health of the body, such as growth, reproduction, and resistance to infection. They differ in physical and chemical properties and in biological functions. Vitamins function in highly specific metabolic processes. They cannot be synthesized in sufficient quantity by the body alone, and must therefore be obtained from the diet, from fortified foods and supplements and, in the case of vitamin D, from skin exposure to the sun. Vitamin C is readily available in diets including regular and adequate amounts of fruit and vegetable intake at all ages but this is not universally available nor part of all dietary cultures.

Many diets in low-, medium-, and high-income countries are in fact deficient in more than one of these needed elements and, along with trace minerals, should be added to foods commonly eaten by most people such as flour, rice, cooking oils, milk, salt, and sugar. Fortification of common basic foods has become increasingly justified in science and in practice over the past century with successful experience in fortification of basic foods with iodine, iron, vitamin B complex including folic acid, vitamin D and others to prevent many micronutrient deficiency conditions. Moreover, supplements are essential for certain groups in the population who need higher doses than that made available by food fortification.

Vitamin C is the primary antioxidant in the diet. It is available in balanced diets with vegetables and fruit, but can be deficient in the usual diets of many persons. A dietary lack of vitamin C adversely affects the general health of individuals, especially when under stress of infections such as the common cold or chronic illness.

Vitamin C is water-soluble and not synthesized in the human body thus adequate dietary intake is essential for maintaining health, especially for children, pregnant women, chronically ill and elderly people. As an antioxidant it is essential for absorption of iron and for collagen formation to maintain the skin and connective tissue, as well as for bones, blood vessels, wound healing, and facilitating recovery from burns. Vitamin C is widely available in fruit (especially grapefruit, lemons, limes, blackcurrants, oranges, berries and kiwi fruit) and vegetables (e.g., broccoli, green and red peppers, tomatoes, cabbage, sprouts, and sweet potatoes). It is also found in milk, fish, and some meats, such as liver.

Vitamin C deficiency still occurs as part of the general problem of undernutrition, associated with trauma and surgical care, refugee and migrant populations, people living in isolation, persons with chronic disease, poor nutrient absorption (such as with smoking, alcoholism, gastroenteric diseases), and inadequate nutrition among people living in high-, medium- and low-income countries. Symptoms include fatigue, lethargy, depression, gingivitis, and bleeding from the gums, skin petechiae (rash), internal bleeding, reduced resistance to infections, impaired wound healing, and mental illness. Patients on renal dialysis and anticoagulation therapy require vitamin C supplements. The required amount of vitamin C varies with the state of health and thus supplements are recommended to prevent or shorten the duration of common acute illnesses and are necessary in long-term illnesses such as for cancer patients, HIV/AIDS, and others.

People in categories considered at risk for deficiency, and therefore requiring regular vitamin C intake, include infants fed on cow's milk only; cigarette smokers; pregnant and lactating women; anorexia nervosa and bulimic patients; type 1 diabetes; immune-deficient patients; chronically ill patients; patients with enteric diseases and malabsorption such as celiac disease; and patients on restrictive diets due to allergies. Others at risk include a wide variety of people who lack regular access to fresh fruit and vegetables including elderly people living on poor diets ("tea and toast syndrome"); residents of remote, geographically isolated locations without access to diverse foods needed for healthy diets; poor families without financial or physical access to fresh fruit and vegetables; people eating primarily at fast food restaurants; alcoholics; refugees dependant on food donations; homeless people; drug addicts; institutionalized patients with poor eating habits; and people who have extreme dietary practices. Other groups in need of vitamin C and micronutrient support needs are HIV/AIDS and cancer patients, as well as patients on chronic renal dialysis or coumadin anticoagulation therapy. In total, these groups constitute a substantial segment of societies, even in high-income countries.

Scurvy prevention and control is a vital consideration in major emergency situations, such as following natural or man-made disasters with mass refugee situations, or homeless populations. Prevention of vitamin C deficiency along with prevention of thiamine deficiency, pellagra, and iron deficiency anemia are vital measures for disaster preparation and management with nutritional support policies for supplements, especially for infants, pregnant women and other vulnerable groups.

Vitamin C deficiency may be a comorbid condition among patients with other MNDs (e.g., iodine deficiency, iron deficiency/anemia, rickets), and those with psychotic and mental illness, chronic renal failure, cancer, and chronic illness. Refugees, minorities, and aboriginal populations are vulnerable to vitamin C and other multiple micronutrient deficiency conditions. The use of vitamin C and other antioxidants to treat severe trauma and burn patients is an ongoing area of clinical research. Additionally, many other potential benefits have been claimed and are under continuing review.

Vitamin C deficiency is still a global problem, with recognition that MNDs usually include more than a single vitamin or mineral. Deficiencies of iodine, iron, selenium, and vitamins B, C, D, and others are now considered to be multifactorial. From treating poorly fed pregnant women with iron and folic acid as practiced for decades we are now also recognizing the need for iodine, selenium, zinc, magnesium, vitamins A, B group, C, D and B12. The public health issue of improving pregnancy and neonatal outcomes will require multivitamin supplementation as well as fortification of basic foods.

ETHICAL ISSUES

The importance of vitamin C deprivation must be taken into account for ethical health policies. Undernutrition with MNDs and calorie deprivation are worldwide issues. Underlying morbidity and mortality are frequently associated with poverty and social deprivation. Vitamin C deficiency is a special problem for vulnerable groups of people in every society, including:

- the elderly and other groups unable to maintain a healthful diet in poor health, or due to lack of access to healthful foods for social and economic reasons;
- people with acute trauma, fractures, burns;
- people with chronic medical conditions;
- people with dependency on smoking, alcohol, and drugs;

- people with low income; and
- people with mental illness.

Yet interventions to reduce the high prevalence of subclinical MNDs, such as vitamin C, are not sufficiently recognized and promoted as national and international public health priorities. Routine supplementation of chronically ill and other high-risk groups is sporadic, and fortification of basic foods with vitamin C and other micronutrients is essential for population health. This applies in high-income as well as in medium- and low-income countries.

The lessons learned from Lind's study, and many others who followed in nutritional epidemiology, should lead those who deal with population health policy to address MNDs. This should be considered in modern times as part of clinical care and population health, and in disaster situations, including those in which people are displaced as a result of conflict in regions or countries in wartime conditions, and suffer from physical harm and nutritional deprivation. In disaster situations with uncertainty of healthful food supplies it is even more important to ensure vitamin C and other micronutrient adequacy. Scurvy is uncommon, but can occur in chronically ill and debilitated people; but subclinical vitamin C deficiency is occurring in vulnerable population groups on a global basis.

Ascorbic acid is an "antioxidant" that seems to have protective effects against "free radicals," which are potentially harmful derivatives of food and environmental factors. Antioxidants include vitamin C, beta carotene, selenium, vitamin E, and others. Free radicals can damage strands of DNA, leading to effects such as assisting absorption of low-density lipoprotein (LDL, i.e., "bad" cholesterol) molecules into artery walls, causing atherosclerosis. Moreover, this DNA damage may contribute to cancer and other chronic conditions. The protective effects of antioxidants are under intense research scrutiny since the 1990s but have not been definitively proven to be as effective in disease prevention as originally thought. However, high fruit and vegetable intake are highly recommended as important measures to reduce risk of cardiovascular diseases and cancer as seen in lower mortality from cardiovascular disease and cancer of the lung in a high fruit and vegetable consuming country such as Italy, Greece and Israel.

The World Health Organization (WHO) recommends a daily intake of 45 mg of vitamin C for healthy adults and 25−30 mg for infants. The US National Institutes of Health (NIH) recommend between 40−50 mg/day for infants, 15−75 mg/day for toddlers to adolescents, and 75−90 mg/day for adults, depending on age, gender, pregnancy status, and up to 120 mg/day for lactating mothers.

Some advocates, including Linus Pauling, a 1954 Nobel Prize laureate for chemistry, promoted mega doses of vitamin C for prevention of many diseases. This advocacy has fallen out of acceptability, with evidence of harmful effects of massive overdosage.

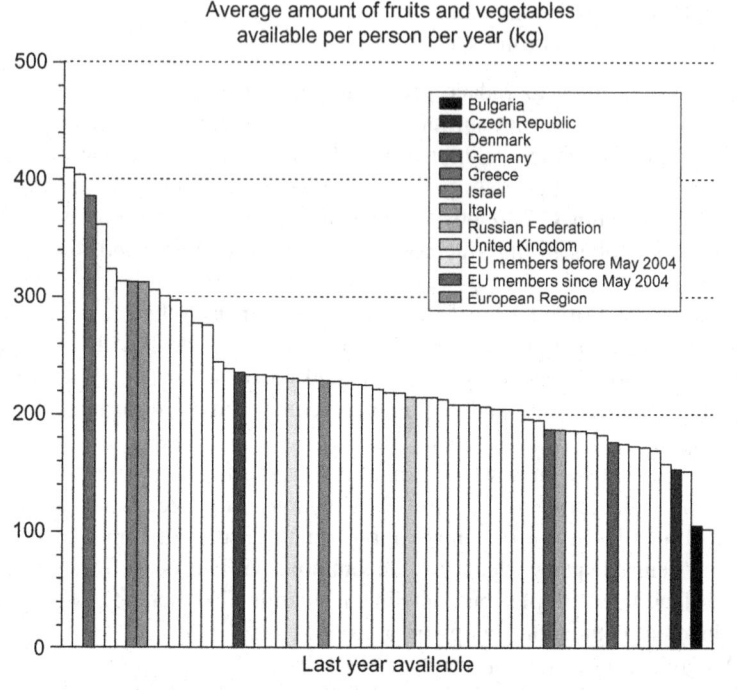

FIGURE 1.1   Average amount of fruit and vegetables available per person per year (kg) in selected European countries. Source: *World Health Organization European Region. Health for All Data Base, July 2016. Available at: http://data.euro.who.int/hfadb/ (accessed 24 June 2017).*

While frank scurvy is rare, except in severe environmental or national disaster situations, the prevalence of mild deficiency worldwide may be high. Data from the US National Health and Nutrition Examination Survey (NHANES) of 1988−94 indicated marginal deficiency in 9 percent of women and 13 percent in men, resulting from dietary deficiency in vegetable intake and chronic disease conditions.

Defining which foods belong to fruits and which ones to vegetables varies between European countries and no common definition exists, leading to difficulties in comparisons of the member countries. The United Nations Food and Agriculture Organization (FAO) provides data that indicate a marked north-south gradient in fruit and vegetable consumption in Europe. Countries in northern and eastern Europe have low consumption of vitamin C, while southern European countries, such as Italy, Greece, and Israel have high levels of vitamin C in the "Mediterranean diet." The European Region of the WHO reports that fruit and vegetable consumption can vary widely and affect population health such as between European Region countries, as seen in Figure 1.1.

ECONOMIC ISSUES

MNDs rarely occur alone and are often associated and interactive with chronic illness, thus adversely effecting treatment outcomes and associated costs, such as in patients with cancer, AIDS, renal dialysis, and others. The economic consequences of MNDs, including vitamin C deficiency, are also related to low work capacity and productivity. Economic growth requires improved health of adults in work, children in development, and education capacity. The World Bank and other economic agencies place nutritional security high in priority for economic progress in low- and medium-income countries. The Food and Agriculture Organization of the United Nations (FAO) suggests that *"investing US$1.2 billion annually in micronutrient supplements, food fortification and biofortification of staple crops for five years would generate annual benefits of US$15.3 billion, a benefit-to-cost ratio of almost 13 to 1."* (FAO, 2017). The benefits from investing in micronutrient supplements, food fortification, and biofortification of staple crops would generate better health, fewer deaths, and increased economic growth.

Agriculture policies in high-income countries, where farmers' unions and corporate farming are politically powerful, provide high levels of subsidies to the traditional "commodity crops", mainly wheat, corn, beans, cotton, dairy, sugar and meat agriculture. Support for "specialty crops" which include fruit and vegetables are much more limited, for specific programs such as crop insurance, disaster assistance, pest and disease protection, and research. These policies, common in the United States, Canada, and Europe, provide subsidies to the least healthful foods. But much less support is available for fruit and vegetables, the healthiest component for national consumption. This limits availability at affordable costs for large sectors of the population even in high income countries. Such policies are counterproductive for health; they promote low nutritional value products at low cost increasing their consumption, while deterring healthful nutrition by cost and availability factors. This policy paradox is a contributor to growing obesity especially among the poorer sectors of society.

Malnourishment includes subclinical conditions where one or multiple vitamins and essential minerals are missing from the regular diet or, in the case of vitamin D, when sunlight exposure is inadequate to produce sufficient amounts of this essential vitamin in the skin to meet the needs of bone health. Lowered vitamin C intake can occur in the elderly and chronically ill with cancer, AIDS, renal disease, or in common situations where there are low levels of vegetable and fruit consumption. Chronic illness aggravated by lethargy, poor appetite and difficulty in chewing vegetables can be a factor for susceptibility to infection and avoidable prolongation of lengthy and costly stay in acute care hospitals.

WHO addresses scurvy, along with pellagra and thiamine deficiency, as serious problems in emergency situations, where adequate nutrition is not available or absorbed. Fortification of basic foods is a widely practiced public health measure to protect vulnerable populations or situations. National and international aid agencies need to recognize multivitamin supply as crucial for preventive care in refugee, disaster, and war situations. International refugee agencies, donors, and national governments should prioritize nutritional support for the most vulnerable i.e., pregnant women, infants, and children with essential vitamin and mineral supplements. This is a major global ethical challenge when donor fatigue is reducing resources available, and refugee populations have soared to reach 66 million persons globally in 2017.

CONCLUSION

Lind's pioneering study showed that citrus fruit in the diet cures and prevents scurvy. As a result, this practice was adopted as a standard method of preserving the health of late 18th century British sailors on long voyages. As knowledge of nutrition gained momentum in the 20th century, vitamin C in adequate amounts was found to be an important component of health promotion. Healthy diets with regular consumption of vegetables and fruit prevent vitamin C deficiency and frank scurvy. But low levels of vitamin C can be masked, especially in vulnerable populations, and may cause serious manifestations after 2–3 months. Frank scurvy in adults manifests symptoms such as lassitude, weakness and irritability, swollen bleeding gums, vague muscle or joints pain in legs and feet, weight loss, peripheral edema, and impaired work capacity. Moreover, internal bleeding can be fatal. In infants, scurvy leads to irritability, leg tenderness, and paralysis. Additionally, vitamin C deficiency impairs resistance to infections.

Cultural and traditional dietary patterns are important factors in the epidemiology of many important health conditions such as stroke, coronary heart disease, and cancer of lung and other cancers. Vegetable and fruit consumption are one of the key factors in the health benefits of the Mediterranean diet, compared to many traditional and current diets in Eastern Europe, or in the southern region of the United States sometimes called "the Stroke Belt".

Prevention of vitamin C deficiency depends on a healthful diet of vegetables and fruits, which are also effective in preventing cardiovascular diseases and cancer. Along with regular exercise, regular vegetable and fruit consumption is considered among the most effective public health measures of self-care and population health.

Lind's pioneering investigation opened policy issues around the prevention of a specific dietary deficiency disease that led to new energies, explorations, studies, and recognition of nutritional sciences, epidemiology and policy. With 2 billion people estimated to have hidden hunger with MNDs globally, the public health challenges are enormous, but thanks to Lind and his successors we have the knowledge to reduce this burden on global health.

Food and nutrition security is not only an individual problem but also a national and global issue. FAO and WHO emphasize that the societal cost of undernutrition (and overnutrition) in terms of health, societal, and economic is high. Investing in solutions can improve long-term nutritional outcomes. Improved policies for education, monitoring and food systems of production, and marketing can greatly improve nutritional security as part of the food security. National agricultural policies and subsidies to promote low cost fruit and vegetable production at least comparable to farm subsidies to dairy, meat and sugar production are important to increase their affordability, popularity and consumption. This not only requires both physical and financial access to nutritious foods at affordable prices but also enhanced nutritional value of basic foods and supplementation of essential vitamins and minerals to vulnerable populations. Many of these food system changes must be directed by well-coordinated nutrition policies from governments, the private sector, and families themselves. Today, there is wide knowledge and many tools are available such as community-wide education for better dietary practices, in schools, homes, workplaces, institutional settings and others. Poverty reduction to improve access to healthy diets, essential micronutrient supplements, and fortification of basic foods are vital public health policy issues globally.

RECOMMENDATIONS

International organizations, national, state and local governments, private donor agencies and the private sector should undertake population based nutrition policies for implementation globally:

1. Promote fruit and vegetable consumption in home, school, work, catering, public eating places, and institutional settings.
2. Promote education for fruit and vegetable consumption in education and health system programs.
3. Promote policies and implementation of well regulated fortification of basic foods with vitamin C and other essential micronutrients, including iron, iodine, magnesium, selenium, folic acid, vitamin B complex, vitamin D and others.
4. Promote adoption of policies and implementation of vitamin C and multivitamins supplements for high-risk population groups such as pregnant and lactating women, infants and toddlers, chronically ill persons, homeless and other deprived or institutionalized groups.
5. Promote fruit and vegetable marketing in poor urban neighborhoods and isolated remote communities.
6. Promote national and international agriculture policies with subsidies to encourage fruit and vegetable production and marketing at low cost in

preference or at least as are provided to other agriculture sectors such as dairy, sugar and meat production.

7. Promote surveys on fruit and vegetable consumption as a regular component of nutrition monitoring.

8. Disaster preparation should include provision of vitamin C and multivitamins for situations of long-term deprivation of normal societal conditions of supply and home economics.

STUDENT REVIEW QUESTIONS

1. Why is Lind's study of scurvy considered a pioneering epidemiologic study?

2. What is a randomized clinical trial? What are its strengths and weaknesses?

3. Give three examples of current nutritional deficiency conditions in your own country.

4. What are the options for preventing these deficiencies in your country?

5. How does vitamin C deficiency affect people with chronic diseases?

6. Describe a study that could demonstrate an effective intervention to prevent that deficiency condition.

7. Describe high-risk situations in which vitamin C and other micronutrient supplements should be part of health care.

8. Explain why multivitamin supplements are preferred for pregnancy and elderly care rather than a few individual vitamins and minerals.

9. What preparation should be taken for prevention of frank or subclinical micronutrient deficiency conditions in emergency situations?

10. How do agricultural policies affect national fruit and vegetable consumption and relate to population health?

RECOMMENDED READINGS

1.   Aburto NJ, Rogers L, De-Regil LM, Kuruchittham V, Rob G, Arif R, et al. An evaluation of a global vitamin and mineral nutrition surveillance system. Arch Latinoam Nutr. 2013;63(2):105−113. Available at: http://www.alanrevista.org/ediciones/2013/2/?i=art1/ (accessed 19 July 2017).

2.   Allen L, de Benoist B, Dary O, Hurrel R. Guidelines on food fortification with micronutrients. Geneva, Switzerland: WHO, 2006. Available at: http://www.who.int/nutrition/publications/ guide_food_fortification_micronutrients.pdf (accessed 19 July 2017).

3.   American Medical Association Acknowledges the Role of Vitamins for Chronic Disease Prevention in Adults. Available at: http://www.mreassociates.org/pages/ama_speaks_out. html (accessed 14 September 2017).

4.   Arron ST, Liao W, Maurer T. Scurvy: a presenting sign of psychosis. J Am Acad Dermatol. 2007;57(2 Suppl):S8−S10. Available at: http://www.ncbi.nlm.nih.gov/pubmed/17637387 (accessed 25 June 2017).

5. Backstrand JR. The history and future of food fortification in the United States: a public health perspective. Nutr Rev. 2002;60(1):15−26. Available at: http://www.ncbi.nlm.nih.gov/pubmed/11842999 (accessed 25 June 2017).
6. Baron JH. Sailors' scurvy before and after James Lind−a reassessment. Nutr Rev. 2009; 67(6):315−332. Abstract available at: http://www.ncbi.nlm.nih.gov/pubmed/19519673 (accessed 19 July 2017).
7. Berger MM. Antioxidant micronutrients in major trauma and burns: evidence and practice. Nutr Clin Pract. 2006;21(5):438−449. Available at: http://ncp.sagepub.com/content/21/5/438 (accessed 19 July 2017).
8. Biesalski HK. Parenteral ascorbic acid in haemodialysis patients. Curr Opin Clin Nutr Metab Care. 2008;(6), 741−746. Available at: http://www.ncbi.nlm.nih.gov/pubmed/18827578 (accessed 25 June 2017).
9. Carpenter KJ. A short history of nutritional science, part I 1785−1885. J Nutr. 2003; 133(3):638−645. Available at: http://jn.nutrition.org/content/133/3/638.full.pdf + html (accessed 19 July 2017).
10. Carpenter KJ. A short history of nutritional science, part 2. J Nutr. 2003;133 (4):975−984. Available at: http://jn.nutrition.org/content/133/4/975.full.pdf+html (accessed 19 July 2017).
11. Carpenter KJ. A short history of nutritional science: part 3 (1912−1944). J Nutr. 2003; 133(10):3023−3032. Available at: http://jn.nutrition.org/content/133/10/3023.full.pdf+html (accessed 19 July 2017).
12. Carpenter KJ. A short history of nutritional science: part 4 (1945−1985). J Nutr. 2003; 133(11):3331−3342. Available at: http://jn.nutrition.org/content/133/11/3331.full.pdf+html (accessed 19 July 2017).
13. Carpenter KJ. The discovery of vitamin C. Ann Nutr Metab. 2012;61(3):259−264. Available at: http://www.ncbi.nlm.nih.gov/pubmed/23183299 (accessed 19 July 2017).
14. Centers for Disease Control and Prevention. Achievements in public health, 1900−1999: safer and healthier foods. MMWR Morb Mortal Wkly Rep. 1999;48(40):905−913. Available at: http://www.cdc.gov/mmwr/preview/mmwrhtml/mm4840a1.htm (accessed 19 July 2017).
15. Centers for Disease Control and Prevention. Famine-affected, refugee, and displaced populations: recommendations for public health issues. MMWR Morb Mort Wkly Rep. 1992;41(No. RR-13);0001. Available at: https://www.cdc.gov/mmwr/preview/mmwrhtml/00019261.htm (accessed 13 September 2017).
16. Centers for Disease Control and Prevention. International micronutrient malnutrition prevention and control program (IMMPaCt). Available at: http://www.cdc.gov/immpact/index.html (accessed 25 June 2017).
17. Centers for Disease Control and Prevention. National health and nutrition examination survey (NHANES). Available at: http://www.cdc.gov/nchs/nhanes.htm (accessed 25 June 2017).
18. Centers for Disease Control and Prevention. What we eat in America, DHHS-USDA dietary survey integration. Available at: http://www.cdc.gov/nchs/nhanes/wweia.htm (accessed 19 July 2017).
19. Chalmers I. The James Lind initiative. J R Soc Med. 2003;96(12):575−576. Available at: http://www.ncbi.nlm.nih.gov/pmc/articles/PMC539653/ (accessed 19 July 2017).
20. De Tullio MC. Beyond the antioxidant: the double life of vitamin C. Subcell Biochem. 2012;56:49−65. Abstract available at: http://www.ncbi.nlm.nih.gov/pubmed/22116694 (accessed 19 July 2017).

21. European Food Information Council. Fruit and vegetable consumption in Europe — do Europeans get enough? Available at: http://www.eufic.org/article/en/expid/Fruit-vegetable-consumption-Europe/ (accessed 19 July 2017).

22. Fairfield KM, Fletcher RH. Vitamins for chronic disease prevention in adults: scientific review. JAMA. 2002;287:3116−3126. Available at: http://jamanetwork.com/journals/jama/fullarticle/195038 (accessed 13 September 2017).

23. Fletcher RH, Fairfield KM. Vitamins for chronic disease prevention in adults: clinical applications. JAMA. 2002;287:3127−3129. Available at: https://www.ncbi.nlm.nih.gov/pubmed/12069676 (accessed 13 September 2017).

24. Food and Agriculture Organization. Understanding the true cost of malnutrition Available at: http://www.fao.org/zhc/detail-events/en/c/238389/ (accessed 17 October 2015).

25. Gan R, Eintracht S, Hoffer LJ. Vitamin C deficiency in a university teaching hospital. J Am Coll Nutr. 2008;27(3):428−433. Available at: http://www.ncbi.nlm.nih.gov/pubmed/18838532 (accessed 19 July 2017).

26. Geber J, Murphy E. Scurvy in the Great Irish Famine: evidence of vitamin C deficiency from a mid-19th century skeletal population. Am J Phys Anthropol. 2012;148(4):512−524. Available at: http://www.ncbi.nlm.nih.gov/pubmed/22460661 (accessed 19 July 2017).

27. Goebel L, Griffing GT, Wong JJ, Perry V, Schwarzenberger K, Laumann AE, et al. Scurvy. Medscape, update September 23, 2015. Available at: http://emedicine.medscape.com/article/125350-overview#showall (accessed 19 July 2017).

28. Hampl JS, Taylor CA, Johnston CS. Vitamin C deficiency and depletion in the United States: the Third National Health and Nutrition Examination Survey, 1988 to 1994. Am J Public Health. 2004;94(5):870−875. Available at: http://www.ncbi.nlm.nih.gov/pubmed/15117714 (accessed 19 July 2017).

29. Hancock RD, Viola R. Improving the nutritional value of crops through enhancement of L-ascorbic acid (vitamin C) content: rationale and biotechnological opportunities. J Agric Food Chem. 2005;53(13):5248−5257. Available at: http://www.ncbi.nlm.nih.gov/pubmed/15969504 (accessed 19 July 2017).

30. Hansen EP, Metzsche C, Henningsen E, Toft P. Severe scurvy after gastric bypass surgery and a poor postoperative diet. J Clin Med Res. 2012;4(2):135−137. Available at: http://www.ncbi.nlm.nih.gov/pmc/articles/PMC3320124/ (accessed 19 July 2017).

31. Hemilä H, Chalker E. Vitamin C for preventing and treating the common cold. Cochrane Database Syst Rev. 2013;1:CD000980. Abstract available at: http://www.ncbi.nlm.nih.gov/pubmed/23440782 (accessed 19 July 2017).

32. Hercberg S, Preziosi P, Galan P, Devanlay M, Keller H, Bourgeois C, et al. Vitamin status of a healthy French population: dietary intakes and biochemical markers. Int J Vitam Nutr Res. 1994;64(3):220−232. Available at: http://www.ncbi.nlm.nih.gov/pubmed/7814238 (accessed 19 July 2017).

33. Institute of Medicine. Food and Nutrition Board. Dietary reference intakes (DRIs). Available at: http://www.nationalacademies.org/hmd/~/media/Files/Activity%20Files/Nutrition/DRI-Tables/5Summary%20TableTables%2014.pdf?la=en)f6. (accessed 25 June 2017).

34. Jacob RA, Sotoudeh G. Vitamin C function and status in chronic disease. Nutr Clin Care. 2002;5(2):66−74. Available at: http://www.ncbi.nlm.nih.gov/pubmed/12134712 (accessed 19 July 2017).

35. Jenny C. Evaluating infants and young children with multiple fractures. Pediatrics. 2006;118(3):1299−1303. Available at: http://pediatrics.aappublications.org/content/118/3/1299.long (accessed 25 June 2017).

36. Johnson R. Fruits, vegetables, and other specialty crops: selected farm bill and federal programs. Congressional Research Service, 11 July 2014. 7-5700, www.crs.gov R42771. Available at: http://nationalaglawcenter.org/wp-content/uploads/assets/crs/R42771.pdf (accessed 27 September 2017).

37. Kocot J, Luchowska-Kocot D, Kiełczykowska M, Musik I, Kurzepa J. Does vitamin C influence neurodegenerative diseases and psychiatric disorders? Nutrients. 2017;9:659. Available at: https://www.ncbi.nlm.nih.gov/pmc/articles/PMC5537779/ (accessed 26 October 2017).

38. Leger D. Scurvy: reemergence of nutritional deficiencies. Can Fam Physician. 2008;54 (10):1403–1406. Available at: http://www.ncbi.nlm.nih.gov/pubmed/18854467 (accessed 25 June 2017).

39. Lind J. Treatise of the scurvy: in three parts. Containing an inquiry into the nature, causes and cure of that disease. Together with a critical and chronological view of what has been published on the subject. Edinburgh: Printed by Sands, Murray and Cochran for A Kincaid and A Donaldson, 1753. Available at: http://www.jameslindlibrary.org/lind-j-1753/ (accessed 19 July 2017).

40. Martini SA, Phillips M. Nutrition and food commodities in the 20th century. Agric Food Chem. 2009;57(18):8130–8135. Available at: https://doi.org/10.1021/jf9000567. Abstract available at: https://www.ncbi.nlm.nih.gov/pubmed/19719130 (accessed 27 September 2017).

41. Mayland CR, Bennett MI, Allan K. Vitamin C deficiency in cancer patients. Palliat Med. 2005;19(1):17–20. Available at: http://www.ncbi.nlm.nih.gov/pubmed/15690864 (accessed 25 June 2017).

42. Mayo Clinic. Diseases and conditions: vitamin deficiency anemia. Available at: http://www.mayoclinic.org/diseases-conditions/vitamin-deficiency-anemia/basics/causes/con-20019550 (accessed 19 July 2017).

43. Milne I. Who was James Lind, and what exactly did he achieve? James Lind Library. Bulletin: commentaries on the history of treatment evaluation, 2012. Available at: http://www.jameslindlibrary.org/articles/who-was-james-lind-and-what-exactly-did-he-achieve/ (accessed 19 July 2017).

44. Mosdol A, Erens B, Brunner EJ. Estimated prevalence and predictors of vitamin C deficiency within UK's low-income population. J Public Health (Oxf). 2008;30(4):456–460. Available at: http://www.ncbi.nlm.nih.gov/pubmed/18812436 (accessed 19 July 2017).

45. National Health Service. Scurvy. Available at: http://www.nhs.uk/Conditions/Scurvy/Pages/Introduction.aspx (accessed 25 October 2016).

46. National Institutes of Health. Office of Dietary Supplements. Vitamin C fact sheet for health professionals, June 5, 2013. Available at: https://ods.od.nih.gov/factsheets/VitaminC-HealthProfessional/ (accessed 19 July 2017).

47. Nobel Prize for Medicine or Physiology 1937. Albert von Szent-Györgyi Nagyrápolt. Available at: http://www.nobelprize.org/nobel_prizes/medicine/laureates/1937/szent-gyorgyi-facts.html (accessed 19 July 2017).

48. Nobel Prize in Chemistry 1937. Awarded to Walter Norman Haworth for his work on vitamin C along with Paul Karrer for work on carotenoids and flavins, and vitamins A and B2. Available at: http://www.nobelprize.org/nobel_prizes/chemistry/laureates/1937/haworth-facts.html (accessed 19 July 2017).

49. Noble JM, Mandel A, Patterson MC. Scurvy and rickets masked by chronic neurologic illness: revisiting "psychologic malnutrition". Pediatrics. 2007;119(3):e783–e790. Available at: http://www.ncbi.nlm.nih.gov/pubmed/17332193 (accessed 25 June 2017).

50. Olmedo JM, Yiannias JA, Windgassen EB, Gornet MK. Scurvy: a disease almost forgotten. Int J Dermatol. 2006;45(8):909−913. Abstract available at: http://www.ncbi.nlm.nih.gov/pubmed/16911372 (accessed 19 July 2017).

51. Ratanachu-Ek S, Sukswai P, Jeerathanyasakun Y. Scurvy in pediatric patients: a review of 28 cases. J Med Assoc Thai. 2003;86(Suppl 3):S734−S740. Available at: http://www.ncbi.nlm.nih.gov/pubmed/14700174 (accessed 25 June 2017).

52. Rosen G. A history of public health. Revised and expanded edition. Baltimore, MD: The Johns Hopkins University Press, 2015.

53. Singer R, Rhodes HC, Chin G, Kulkarni H, et al. High prevalence of ascorbate deficiency in an Australian peritoneal dialysis population. Nephrology (Carlton). 2008;13(1):17−22. Available at: http://www.ncbi.nlm.nih.gov/pubmed/18199096 (accessed 25 June 2017).

54. Toole MJ, Waldman RJ. Refugees and displaced persons: war, hunger and public health. JAMA. 1993;(5), 600−605. Available at: http://cidbimena.desastres.hn/pdf/eng/doc5704/doc5704-contenido.pdf (accessed 13 September 2017).

55. Toffanello ED, Inelmen EM, Minicuci N, Campigotto F, Sergi G, Coin A, et al. Ten-year trends in vitamin intake in free-living healthy elderly people: the risk of subclinical malnutrition. J Nutr Health Aging. 2011;15(2):99−103. Available at: http://www.ncbi.nlm.nih.gov/pubmed/21365161 (accessed 25 June 2017).

56. Tulchinsky TH, Kalusk DN. Food fortification and risk group supplementation are vital parts of a comprehensive nutrition policy for prevention of chronic diseases. Eur J Public Health. 2004;14:226−228. Available at: http://www.ncbi.nlm.nih.gov/pubmed/15369023 (accessed 25 June 2017).

57. Tulchinsky TH, Varavikova EA. The new public health. 3rd edition. San Diego, CA: Elsevier/Academic Press, 2014. Chapter 8.

58. Tveden-Nyborg P, Lykkesfeldt J. Does vitamin C deficiency result in impaired brain development in infants? Redox Rep. 2009;14(1):2−6. Available at: http://www.ncbi.nlm.nih.gov/pubmed/19161672 (accessed 25 June 2017).

59. World Health Organization. Scurvy and its prevention and control in major emergencies. Geneva, Switzerland: WHO, 1999. Available at http://www.who.int/nutrition/publications/emergencies/WHO_NHD_99.11/en/ (accessed 19 July 2017).

60. World Health Organization. Meeting on WHO recommendations for antenatal care (ANC) focusing on nutrition during pregnancy and implementation considerations. Guideline development panel meetings on WHO antenatal care guidelines, October 27−29, 2015. Available at: http://www.who.int/nutrition/events/2015_meeting_antenatalcare_pregnancy_27to29oct/en/ (accessed 19 July 2017).

Chapter 2

Edward Jenner, Vaccination and Eradication of Smallpox

ABSTRACT

In 1796, Edward Jenner (1749–1823), a country physician in Gloustershire, England, investigated local beliefs that milkmaids were immune to smallpox because of their exposure to cowpox. He took matter from a cowpox pustule of a milkmaid and applied it with scratches to the skin of a young boy named James Phipps, who was later inoculated with smallpox and did not develop the disease. Smallpox continued to be a periodic pandemic worldwide with millions of sufferers and deaths. In 1953 the World Health Assembly (WHA) the governing body of the World Health Organization (WHO) rejected the notion that smallpox should be selected for eradication. But gradual expansion of smallpox vaccination globally during the 20th century led WHO in 1966 to declare eradication of smallpox as a global health target. In 1967 a year with more than 10 million smallpox cases and 2 million deaths in 43 countries, implementation of the eradication campaign was launched. The campaign was conducted by the WHO in cooperation with many agencies and countries, with combined strategies of mass vaccination and focal eradication based on case reporting and localized vaccination to prevent spread of the disease. The campaign was assisted by many innovations and use of volunteer community health workers. The last known case was identified in Somalia in 1977, and the WHO declared that global eradication of smallpox was accomplished in 1980. This enormous achievement has set precedents for global eradication of other infectious diseases including poliomyelitis, measles, and many others.

BACKGROUND

Smallpox, a devastating and disfiguring epidemic disease, ravaged all parts of the world and has been known since the third century BCE (Before the Common Era). Described first by Rhazes, a Persian physician, in the tenth century CE (Common Era), the disease was confused with measles and was widespread in Asia, the Middle East, and Europe during the Middle Ages. It was clearly designated as a cause of death in the London Bills of Mortality in 1629. Smallpox epidemics occurred throughout the 17th, 18th, and 19th centuries primarily as a disease of childhood, with mortality rates between 25 percent and 40 percent or more and disfiguring sequelae. Smallpox was also a key factor in the near elimination of the Aztecs and other societies in

Case Studies in Public Health. DOI: http://dx.doi.org/10.1016/B978-0-12-804571-8.00010-X

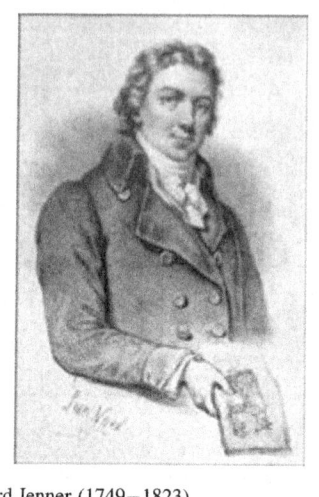

Edward Jenner (1749–1823)
The first experiment to test this theory involved milk-maid Sarah Nelmes and James Phipps, the 8 year-old son of Jenner's gardener. Dr. Jenner took material from a cowpox (variola) sore on her hand and inoculated it into Phipps' arm. Months later, Jenner exposed Phipps a number of times to variola virus, but Phipps never developed smallpox. More experiments followed, and, in 1801, Jenner published his treatise *"On the Origin of the Vaccine Inoculation,"* summarizing his discoveries and expressing hope that *"the annihilation of the smallpox, the most dreadful scourge of the human species, must be the final result of this practice." Source: Photo courtesy of the National Library of Medicine. Available at: https://www.cdc.gov/smallpox/history/history.html (accessed 11 August 2017).*

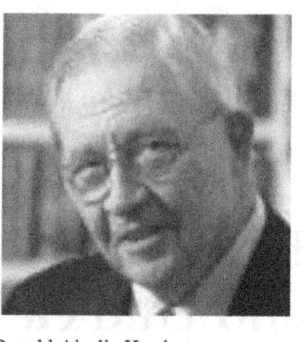

Donald Ainslie Henderson
(1936–2016)
Director of virus surveillance programs at CDC moved to Geneva to lead the WHO global campaign 1966 to 1977 to eradicate smallpox, achieved by 1977. *Source: Donald Ainslie (D. A.) Henderson, MD, MPH (1928–2016) Smallpox Eradication: Leadership and Legacy. J Infect Dis. 2017 Mar 1; 215(5): 673–676. Published online 2017 Feb 7. doi: 10.1093/infdis/jiw640 PMC Open Access, Creative Commons Attribution. Available at: https://www.ncbi.nlm.nih.gov/pmc/articles/PMC5388283/pdf/jiw640.pdf (accessed 28 October 2017.)*

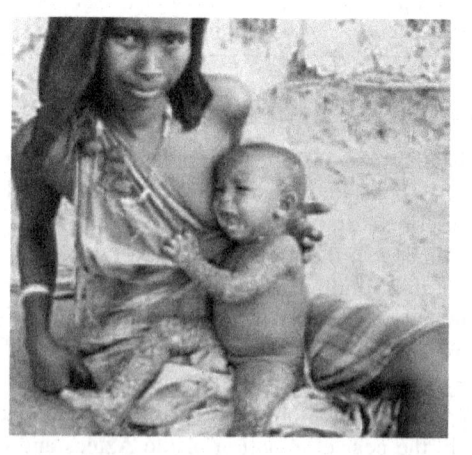

Somalia, 1970s. A mother holds a child whose body is almost entirely covered with smallpox pustules. *Source: World Health Organization.*

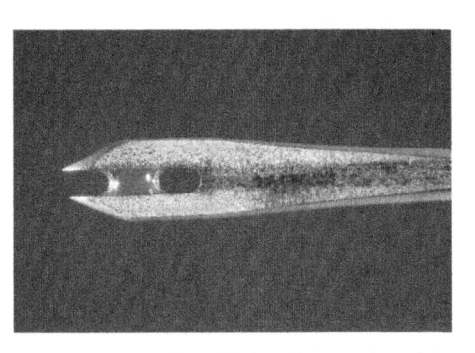

Rubin Bifurcated Needle invented in 1965 enabled rapid expansion of the smallpox eradication. Some vaccine solution can be seen clinging to the tip of the needle, ready to be administered to a vaccine recipient. *Source: Centers for Disease Control and Prevention Public Health Image Library (PHIL) Rubin needle. Available at: https://phil.cdc.gov/phil/details_linked.asp? pid = 2667&permalink = 2667 (accessed 11 August 2017).*

Central and South America following the Spanish invasion. The disease was spread deliberately as an act of war in North America in the late 18th century and naturally by person to person transmission and on contaminated personal contact materials such as bedding.

Prevention of this disease by inoculation (variolation) or transmission of the disease to healthy persons to prevent them from a more virulent form during epidemics was reported in ancient China. Variolation was mostly practiced among children, but was a dangerous procedure with a substantial mortality rate. The practice of variolation was brought to England in 1721 by Lady Mary Montagu, wife of the British ambassador to Constantinople, where this was a common practice. It was widely adopted in England in the mid-18th century, when the disease affected millions of people in Europe alone. Catherine the Great in Russia had her son inoculated by variolation by a leading English practitioner.

Edward Jenner (1749–1823) was born in Berkeley, Gloucestershire, England, son of the local vicar. At the age of 14, he was apprenticed to a local surgeon and then trained in London. In 1772, he returned to Berkeley and spent most of the rest of his career as a doctor in his native town. In 1796, Jenner investigated local folklore that milkmaids were immune to smallpox because of their exposure to cowpox. In 1796, at age 47, he took matter from a cowpox pustule of a milkmaid named Sarah Nelmes and applied it with scratches to the skin of an eight year old boy named James Phipps, who was later inoculated with smallpox and did not develop the disease. This was the first successful vaccination against an infectious disease.

In 1798, Jenner published his book, *An Inquiry Into the Causes and Effects of the Variolae Vaccinae (Cowpox)*, describing his widescale vaccination experience and its successful protection against smallpox. Jenner

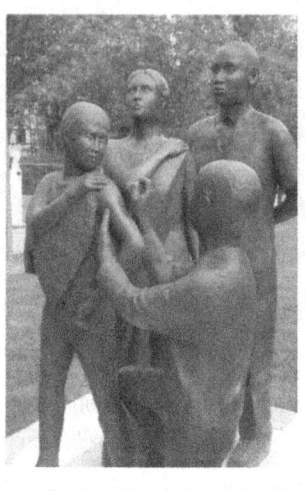

Statue commemorates smallpox eradication. Unveiled on May 17, 2010 commemorating the 30th anniversary of the eradication of smallpox located in front of the World Health Organization (WHO) headquarters. Sculptor Martin William. *Source: World Health Organization. Statue commemorates smallpox eradication. Available at: http://www.who.int/mediacentre/news/notes/2010/ smallpox_20100517/en/ Donald Ainslie (DA) Henderson, MD, MPH (1928–2016) Smallpox Eradication: Leadership and Legacy. J Infect Dis. 2017 Mar 1; 215(5): 673–676. Published online 2017 Feb 7. doi: 10.1093/infdis/jiw640 Available at: https://www.ncbi.nlm.nih.gov/pmc/ articles/PMC5388283/pdf/jiw640.pdf (accessed 28 October 2017.)*

prophesized that "*this practice would wipe out this scourge from the face of the earth*," forecasting the concept of global disease eradication. His report was translated into many languages within a few years.

Because variolation exposure of people to the pustular matter of cases of smallpox was practiced widely in the 18th century and constituted a very lucrative medical business, opposition to vaccination was intense. Jenner's contribution was ignored by the scientific and medical establishment of the day, but the importance of this discovery was soon recognized and rewarded in 1802 by the British Parliament, which granted him the sum of £10,000, and 5 years later again rewarded him with £20,000 more.

In 1800, vaccination was adopted by the British armed forces, and the practice spread to Europe, the Americas, and the British Empire. Denmark made vaccination mandatory in the early 19th century and soon eradicated smallpox locally. Despite some professional opposition, the practice spread rapidly from the upper classes and voluntary groups to the common people because of the fear of smallpox. Vaccination later became compulsory in many countries, with the ultimate public health achievement of global eradication in the late 20th century.

Halfdan Mahler, Director General of WHO, describes the process: "*The World Health Organization was established in 1948 and from its inception successive World Health Assemblies urged Member States to take all* *measures to control smallpox. In 1953 the first Director General, Dr. Brock Chisholm, made an unsuccessful attempt to persuade the World Health Assembly to undertake a global smallpox eradication programme. But only minimal funds were provided, and although by 1967 the disease was eliminated from some thirty countries in Asia, Africa and South America, the hard core of the problem - the Indian sub-continent and most countries in sub-Saharan Africa - were largely unaffected. In 1966 the World Health Assembly decided that this situation was intolerable, and established an Intensified Smallpox Eradication Programme, with an annual allocation of $2.4 million from the WHO regular budget and the declared goal of global eradication within 10 years. Thanks to the efforts of numberless national health staff in the endemic countries, the enthusiastic devotion of international workers, and the masterly coordination of the effort by the WHO Smallpox Eradication Unit, the goal of global eradication was achieved in just over 10 years." (Fenner F, et al.; WHO, 1988).*

The World Health Assembly (WHA) in 1953 first discussed the feasibility that smallpox could be eradicated, but with then current emphasis on malaria control, there was little support and the idea was rejected. In 1958, Viktor Zhdanov of the USSR proposed smallpox eradication as a global health target to the WHA. Based on success in eradicating smallpox in the USSR since the 1930s and vast production facilities for the vaccine, the USSR WHA delegation offered to donate 140 million doses of vaccine annually, approximately 50 percent of the amount of vaccine needed yearly for the at-risk population worldwide. In 1965, President Lyndon Johnson announced full US support for a program to eradicate smallpox in 20 countries of West and Central Africa and backed the idea of global smallpox eradication. In 1966, he sent one of the country's top epidemiologists, Dr. Donald A. Henderson of the US Centers for Disease Control (CDC), to Geneva to head WHO's smallpox eradication unit.

In 1966−67 the WHO adopted and implemented a program targeted at achieving smallpox eradication at a time when smallpox vaccination coverage was 80 percent in endemic countries. The program was controversial among infectious disease experts promoting eradication of malaria, but the smallpox initiative was successful with the partnership of the United States and the Soviet Union and cooperative leadership during the Cold War. Henderson was appointed head of the WHO eradication program with concurrence of the USSR.

In 1967, smallpox cases were reported in 44 countries (33 endemic and 11 imported), which declined by 1970 and 1973 to 17 and 6 countries, respectively. In 1973 the program implemented a new strategy to complement the mass vaccination approach by adding a case control-targeted approach with intensive surveillance, case contact follow-up, and vaccination. This was successful in helping achieve a case incidence of under 5/100,000 population. The program then moved into a consolidation and maintenance phase with vaccination of newborns and new residents.

Efforts in the 1920s and 1930s to standardize and attenuate the various strains of smallpox reduced complication rates in vaccines. Technical innovations in the 1950s such as development of lyophilization (freeze drying) of vaccine in England and the bifurcated needle in the United States allowed for easier and more widespread vaccination in tropical countries with lesser-trained personnel in more remote areas. The bifurcated needle invented by Benjamin Rubin, of Wyeth Laboratories required one-fourth the amount of vaccine needed with previous methods and was simpler to perform. The dry powdered vaccine was not heat sensitive and could be reconstituted at the time of use. These two innovations greatly eased the supply and administration of vaccination including by community health workers and thus enhancing the feasibility of eradication. These measures along with isolation of cases and aggressive follow-up of contacts increased community awareness. Under the leadership of Donald Henderson, ably assisted by William Foege (later director of the CDC) and an international team, effective strategies evolved. Mass vaccination campaigns increased herd immunity in the population, and community surveillance led to containment of local cases as potential "hotspots" by isolating the virus to stop its spread by a "cordon sanitaire" of immunized family, friends, neighbors and adjacent communities led to increased herd immunity among the population. All these strategies were used to combat the disease.

CURRENT RELEVANCE

In 1977, the last case of naturally occurring smallpox was identified in Somalia, a cook aged 23 who was not vaccinated, despite being a part-time vaccinationist. He was exposed to two children with smallpox in a Somali refugee camp in October 1977. He developed a rash initially thought to be chicken pox, but with other symptoms it was gradually recognized as smallpox. A vaccination campaign was carried out on his family, and surrounding homes for a total of nearly 55 thousand people. No further cases of natural transmission of smallpox have occurred since and he is designated as the last one. Several laboratory-related cases happened in a 1978 laboratory accident in the United Kingdom.

Eradication of smallpox was declared by the WHO in 1980. The eradication program cost US$ 112 million ($8 million annually), with an estimated direct savings of tens of billions of US dollars as well as saving millions of lives and complications from smallpox. In contrast, the annual cost of malaria is estimated at US$ 100 billion of lost gross domestic product much of which could be reduced with cost-effective interventions such as insecticide impregnated bednets and vector control efforts as well as development of effective vaccines.

Eradication of smallpox was declared by the WHO in 1980. The 1999 WHA recommendation to destroy the remaining government approved stocks of smallpox virus in the United States and Russia has not been achieved. There is ongoing concern that the virus could be potentially used as a weapon of mass destruction (WMD). Others suggest the virus should be kept for immunization as part of disaster management plans, further research, and for genomic biology. As of 2017, the remaining stocks are still held at the WHO Collaborating Centers in Russia and the United States.

Because of concern that the variola smallpox virus could be retrieved and developed by terrorist groups as a biological weapon, the CDC has prepared diagnostic tests and specialized laboratories for an emergency situation. In February 2017, the CDC Poxvirus and Rabies Branch received US Food and Drug Administration (USFDA) clearance for a new diagnostic test to detect the smallpox variola virus. The new Variola Virus Real-time PCR Assay is designed to increase sensitivity and specificity and will replace the previous test deployed to Laboratory Response Network (LRN) laboratories. The new variola test enhances US government preparedness efforts to quickly detect and respond in case of a biological attack.

The possibility of the smallpox virus being used as a WMD has been discussed by various authorities and researchers. Precautionary measures with vaccination of first responders, including police and medical personnel, was also suggested in 2003, following the terrorist destruction of the Twin Towers in New York City on September 11, 2001. There is concern that the smallpox virus stocks could fall into the hands of rogue scientists, potentially threatening the largely vulnerable world population. Current doctors have no experience with this disease and there are very limited stocks of vaccine. This has led to consideration of emergency response plans, increasing stocks of vaccine, and vaccination of first responders.

Jenner's experiment and its documentation was the scientific breakthrough that led to an enormous public health achievement in eradication of a horrendous disease that killed millions even in the 20th century. It also provided a basis for strategies and tactics to eradicate other infectious and noninfectious diseases such as poliomyelitis, leprosy, and even noncommunicable conditions, e.g., micronutrient deficiency conditions such as iodine deficiency disorders. The eradication of smallpox, one of the most common and deadliest diseases of mankind was finally achieved in 1977, based on Jenner's discovery of vaccination nearly two hundred years earlier.

ETHICAL ISSUES

Vaccination and eradication of smallpox is one of the great societal achievements in history and has helped control or eliminate many diseases. Opposition to vaccination following Jenner's report was intense mainly from doctors protecting their lucrative variola inoculation practices. Vaccination was made compulsory in England in 1853, but later with loophole escape

clauses, was essentially repealed in 1907. Compulsory vaccination was introduced in the United States in Massachusetts in 1809, followed by other states
and later repealed. The US Supreme Court ruled in a landmark case in 1905
(Jacobson vs Massachusetts) that the public good sometimes overrides the
private right of refusal in the case of vaccination. Discussions of this case
100 years later divide those who believe public health must work only by
credibility and persuasion, as opposed to those who believe that public health
still requires regulatory powers mandating public health standards, including
immunization (see Chapters 13,17,19, and 20 for more discussion of legal
and ethical issues in public health.)

Opposition to vaccination continued in the late 20th and early 21st centuries with small but growing reluctance and refusal of vaccination by parents
based on false information and ideological issues. While mandatory vaccination for smallpox was a success and mandatory requirements of proof of
complete vaccination for school attendance in the United States has been in
effect for many years, with exemptions based on ideological viewpoints are
still allowed.

The 2014−2017 measles epidemic in the United States following importation from a mass epidemic in Europe during 2010 brought the mandatory
immunization issue into open discussion. In 2015, the US state of California
enacted legislation banning personal and religious exemptions for immunization among public schoolchildren, although exemptions may be permitted for
medical grounds. This issue will be debated for years to come along with
other public health measures, but as seen in the case of smallpox egregious
opposition can be overcome by sustained professional dedication to disease
prevention and health promotion. In 2017, mandatory immunization for the
basic childhood disease is under consideration in France and in Germany
with fines for non compliance.

ECONOMIC ISSUES

Massive epidemics of smallpox in the 17th to the 20th centuries killed
millions of people and maimed millions more. Smallpox was an example of
a viral disease that could be and was eradicated, and there are many others
that we can now control or eliminate to help build healthier societies for economic and social progress.

Vaccination has proven to be one of the most cost-effective public health
measures to advance health and societal development. Successes in vast
reductions of mortality and morbidity of vaccine-preventable diseases are
encouraging for low- and middle-income countries in the 21st century.
Increasing coverage from some 80 percent globally to over 90 percent will
produce rapid advancement in the health of children particularly if accompanied by other advances in nutrition, universal education for both boys and

girls, and reduced inequality for of economically disadvantaged segments of the population consistent with the United Nations Millennium Development Goals (MDGs) and the successor Sustainable Development Goals (SDGs).

WHO has played a leading role in promoting the Expanded Programme on Immunization and the expansion of public health networks in low- and middle-income countries, targeting strengthening of routine immunization and eradication of rubella, poliomyelitis, measles and other vaccine preventable diseases (see Chapters 12,15 and 19). Since 1993, the World Bank has recognized that freedom from preventable diseases is one of the basic contributors to economic growth. Major international donors such as the Bill and Melinda Gates Foundation and the Global Alliance for Vaccination Initiatives (GAVI) as well as donor countries, along with other charitable societies such as the Rotary Club have provided essential funding and leadership to help implement advanced vaccination programs in low- and middle-income countries.

Expanding vaccination programs is an ongoing challenge as new vaccines are developed, proven safe and effective for many childhood and adult infectious diseases in preventing diseases such as measles, rubella, mumps, and cancer-causing microorganisms such as hepatitis B and human papillomavirus.

CONCLUSION

Edward Jenner discovered the use of vaccination and correctly predicted this could lead to eradication of smallpox which occurred by 1980. This stands as one of the great achievements of human civilization, preventing great suffering and countless deaths globally. Smallpox eradication set a strategic precedent and tactical methodologies for addressing other important diseases including those within sight, poliomyelitis, and measles. Control and eradication of infectious disease and over the longer-term tropical diseases and the common causes of respiratory and waterborne disease are vital issues for the second and third decades of the 21st century.

Similar potential exists for other important infectious and chronic diseases caused by infections, such as cervical and gastric cancers, and congenital rubella syndrome (CRS). Nutritional disorders such as iodine deficiency or neural tube defects caused by folic acid deficiency in the first weeks of pregnancy can be controlled, or largely eliminated by currently available public health methods.

Scientific breakthroughs will permit development of new vaccines and immunologic prevention of some cancers and other chronic conditions, as well as micronutrient deficiency conditions such as iodine deficiency and many birth defects by screening, food fortification and genetic counseling (see Chapters 3: Case: From Panum to Eradication of Measles, Chapter 10: Case: Endemic Goiter and Eradication of Iodine Deficiency Disorders, Chapter 17: Case: Mandatory Vitamin K Injection for Newborns to Prevent

Vitamin K Deficiency Bleeding Disorder (Previously Hemorrhagic Disease of the Newborn), Chapter 18: Case: Eliminating Beta-Thalassemia Major and Other Birth Disorders, and Chapter 20: Case: Robert Guthrie and Nicholas Wald: Screening and Preventing for Birth Defects).

Eradication of each specific targeted infectious and noninfectious disease requires strategies and tactics depending on characteristics of the disease and available modalities of prevention whether through vaccines, environmental change, or change in human behavior or combinations of these elements.

These diseases will not go away by themselves. A decision to focus on such targets requires political and societal commitment, adequate funding, and a well-trained organized public health workforce. Targeting groups of diseases, such as measles, mumps, and rubella, can be undertaken together because of the availability of combined effective and affordable vaccines. Other interventions such as combating smoking, opioid addiction, unsafe driving conditions, and unhealthy diets can achieve important reductions in morbidity and mortality even if not totally. Monitoring the incidence and prevalence of diseases provides the information needed to select appropriate control-elimination-eradication methods. This requires strong reporting systems with well-trained personnel capable of epidemiologic situation analysis. Strategies such as raising herd immunity to over 95% of the population, for example, must be supported by containment of local outbreaks by creating a *cordon sanitaire* of protected populations. The response system must be flexible and immediate for step-by-step containment and elimination. Reducing the condition and its elimination may need to focus on specific regions or population groups.

Multinational efforts and global health targets such as those selected in the United Nations initiated Millennium Development Goals (2000−15 MDGs) have produced impressive achievements in health, poverty reduction, and improved education. The process stimulated international political commitment to undertake such health objectives, with specific focus on maternal and child health, infectious diseases and environmental health issues. The follow-up Sustainable Development Goals (SDGs) have broadened the objectives and will hopefully bring reduced inequality and wide success in reducing the prevalence of important population health issues.

Health is not a luxury but a basis for societal success in the potential of human development. Programs for disease reduction, elimination, or eradication require a sufficiently robust political, economic, ethical, and professional commitment. Promoting public support and participation is an ongoing challenge as skepticism and outright opposition to immunization and other measures are promoted by lobby groups, with extensive use of electronic social media. Disinformation and unfounded allegations of harm from vaccines, or from food fortification are directed through abuse of the social media reaching hundreds of millions of people with enormous success and resulting in economically damaging and costly care for preventable diseases. The legacy of Edward Jenner, of Donald Henderson and many others who contributed to global eradication of the horrific disease, provides a model for eliminating or eradicating many other scourges of mankind.

Health monitoring and public health structures require political and public support, well-developed human resources to achieve goals of disease containment as well as elimination and, when feasible disease eradication. Community-based surveillance and education are vital to control communicable disease. Control, elimination, and even eradication of noncommunicable diseases depend on diverse factors such as the culture of societal and individual behavior regarding the relevant risk factors in the epidemic.

RECOMMENDATIONS

Smallpox eradication should be followed by polio eradication, measles and rubella elimination to eradication in the nearest future.

Eradication of infectious and noninfectious diseases are increasingly feasible, and should be targeted based on objective criteria of feasibility, time and resources required, adequacy of public health infrastructure and human resources available.

1. Political support by international and national governments is crucial to this process, so that specific targets should be included in SDGs momentum now in progress (2015−30). Specifically, these include SDG Goal 3 Targets of: "Support the research and development of vaccines and medicines for the communicable and noncommunicable diseases that primarily affect developing countries, provide access to affordable essential medicines and vaccines, . . .the right of developing countries to use to the full the provisions in the Agreement on Trade Related Aspects of Intellectual Property Rights regarding flexibilities to protect public health, and, in particular, provide access to medicines for all":

2. "Substantially increase health financing and the recruitment, development, training and retention of the health workforce in developing countries, especially in least developed countries and small island developing States";

3. "Strengthen the capacity of all countries, in particular developing countries, for early warning, risk reduction and management of national and global health risks"

4. Close monitoring of international and national preparation for the possibility of terrorist or organized national or militia armed forces use of restored smallpox virus in mass terror warfare. This includes continued research in rapid diagnostic facilities, improved vaccine production capacity at short notice and storage of vaccine supplies for strategic deployment. Education of health workers in this possibility should be included in disaster preparation programs at national and state levels of government.

5. Public health should be strengthened and promoted in public policy with political, financial and moral support globally and by national and local government.
6. Nongovernmental organizations, advocacy, and financial support should be promoted as vital partners in public health progress.
7. Public health and its achievements should be part of general education in primary, secondary, and higher education levels.
8. The public health academic and professional communities share in the responsibility and accountability for recognition and implementation of prevention and early health care to enhance population health to its highest potential in practice.
9. Workforce strengthening by schools of public health should be promoted in high-, medium-, and low-income countries, preferably distinct from medical faculties, to strengthen workforce capacity through well accredited undergraduate as well as graduate studies programs for the public health workforce.
10. Development and implementation of disease eradication programs require partnering in network organizations, such as GAVI, with academic, medical, social, private sector and governmental bodies and included as part of public health workforce orientation and skill development; this includes increasing the depth of the public health workforce to address the challenges of disease control and where feasible eradication, strengthening of the multidisciplinary public health workforce including community health workers (*Promatores*) to expand capacity in health promotion and prevention programs.

STUDENT REVIEW QUESTIONS

1. What lessons can be learned from the smallpox eradication effort in current public health practice?
2. What is the importance of *mass vaccination* and *case-control vaccination* policies and how do they complement each other?
3. What are the arguments for and against destroying the remaining smallpox virus stocks in the WHO Collaborating Centers at the Centers for Disease Control and Prevention in the Atlanta and Moscow laboratories?
4. What other infectious diseases can be considered for global eradication?
5. What non-infectious diseases can be considered for elimination as public health problems?
6. Why is there opposition to vaccination and how can it be addressed?
7. Which cancers can currently be reduced by control and/or eradication of the infectious agent?
8. Can smallpox be reconstituted as a terrorist or biological warfare weapon?

RECOMMENDED READINGS

1. Aylward B, Hennessey KA, Zagaria N, Olivé J-M, Cochi S, Agency for Healthcare Research and Quality. When is a disease eradicable? 100 years of lessons learned. Am J Public Health. 2000;90(10):1515−1520. Available at: http://ajph.aphapublications.org/doi/pdf/10.2105/AJPH.90.10.1515 (accessed 11 July 2017).
2. Agency for Healthcare Research and Quality. Addressing the smallpox threat: issues, strategies, and tools: bioterrorism and health system reparedness, Issue Brief No. 1. Available at: https://archive.ahrq.gov/news/ulp/btbriefs/btbrief1.pdf (accessed 11 July 2017).
3. Carter Center. International task force for disease eradication. Available at: http://www.cartercenter.org/health/itfde/index.html (accessed).
4. Centers for Disease Control and Prevention. National Center for Immunization and Respiratory Diseases, Global Immunization Division. Global immunization strategic framework 2011−2015. Available at: http://www.cdc.gov/globalhealth/immunization/docs/gidstrat-framewk.pdf (accessed 11 July 2017).
5. Centers for Disease Control and Prevention. A CDC framework for preventing infectious diseases: sustaining the essentials and innovating for the future. Atlanta, GA: Centers for Disease Control and Prevention, 2011. Available at: http://www.cdc.gov/oid/docs/ID-Framework.pdf (accessed 11 July 2017).
6. Centers for Disease Control and Prevention. Progress report on a CDC's framework for preventing infectious diseases: sustaining the essentials and innovating for the future, October 2011−May 2013. Atlanta, GA: Centers for Disease Control, 2013. Available at: http://www.cdc.gov/oid/docs/id-framework-progress-report.pdf (accessed 11 July 2017).
7. Centers for Disease Control and Prevention. Achievements in public health, 1900−1999: control of infectious diseases. MMWR Morb Mortal Wkly Rep. 1999;48(29):621. Available at: http://www.cdc.gov/mmwr/preview/mmwrhtml/mm4829a1.htm (accessed 11 July 2017).
8. Centers for Disease Control and Prevention. Achievements in public health, 1900−1999. Impact of vaccines universally recommended for children—United States, 1990−1998. MMWR Morbid Mortal Wkly Rep. 1999;48(29):243−248. Available at: http://www.cdc.gov/mmwr/preview/mmwrhtml/00056803.htm (accessed 11 July 2017).
9. Centers for Disease Control and Prevention. Addressing emerging infectious disease threats: a prevention strategy for the United States executive summary. MMWR Recomm Rep. 1994;43(RR-5):1−18. Available at: http://www.cdc.gov/mmwr/preview/mmwrhtml/00031393.htm (accessed 11 July 2017).
10. Centers for Disease Control and Prevention. Case definition for infectious conditions under public health surveillance. MMWR Recomm Rep. 1997;46(RR10):1−55. Available at: http://www.cdc.gov/mmwr/preview/mmwrhtml/00047449.htm (accessed 18 October 2015).
11. Centers for Disease Control and Prevention. Global routine vaccination coverage, 2009. MMWR Morb Mortal Wkly Rep. 2010;59(42):1367−1371. Available at: http://www.cdc.gov/mmwr/preview/mmwrhtml/mm5942a3.htm (accessed 18 October 2015).
12. Centers for Disease Control and Prevention. Parasites—onchocerciasis (also known as river blindness). updated August 2015. Available at: http://www.cdc.gov/parasites/onchocerciasis/ (accessed 11 July 2017).
13 Centers for Disease Control and Prevention. History of smallpox, 30 August 2016. Available at: https://www.cdc.gov/smallpox/history/history.html (accessed 11 August 2017).

14. Centers for Disease Control and Prevention. Our work 2017, 5 May 2017. New test to detect smallpox. Available at: https://www.cdc.gov/ncezid/what-we-do/recent-work.html#topic3apr2017 (accessed 26 May 2017).
15. Centers for Disease Control and Prevention. Progress toward global eradication of dracunculiasis, January 2011–June 2012. MMWR Morb Mortal Wkly Rep. 2012;61(42):854–857. Available at http://www.cdc.gov/mmwr/preview/mmwrhtml/mm6142a2.htm (accessed 11 July 2017).
16. Centers for Disease Control and Prevention. Progress toward introduction of *Haemophilus influenzae* type b vaccine in low-income countries—worldwide, 2004–2007. MMWR Morb Mortal Wkly Rep. 2008;57(06):148–151. Available at: http://www.cdc.gov/mmwr/preview/mmwrhtml/mm5706a3.htm (accessed 11 July 2017).
17. Centers for Disease Control and Prevention. Recommendations of the International Task Force for Disease Eradication. MMWR Recomm Rep. 1993;42(RR16):1–39. Available at: http://www.cartercenter.org/documents/1184.pdf (accessed 11 July 2017).
18. Centers for Disease Control and Prevention. Vaccination coverage among children in kindergarten—United States, 2011–12 school year. MMWR Morb Mortal Wkly Rep. 2012;61(33):647–652. Available at: http://www.cdc.gov/mmwr/preview/mmwrhtml/mm6133a2.htm (accessed 11 July 2017).
19. Centers for Disease Control and Prevention. Vaccination coverage among children in kindergarten—United States, 2014–15 school year. MMWR Morb Mortal Wkly Rep. 2015;64(33):897–904. Available at: http://www.cdc.gov/mmwr/preview/mmwrhtml/mm6433a2.htm (accessed 11 July 2017).
20. Center for Global Development. Available at: http://www.cgdev.org/doc/millions/MScase1.pdf (accessed 11 July 2017).
21. Colgrove J, Bayer R. Manifold restraints: liberty, public health, and the legacy of *Jacobson v Massachusetts*. Am J Public Health. 2005;95(4):571–576. http://dx.doiorg/10.2105/AJPH.2004.055145. Available at: http://ajph.aphapublications.org/doi/10.2105/AJPH.2004.055145 (accessed 11 July 2017).
22. Henderson DA. Who led effort to eradicate smallpox, dies at 87. Medscape. August 22, 2016. Available at: http://www.medscape.com/viewarticle/867702?nlid=109028_2243&src=WNL_mdplsnews_160826_mscpedit_infd&uac=107534HX&spon=3&impID=1186179&faf=1 (accessed 23 October 2017).
23. Editorial team. Measles once again endemic in the United Kingdom. Euro Surveill. 2008;13(27):pii-18919. Available at: http://www.eurosurveillance.org/viewarticle.aspx?articleid=18919 (accessed 11 July 2017).
24. Fenner F, Henderson DA, Arita I, Ježek Z, Ladnyi ID. Smallpox and its eradication. Geneva: World Health Organization, 1988. Available at: http://apps.who.int/iris/handle/10665/39485 (accessed 3 July 2017).
25. Henderson D. International partnerships: smallpox eradication —a cold war victory. World Health Forum. 1998;19:113–119. Available at: http://apps.who.int/iris/handle/10665/55594 (accessed 18 October 2015).
26. Henderson DA, Klepac P. Lessons from the eradication of smallpox: an interview with D. A. Henderson. Philos Trans R Soc Lond B Biol Sci. 2013;368(1623):20130113. doi:10.1098/rstb.2013.0113. Available at: http://www.ncbi.nlm.nih.gov/pmc/articles/PMC3720050/ (accessed 11 July 2017).
27. Henderson DA. Eradication: lessons from the past. MMWR Morb Mort Wkly Rep Suppl. 1999;48(SU01):16–22. Available at: http://www.cdc.gov/mmwr/preview/mmwrhtml/su48a6.htm (accessed 11 July 2017).

28. Henderson DA, Arita I. The smallpox threat: a time to reconsider global policy. Biosecur Bioterror. 2014;12(3):117−121. Available at: http://www.centerforhealthsecurity.org/our-work/publications/the-smallpox-threat-a-time-to-reconsider-global-policy (accessed 11 July 2017).

29. Hopkins DR. Global health: disease eradication. N Engl J Med. 2013;368:54−63. Available at: http://www.nejm.org/doi/full/10.1056/NEJMra1200391 (accessed 11 July 2017).

30. Institute of Medicine (US). Forum on emerging infections. In: Knobler S, Lederberg J, Pray LA, editors. Considerations for viral disease eradication: lessons learned and future strategies: workshop summary. Washington, DC: National Academies Press, 2002. Available at: https://www.nap.edu/catalog/10424/considerations-for-viral-disease-eradication-lessons-learned-and-future-strategies (accessed 8 July 2017).

31. Institute for Vaccine Safety. Johns Hopkins University. Summary: bifurcated needle workshop, 2001. Available at: http://www.vaccinesafety.edu/Summary-BifurcatedNeedles.pdf (accessed 18 June 2017).

32. Klepac P, Metcalf CJE, McLean AR, Hampson K. Towards the endgame and beyond: complexities and challenges for the elimination of infectious diseases. Phil Trans R Soc B. 2013;368:20120137. Available at: http://rstb.royalsocietypublishing.org/content/royptb/368/1623/20120137.full.pdf (accessed 2 November 2016).

33. McNeil A.G.D.A. Henderson, doctor who helped end smallpox scourge, dies at 87. New York Times. August 21, 2016. Available at: https://www.nytimes.com/2016/08/22/us/dr-donald-a-henderson-who-helped-end-smallpox-dies-at-87.html (accessed 3 July 2017).

34. Mariner WK, Annas GJ, Glantz LH. Jacobson v Massachusetts: it's not your great-great-grandfather's public health law. Am J Public Health. 2005;95(4):581−590. Available at: http://dx.doi.org/10.2105/AJPH.2004.055160. Available at: https://www.ncbi.nlm.nih.gov/pmc/articles/PMC1449224/pdf/0950581.pdf (accessed 24 September 2017).

35. Mariner WK, Annas GJ, Glantz LH. *Jacobson v Massachusetts*: It's not your great-great-grandfather's public health law. Am J Public Health. 2005;95(4):581−590. http://dx.doi.org/10.2105/AJPH.2004.055160. Available at: https://www.ncbi.nlm.nih.gov/pmc/articles/PMC1449224/ (accessed 11 July 2017).

36. National Institutes of Health. US National Library of Medicine. Smallpox a great and terrible scourge, updated 2013. Available at: https://www.nlm.nih.gov/exhibition/smallpox/ (accessed 11 July 2017).

37. National Vaccine Information Center. State of California. California State vaccine requirements. Available at: http://www.nvic.org/Vaccine-Laws/state-vaccine-requirements/california.aspx (accessed 11 July 2017).

38. Obituary. Donald Ainslie D.A. Henderson, MD, MPH (1928−2016). Smallpox eradication: leadership and legacy. J Inf Dis. 2017;215(5):673-676. doi:10.1093/infdis/jiw640. Available at: https://www.ncbi.nlm.nih.gov/pmc/articles/PMC5388283/ (accessed 17 May 2017).

39. Plotkin SA, Orenstein WA, Offit PA, editors. Vaccines. 6th edition. Philadelphia, PA: Elsevier Saunders, 2013. Available at: http://www.sciencedirect.com/science/article/pii/B9781455700905000872 (accessed 9 July 2017).

40. Riedel S. Edward Jenner and the history of smallpox and vaccination. Proc Baylor Univ Med Center. 2005;18(1):21−25. Available at: http://www.ncbi.nlm.nih.gov/pmc/articles/PMC1200696/ (accessed 18 October 2016).

41. Riedel S. Smallpox and biological warfare: a disease revisited. Proc (Baylor Univ Med Center). 2005;18(1):13–20. Available at: https://www.ncbi.nlm.nih.gov/pmc/articles/PMC1200695/pdf/bumc0018-0013.pdf (accessed 3 November 2017).

42. Rosen G. A history of public health. Revised expanded edition. Baltimore, MD: Johns Hopkins University Press, 1993. Available at: http://www.amazon.com/History-Public-Health-George-Rosen/dp/1421416018 (accessed 11 July 2017).

43. Small PA. Books and Media: Smallpox: The death of a disease and house on fire: The fight to eradicate smallpox. Emerg Infect Dis. 2011;17(11):2085–2086. Available at: https://wwwnc.cdc.gov/eid/article/17/11/11-1229_article (accessed 4 July 2017).

44. Smith KF, Sax DF, Gaines SD, Guernier V, Guégan JF. Globalization of human infectious disease. Ecology. 2007;88:1903–1910. Available at: http://www.ncbi.nlm.nih.gov/pubmed/17824419 (accessed 11 July 2017).

45. The College of Physicians of Philadelphia. The history of vaccines; history of anti-vaccination movements. Available at: http://www.historyofvaccines.org/content/articles/history-anti-vaccination-movements (accessed 11 July 2017).

46. Tulchinsky TH, Varavikova EA. The new public health. 3rd edition. San Diego, CA: Elsevier/Academic Press, 2014. Chapter 4.

47. United Nations. Sustainable Development Goals. Goal 3: Ensure healthy lives and promote well-being for all at all ages. Available at: http://www.un.org/sustainabledevelopment/health/ (accessed 7 November 2017).

48. Wisner B, Adams J. Environmental health in disasters and emergencies: a practical guide. Geneva, Switzerland: WHO, 2002. Available at: http://apps.who.int/iris/handle/10665/42561 (accessed 9 July 2017).

49. World Health Organization. Global measles and rubella strategic plan: 2012–2020. Geneva, Switzerland: WHO, 2012. Available at: http://apps.who.int/iris/bitstream/10665/44855/1/9789241503396_eng.pdf (accessed 11 July 2017).

50. World Health Organization. The smallpox eradication programme—SEP (1966–1980). Available at: http://www.who.int/features/2010/smallpox/en/ (accessed 11 July 2017).

51. World Health Organization. WHO statue commemorates smallpox eradication 2010. Available at: http://www.who.int/mediacentre/news/notes/2010/smallpox_20100517/en/ (accessed 11 July 2017).

52. World Health Organization Europe. Health 21: an introduction to the health for all policy framework for the WHO European Region. Geneva, Switzerland: WHO, 1998. Available at: http://www.euro.who.int/__data/assets/pdf_file/0003/88590/EHFA5-E.pdf?ua = 1 (accessed 11 July 2017).

53. World Health Organization. Human African trypanosomiasis: number of new cases drops to historically low level in 50 years. Geneva, Switzerland: WHO, 2010. Available at: http://www.who.int/neglected_diseases/integrated_media/integrated_media_hat_june_2010/en/ (accessed 11 July 2017).

54. World Health Organization. Hepatitis B, updated 12 July 2013. Available at: http://www.who.int/immunization/topics/hepatitis_b/en/ (accessed 11 July 2017).

55. World Health Organization. Leprosy, Fact sheet. updated February 2017. Available at: http://www.who.int/mediacentre/factsheets/fs101/en/ (accessed 11 July 2017).

56. World Health Organization. Meeting of the International Task Force for Disease Eradication, April 2015. Wkly Epidemiol Rec. 2015;90:381–382. Available at: http://www.who.int/wer/2015/wer9031.pdf (accessed 11 July 2017).

57. World Health Organization. Meeting of the International Task Force for Disease Eradication, 11 January 2007. Wkly Epidemiol Rec. 2007;82:197–208. Available at: http://www.who.int/wer/2007/wer8222_23.pdf (accessed 11 July 2017).
58. World Health Organization. The smallpox eradication program—SEP (1966–1980). Available at: http://www.who.int/features/2010/smallpox/en/ (accessed 18 June 2017).
59. World Health Organization. The global eradication campaign: dracunculiasis is the first parasitic disease set for eradication.n. Available at: http://www.who.int/dracunculiasis/eradication/en/ (accessed 11 July 2017).
60. World Health Organization. Bugs, drugs and smoke: stories from public health. - Smallpox: eradicating an ancient scourge. Geneva, Switzerland: WHO, 2011. Available at: http://www.who.int/about/history/publications/public_health_stories/en/ (accessed 11July 2017).

Chapter 3

From Panum to Eradication of Measles

ABSTRACT

A young doctor, Peter Panum was sent by the Danish government to investigate an epidemic of measles in the Faroe Islands in 1846. With an outstanding epidemiologic investigation he found that 6,000 of the 7,782 islanders were stricken with measles, leading to 102 deaths from the disease or its complications. He concluded that measles is a highly contagious disease that spreads from person to person (supporting the controversial Germ theory of disease over the Miasma concept) and that measles infection provides lifelong immunity.

Measles remained a global endemic disease with a low level of public concern as it was considered a normal rite of passage in childhood. But measles has severe complications and a high mortality rate, especially in poorly nourished children in developing countries. In the United States before the introduction of the first measles vaccine in 1963, 90 percent of children contracted measles before age 15, with epidemic cycles occurring every 2–3 years, and close to 500,000 cases, 48,000 hospitalizations and up to 500 deaths reported annually reported annually. However, peak incidence occurred every 5–9 years with estimates of the actual number of cases as high as 4 million.

Following introduction of a safe, effective, and low-cost vaccine, the number of measles cases fell rapidly in industrialized countries. Following the success of eradication of smallpox, optimism focused on polio and then measles for potential eradication. Some regions of the World Health Organization (WHO), such as the Pan American Health Organization (PAHO), and European Regions were later declared measles free. Measles deaths declined globally from an estimated 651,600 deaths in 2000 to 134,200 in 2015, mostly in children under age 5.

Despite growing optimism of declining rates globally, measles returned in the 21st century to Europe and transmitted by travelers to the Americas. This was facilitated by failure of the "one-dose policy," coupled with incomplete vaccine implementation and some public resistance to vaccination. These factors have made eradication a more distant goal. In 2012, the 2005 WHO proposal to eliminate measles by 2015 was adjusted to 2020. Parental refusal of vaccination is stimulated by and disproven claims of association with autism presenting legal and ethical problems. However, with sustained global effort, the goal of measles eradication can be achieved in the coming decade. This will be an enormous achievement for global health.

Case Studies in Public Health. DOI: http://dx.doi.org/10.1016/B978-0-12-804571-8.00005-6

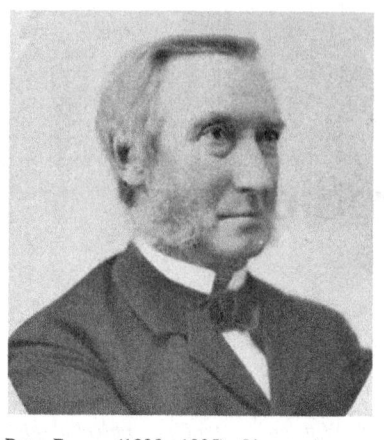

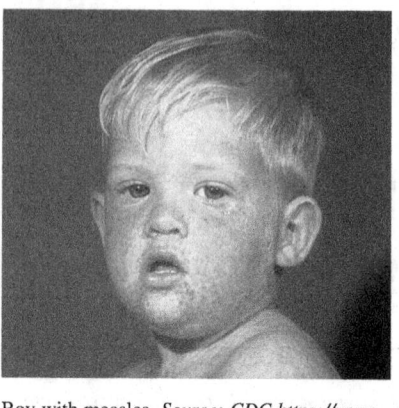

Boy with measles. *Source: CDC https://www. historyofvaccines.org/content/boy-measles.*

Peter Panum (1820—1885); Observations made during the epidemic of measles on the Faroe Islands in the year 1846. *Source: Bibliotek Laeger, Copenhagen, 1847. https://www.historyofvaccines.org/content/ portrait-peter-panum.*

BACKGROUND

Measles is an acute infectious disease caused by a virus of the *Paramyxovirus* family. It is one of the most highly infectious diseases, with a very high ratio of clinical to subclinical cases (99 to 1). Mortality rates are high in young children, especially those with compromised nutritional status, particularly those with vitamin A deficiency. The measles virus evolved from a virus disease of cattle (rinderpest) some 3,000—5,000 years ago. In the pre-vaccine era, measles was endemic worldwide, and it remains a major childhood infectious disease. Despite a major decline in deaths from millions per year in the pre-vaccine period, WHO reports 90,000 measles deaths globally in 2016, as compared to 550,000 deaths in 2000. Yet, epidemics are current in Europe and other parts of the world.

In 1846 at the age of 26, Peter Ludwig Panum, a newly graduated Danish medical doctor, was sent to the Faroe Islands by the Danish government to investigate an outbreak of measles. It was the first local outbreak since 1781. He actively traced the chain of transmission throughout the island as well as the immunity of those exposed to the previous epidemic. His report was entitled *Observations Made During The Epidemic Of Measles On The Faroe Islands In The Year 1846*. From his observation, he concluded that the disease was transmitted from person to person and from village to village by contagion (i.e., the Germ theory), contrary to the prevailing medical opinion that the measles was spread by bad air (i.e., the Miasma concept).

He also concluded that one attack provides lifelong immunity. In his own words, Panum described the measles epidemic of the Faroe Islands as follows:

"If among the 6,000 cases, of which I myself observed and treated about 1,000, not one was found in which it would be justifiable, on any grounds whatever, to suppose a miasmatic origin of the measles, because it was absolutely clear that the disease was transmitted from man to man and from village to village by contagion, whether the latter was received by immediate contact with a sick person or was conveyed to the infected person by clothes, or the like, it is certainly reasonable to entertain a considerable degree of doubt as to the miasmatic nature of the disease ... For if people think that the cases of the disease must be sought for as generally dispersed in the atmosphere, they can have no hope of protecting themselves against it, and will not be disposed to institute measures in this respect, since such measures must be regarded as vain; but if it is considered as settled that the measles is transmitted only to such individuals as are susceptible to the infectious material which every measles patient carries ... there may be hope of setting limits to the propagation of the disease ... Since people were convinced that the seeds of the disease could be carried through the air from house to house, from village to village, and from island to island, they did not think the trouble worthwhile to undertake isolation, whereby the disease would probably have been limited to quite a few houses. Experience had, however, taught a part of the inhabitants in 1781 that the spread of measles could be hindered by isolating places or even houses; and the old people, who had preserved recollection of this from their youth, effected in many places, on their own responsibility a sort of quarantine, whereby the places concerned were entirely or partially spared. Not until later on, when experience also taught the physicians of the country that the infection is quite obviously carried from place to place, and does not jump about, did they, too, begin to dissuade from communication with the infected houses and places, but the disease had by then already been spread over the entire country, and it was too late from the public viewpoint to institute serious measures toward isolation. Experience in regard to the fact that the measles is not miasmatic but prey contagious in character has been so dearly bought on the Faroe Islands ... that it is correct in practice, to consider the measles as contagious and not a miasmatic nor miasmatic-contagious disease."

Source: Panum PL. Observations made during the epidemic of measles on the Faroe Islands in the year 1846. In: Roueche B, editor. Curiosities of medicine: an assembly of medical diversions, 1552–1962. London: Victor Gollancz Ltd, 1963, pp. 210–236. Available at: http://www.deltaomega.org/documents/PanumFaroeIslands.pdf (accessed 19 February 2017).

In this description, Panum provides evidence of case-to-case transmission of the disease, thereby strengthening the Germ theory and discrediting the

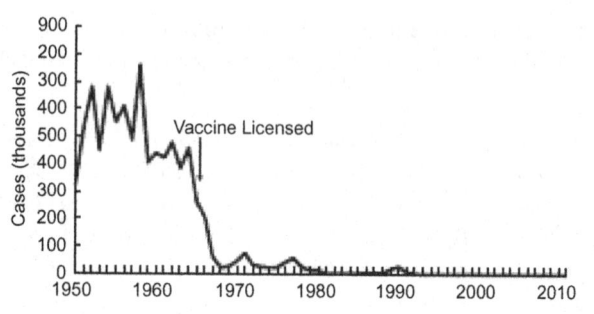

FIGURE 3.1 Measles cases, United States 1950–2011. *Source: Centers for Disease Control and Prevention. Pink Book, Measles. Available at https://www.cdc.gov/vaccines/pubs/pinkbook/ meas.html (accessed 4 September 2017).*

Miasma concept. His scientific contribution includes the description of case transmission, incubation period, immunity from previous infection, and the clinical aspects of measles, and his epidemiologic investigative approach is still in practice today.

Prior to the advent of effective and widespread use of vaccines for measles in the 1960s, nearly everyone contracted the disease during childhood. Estimates of annual incidence of measles were as high as 100–120 million cases, with 6 to 8 million deaths occurring each year globally. Measles also has high rates of complications such as pneumonia, encephalitis, and death. Mortality rates from measles typically vary from 0.1 percent to 10 percent but can be as high as 30 percent in some locations, depending largely on the nutrition and general health of children.

The advent of effective, safe, and inexpensive vaccines presented new challenges and opportunities for public and global health. The measles virus was first isolated by Thomas Peebles in Boston in 1954. Along with Samuel Katz, Peebles developed a vaccine that produced antibodies but required further attenuation to reduce associated symptoms of mild measles. An improved vaccine was developed by Maurice Hilleman using a strain of measles isolated by John Enders (who received a Nobel Prize in Medicine in 1954) called the Moraten (More attenuated Enders) strain. This is the only measles strain used in the United States since its licensing in 1967. The measles vaccine is included in the MMR (measles, mumps, and rubella) vaccine used globally. One dose of measles-containing vaccine at 9 months of age provides 85 percent of children protective antibodies, and gives immunity to 95 percent of children by 12 months of age. It is one of the safest and most cost-effective and immunogenic vaccines. See Figure 3.1 showing the dramatic decline in measles cases in the US from 1963 to 2011 following the licensing of the 1963 measles vaccine.

In the United States, the Centers for Disease Control and Prevention (CDC) estimates that before measles vaccination was introduced in the 1960s, some 3 to 4 million people suffered from measles annually, with some 48,000 hospitalizations, 4,000 cases of encephalitis, and 500 deaths. Serious complications and death rates vary in relation to the prior health and nutrition status to the extent that vitamin and mineral supplementation—especially vitamin A—is a vital part of care for children with measles. In addition, a rapidly fatal neurological degenerative condition called Subacute Sclerosing Pan Encepahalitis (SSPE) can occur in a minority of children for up to a decade following an episode of measles.

Despite its serious morbidity and mortality rates, measles is still commonly thought of as a mild illness and as a normal rite of passage of children. This perception, in combination with marketing by vaccine manufacturers, which assured the public and health professionals of lifelong protection from one dose of the vaccine, has led to policy errors. As many as four percent of immunizations fail to produce protective antibodies when administered, depending on the child's age, and it is difficult to achieve full herd immunity, which requires over 95 percent immunization coverage. Together, failure to reach all children for vaccination, failure of uptake of the vaccine, and a decline in immunity levels leads to a buildup of a susceptible population to this easily transmitted virus and to periodic measles outbreaks continuing well into the 21st century.

Concerns about the spread of measles led to the adoption and implementation of the "two-dose policy" by the US Advisory Committee on Immunization Practices (ACIP) and the American Academy of Pediatrics (AAP) in 1989. Later, international organizations also adopted the two-dose policy, extending coverage to children and young adults to ensure both individual protection and herd immunity. The two-dose policy was adopted late in many countries, and so it took time for the circulation of the virus to come under control. However, its long-term results have been positive, even leading to the elimination of the virus and its disease in some regions but importation and local circulation among susceptible persons still occurs.

CURRENT RELEVANCE

In the 1980s before measles vaccination was widespread globally, measles was responsible for nearly 2.6 million child deaths each year. With increasing use of the vaccine, there was a drastic reduction in measles cases and deaths. However, large pockets of susceptible populations remain vulnerable to this highly communicable, but preventable disease.

In 2010, the 63rd World Health Assembly (WHA) endorsed a global initiative toward the eventual eradication of measles but without a specific target date. At the time, the WHO Region of the Americas was declared measles free, and the Western Pacific Region (WPR) was approaching measles-free status. Measles elimination is defined as the absence of endemic measles virus transmission in a region or other defined geographical area for ≥ 12 months, in the presence of a well-performing surveillance system. However, other WHO Regions, including the European Region, still had large outbreaks. Globally, measles cases declined from 146 per million population in 2000 to 40 per million in 2013. Global measles mortality declined by 75 percent from more than 544,200 in 2000 to 145,700 in 2013, preventing an estimated 13.8 million deaths between 2000 and 2013.

Despite the global decline in measles cases since 2010, measles outbreaks resurged in Europe, the Americas, and globally, and in 2012, the WHO moved the target for eradication from 2015 to 2020. The WHO Region of the Americas is on track to achieve measles eradication, and the WPR is approaching the target. However, the WHO European, Eastern Mediterranean, South-East Asian, and African Regions are some distance from achieving this goal. The WHO also reports that global routine measles immunization coverage remains steady at 84 percent, and 145 countries have adopted the two-dose policy. In addition, mass immunization campaigns are conducted, reaching 145 million children in 2012 alone and more than 1 billion since 2000 as part of the global Measles & Rubella Initiative.

The measles case-fatality rate can be as high as 10 percent in developed nations but can be as high as 30 percent in child populations with high levels of malnutrition, weakened immune systems (e.g., from HIV/AIDS), and a lack of adequate health care. The live vaccine licensed in 1963 has been replaced by a more effective and heat-stable vaccine. However, a primary vaccination failure rate can be as high as eight percent, with about four percent losing protection over time. In an effort to eradicate measles, the two-dose policy was essential with the second booster dose increasing immunity levels. In 2000, 72 percent of the world population received a first dose of a measles-containing vaccine (MCV); by 2010, coverage increased to 85 percent, with regional variation (Figure 3.2).

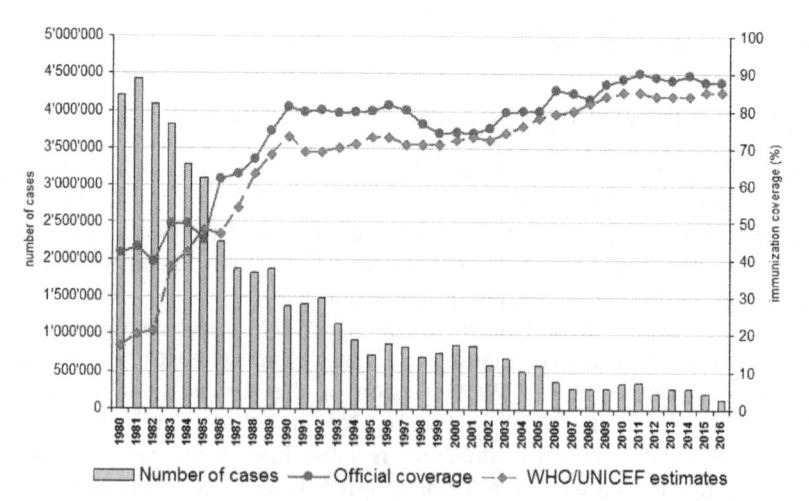

FIGURE 3.2 Global Measles cases and vaccination coverage, first dose (MCV), 1980–2016. *Source: World Health Organization. Immunization, Vaccines and Biologicals. Measles. 9 August 2017. Available at: http://www.who.int/immunization/monitoring_surveillance/burden/vpd/ surveillance_type/active/measles/en/ (accessed 12 August 2017).*

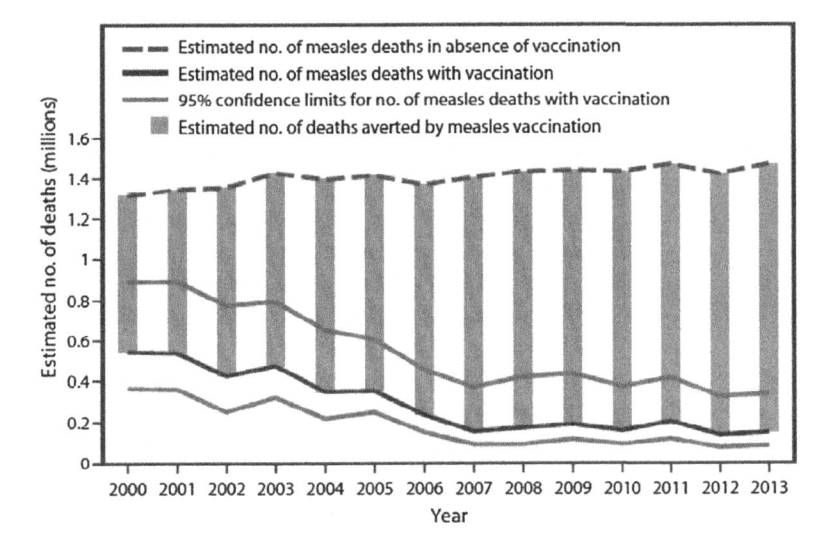

FIGURE 3.3   Estimated global measles deaths averted by vaccination, 2000–2013. *Source: Centers for Disease Control and Prevention. Deaths and deaths averted 2000–2013: global control and regional elimination of measles, 2000–2013. Morb Mortal Wkly Rep. 2014;63 (05):103–107.* Available at: *http://www.cdc.gov/mmwr/preview/mmwrhtml/mm6305a5.htm (accessed 19 February 2017).*

As shown in Figure 3.3 measles, vaccination prevented an estimated 13.8 million deaths globally compared to actual deaths with no vaccination during the period 2000 to 2012 (Figure 3.3).

In the early 1990s, measles led to over 1 million deaths globally, with high rates among poorly nourished children; half of these deaths were in Africa. Between 1989 and 1991, more than 55,000 measles cases were reported in the United States, with over 100 deaths. With widespread vaccination in the United States, measles cases declined from about 4 million to fewer than 100 cases, most of which were imported but with some spreading locally among inadequately immunized persons. The importation of measles into the United States has led to an increase of measles cases in children, especially in children under the 9–12 month recommended age for immunization, in immunocompromised persons, in older children or young adults not appropriately immunized, and in those with primary failure of vaccine uptake or a decline in antibody levels. The US has experienced an upsurge of measles cases since 2010, with 63 cases in 2010, 220 in 2011, 55 in 2012, 187 in 2013, 667 in 2014, 188 in 2015, 86 in 2016, and 120 in 2017 (to October) based on imported cases and spread to contacts.

Complacency and vaccine denial among both parents and medical/public health service providers led to measles outbreaks in countries that had not seen major outbreaks for many years. A number of large-scale outbreaks occurred in Europe as a result of public indifference, lax policies, and resistance to immunization. While measles was no longer considered to be endemic in the Americas as of 2002, many countries in the Americas, including the United States, experienced localized outbreaks as a result of contacts with cases imported from other countries. Low-income countries with weak health systems continued to struggle with the disease despite major assistance from international donors.

Waves of measles outbreaks occurred in Western Europe during the 1990s and between 2005 and 2014, with increases in measles cases across the region. Large outbreaks of 44,000 notified cases occurred in the Ukraine from 2005 to 2006, 1,400 cases in Switzerland from 2006 to 2008, and 200 cases in Austria in 2008. These outbreaks contributed to a rise in the global number of measles cases reported, from 7,499 in 2009 to 30,625 in 2010. Most cases occurred among unimmunized populations due to complacency among policymakers, a lack of harmonization of immunization schedules in Europe, large-scale movement of people across the European Union (EU), and where the influence of antivaccination groups was increasing. Large measles outbreaks in France, Bulgaria, and Ukraine accounted for the majority of cases between 2010 and 2012. Between January and November 2012, France, Italy, Romania, Spain, and the United Kingdom accounted for 87 percent of all reported measles cases in Europe, with seven cases complicated by measles-related encephalitis but no measles deaths. In 2013, measles outbreaks and reported cases also increased in Azerbaijan, Georgia, and Turkey. The European Centre for Disease Prevention and Control reports that cases of measles in Europe increased by 50 percent in the first five months of 2017, with total cases equivalent to all of 2016. (see Box 3.1).

International transmission of the virus has led to epidemics in countries thought to have achieved eradication. Despite earlier assessments that Europe was measles free, 4,224 cases were reported by 30 EU members and access states between July 2014 and July 2015—over 63 percent of which were laboratory confirmed. Germany accounted for 58 percent of cases, with outbreaks also occurring in Austria, Denmark, Norway, France, United Kingdom, Sweden, Belgium, Lithuania, and Belarus. Ten countries reported rates below one case per million and six reported zero cases. Children under 5 years of age accounted for one quarter of cases, of whom 77 percent were unvaccinated while 84 percent of total cases were unvaccinated. The age group over 30 years accounted for 23 percent of total cases. In this period, acute measles encephalitis occurred in eight cases, with one reported death.

The United Kingdom experienced a decline in measles coverage and large-scale measles outbreaks during the late 1990s resulting from fraudulent and disproven allegations of measles vaccination being associated with autism ("the Wakefield Effect"). As a result, measles epidemics occurred throughout the United Kingdom including England, Wales, and Scotland. In England, measles vaccination coverage fell below 85 percent in children aged 5 years from 2001 to 2005, with measles outbreaks occurring from

BOX 3.1 Measles in Europe

In 2013, Germany experienced a measles outbreak of more than 1,600 cases. There are differences in immunization schedules, which are independent in each state. In Germany, a review of outbreaks in two populous districts showed that in about 23 percent of cases family doctors either did not offer, and in some cases recommended against, immunization.

In 4 months of 2017, Milan Italy reported 233 suspected cases of measles; 87 percent laboratory-confirmed cases; 60 percent were individuals aged 15—39 years; 6 percent were ≤ 1 year of age; 88 percent were not vaccinated and 12 percent vaccinated; 108 of 203 were sporadic cases and 95 were related to 47 clusters. From the beginning of 2017 to 6 August, the Italian Ministry of Health reported 4,087 cases of measles and three deaths nationally.

In 2016, several other European Union / European Economic Area (EU/EEA) countries reported measles outbreaks and an increase in the number of cases continues to be observed in 2017. Some previous and ongoing measles outbreaks in other EU/EEA countries have been epidemiologically linked to the current outbreak in Romania. Nosocomial outbreaks highlight the importance of improving measles vaccination coverage of healthcare workers. In 2016, several other EU/EEA countries reported measles outbreaks and an increase in the number of cases continues to be observed in 2017, possibly linked to the current outbreak in Romania. Overall, more than 14,000 cases have been reported in the EU/EEA since January 2016, including 35 deaths.

The measles outbreak in Italy from January to August 2017 included over 4,400 cases reported in 20 Regions. The median age was 27 years; 88 percent of the cases were unvaccinated. The highest incidence was in infants below one year of age and 7 percent of cases occurred among healthcare workers. Three deaths and two cases of encephalitis were reported. Wide immunity gaps and nosocomial transmission are major challenges to measles elimination in Italy.

Sources: European Centre for Disease Control and Prevention. Surveillance and disease data: main developments, updated 11 October 2016. Available at: http://ecdc.europa.eu/en/healthtopics/ measles/epidemiological_data/pages/annual_epidemiological_reports.aspx (accessed 19 February 2017). Amendola A, Bianchi S, Frati ER, Ciceri G, Faccini M, Senatore S, et al. Ongoing large measles outbreak with nosocomial transmission in Milan, northern Italy, March—August 2017. Euro Surveill. 2017;22(33). Available at: http://www.eurosurveillance.org/ViewArticle.aspx? ArticleId = 22858 (accessed 20 August 2017). European Centre for Disease Prevention and Control. Epidemiological update: Measles - monitoring European outbreaks, 7 July 2017. Available at: https://ecdc.europa.eu/en/news-events/epidemiological-update-measles-monitoring-european- outbreaks-7-july-2017 (accessed 20 August 2017). Del Manso M, Baggieri M, Magurano F, Rota MC. Ongoing outbreak with well over 4,000 measles cases in Italy from January to end of August 2017: what is making elimination so difficult? Euro Surveill. 2017;22(37):pii=30614. DOI: http:// dx.doi.org/10.2807/1560-7917.ES.2017.22.37.30614. Available at: http://www.eurosurveillance. org/ViewArticle.aspx?ArticleId=22876 (accessed 14 September 2017).

2006 to 2008 throughout the United Kingdom, and again in 2012 and 2013. Many cases were in the north-west and north-east regions among infants younger than the recommended immunization age and among children between the ages of 7 and 16. Measles showed signs of coming under control by 2014, with England reporting only 103 laboratory confirmed cases compared to 1413 in 2013.

The European Center for Disease Control (ECDC) reported that between November 2015 and October 2016, 30 European Union and potential new members (EU/EEA) reported 3,037 cases of measles. The highest numbers of cases were reported by Romania (1,011), Italy (728), and the United Kingdom (569), accounting respectively for 33, 24, and 19 percent of the EU/EEA cases in the 12-month period. Measles is targeted for elimination in Europe but the measles notification rate was below the elimination target of one case per million population in 17 of 30 reporting countries; nine countries reported zero cases. The highest notification rates were Romania (50.9), Italy (12.0), and Ireland (11.0). The diagnosis of measles was confirmed by positive laboratory results (serology, virus detection, or isolation) in 72 percent of all cases. Of all 3,301 cases with known ages, 1,213 (40%) were children under 5 years of age, but 892 (29%) were aged 20 years or over. The highest incidence rates reported were children below 1 year of age (55.4 per million) and children between 1 and 4 years of age (43.6 per million). Romania reported more than 3,400 cases and 17 deaths from January 2016 to April 2017, and calls for a revamping of the national immunization program (see Box 3.1).

While increased vaccination rates have helped incidence rates to decline, over 95 percent of deaths from measles continue to occur in low-income countries with weak health systems, high levels of undernutrition, and relatively poor immunization coverage. In sub-Saharan Africa, measles incidence declined from 838 to 238 per million persons between 2000 and 2010, and vaccination with one dose of MCV reached a coverage rate of 83 percent in 2009, remaining at that level until 2016. Even with improvements in coverage, the African Region experienced a widespread resurgence of measles from 2009 to 2010, with more than 250,000 cases and 1,500 deaths in 28 sub-Saharan Africa countries. In 2011, Nigeria reported 30,000 cases with 122 deaths, and the Democratic Republic of the Congo reported 16,000 cases and 107 deaths between January and February 2011 alone. In the Eastern Mediterranean Region (EMR), about 35 percent of the population live in Afghanistan, Sudan, Somalia, Djibouti, and Pakistan where measles immunization rates remain below 60 percent and annual deaths are estimated at 81,000 among children under 5. The WHO reports that in 2015, global figures for measles included just under 200,000 reported cases, 134,000 deaths, and 85 percent global coverage (one dose of measles continuing vaccine, with 16 percent of countries reaching over 90 percent child coverage) (Figure 3.2).

Despite success in vaccination with one dose and increasing subsequently to two doses, the failure to eradicate measles is one of policy and implementation. Priority has been given to polio eradication—a far less lethal disease—largely because of its fearsome crippling effects and the popular drama of effective vaccination programs capturing public attention. Control, elimination, and potential eradication of measles will require more intense efforts to increase basic coverage, as well as catch-up campaigns to implement the two-dose policy. New strategies are needed to influence global public perception of vaccine safety and to convey the vital importance of immunization in protecting children and preventing the spread of disease among children who may be at risk due to immune suppression due to disease or cancer treatment.

Globally, in 2013, about 85 percent of the world's children received one dose of measles vaccine by their first birthday through routine health services compared to 72 percent in 2000. Also, the number of deaths from measles has been shown to be reduced by 50 percent with the use of vitamin A supplementation, which helps to improve nutrition and to prevent measles eye damage and blindness. Measles contributes to an increase in the severity of prior malnutrition contributing to kwashiorkor and other forms of protein-energy malnutrition in severe poverty areas of the world. In refugee situations, measles immunization regardless of previous immunization is an essential part of life-saving support systems.

Measles elimination is an important factor in achieving Sustainable Development Goal (SDG) 3 for ending preventable deaths of newborns and children under 5. Currently, the WHO aims to achieve measles eradication in at least five regions by 2020. In 2012, the WHO launched a new initiative combining measles and rubella vaccination and promoted MMR so that rubella and mumps and their complications can also be eliminated. Also, the WHO extended the priority it gave to polio eradication to measles, and subsequently also to rubella, due to the availability and success of the MMR vaccine (see Chapter 19).

High immunization rates in developed and developing countries are essential to achieve and sustain global measles control goals. Measles protection requires high levels of routine immunization, with two doses for over 95 percent of a population, to avoid buildup of a susceptible population easily infected when exposed to even minimal transient exposure, such as occurred in the United States in Disneyland in 2014 and spreading to other parts of California. The two-dose measles policy needs greater emphasis to increase coverage from 87 percent to reach the goal of 95 percent herd immunity level. To accomplish this goal, a range of improved strategic efforts is needed that include: the identification of barriers to obtaining immunization, particularly for high-risk populations; enhanced education of service providers; and strengthened surveillance systems. Catch-up campaigns should include adults up to age 45 who may not have received 2 doses of a measles containing vaccine or none at all. The biggest challenge is to reduce the number of parental refusals on grounds of misinformation spread through the Internet. In Europe, a pan-European strategy is needed for the sustainable elimination of measles.

The PAHO recommended: "catch-up," "keep-up," and "follow-up" vaccination strategies, have succeeded in interrupting measles transmission in the Americas. In practice, this meant one-time nationwide campaigns targeting 1- to 14-year-old children; promoting routine vaccination among 1-year-olds; and nationwide campaigns conducted every 4 years targeting all 1–4 year olds, along with active integrated surveillance. Long-term elimination of indigenous measles cases is achievable, indicating that global eradication is achievable with implementation of appropriate strategies to save many thousands of lives. However, in recent years, measles cases in the Americas have been imported from other countries and spread locally, in some cases becoming endemic once again.

The 1998 UK fraudulent allegations of measles vaccine causing autism is still a widely held view that continues to spread on social media, despite being disproven. Misinformation on the Internet and other social media promoting widespread opposition to immunization is not uncommon, even among well-educated and prosperous families, largely due to the spread of antivaccination ideological beliefs and conspiracy theories of poisoning. Competing public health priorities, along with a lack of strong advocacy for the public in most countries, has resulted in a lack of visibility and active attention to investment in and the implementation of measles eradication strategies.

Voluntary vaccination policies downplay the importance of child immunization in reducing the incidence of communicable diseases such as measles. They risk reducing herd immunity to below 95 percent coverage, given the 5 percent failure rate of vaccine uptake and waning immunity, which were the essential factors justifying the two-dose policy. Public concern over misreported potential risks of adverse vaccine reactions has contributed to reduction in vaccine coverage rates, making it more difficult to achieve eradication.

Globally, measles continues to cause death and severe disease in children. Almost every organ of the body can be affected by complications of measles. Common causes of death include pneumonia, croup, and encephalitis, which can result in long-term disability. Measles is also a common cause of blindness in developing countries. Immune deficiency disorders, malnutrition, vitamin A deficiency, intense exposures to measles, and lack of previous measles vaccination increase the occurrence of complications. Improvements in socioeconomic status can also decrease case-fatality rates.

In situations of natural or man-made disaster, measles and other infectious diseases can greatly extend the disaster's long-term consequences. The 2004 Indian Ocean earthquake and tsunami disaster are further examples of the importance of measles vaccination in disaster situations when refugees are living in crowded situations. Measles outbreaks can easily occur but are preventable if the disaster management plans include childhood immunization along with vitamin A and nutritional support to reduce case-fatality rates. A follow-up report of the tsunami noted that about 1.2 million children received measles immunization along with more than 3 million children who received vitamin A supplementation and other measures aimed at prevention of disease outbreaks (e.g., nutrition support and safe water supplies).

Panum's important epidemiological analysis helped to establish the Germ theory as the predominant factor in infectious disease epidemiology. In the 20th century a new cofactor was added in that nutritional deficiency was found to be a factor in fatality rates from measles. Vitamin A supplementation became part of the global program of measles and prevention of child mortality in general. Despite enormous progress in control of the disease, eradication is still elusive and subject to distractions that can delay eradication. The sad fact remains that millions of children will die as a result of the inadequacies of focus and implementation of control measures to eradicate this preventable disease.

ETHICAL ISSUES

Public health routinely relies on persuasion to achieve compliance with immunization schedules. The United States and other countries have established vaccine-adverse events legislation, standardizing the reporting of adverse vaccination situations. The UK experience over several decades suggests that public media scares can influence the public's perception of the "dangers" associated with vaccines, which led to a significant reduction in immunization coverage and to the return of pertussis in the 1980s and measles in the 1990s. Namely, the "Wakefield Effect" was the result of a fraudulent "study" in the United Kingdom published in Lancet in 1998 alleging that measles serum in MMR vaccine causes autism. This report created a great deal of publicity, anxiety, and loss of confidence, promoting parental refusal and declining acceptance of measles vaccine use. This resulted in a resurgence of measles in the United Kingdom and other countries and a reduction in herd immunity. The Internet is laden with conspiracy theories on vaccines and the disproven alleged relationship of measles vaccine and autism is a common reason given by mothers refusing vaccinations for their children especially, but not only, for MMR.

The influence of latter-day antivaccinationists has raised questions about who should be responsible for vaccination policy and implementation and also about the rights of parents and children in refusing vaccination. Much of the measles epidemic in Europe is school-related, occurring among the underimmunized age group between the ages of 10 and 16 years. As previously mentioned, authorities in California, in the United States, became alarmed over an outbreak of about 100 cases of measles thought to have originated in Disneyland traced to an imported case in 2014. The subsequent investigation led to the discovery that there was a 67 percent increase in the invocation of the "personal belief exemption (PBE)" for vaccination in the previous 10 years, leading to a decline in herd immunity. Ultimately, this led to a 2015 California statute that banned vaccination exemptions for nonmedical reasons. A study of PBE by Brennan et al, 2017 of personal exemption rates for school attendance in California showed private schools had rates over four times higher than those of public school children (8.7 vs. 2.1 percent) and rates in one group of private schools as high as 45 percent, 19 times higher than rates in public schools, with increasing trends of PBE in many private school networks.

Vaccination is a moral, social, and in the United States a legal obligation to protect those who cannot be immunized. The failure to vaccinate poses health risks to any child, but more so to those who are particularly vulnerable to infectious diseases such as children below age 12 months who are unable to receive the MMR vaccine and also to immune-compromised patients of any age. Herd immunity is crucial for protection and to eliminate this important disease.

ECONOMIC ISSUES

In the United States, the 2011 measles outbreak of 107 cases cost $5.3 million. Between 1989 and 1991, measles resulted in more than 100 deaths, with over 55,000 cases reported. This was followed by a return of SSPE, a rare but fatal neurological complication of measles in children in the United States. SSPE is extremely costly for care needs, and had largely disappeared after the measles vaccine became widely used.

On a global scale, shortfalls in national funding and weak public health systems contribute to delays in supplementary immunization activities despite major funding by bilateral and international donors. Inadequate immunization coverage and disease outbreaks in Africa and in India impact the achievement of SDG 3, including the target to end the preventable death of newborns and children up to 5 years of age. The WHO notes that decreases in financial resources and a lack of political commitments have substantial implications for measles morbidity and mortality, which could increase in the future beyond current morbidity rates.

The two dose policy was rare in the 1980s but gradually adopted since then in high-income countries, but slowly in medium- and low-income countries. A Canadian study in the 1990s showed that the two-dose policy was cost effective in reducing and preventing measles and its complications. Other analyses in the 1990s indicated an economic as well as a public health benefit of the two-dose policy, which has been adopted as the "gold standard" of measles immunization strategies.

According to the WHO, measles vaccination, at a cost of $1 per dose with a two-dose policy, provides cost benefits as high as US$10 billion. In 2006, Germany reported that the per case cost was €317 for 614 measles cases. GAVI, the Vaccine Alliance funds improved vaccine programs in low-income countries, including two doses of measles vaccine, outbreak preparedness and rapid response, research to improve diagnostics, and communication strategies.

While the cost of MMR vaccine has been dramatically reduced, research and development has made vaccines more easily transported and administered and is ongoing. Heat-stable vaccines, for example, can reduce the cumbersome and costly cold-chain requirements. Well-trained and supervised community health workers can ease the difficulties in vaccination coverage in hard-to-reach communities. Completion of vaccination in remote areas using community health workers along with simpler and inexpensive methods of distribution and administration will help to meet the goal of 95 percent herd immunity. Political and health leaders as well as providers should do all they can to promote vaccination and reduce fears of vaccine safety.

CONCLUSION

Measles vaccination is one of the great tools for advancing public health globally. Measles eradication is still achievable but will require sustained efforts and resources.

Control, elimination, and potential eradication of measles globally will require more years of intense effort to increase basic coverage with two doses of the vaccine as well as catch-up campaigns for young adults who have been shown to be vulnerable due to past immunization policies. A sustained two-dose policy with high priority globally, supplemented by catch-up campaigns for older children and young adults, and outbreak control that includes epidemiologic investigation and continuous surveillance is required. Achieving the recommended over 95 percent measles vaccine coverage for adequate herd immunity is a difficult target for many nations even for a one-dose policy, but for two doses even more so. The refusal of immunization among educated sectors of society remains a problem that raises ethical and legal issues which are currently being debated in the United States, in Europe and elsewhere.

Measles eradication is and should remain one of the central targets on the global public health community agenda for SDG attainment of health targets. The WHO Global Measles and Rubella Strategic Plan, 2012–20, is built on successes in reducing morbidity and mortality globally and on the elimination of indigenous transmission of measles in some regions. But the recurrence of measles from imported cases has made eradication a challenge. Importation and spread by an imported index case can lead to epidemics, which can spread, become endemic and hinder goal achievement. An increased focus on health promotion and education, is needed with community involvement, as well as political leadership. Surveillance and case-based outbreak control are important components of measles elimination activities. Measles elimination efforts should be joined with polio end-stage and rubella eradication strategies. The WHO Strategic Advisory Committee (SAGE) in January 2016 concluded that the target date for measles eradication will vary by region, but the global eradication target will be put off until after 2020 due to slower than anticipated progress in routine vaccination in many low-income countries.

Improvements in the determinants of health such as living standards, adequate housing, nutrition, and extension and improvement of quality healthcare services are important measures for improving population health in addition to a focus on communicable diseases, such as measles. For example, prevention of vulnerability and comorbidity by vitamin A supplements and malaria bednets have been shown to be effective in reducing measles case fatality among high-risk populations. Successful control of measles also requires broad-based cooperative efforts across sectors and at all levels of society: governments, communities, voluntary agencies, and service providers. Using MMR vaccine for measles control brings the added benefit of reducing rubella, congenital rubella syndrome, and mumps.

The decline in immunization coverage with the MMR vaccine in the United Kingdom in the late 1990s was a result of widespread publicity and concerns from a fraudulent and disproven allegation of an autism association (the "Wakefield Effect"). Many children were left unimmunized and, consequently, unprotected, as a result of parental fears of MMR vaccine complications. It also leaves individuals who are unable to receive the vaccine due to an increased risk of potential complications at increased risk, such as those with chronic diseases (e.g., sickle cell anemia, HIV or leukemia). Inadequate herd immunity endangers unimmunized infants, older children, and young adults with large-scale outbreaks, increasing the risk of disease even among adequately immunized children and threatening those with impaired immune systems with the disease and even death.

Measles eradication is possible, but it requires resources and high-level political and financial support. The international commitment to measles eradication is achievable in all countries by using measures to attain over 95 percent immunization coverage and reducing refusals of immunization. It will also require commitment to financing and infrastructure development. Technological changes such as freeze-dried vaccines, which can be applied by nasal spray, don't require cold-chain resources and with administration by nurses or community health workers, are on the horizon.

The challenge is manageable for the world health community over the next decade, thus fulfilling the promise first recognized in Panum's work. Political commitment and leadership through both the governmental and private sectors are also needed to enhance efforts to eliminate measles, which is also crucial to achieving the SDGs. The eradication of measles to be achievable will require steady expansion of routine immunization coverage with adequate financial support and strengthened human resource infrastructure.

It will be an achievement of humanity no less important than eradication of poliomyelitis, both of which are no less challenging than landing a man on the moon.

RECOMMENDATIONS

1. Vaccination coverage of over 95 percent with two doses of MCVs should be promoted financially and organizationally in all countries as an integral part of national immunization programs.
2. A two-dose measles vaccination policy is vital, along with special supplementary campaigns as standard national policy in all countries, preferably using MMR, in order to also eliminate circulation of measles as well as mumps and rubella.
3. Integrated, targeted, and documented performance indicators are key components of the type of case-based surveillance and outbreak control program needed in all countries. This is of major importance in populations experiencing civil unrest of conflicts.
4. Parental discretion should be seen from the perspective that an unimmunized child puts other children at risk; mandatory immunization for school attendance is needed as in the 2015 California and European initiatives, to produce a documented medical reason to avoid giving MMR vaccine. This is as important for child safety as with parental responsibility for mandatory child safety car seats or bicycle rider helmets as required by law in many countries.
5. Low- and middle-income countries need sustainable measures to increase internal efforts and resources for child programs with decreased reliance on support from international agencies and governments.
6. National efforts to enhance community-based health promotion to increase understanding and support for integrated immunization programs would assist in meeting the elimination or eradication challenge of measles.

STUDENT REVIEW QUESTIONS

1. How do the Miasma and Germ Theories conflict? How do they complement each other?
2. How did Panum's epidemiologic investigation help resolve the conflict between these two theories?
3. What is the relevance of Panum's work to public health today?
4. What is the "Two-Dose Policy" for measles and why is it important?
5. What are the policy issues for global health in measles eradication?
6. What are the key factors of widespread parental refusal or failure to vaccinate children?

7. How did measles reappear in regions thought to have eliminated the virus?
8. What is required in order to achieve global eradication of measles?
9. What other infectious and non-infectious diseases are planned for eradication?
10. Why does vaccination policy require continuous epidemiologic and laboratory monitoring?

RECOMMENDED READINGS

1. Amendola A, Bianchi S, Frati ER, Ciceri G, Faccini M, Senatore S, et al. Ongoing large measles outbreak with nosocomial transmission in Milan, northern Italy, March–August 2017. Euro Surveill. 2017;22(33):30596. Available at: http://www.eurosurveillance.org/ViewArticle.aspx?ArticleId=22858 (accessed 20 August 2017).

2. Aylward B, Hennessey KA, Zagaria N, Olivé J-M, Cochi S. When is a disease eradicable? 100 years of lessons learned. Am J Public Health. 2000;90(10):1515–1520. Available at: https://www.ncbi.nlm.nih.gov/pmc/articles/PMC1446384/ (accessed 14 February 2017).

3. Bauch CT, Earn DJ. Vaccination and the theory of games. Proc Natl Acad Sci USA. 2004;101:13391–13394. Available at: http://www.ncbi.nlm.nih.gov/pubmed/15329411 (accessed 19 February 2017).

4. Bino S, Kakarriqi E, Xibinaku M, Ion-Nedelcu N, Bukli M, Emiroglu N, et al. Measles-rubella mass immunization campaign in Albania, November 2000. J Infect Dis. 2003;187 (Suppl1):S223–S229. Available at: http://jid.oxfordjournals.org/content/187/Supplement_1/S223.long (accessed 19 February 2017).

5. Brennan JM, Bednarczyk RA, Richards JL, Allen KE, Warraich GJ, Omer S. Trends in personal belief exemption rates among alternative private schools: Waldorf, Montessori and Holistic kindergardens in California, 2000–2014. Am J Public Health. 2017;107:108–112. Abstract available at: https://www.ncbi.nlm.nih.gov/pubmed/27854520 (accessed 7 September 2017).

6. Carter Center. International task force for disease eradication. Available at: http://www.cartercenter.org/health/itfde/index.html (accessed 19 February 2017).

7. Castillo-Solorzano C, Marsigli C, Danovaro-Holliday MC, Ruiz-Matus C, Tambini G, Andrus JK. Measles and rubella elimination initiatives in the Americas: lessons learned and best practices. J Infect Dis. 2011;204(Suppl 1):S27983. Available at: http://jid.oxfordjournals.org/content/204/suppl_1/S279.long (accessed 19 February 2017).

8. Centers for Disease Control and Prevention. Achievements in public health, 1900–1999: control of infectious diseases. Morb Mortal Wkly Rep. 1999;48(29):621–629. Available at: https://www.cdc.gov/mmwr/preview/mmwrhtml/mm4829a1.htm (accessed 19 February 2017).

9. Centers for Disease Control and Prevention Advisory Committee on Immunization Practices (ACIP). Recommended immunization schedule for persons aged 0 through 18 years—United States, updated February 6, 2017. Available at: http://www.cdc.gov/vaccines/schedules/ (accessed 19 February 2017).

10. Centers for Disease Control and Prevention. Ten great public health achievements—United States, 2001–2010. Morb Mortal Wkly Rep. 2011;60:619–623. Available at: http://www.cdc.gov/mmwr/preview/mmwrhtml/mm6019a5.htm (accessed 19 July 2015).

11. Centers for Disease Control and Prevention. Ten great public health achievements—worldwide, 2001–2010. Morb Mortal Wkly Rep. 2011;60:814–818. Available at: http://www.cdc.gov/mmwr/preview/mmwrhtml/mm6024a4.htm (accessed 14 February 2017).

12. Centers for Disease Control and Prevention. Measles—United States, 2011. Morb Mortal Wkly Rep. 2012;61:253–257. Available at: http://www.cdc.gov/mmwr/preview/mmwrhtml/mm6115a1.htm (accessed 14 February 2017).

13. Centers for Disease Control and Prevention. Increased transmission and outbreaks of measles, European Region, 2011. Available at: http://www.cdc.gov/mmwr/preview/mmwrhtml/mm6047a1.htm (accessed 14 February 2017).

14. Centers for Disease Control and Prevention. Immunization schedules: Birth–18 Years & "Catch-up" immunization schedules United States 2015: details for health care professionals. Available at: http://www.cdc.gov/vaccines/schedules/hcp/child-adolescent.html (accessed 14 July 2015).

15. Centers for Disease Control and Prevention. Global control and regional elimination of measles, 2000–2012. Morb Mortal Wkly Rep. 2014;63(05):103–107. Available at: http://www.cdc.gov/mmwr/preview/mmwrhtml/mm6305a5.htm (accessed 11 February 2017).

16. Centers for Disease Control and Prevention. Measles cases and outbreaks. Page last updated 23 August 2017. Available at: https://www.cdc.gov/measles/cases-outbreaks.html (accessed 7 September 2017).

17. Centers for Disease Control and Prevention. Pink Book, Measles. Available at: https://www.cdc.gov/vaccines/pubs/pinkbook/images/meas-fig-02.jpg (accessed 4 September 2017).

18. College of Physicians of Philadelphia. History of anti-vaccination movements. Vaccines, 2013. Available at: http://www.historyofvaccines.org/content/articles/history-anti-vaccination-movements (accessed 19 February 2017).

19. College of Physicians of Philadelphia. Vaccines: vaccine development and licensing events. Available at: http://www.historyofvaccines.org/content/articles/vaccine-development-licensing-events (accessed 14 February 2017).

20. Delamater PL, Leslie TF, Yang YT. Change in medical exemptions from immunization in California after elimination of personal belief exemptions. JAMA. 2017;318(9):863–864. doi:10.1001/jama.2017.9242. Abstract available at: http://jamanetwork.com/journals/jama/article-abstract/2652640 (accessed 8 September 2017).

21. de Quadros CA. Can measles be eradicated globally? Bull World Health Organ. 2004;82 (2):134–138. Available at: https://www.ncbi.nlm.nih.gov/pmc/articles/PMC2585902/pdf/15042236.pdf (accessed 19 February 2017).

22. de Quadros CA, Andrus JK, Danovaro-Holliday MC, Castillo-Solórzano C. Feasibility of global measles eradication after interruption of transmission in the Americas. Expert Rev Vaccines. 2008;7(3):355–362. Available at: http://www.measlesrubellainitiative.org/wp-content/uploads/2013/06/Feasibility-global-eradication.pdf (accessed 14 February 2017).

23. Dowdle WR. The principles of disease elimination and eradication. Morb Mortal Wkly Rep. 1999;48:23–27. Available at: http://www.cdc.gov/mmwr/preview/mmwrhtml/su48a7.htm (accessed 19 February 2017).

24. European Centre for Disease Control and Prevention. Surveillance and disease data: main developments, updated 11 October 2016. Available at: http://ecdc.europa.eu/en/healthtopics/measles/epidemiological_data/pages/annual_epidemiological_reports.aspx (accessed 19 February 2017).

25. Gaafar T, Moshni E, Lievano F. The challenge of achieving measles elimination in the eastern Mediterranean region by 2010. J Infect Dis. 2003;187:S164–S171. Available at: http://jid.oxfordjournals.org/content/187/Supplement_1/S164.full.pdf + html (accessed 14 February 2017).

26. Garon J, Orenstein W. Improving the science of measles prevention—will it make for a better immunization program? PLoS Med. 2016;13(10):e1002145. doi:10.1371/journal. pmed.1002145. Available at: https://open.library.emory.edu/publications/emory%3Ars257/ (accessed 19 February 2017).

27. General Medical Council Great Britain. Dr Andrew Jeremy Wakefield determination on serious professional misconduct (SPM) and sanction, 2010. Available at: http://briandeer. com/solved/gmc-wakefield-sentence.pdf (accessed 14 February 2017).

28. Ginsberg GM, Tulchinsky TH. Costs and benefits of a second measles inoculation of children in Israel, the West Bank and Gaza. J Epidemiol Commun Health. 1990;44:274–280. Available at: https://www.researchgate.net/publication/21030061_Costs_and_benefits_of_a_ second_measles_inoculation_of_children_in_Israel_the_West_Bank_and_Gaza (accessed 14 February 2017).

29. Goodman RA, Foster KL, Trowbridge FL, Figueroa JP. Global disease elimination and eradication as public health strategies. Morb Mortal Wkly Rep. 1999;48(Suppl):1–309. Available at: ftp://ftp.cdc.gov/pub/Publications/mmwr/other/suppl48.pdf (accessed 14 February 2017).

30. Gostin LO. Law, ethics, and public health in the vaccination debates: politics of the measles outbreak. JAMA Online. 2015. Available at: http://scholarship.law.georgetown.edu/cgi/ viewcontent.cgi?article = 2472&context = facpub (accessed 14 February 2017).

31. Guide to Community Preventive Services. Vaccination program requirements for child care, school, and college attendance: summary of task force findings, 2016. Available at: https://www.thecommunityguide.org/findings/vaccination-programs-requirements-child-care-school-and-college-attendance (accessed 19 February 2017).

32. Health Protection Agency, UK. Increase in measles cases in 2006, in England and Wales. Available at: www.gov.uk/government/publications/measles-confirmed-cases/confirmed-cases-of-measles-mumps-and-rubella-in-england-and-wales-2012-to-2013 (accessed 14 February 2017).

33. Hendriks J, Blume S. Measles vaccination before the Measles-Mumps-Rubella Vaccine. Am J Public Health. 2013;103(8):1393–1401. https://doi.org10.2105/AJPH.2012.301075. Available at: https://www.ncbi.nlm.nih.gov/pmc/articles/PMC4007870/pdf/AJPH.2012.301 075.pdf (accessed 4 September 2017).

34. Hellenbrand W, Siedler A, Tischer A, Meyer C, Reiter S, et al. Progress towards measles elimination in Germany. J Infect Dis. 2003;187(Suppl 1):S208–S216. Available at: http:// jid.oxfordjournals.org/content/187/Supplement_1/S208.long (accessed 14 February 2017).

35. Heymann DL. Control of communicable diseases manual. 20th edition. Washington, DC: American Public Health Association, 2014. Available at: http://secure.apha.org/imis/ ItemDetail?iProductCode = 978-087553-0185&CATEGORY = BK (accessed 14 February 2017).

36. Hopkins DR. Disease eradication. N Engl J Med. 2013;368:54–63. Available at: http:// www.nejm.org/doi/full/10.1056/NEJMra1200391 (accessed 14 February 2017).

37. Hugh-Jones ME. Overview of anthrax. Merck MSD Veterinary Manual, 2016. Available at: http://www.msdvetmanual.com/generalized-conditions/anthrax/overview-of-anthrax (accessed 11 September 2017).

38. Levin A, Burgess C, Garrison LP, Bauch C, Babigumira J, Simons E, et al. Global eradication of measles: an epidemiologic and economic evaluation. J Infect Dis. 2011;204(Suppl 1):S98−S106. Available at: http://jid.oxfordjournals.org/content/204/suppl_1/S98.full (accessed 19 February 2017).

39. McLean HQ, Fiebelkorn AP, Temte JL, Wallace GS, Centers for Disease Control and Prevention. Prevention of measles, rubella, congenital rubella syndrome, and mumps, 2013: summary recommendations of the Advisory Committee on Immunization Practices (ACIP). MMWR Recomm Rep. 2013;62(RR-04):1−34. Available at: http://www.ncbi.nlm.nih.gov/pubmed/23760231 (accessed 14 February 2017).

40. Measles and Rubella Initiative. Substantial decline in global measles deaths, but disease still kills 90 000 per year. Joint news release CDC/GAVI/UNICEF/WHO, 26 October 2017. Available at: https://measlesrubellainitiative.org/measles-news/substantial-decline-global-measles-deaths-disease-still-kills-90-000-per-year/ (accessed 9 November 2017).

41. Meissner HC, Strebel PM, Orenstein WA. Measles vaccines and the potential for worldwide eradication of measles. Pediatrics. 2004 Oct;114(4):1065−1069. Available at: http://www.ncbi.nlm.nih.gov/pubmed/15466106 (accessed 14 July 2015).

42. Muscat M, Shefer A, Ben Mamou M, Spataru R, Jankovic D, Deshevoy S, et al. The state of measles and rubella in the WHO European Region, 2013. Clin Microbiol Infect. 2014; (Suppl 5), 12−18. Available at: http://onlinelibrary.wiley.com/doi/10.1111/1469-0691.12584/pdf (accessed 14 FEbruary 2017).

43. National Vaccine Information Center. California State vaccine requirements. Posted 11 August 2015. Available at: http://www.nvic.org/Vaccine-Laws/state-vaccine-requirements/california.aspx (accessed 19 February 2017).

44. Orenstein WA, Papania MJ, Wharton ME. Measles elimination in the United States. J Infect Dis. 2004;189(Suppl 1):S1−S3. Available at: https://academic.oup.com/jid/article/189/Supplement_1/S1/820569/Measles-Elimination-in-the-United-States (accessed 19 February 2017).

45. Panum PL. Observations made during the epidemic of measles on the Faroe Islands in the year 1846. In: Roueche B, editor. Curiosities of medicine: an assembly of medical diversions, 1552−1962. London: Victor Gollancz Ltd, 1963210−236. Available at: http://www.deltaomega.org/documents/PanumFaroeIslands.pdf (accessed 19 February 2017).

46. Ramsay ME, Jin L, White J, Litton P, Cohen B, Brown D. The elimination of indigenous measles transmission in England and Wales. J Infect Dis. 2003;187:S198−S207. Abstract available at: http://www.ncbi.nlm.nih.gov/pubmed/12721914 (accessed 14 February 2017).

47. Riviere M, Tretiak R, Carey L, Fitzsimmon C, Leclerc C. Economic benefits of a routine second dose of combined measles, mumps and rubella vaccine in Canada. Can J Inf Dis. 1997;8(5):257−264. Available at: http://www.ncbi.nlm.nih.gov/pmc/articles/PMC3250895/ (accessed 14 February 2017).

48. Rosen G. A history of public health. Expanded edition. Baltimore MD: Johns Hopkins University Press, 1993.

49. Smeeth L, Cook C, Fombonne E, Heavey L, Rodrigues LC, Smith PG, et al. MMR vaccination and pervasive developmental disorders: a case−control study. Lancet. 2004;364 (9438):963−969. Available at: http://www.ncbi.nlm.nih.gov/pubmed/15364187 (accessed 19 February 2017).

50. Takla A, Wichmann O, Rieck, Matysiak-Klose D. Measles incidence and reporting trends in Germany 2007−2011. Bull World Health Organ. 2014;92:742−749. Available at: http://www.who.int/bulletin/volumes/92/10/13-135145/en (accessed 14 February 2017).

51. Tulchinsky TH, Ginsberg GM, Abed Y, Angeles MT, Akukwe C, Bonn J. Measles control in developing and developed countries: the case for a two-dose policy. Bull World Health Organ. 1993;71:93−103. Available at: https://www.ncbi.nlm.nih.gov/pmc/articles/PMC2393424/pdf/bullwho00035-0105.pdf (accessed 14 February 2017).

52. Werber D, Hoffmann A, Santibanez S, Mankertz A, Sagebiel D. Large measles outbreak introduced by asylum seekers and spread among the insufficiently vaccinated resident population, Berlin, October 2014 to August 2015. Euro Surveill. 2017;22(34). PII=30599. https://doi.org/10.2807/1560-7917.ES.2017.22.34.30599. Available at: http://www.eurosurveillance.org/ViewArticle.aspx?ArticleId=22861 (accessed 25 August 2017).

53. World Health Organization. Meeting of the International Task Force for Disease Eradication, April 2011. Wkly Epidemiol Rec. 2011;86:341−352. Available at: http://www.who.int/wer/2011/wer8632.pdf (accessed 19 February 2017).

54. World Health Organization. Global Measles and Rubella Strategic Plan: 2012−2020. Geneva: WHO, 2012. Available at: http://www.who.int/immunization/newsroom/Measles_Rubella_StrategicPlan_2012_2020.pdf (accessed 14 February 2017).

55. World Health Organization. WHO Fact sheet 286, reviewed November 2016. Available at: http://www.who.int/mediacentre/factsheets/fs286/en/ (accessed 19 February 2017).

56. World Health Organization. World Health Organization: SAGE endorses mid-term review of global strategy, 21 October 2016. Available at: http://measlesrubellainitiative.org/sage-endorses-measles-rubella-global-strategy/ (accessed 19 February 2017).

57. World Health Organization. Immunization, vaccines and biologicals. Measles, last updated October 2017. Available at: http://www.who.int/immunization/monitoring_surveillance/burden/vpd/surveillance_type/active/measles/en/ (accessed 19 August 2017).

Chapter 4

Semmelweis, Credé, Lister, and Nightingale: Pioneers in Controlling Hospital Infections

ABSTRACT

In the 1850s–1860s infections were the cause of death in surgical practice in high percentages of patients even in the most prestigious hospitals. In the 1850s, Semmelweis in Vienna observed differences in mortality from childbed fever following delivery of poor women in one clinic where doctors and students examined women after autopsies of puerperal fever cases while women attended by midwives had far fewer cases. Semmelweis asked doctors and students to wash their hands before examining pregnant women followed by a dramatic reduction in puerperal fever deaths. Carl Credé in Leipzig demonstrated that silver nitrate drops in the eyes of newborns prevented blindness from ophthalmia neonatorum from exposure to gonorrheal infection during birth. Florence Nightingale returned to England from the chaos of medical services in the Crimean War. She strongly influenced public health, vital statistics, hospital design, and administration with concepts of sanitation and good hygiene to prevent infections in hospitalized patients. In the mid-1860s, Joseph Lister, Professor of Surgery in Edinburgh, under the influence of Pasteur in France and Semmelweis in Vienna, developed a theory of "antisepsis." Lister's work on chemical disinfection for surgery in 1865 was a pragmatic development that led to major advances in surgical practice. He persisted with his antisepsis theory and his results became accepted so that sterile surgery became standard practice. Credé, Semmelweis, Nightingale, and Lister changed the world with safer hospital, obstetric, neonatal, and surgical care resulting in saving countless lives globally. Yet in the 21st century, maternal mortality remains a global crisis due to lack of hygienic safe delivery care in many countries. Health care acquired infections constitute a major public health clinical and ethical problem in high-, medium-, and low-income countries.

The epidemiology of health care-related infections includes increasing antimicrobial resistance, suboptimal assays for the microbiologic screening of organ donors, and virus-associated malignancies. Medical treatments with immunosuppressive agents which lower resistance to infections are increasingly common in health care.

Case Studies in Public Health. DOI: http://dx.doi.org/10.1016/B978-0-12-804571-8.00025-1

Quality improvement initiatives have decreased HAI incidence and cost, and hospitals are encouraged to invest in prevention strategies to realize savings from the prevention of these complications rather than being penalized through recent payment reforms of insurance systems.

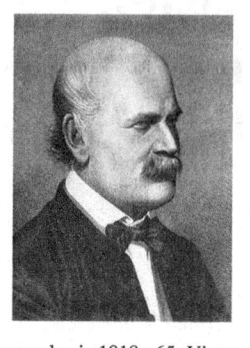

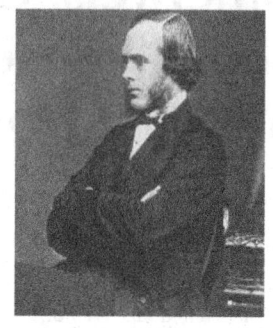

Ignaz Semmelweis 1818–65. Vienna, Budapest. Pioneered handwashing to prevent puerperal fever. *Source: https://en.wikipedia.org/wiki/Ignaz_SemmelweisPuerperal fever.*

Joseph Lister 1827–1912. Edinburgh. Promoted antisepsic pracices for surgery. *Courtesy: Science Museum, UK*

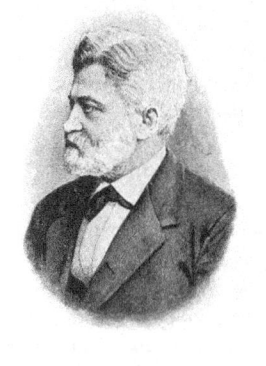

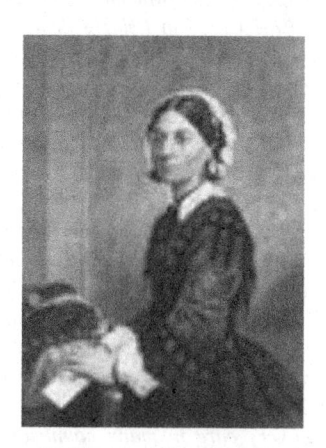

Carl Siegmund Franz Credé, 1819–92. Leipzig. Prevention of gonorrheal ophthalmia blindness in newborns. *Courtesy: Wellcome Foundation.*

Florence Nightingale, 1820–1910. London. Founder of the nursing profession and hospital hygiene. *Courtesy: Wellcome Foundation.*

BACKGROUND

The prevailing concept of the basis of infection remained firmly entrenched in the "Miasma Theory," until the late 19th century despite growing evidence to the contrary by pioneers of microbiology and immunology. The Miasma Theory can be traced back to Greek and Roman medicine and the concepts of Hippocrates and Galen that infection was the result of noxious mists or vapors emanating from filth and refuse in towns. Surgeons in the time of Galen in Ancient Rome considered infection to be part of the process of wound healing, hence the concept "laudable pus" persisted until late in the 19th century. During the Crimean War (1853–1956) and the American Civil War (1861–1965), wounded soldiers with limb amputations would frequently die at rates of 20–100 percent depending on the site of amputation from gangrene following infection.

The contagion theory of disease regarding syphilis was described by Girolamo Fracastoro (1478–1553) in 1530. Syphilis was thought to have been brought to Europe by sailors who were part of the Columbus expeditions, returning from the Americas and spread by mercenary armies across Europe. Initially, the Germ Theory was strengthened by the invention of the microscope in the 1600s, but more definitively the Germ Theory of disease would not be well established until 1870s and Koch's postulates in 1890. The ground-breaking work in the 19th century by John Snow, Oliver Holmes, Carl Credé, Ignaz Semmelweis, Louis Pasteur, Robert Koch, Joseph Lister, and Florence Nightingale, among others, provided the cumulative science and practical experience for fighting infection. Their innovative ideas faced resistance and hostility by the medical profession and others deemed to be experts in these fields. Despite the obstacles to advancement, the evidence of the scientific basis of the Germ—or contagion—Theory finally prevailed.

In the 1840s, puerperal fever was a major cause of death in childbirth, and was the subject of investigation by Oliver Wendell Holmes, a prominent Boston physician. In 1843, he published *On the Contagiousness of Childbed Fever*, and argued that this was transferred from patient to patient by doctors or nurses. As a result of the continued rejection of his arguments by the medical establishment, Holmes gave up on his efforts to establish the contagion theory in relation to the spread of diseases.

Ignaz Philipp Semmelweis (1818–65) was born in Budapest. After studying for two years at the University of Pest in his native Hungary, he moved to Vienna to the Law Faculty and then went back to medicine. He received his medical degree in 1844, specialized in midwifery, and became an assistant to the director of the First Obstetric Clinic in the large Vienna Lying-In Hospital. He was distressed to observe that puerperal fever occurred within a few hours after delivery, with one out of ten mothers dying as a result of infection. The hospital was divided into two clinics: one was for the instruction of medical students and had high rates of puerperal fever (an average 10%); the second clinic was for training midwives and had much lower rates of puerperal fever (an average 4%). Semmelweis also observed that death rates among the hospitalized women were 25–30 percent higher than home- or street-births. He suspected that the traditional idea of puerperal fever being due to miasmas or odors was not true, reasoning that if puerperal fever was due to miasmas, the rates of puerperal fever would be similar in both clinics. Overcrowding was also suggested. However, the midwife clinic was ordinarily more crowded than the clinic run by medical students and teachers who also did autopsies while the midwives did not perform autopsies.

His suspicion of contamination as the cause of puerperal fever was reinforced when a medical colleague and close friend died in 1847 of a severe infection similar to puerperal fever after having been cut during an autopsy of a puerperal fever case. Semmelweis theorized that doctors and medical students could carry contamination with infectious particles from the cadavers to the women in childbirth. He instructed physicians and students doing autopsies to wash their hands with a solution of chlorinated lime before examining pregnant women in labor. As a result, during 1848 the mortality of the first (medical) clinic fell to less than that of the second (midwife) clinic. This focus on the importance of person-to-person transmission of infectious material of puerperal sepsis made an important contribution to the struggles between the germ and miasma theories of disease. His work, although carefully documented, was considered extreme at the time; his idea of cleanliness was largely ignored, rejected or ridiculed, and was strongly opposed by the medical community. It took almost 40 years for his theory to be adopted.

The hostile response of medical staff to his ideas, led to Semmelweis being forced out of his position in Vienna in 1850 and he returned to Budapest as a Professor of Obstetrics. There his ideas were accepted and he developed a private practice. He married and had a family, but two of his five children died. In 1861 he published his great work *The Etiology, Concept, and Prophylaxis of Childbed Fever*. A large proportion of the medical community continued its resistance and hostility, and his theory was rejected by the miasma theory proponents dominated by Rudolf Virchow in Germany, the leading proponent of social medicine. This rejection by the medical community and the death of two of his children drove Semmelweis to despair. Outraged by the indifference or outright rejection of the medical profession he wrote increasingly angry open letters to prominent European obstetricians, including calling them irresponsible murderers. His contemporaries, including his wife, believed he was losing his mind, now thought to be due to early Alzheimers disease; in 1865 he was committed to an insane asylum with brutal treatment where he died 14 days later, suspected to be the result of a severe beating by guards.

His influence on the knowledge and control of infection was extolled by Lister and Pasteur. Semmelweis's clean delivery methods were gradually accepted and his findings were eventually explained with Pasteur's Germ Theory. Even leading hospitals took years to adopt his methods of antisepsis which he had developed decades before in Vienna. Semmelweis is now recognized as a brave and tragic pioneer of antiseptic procedures and the role of observations in clinical practice, which has led the way to subsequent vast effects in public health. His pioneering investigation of childbed fever (streptococcal infection in childbirth) in Vienna contributed to support for the Germ Theory, leading to vast improvement in obstetric practices and reduced maternal mortality.

Surgery in the 19th century was characterized with high morbidity and mortality rates largely due to postsurgery infections. The problem was thought to be linked to foul odors of old buildings, and so the solution proposed to stop the "epidemic" was to destroy existing hospital buildings and build them anew. Traumatic and surgical wounds were accompanied by the presence of suppuration and inflammation, thought of as "laudable pus"— infection considered essential to the normal healing process of wound repair. Septic death rates following surgery ranged between 60 and 90 percent, often accompanied by tetanus, streptococcal infection, gangrene, and septicemia.

Joseph Lister (1827–1912), was born in Upton, England. He studied at University College in London and received his Bachelor of Arts degree in 1847, and in 1852 his Bachelor of Medicine with honors. He became a fellow of the Royal College of Surgeons and a house surgeon at University College Hospital. He moved to Edinburgh, Scotland, in 1853 to study surgery at the Edinburgh Royal Infirmary and began his surgical practice. He became concerned with the tremendous mortality rates associated with surgical and traumatic wounds. In 1856, he traveled to Vienna and met with former colleagues of Semmelweis. He became motivated to seek ways to apply their ideas for safe obstetrics to surgical practice. Lister became a professor of surgery at the Royal Infirmary in Glasgow in 1860. In 1864, Louis Pasteur delivered his world-changing paper on fermentation and spoilage of beer, wine, and milk caused by micro-organisms and a description of methods for eliminating micro-organisms by exposure to heat or chemical solutions.

Lister heard of Pasteur's work on putrefaction in 1865, and realized the applicability of the Germ Theory to surgical practice. He tested "antiseptic" techniques to prevent wound infections. In 1867 he published a series of articles in Lancet, including his first study comparing morbidity and mortality between simple and compound fractures—i.e., those with unbroken skin versus those with bones protruding through an opening in the skin. The first report entitled, "On a New Method of Treating Compound Fractures, Abscesses etc. with Observation on the Condition of Suppuration." This led to his growing conviction of the need for antisepsis including sterilizing instruments, carbolic acid, hand-washing, and clean dressings for safer surgical practice. He sought to improve antiseptic techniques and adopted the use of carbolic acid (phenol) to "sterilize" surgical instruments inspired by phenol's previous use to treat sewage which had resulted in a reduction in diseases in Carlisle, England. Lister's 1867 publication *On the Antiseptic Principle in the Practice of Surgery*" described using carbolic acid to spray operating theaters and to cleanse surgical wounds, so applying the Germ Theory with significant benefit to surgical outcome.

Lister expressed his ideas as follows:

"... how the atmosphere produces decomposition of organic substances, we find that a flood of light has been thrown upon this most important question by the philosophic researches of M. Pasteur, who has demonstrated by thoroughly convincing evidence that it is not to its oxygen or to any of its gaseous constituents that the air owes this property, but to minute particles suspended in it, which are the germs of various low forms of life, long since revealed by the microscope, and regarded as merely accidental concomitants of putrescence, but now shown by Pasteur to be its essential cause ...

Applying these principles to the treatment of compound fracture, bearing in mind that it is from the vitality of the atmospheric particles that all the mischief arises, it appears that all that is requisite is to dress the wound with some material capable of killing these septic germs ... "

The next question Lister asked himself was what material would suffice.

"In the course of the year 1864, I was much struck with an account of the remarkable effects produced by carbolic acid upon the sewage of the town of Carlisle ... not only preventing all odour from the lands irrigated with the refuse material, but ... destroying the protozoan which usually infest cattle fed upon such pastures ... The applicability of carbolic acid for the treatment of compound fracture occurred to me ..."

In his 1867 paper *"On the Antiseptic Principle of the Practice of Surgery,"* Lister continued his case reports of the successes of his technique, including specific instructions on exact methodology. In his opening statement, Lister wrote: *"To prevent the occurrence of suppuration with all its attendant risks was an object manifestly desirable, but till lately apparently unattainable, since it seemed hopeless to attempt to exclude the oxygen which was universally regarded as the agent by which putrefaction was affected ..."* However his application of antisepsis to compound fractures saw the revelation that, *"... these evils are entirely avoided by the antiseptic treatment so that limbs otherwise condemned to amputation may be retained."* Lister then went on to discuss the application of his principles to severe traumatic wounds, abscesses, septic arthritis, contused wounds, and incised wounds. He also commenced all operations with an antiseptic cleansing of the patient.

Before Lister, the importance of cleanliness in surgery was not recognized nor practiced widely and a surgeon's prestige was enhanced by wearing blood- and pus-stained clothing. Lister's unique contribution was the application of the contagion or Germ Theory to surgery and the realization that everything contacting a wound should be free of germs, thus leading to development of techniques of antisepsis. Antisepsis was contingent on acceptance of the Germ Theory, which was still widely resisted by medical professionals in America as well as in Europe. Lister's work, in conjunction with that of Semmelweis and Pasteur in particular, led to acceptance of the Germ Theory in microbiology, immunology, and, gradually, in medical practice.

Lister's sterility methods were to have an enormous impact not only on surgery, but also revolutionized the practice of medicine. He demonstrated large reductions in post-surgical rates of infection and deaths from sepsis. In nine months of follow-up after the introduction of antiseptic practices in Lister's hospital, there were no cases of generalized infection, gangrene, or erysipelas. Lister concluded: "*As there appears to be no doubt regarding the cause of this change, the importance of the fact can hardly be exaggerated.*" His methods were gradually adopted by the medical community after 1870, and over the next 20 years antiseptic methods in surgery became almost universal.

Antiseptic techniques remain a cornerstone of surgical and clinical practice across all disciplines, health settings, and patient populations. This includes wound treatment, but more profoundly, fundamental changes in surgical practice, hospitals, and maternity units. Lord Lister died aged 84 after receiving many honors and recognition in Britain and the western world.

During the period 1854−60, another hygienic breakthrough in hospitals was achieved through the work of Carl Franz Credé (1819−92), a professor of obstetrics at the University of Leipzig. Gonorrhea was common in all levels of society in 19th century Europe. Ophthalmic infection of newborns was a widespread cause of infection, scarring, and blindness due to gonococcal infections acquired during the birth process from an infected mother. Credé attempted to treat neonatal gonococcal ophthalmic infection with many medications. He discovered the use of silver nitrate as an effective prophylactic treatment and introduced its use as a routine preventive measure during the period 1854−60 with astonishing success. Prophylactic use of silver nitrate spread rapidly hospital by hospital, but due to widespread medical opposition to this innovation, decades passed before it was mandated widely. It was only in 1879 that the gonococcus organism was discovered by Albert Ludwig Neisser (1855−1916). Estimates of children saved from blindness by this procedure in Europe during the 19th century are as high as one million cases. Credé's impact is still the standard for newborn care recommended nearly universally.

Florence Nightingale is mostly recognized for momentous work in nursing and hospital administration during the Crimean War (1854−56) and returning subsequently to England with the respect of the nation and a national heroine. This enabled her to establish nursing as a profession and in her subsequent and successful campaigns initiated improved standards of military medicine, hospital hygiene, planning, supply services and management, hospital statistics, and community health nursing. Her outstanding contributions resulted in the development of modern, organized health care for soldiers, and for civilian hospital sanitation and hygiene. Nightingale was a believer in the Miasma Theory of disease, but in practice her stress was on sanitation, hygiene, and good nursing care contributed greatly to making public health, hospital care, and tending to wounded soldiers much more efficient and safe.

Nightingale sought to introduce professional nursing into the dreaded workhouse infirmaries and to eliminate abuses, working with the Association for the Improvement of the London Workhouse Infirmaries, for which she sought reform and improvements. She believed in statistics and the importance of quantitative data to prove the case for hospital reform. When she returned from the Crimea as a national hero, she spent her efforts on developing nursing as a profession, but equally on promoting social reform in Britain and India.

Her vision was of a public health care system within a broader system of social welfare, including basic public sanitation. She used her celebrity status to influence the political elite to achieve change. She also utilized social opportunities to convince political leaders of the need for reform, using the media and keeping her focus on saving lives. Her vision included broad reform of the socioeconomic system in an early conceptualization of the welfare state. In opposition to conservatism and Marxism of the day, she favored the private sector largely running the economy, but vigorously promoted strong social measures for income security, savings and pensions, employment stimulation, better housing, with provision for the disabled, aged and chronically ill, and a whole system of public health care.

CURRENT RELEVANCE

Hospital or health care associated (HAI) infections, their causes and measures to prevent them, are all current concerns to health systems, not only for the danger they pose to the lives of patients but also for the economic consequences of infection effects, and their prevention. Linking historical cases to modern-day public health issues underlines the importance of the game-changing pioneers whose insights and bravery to stand up to hostile medical traditionalists led to their contribution to population- and individual health.

WHO reports that infections acquired in health care settings are "the most frequent adverse event in health care delivery worldwide" affecting hundreds of millions of patients each year, with significant mortality and financial loss for health systems. In developing countries, seven to ten of every 100 hospitalized patients will acquire at least one health care-associated infection. This is particularly significant in low- and middle-income countries for patients in intensive care units, and is a major factor in high rates of neonatal mortality. Surgical site infection is the leading infection in poor country settings with limited resources, affecting up to one-third of patients post-operation. In high-income countries, approximately 30 percent of patients in intensive care units (ICU) are affected by at least one health care-associated infection.

In low-income countries, the key factors for nosocomial infections include inadequate facilities and hygienic conditions, understaffing, overcrowding, insufficient equipment, and poor training in basic infection control measures, including injection and blood transfusion safety. National and local guidelines for infection control and policies are lacking and greatly contribute to hazards for patient care and survival. Newborns are especially at high risk of acquiring health care-associated infection in developing countries.

The European Centers for Disease Control and Prevention (ECDC) reports health care-associated infection prevalence of 7.1 percent, with estimates that approximately 4.5 million episodes of health care-associated infection occur yearly in Europe. The United States CDC's National Nosocomial Infection Surveillance (NNIS) unit monitors these types of infections as well as the efforts to prevent them. The British National Health Service (NHS) is extremely concerned with methicillin-resistant Staphylococcus aureus (MRSA) becoming a major public issue of the "negligence of the government" in maintaining the NHS, and a subject of parliamentary and public debate.

Nosocomial infections remain an important cause of both morbidity and mortality across all spectrums of inpatient care, nursing homes and other settings with confined conditions—such as prisons—and throughout the world represent enormous costs to a system facing growing financial constraints and organizational reform. A recent report from Britain states that around 21,000 cases of severe sepsis occur each year in England and Wales, accounting for an estimated 27 percent of admissions to intensive care units and 46 percent of all bed days in such units. Despite advances in critical care, failing to prevent severe sepsis remains a frequent cause of mortality.

Health care-associated infections are an increasing hospital problem with significant harmful effects on patient morbidity and mortality. Population aging, medical and surgical interventions, implanted foreign bodies, organ transplantations, problematic air exchange systems, and inadequate handwashing by staff, are all factors that increase risks during hospitalization. Renovation of aging hospitals increases the risk of airborne fungal and other infections. Gram-negative bacilli—either intrinsically resistant to antimicrobials or acquiring antimicrobial resistance—are linked to increasingly multidrug-resistant hospital-acquired infections. Because of limited options for treatment, multi drug-resistant infections represent a serious public health issue requiring a stronger emphasis in preventive measures in hospitals and long term care facilities.

Prevention and control measures are increasingly accepted as vital to address emerging health care facility infections with strong institutional and national surveillance and prevention. New methods of sterilization and development of noninvasive infection-resistant methods are important as financing systems introduce financial penalties for excessive rates of hospital infections. Most important is the education of health care workers on the strict implementation of hand-washing, catheter infection control measures, and other decontamination procedures—which are effective even in low-income countries.

Health care facility infection control multidimensional approaches include outcome and process surveillance, feedback on catheter-associated urinary tract infection rates, on performance, education, and a well planned program of preventive measures. Patient safety can be compromised with long term ventilator-associated pneumonia, central line blood stream infection, catheters, intravenous lines, unscreened blood transfusions, inadequately sterilized endoscopes, and many other hospital-based events. Transmission of infectious diseases is not only a problem for hospital inpatient-, surgical-, dialysis-, and outpatient departments, but also in dental clinics and long -term care facilities.

The issue of health care personnel transmission of infections also has a modern application in the case of vaccine-preventable diseases from health personnel to patients, and from patients to their families, and to the community. Measles transmission is a case in point, with imported or epidemic measles—as occurred in Europe—easily transmitted in medical clinic waiting rooms to other patients, as well as by care givers in kindergartens, schools, and other communal settings. Inadequately or unimmunized health care staff for diseases thought to be under control, can place patients at risk, therefore, immunization status of health care personnel should be continuously reviewed.

Credé's ocular prophylaxis with 2 percent silver nitrate at birth resulted in a dramatic reduction in incidents of neonatal gonococcal conjunctivitis from 10 percent to 0.3 percent. In recent years, this has been under debate as possibly no longer being needed, given that the prevalence of sexually transmitted infections has declined, treatment of ophthalmia neonatorum has improved, and due to ocular prophylaxis carrying the risk of developing antibiotic resistance. As a result, ocular prophylaxis has fallen out of practice in some countries in the developed world, which has led to the reemergence of sight-threatening infections. Since sexually transmitted diseases—including gonorrhea—are recurring, the evidence supports the continuation of neonatal ocular prophylaxis remaining the standard of care for all newborns, with one percent silver nitrate, 0.5 percent erythromycin ointment, or one percent tetracycline alternative.

Awareness of poor hand hygiene is being promoted by WHO as causing germ transmission, including organisms resistant to most or all available antibiotics, which risks patients' lives from heath care-associated infections. In some facilities, 90 percent of health care workers do not clean their hands effectively. The epidemiology of health care-related infections includes increasing antimicrobial resistance, suboptimal assays for the microbiologic screening of organ donors, and virus-associated malignancies. Medical treatments with immunosuppressive agents which lower resistance to infections are increasingly common in healthcare.

ETHICAL ISSUES

Health care-associated infection is an ethical issue of hygiene as well as a political, economic, and professional one. National governments are responsible for the health of their population. Priorities of resource allocation do not adequately address education and preventive measures of sanitation, hygiene, and health facility safety for patients.

Hospital infections are among the most important public health issues of the 21st century with the rise of multidrug-resistant organisms. The issue is further complicated by resistance of hospital staff to being immunized against influenza (annually), pneumococcal pneumonia, and other vaccine-preventable diseases, which can readily spread and cause serious consequences to vulnerable persons, the elderly, or seriously ill hospitalized patients. Another complication is the issue of a problematic standards of personal hygienic techniques while working with patients.

Health care facilities in the US are increasingly requiring health care workers, often despite strong objections on the grounds of civil rights, to be vaccinated for infectious diseases in an effort to reduce outbreaks of vaccine-preventable diseases. In some instances, facilities have established these requirements due to mandates in State statutes and regulations. These State health care facility vaccination laws include vaccine-preventable diseases such as varicella, pertussis, pneumococcal pneumonia, hepatitis A and B, and influenza. Pregnant women are encouraged to immunize against diphtheria, pertussis, and influenza during pregnancy to protect their newborns during the early months before the baby's routine infant immunization program starts.

Promotion of hand-washing has been shown to be effective in child daycare facilities or schools in high-income countries (HICs) which prevents some 30 percent of diarrhea episodes, and a similar proportion in schools in low- and middle- income countries (LMICs), as well as around 28 percent in community-based studies. A hospital-based trial included in a Cochrane Review in 2015 showed that hand-washing promotion also resulted in reduction in the rate of episodes of diarrhea. Diarrheal and respiratory infectious diseases are still significant in LMICs and HICs with around 1.8 million deaths mostly of children under five years of age annually. Diarrhea also contributes significantly to malnutrition in children.

Hygiene is still very much a contemporary global issue affecting progress in reducing maternal and neonatal mortality. Child mortality from diarrhea and respiratory diseases during the Millennium Development Goals (MDGs) initiative has been enhanced by increased use of oral rehydration and vaccines—such as rotavirus and pneumococcal pneumonia. But much more can be done for prevention through education and improved basics of hygiene—including the safe disposal of human waste—but even more by the simple measure of promoting hand-washing in communities and in health care facilities.

Maternal mortality rates (MMR) remain a global professional and ethical health issue. The Millennium Development Goals (MDGs) defined target was for maternal mortality rates to be reduced by three quarters between 1990 and 2015, and to achieve universal access to reproductive health. Globally, maternal mortality declined by 45 percent from levels in 1990 with an estimated 289,000 women dying during or following pregnancy and childbirth in 2013. In low-income countries, a high proportion of deliveries take place in poor rural homes with no professional attendants, except perhaps traditional midwives. The mothers are often very young, poorly nourished, and at high risk.

The link between poverty and maternal health has been clear for more than a century, with extensive evidence from rich and poor countries where rural versus urban gradients are especially high. High-risk pregnancies for maternal and infant morbidity and mortality include previous maternity history, educational and nutritional status, early or advanced age of mothers, marital status, number of previous pregnancies (first or multiple), previous infant deaths, and underlying diseases such as hypertension and HIV/AIDS. Socioeconomic factors, ethnicity, social standing, self-esteem, and psychosocial stress, are all factors specific to individuals. Others are systemic such as lack of family planning, spacing of pregnancies, and poor access to professional care before, during, and following delivery. Lack of prenatal care and delivery at home or in a nonmedical setting without professional care are also major risk factors. In a systematic review of studies of maternal mortality by WHO, severe bleeding, hypertensive diseases, and infections were the dominant causes of deaths. Unsafe abortion associated with infection is a high risk factor where illegal abortions are common especially in poor countries or populations. Transmission of HIV, hepatitis B and C, syphilis, chlamydia, and other sexually transmitted diseases are being reduced by earlier diagnosis and treatment of mothers to protect newborns.

Globally, the main direct causes of neonatal death are preterm or low birth-weight newborns (28%), severe infections (26%), and asphyxia (23%). Neonatal tetanus accounts for a smaller proportion of deaths (7%), but is preventable by immunization of mothers during pregnancy. Maternal complications in labor also carry a high risk of neonatal death. Poverty is strongly associated with increased risk. There is still high neonatal and child mortality in many countries. Infection as a cause of maternal- and infant-mortality remains a challenge to global public health, as it was to Semmelweis in the 19th century.

In the 21st century, health care-associated infections have become a major factor in administration and care services in hospitals, outpatient facilities, long-term care facilities, home-based care, and other community health services, as well as in medical and dental clinics. The problem of multidrug-resistant organisms is dominating medical practice in the health care setting and in communities. Combating this phenomenon and dealing with other pathogenic organisms including viruses and parasites, challenge clinical care, management of cleaning services, design of medical equipment, and put patient-safety and quality-of-care at risk.

Organisms drug-resistant to available antibiotics are a looming public health and clinical disaster. Pathogens may affect patients by transmission from visitors, health care staff, other patients, as well as through contaminated medical equipment, health worker clothing, and unwashed hands coming into contact with patients. Offending organisms include bacteria, viruses, and parasites which can linger on clothing or bedside tables for days, weeks, and even years. Hepatitis B can last a week, clostridium a year, MSRA from seven days to seven months, and norovirus from eight hours to seven days.

The classic epidemiologic triangle of host/agent/environment is a practical model for understanding prevention, addressing each of the key factors in a comprehensive approach. The host may be the patient, neighboring patients, staff or visitors, and vice versa in person-to-person transmission. Influenza is currently a major example, which underlies efforts to immunize staff and the majority of the general population to promote herd immunity to influenza transmission especially in treatment settings. Equipment manufacturers, hospital architects, and maintenance and cleaning staff are all part of the problem, and the solution.

Risk recognition has been compared to defensive driving, but it relies much more on teamwork staff with proactive approaches to recognize hazards and mitigate risks. Even the simple procedure of taking blood (phlebotomy) can be hazardous to a patient or phlebotomist—e.g., the possibility of accidental transmission of hepatitis B and C, or HIV. Intensive care units using ventilator suction are also hazardous situations. Similar standards apply to home-based care, assisted living homes, medical and dental clinics, or outpatient departments with, for example, cancer patients on chemotherapy having reduced resistance to viral and bacterial pneumonias.

Vaccine preventable diseases, such as influenza, measles, and others, are dangers to patients, visitors, and staff of hospital and other care facilities so that the public health function of achieving sufficient herd immunity is an important protection for vulnerable people in health care. Measles, for example, can be easily transmitted and spread to the community from medical waiting rooms. Other sources of infection include pathogens in water released from contamination sites during renovation and equipment/furnishings contamination. Medical equipment includes stethoscopes, thermometers, catheters, endoscopes and many more objects—such as toys in pediatric wards, bedside furniture, cleaning equipment and many other common objects—and, most importantly, unwashed hands of care givers are prone to carry infective as organisms. These are all factors that would be recognizable to Semmelweis, Nightingale, Crede, and Lister if they were present today because of in the mid-19th century.

ECONOMIC ISSUES

In the US, implementation of quality improvement initiatives have been promoted in recent years. A 2013 study of health care-associated infections (HAIs) carried out from 2011 to 2013 in the US reported that the total annual cost for the five major infections was $9.8 billion. Surgical site infections (SSI) contributed to one third of overall cost, followed closely by ventilator-associated pneumonia (31.6%), central line-associated bloodstream infections (18.9%), *Clostridium difficile* infections (15.4%), and catheter-associated urinary tract infections (<1%). Quality improvement initiatives have decreased HAI incidence and cost, and hospitals are encouraged to invest in prevention strategies to realize savings from the prevention of these complications rather than being penalized through recent payment reforms of insurance systems.

Progress is being made. The CDC reports that in 2014, one in 25 hospital patients has at least one health care-associated infection. CDC's annual *National and State Healthcare-Associated Infections Progress Report* (HAI Progress Report, 2014 data, published 2016) describes national and state progress in preventing HAIs. Among national acute-care hospitals, they found a 50 percent decrease in central line-associated bloodstream infections between 2008 and 2014, but no change in overall catheter-associated urinary tract infections between 2009 and 2014. However, there was progress between 2009 and 2014 with a 17 percent decrease in SSI related to the 10 selected tracked procedures.

Modern issues of nosocomial infections include the safety of blood transfusions by screening blood in blood banks. Life-saving blood transfusions are used daily in hospitals and emergency treatment facilities across the US. There are more than 9.5 million blood donors in the US and an estimated five million patients who receive blood annually, resulting in a total of 14.6 million transfusions per year. Although the US blood supply is safer than ever before, the practice of paying donors increases the risk of contaminated blood provided by prison inmates, drug addicts, and HIV carriers. The fact that some bacteria, viruses, prions, and parasites can be transmitted by unscreened blood transfusions has led to tragedies in the past with transmission of HIV and hepatitis C through contaminated blood. Each blood donor is screened for risk of transmissible disease by a questionnaire, and each unit of blood donated in the US is routinely screened for various infectious disease pathogens, including six transfusion-transmitted infective agents—i.e., syphilis, hepatitis B and C, HIV, Zika Virus, Human T-Lymphotropic Virus Types I and II, and West Nile Virus—using nine laboratory tests. In some situations, Chagas disease and cytomegalovirus are also screened. But still there are issues of the potential transmission of HIV and Hepatitis C that are possibly missed on screening tests, resulting in the exclusion of some groups from blood donation.

CONCLUSION

The concepts of hygiene and antisepsis in relation to surgical care arose from separate areas of care and in different countries, at approximately the same time in history.

Semmelweis, Lister, Credé, and Nightingale greatly contributed to the knowledge and application of the Germ Theory of disease while reducing neonatal infections, hospital infection rates, and maternal mortality which are still major public health problems all over the world. These contributions to hospital care were supported by the work of giant figures of science led by Louis Pasteur and Robert Koch in establishing the Germ Theory and Semmelweis, Nightingale. Lister and Credé who pioneered its practical applications. These people are rightly placed among the great innovators of modern public health with major influences on antisepsis, the Germ Theory, and hygiene, with enormous benefits for civil society globally. If they were alive today, they would understand the modern versions of risks in health care-acquired infections and maternal mortality which they addressed in the 19th century and are still present in old and new forms. Today, the evidence is clear that personal, institutional, and community hygiene produce a sustained positive effect on reducing infections, but infectious diseases remain a major public health- and health facility problems globally.

RECOMMENDATIONS

1. Recognizing the importance of health care-associated infections, the education of students in health profession studies should include the topic within basic education and continuing education.
2. Recognizing the importance of safe hospital care in the context of a comprehensive system of population health, economic incentives to promote health care system efficiency and quality, monitoring of health care-associated infections should receive high priority in health system data monitoring.
3. Recognizing the importance of socioeconomic reform for population health including strong public health systems and universal access to health care, national governments need to address these needs side by side, including:

    a. Promoting basic hygiene with safe water supplies, sewage disposal, air quality, and other aspects of health protection.

    b. Promoting basic preventive care through universal immunization and screening programs for cancer and infectious diseases, rehabilitation and long-term care services.

    c. Promoting health promotion to reduce unnecessary hospitalization by improved population health, through activities directed to smoking reduction, healthy diets, fortification of flour, salt, and milk to reduce micronutrient deficiencies which affect many population groups in low-, medium-, and high-income populations.

4. Recognizing the importance of developing new technology for preventing health care-associated infections, financial and organizational efforts should be fostered to promote scientific research for new vaccines and antibiotics which can strengthen prevention and treatment of infectious diseases associated with health care.

5. Promotion of public awareness of the importance of infectious disease, including health care providers who, without prevention of infections, can serve as carriers to infect patients in their care, or bring diseases home to their families. This requires:

    a. Education of the importance of health care infections and ethical responsibilities for risk recognition and staff awareness and organizational commitment to prevention.

    b. Mandatory requirements for immunizations against influenza, diphtheria, pertussis, measles, mumps, rubella, hepatitis, and other disease entities.

6. Prevention of HAIs is vital in training, supervision, and monitoring in home-based care, long-term care, community health services including medical and dental clinics where transmission of infection is a threat to patient safety, to other patients, and to health care workers.

7. Ensuring that the history and current epidemiology of health care-associated infections is a prominent topic for medical, nursing, paramedical, public health, health policy, management study programs, and continuing education.

STUDENT REVIEW QUESTIONS

1. What is the importance of Semmelweis's work in proving the "Germ Theory" versus the "Miasma Theory" of disease?

2. What is the importance of Lister's work in proving the "Germ Theory" versus the "Miasma Theory" of disease?

3. What are the factors associated with nosocomial infections in modern health care facilities and what factors have led to the rise of these despite the work of Lister and others?

4. What lessons can be learned from Credé's work in infant care for routine preventive care of ophthalmia neonatourm in Leipzig in the 19th century?

5. What lessons can be learned from Lister's work for present-day medical and nursing practice?

6. How was Florence Nightingale, as a believer in the Miasma Theory, influential in advancing public health in 19th century England?

7. What are the public health issues of nosocomial infections occurring in the present era?

8. Discuss ethical issues related to health facility-acquired infections.

9. Discuss economic issues related to nosocomial infections.

10. What has been shown in studies that hand-washing promotion can reduce diarrheal and respiratory diseases?

11. What is the impact of sexually transmitted disease in newborn care needs?

12. What is the impact of screening and management of maternal care for mothers with high risk factors in reducing maternal mortality due to infections?

RECOMMENDED READINGS

1. Aiello A, Larson EL. What is the evidence for a causal link between hygiene and infections? Lancet Infectious Dis. 2002;2(2):103−110. Available at: http://zadereyko.info/downloads/Hygiene + disease + Lancet.pdf (accessed 24 April 2017).

2. Black RW, Dykes AC, Anderson KE, Wells JG, Sinclair SP, Gary GW, et al. Handwashing to prevent diarrhea in day-care centers. Am J Epidemiol. 1981;113:445−451.

3. Boyce JM, Pittet D. Guideline for hand hygiene in health-care settings: recommendations of the Healthcare Infection Control Practices Advisory Committee and the HICPAC/SHEA/APIC/IDSA Hand Hygiene Task Force Reports and Recommendation. MMWR Recomm Rep. 2002;51(RR16):1−44. Available at: https://www.ncbi.nlm.nih.gov/pubmed/12418624 (accessed 23 April 2017).

4. Cooper BS, Stone SP, Kibbler CC, Cookson BD, Roberts JA, Medley GF, et al. Isolation measures in the hospital management of methicillin resistant *Staphylococcus aureus* (MRSA): systematic review of the literature. BMJ. 2004;329(7465):533. Available at: https://www.ncbi.nlm.nih.gov/pubmed/15345626 (accessed 23 April 2017).

5. Centers for Disease Control and Prevention. Healthcare-associated infections (HAI) progress report, 3 March 2016. Available at: https://www.cdc.gov/hai/surveillance/progress-report/index.html (accessed 1 March 2017).

6. Centers for Disease Control and Prevention. Healthcare-associated infections (HAI) data and statistics. October 2016. Available at: https://www.cdc.gov/hai/surveillance/index.html (accessed 1 March 2017).

7. Centers for Disease Control and Prevention. Public health law program: vaccination laws. Updated 3 October 2016. Available at: https://www.cdc.gov/phlp/publications/topic/vaccinationlaws.html (accessed 1 March 2017).

8. Centers for Disease Control and Prevention. Blood safety. Updated 31 January 2013. Available at: https://www.cdc.gov/bloodsafety/basics.html (accessed 1 March 2017).

9. Centers for Disease Control and Prevention/National Healthcare Safety Network (NHSN). National and state healthcare-associated infections (HAI) progress report, 2014 data, published 2016. Available at: https://elbiruniblogspotcom.blogspot.co.il/2016/03/healthcare-associated-infections-hai.html (accessed 24 April 2017).

10. Centers for Disease Control and Prevention. Healthcare-associated infection. Available at https://www.cdc.gov/hai/ (accessed 27 April 2017).

11. Editorial. Preventing the spread of MRSA: Common sense and observational studies are of benefit. BMJ. 2004;329(7465):521. Available at: https://www.ncbi.nlm.nih.gov/pmc/articles/PMC516089/ (accessed 23 April 2017).

12. Ejemot-Nwadiaro RI, Ehiri JE, Arikpo D, Meremikwu MM, Critchley JA. Hand washing promotion for preventing diarrhoea. Cochrane Database System Rev. 2015;(9), 1–95. http://dx.doi.org/10.1002/14651858.CD004265.pub3. Available at: https://www.ncbi.nlm.nih.gov/pmc/articles/PMC4563982/ (accessed 24 April 2017).

13. Encyclopedia of World Biography. Florence Nightingale biography, 2017. Available at: http://www.notablebiographies.com/Mo-Ni/Nightingale-Florence.html (accessed 3 March 2017).

14. European Centre for Disease Prevention and Control. European surveillance of health care associated infections in intensive care units—HAI-Net ICU protocol, version 1.02. ECDC, 2015, Stockholm. Available at: http://ecdc.europa.eu/en/publications/Publications/healthcare-associated-infections-HAI-ICU-protocol.pdf (accessed 24 March 2017).

15. Faqs.org. Carl Siegmund Franz Credé Biography (1819–1892), 2017. Available at: http://www.faqs.org/health/bios/80/Carl-Siegmund-Franz-Cred.html (accessed 23 March 2017).

16. Florence Nightingale Museum. Florence Nightingale biography. St Thomas Hospital London. Available at: http://www.florence-nightingale.co.uk/resources/biography/?v=3e8d115eb4b3 (accessed 23 March 2017).

17. HealthyPeople.gov. Healthcare-associated infections, new updated 18 May 2017. Available at: https://www.healthypeople.gov/2020/topics-objectives/topic/healthcare-associated-infections (accessed 21 May 2017).

18. Khan MU. Interruption of shigellosis by hand washing. Trans Roy Soc Trop Med Hyg. 1982;76:164–168. Available at: http://www.sciencedirect.com/science/article/pii/S0196655388800051 (accessed 27 April 2017).

19. Larson E. Innovations in health care: antisepsis as a case study. Am J Public Health. 1989;79:92–99. Available at: https://www.ncbi.nlm.nih.gov/pmc/articles/PMC1349481/pdf/amjph00227-0094.pdf (accessed 24 April 2017).

20. Lawn JE, Cousens S, Zupan J, et al. 4 million neonatal deaths: When? Where? Why? Lancet. 2005;365(9462):891–900. Available at: http://www.thelancet.com/journals/lancet/article/PIIS0140-6736(05)71048-5/fulltext (accessed 24 April 2017).

21. Leavitt JW. Book review of Loudon I. The tragedy of childbed fever. New York: Oxford University Press, 2000. Available at: http://www.nejm.org/doi/full/10.1056/NEJM200008243430819 (accessed 3 March 2017).

22. Major S. NICE issues guidance on sepsis. BMJ. 2004;329:758. Available at: http://www.bmj.com/content/329/7469/758.2 (accessed 23 April 2017).

23. Matejcek A, Goldman RD. Treatment and prevention of ophthalmia neonatorum. Canad Fam Physician. 2013;59(11):1187–1190. Available at: https://www.ncbi.nlm.nih.gov/pmc/articles/PMC3828094/ (accessed 27 April 2017).

24. McDonald L. Florence Nightingale as a social reformer. History Today, 200656. Available at: http://www.historytoday.com/lynn-mcdonald/florence-nightingale-social-reformer (accessed 29 April 2017).

25. McFarland LV, Mulligan ME, Kwok RYY, Stamm WE. Nosocomial acquisition of *Clostridium difficile* infection. N Engl J Med. 1989;320:204–210. http://dx.doi.org.10.1056/NEJM198901263200402. Available at: http://www.nejm.org/doi/pdf/10.1056/NEJM198901263200402 (accessed 30 April 2017).

26. Murray CK, Hinkle MK, Yun HC. History of infections associated with combat-related injuries. J Trauma. 2008;64:S221–S231. Available at: http://afids.org/publications/PDF/CRI/Prevention%20and%20Management%20of%20CRI%20-4-%20-%20History.pdf (accessed 26 April 2017).

27. Murray CJL, Vos T, Lozano R, Naghavi M, Flaxman A, Michaud C, et al. Disability-adjusted life years (DALYs) for 291 diseases and injuries in 21 regions, 1990–2010: a systematic analysis for the Global Burden of Disease Study 2010. Lancet. 2012;380 (9859):2197–2223. Available at: https://www.ncbi.nlm.nih.gov/pubmed/23245608 (accessed 24 April 2017).

28. Pitt D, Aubin JM. Joseph Lister: father of modern surgery. Can J Surg. 2012;55(5):E8–E9. Available at: https://www.ncbi.nlm.nih.gov/pmc/articles/PMC3468637/ (accessed 2 March 2017).

29. Pittet D, Hugonnet S, Harbarth S, Mourouga P, Sauvan V, Touveneau S, et al. Effectiveness of a hospital-wide programme to improve compliance with hand hygiene. Lancet. 2000;356:1307–1312. Available at: http://medlineindustriesinc.com/media/assets/pdf/sterillium-comfort-gel/Effectiveness-of-a-hospital-wide-programme-to-improve-compliance-with-hand-hygiene.pdf (accessed 24 April 2017).

30. Pruitt BA. Combat casualty care and surgical progress. Ann Surgery. 2006;243 (6):715–729. http://dx.doi.org/10.1097/01.sla.0000220038.66466.b5. Available at: https://www.ncbi.nlm.nih.gov/pmc/articles/PMC1570575/ (accessed 26 April 2017).

31. Reilly RF. Medical and surgical care during the American Civil War, 1861–1865. Proc (Bayl Univ Med Cent). 2016;29(2):138–142. PMCID: PMC4790547. Available at: https://www.ncbi.nlm.nih.gov/pmc/articles/PMC4790547/ (accessed 26 April 2017).

32. Rosenthal VD, Ramachandran B, Dueñas L, Alvarez-Moreno C, Navoa-Ng JA, Armas-Ruiz A, et al. Findings of the international nosocomial infection control consortium (INICC), Part I: effectiveness of a multidimensional infection control approach on catheter-associated urinary tract infection rates in pediatric intensive care units of 6 developing countries. Infect Control Hosp Epidemiol. 2012;33(7):696–703. doi:10.1086/666341. Abstract available at: https://www.ncbi.nlm.nih.gov/pubmed/22669231 (accessed 24 April 2017).

33. Rudolph Virchow. Famous scientists. Available at: https://www.famousscientists.org/rudolf-virchow/ (accessed 23 May 2017).

34. Semmelweis Society International. Dr. Semmelweis' biography, 2009. Available at: http://semmelweis.org/about/dr-semmelweis-biography/ (accessed 28 May 2017).

35. Semmelweis I. The etiology, concept, and prophylaxis of childbed fever. In: Codell Carter K, editor. Source: Excerpted from Ignaz Semmelweis. The etiology, concept, and prophylaxis of childbed fever. Madison: University of Wisconsin Press, 1983. 46–59. Available at: http://graphics8.nytimes.com/images/blogs/freakonomics/pdf/the%20etiology,%20concept%20and%20prophylaxis%20of%20childbed%20fever.pdf (accessed 24 March 2017) or https://books.google.co.il/books?id=hnezngRghTgC&pg=PA59&source=gbs_toc_r&cad=3#v=onepage&q&f=false (accessed 27 April 2017).

36. Tampa M, Sarbu I, Matei C, Benea V, Georgescu SR. Brief history of syphilis. J Med Life. 2014;7(1):4–10. Available at: https://www.ncbi.nlm.nih.gov/pmc/articles/PMC3956094/ (accessed 28 April 2017).

37. Tinker A, ten Hoope-Bender P, Azfar S, Bustreo F, Bell R. A continuum of care to save newborn lives. Lancet. 2005;365(9462):822−825. Available at: http://www.who.int/maternal_child_adolescent/documents/pdfs/lancet_neonatal_survival_partnerships.pdf?ua=1 (accessed 24 April 2017).
38. Tulchinsky TH, Varavikova EA. The new public health. Chapter one, History of Public Health. third edition. San Diego: Academic Press/Elsevier, 2014; 17−18.
39. Waknine Y. Hospital infections cost billions, study shows. Medscape. 2013. Available at: http://www.medscape.com/viewarticle/810372 (accessed 3 March 2017).
40. Walker CL, Rudan I, Liu L, Nair H, Theodoratou E, Bhutta ZA, et al. Global burden of childhood pneumonia and diarrhoea. Lancet. 2013. 381(9875):1405−1416. doi:10.1016/S0140-6736(13)60222-6. Available at: https://www.ncbi.nlm.nih.gov/pubmed/23582727 (accessed 24 April 2017).
41. Weinstein RA. Nosocomial infection update. Emerg Infect Dis. 1998;4(3):416−420. Available at: https://www.ncbi.nlm.nih.gov/pubmed/9716961 (accessed 23 April 2017).
42. Weinstein RA, Gaynes R, Edwards JR. National nosocomial infections surveillance system; overview of nosocomial infections caused by gram-negative bacilli. Clin Infect Dis. 2005;41(6):848−854. http://dx.doi.org/10.1086/432803. Available at: https://academic.oup.com/cid/article/41/6/848/2022258/Overview-of-Nosocomial-Infections-Caused-by-Gram (accessed 24 April 2017).
43. World Health Organization. Healthcare-associated infections: fact sheet. Available at: http://www.who.int/gpsc/country_work/gpsc_ccisc_fact_sheet_en.pdf (accessed 24 March 2017).
44. World Health Organization. MDG 5: improve maternal health, reviewed May 2015. Available at: http://www.who.int/topics/millennium_development_goals/maternal_health/en/ (accessed 27 April 2017).
45. World Health Organization. Infection prevention and control. Available at: http://who.int/infection-prevention/en/?utm_source = WHO + List&utm_campaign = 07560aeae9-EMAIL_CAMPAIGN_2017_05_04&utm_medium = email&utm_term = 0_823e9e35c1-07560aeae9-266379801 (accessed 5 May 2017).
46. Zimlichman E, Henderson D, Tamir O, Franz C, Song P, Yamin CK, et al. Health care−associated infections: a meta-analysis of costs and financial impact on the US health care system. JAMA Intern Med. 2013;173(22):2039−2046. Available at: http://jamanetwork.com/journals/jamainternalmedicine/fullarticle/1733452 (accessed 23 April 2017).

Chapter 5

John Snow, Cholera, the Broad Street Pump; Waterborne Diseases Then and Now

ABSTRACT

Cholera was a major global scourge in the 19th century, with frequent large-scale epidemics in European cities primarily originating in the Indian subcontinent. John Snow conducted pioneering investigations on cholera epidemics in England and particularly in London in 1854 in which he demonstrated that contaminated water was the key source of the epidemics. His thorough investigation of an epidemic in the Soho district of London led to his conclusion that contaminated water from the Broad Street pump was the source of the disease and, consequently, the removal of the handle led to cessation of the epidemic. He further studied cholera in London homes that were receiving water from two water supply systems; one from the sewage contaminated portion of the Thames River and the other that drew its water upstream from an uncontaminated part of the river. Rates of infection among clients of the distribution system drawing contaminated water far exceeded the, rates among those served by the company whose water intake was from above the contaminated section of the river. This demonstration reinforced the goals of the sanitation movement, which developed sewage drainage systems and water purification systems in cities and towns in the following decades, therewith vastly reducing the threats of cholera, typhoid and many other waterborne diseases. Despite progress being made globally, the public health problems of waterborne disease, including cholera, are by no means gone today, even in high-income countries. The tragic introduction of cholera after the earthquake devastation in Haiti in 2010 resulted in many thousands of cases and deaths from cholera indicating the still-present dangers of diseases spread into disaster situations. Cholera and other waterborne diseases remain some of the heaviest burdens of disease and death in low-income countries, especially after natural disasters or warfare as in Yemen in 2017 and are continuing challenges for global health.

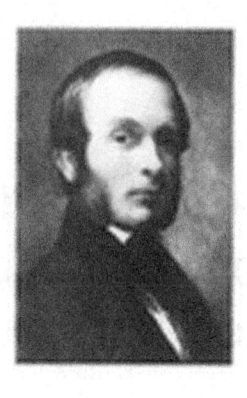

Dr. John Snow (1813–58). London practicing obstetrician/anesthesiologist who conducted a detailed epidemiologic investigation of London cholera epidemic adjacent to the now famous Broad St. pump. *Courtesy: University of California at Los Angeles (UCLA) School of Public Health. Available at: http://www.ph.ucla.edu/epi/snow/snowcricketarticle.html*

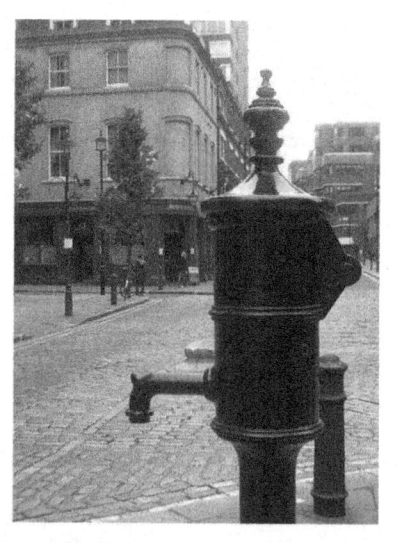

The Broad Street Pump, John Snow memorial, Broadwick Street (formerly Broad Street) in, London. In 1854 an epidemic of cholera affected residents of Soho district. Dr. John Snow surveyed deaths reported in the homes mostly near the pump and used it for their drinking water. His documented evidence suggested that contaminated water from this pump was the source of the epidemic; he caused removal of the handle, and the already declining epidemic due to people leaving the area, ceased entirely. *Source: Creative Commons photograph by Justine.*

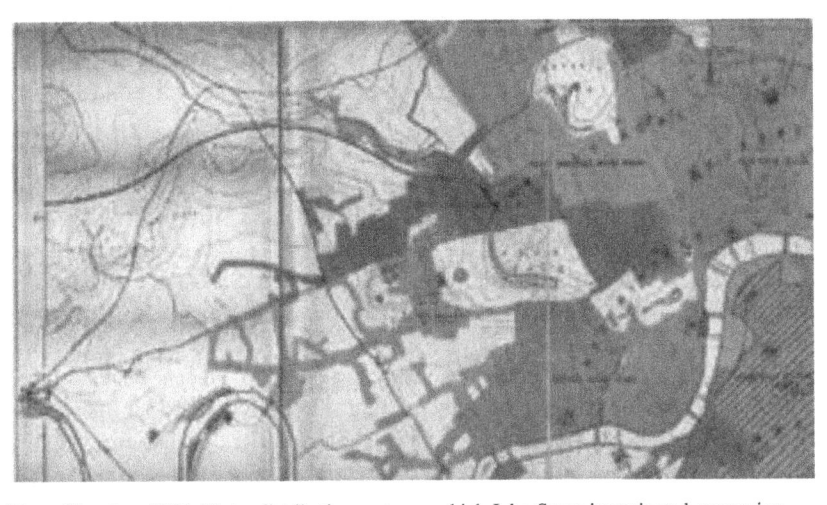

Map of London, 1854. Water-distribution systems, which John Snow investigated comparing cholera cases among consumers of water of two suppliers depending on the site of their water intake from the Thames River. *Courtesy University of California at Los Angeles (UCLA) School of Public Health. Available at: http://www.ph.ucla.edu/epi/snow/snowcricketarticle.html*

BACKGROUND

The $18^{th}-19^{th}$ centuries brought industrialization and large-scale population migration into cities of Europe including London. One result of this demographic shift was overcrowding in poor housing, served by inadequate or nonexistent public water supplies and waste-disposal systems. In London, the introduction of sewers and flushing toilets directly draining into the Thames led it to becoming an open stinking sewer, due to high tides and strong winds pushing seawater upstream. These conditions resulted in repeated outbreaks of water-borne diseases such as cholera, dysentery, tuberculosis, typhoid fever, influenza, yellow fever, and malaria, and other infectious diseases, as well as the loss of the fishing industry.

Cholera is an acute diarrhea caused by infection with the bacterium, *Vibrato cholera*. It is endemic in over 50 countries and also the cause of large epidemics. Since 1817, cholera spread rapidly throughout the world largely due to inadvertent transport of bilge water in ships mainly from the Bay of Bengal. The Indian subcontinent has been a long-term focus of cholera and the source of six worldwide epidemics between 1817 and 1923. The seventh cholera pandemic, which began in 1961, affects on an average 3−5 million people annually, with 120,000 deaths with large scale epidemics in Haiti, Yemen and in central Africa in the second decade of the 21st century.

Between 1848 and 1854, a series of cholera outbreaks occurred in London with large-scale loss of life. One epidemic of cholera occurred in the area of Broad Street, Golden Square, in Soho, a poor district of central London with unhygienic industries and housing.

John Snow was born in 1813 in York, England, the first of nine children. His father was a laborer and later a farmer. John saw unsanitary conditions in his hometown with a river contaminated by town sewage. As a medical apprentice from age 14, he experienced a cholera epidemic in a coal-mining village. Snow vowed to resist drink, gambling and marriage, and became a vegetarian. At age 23 he began medical studies and graduated from the University of London in 1844. John Snow, a physician now considered a founding father of modern epidemiology was the personal anesthetist to Queen Victoria and founding member of the London Epidemiological Society. In 1848, Snow was developing his anesthesia practice in the cholera afflicted district when he undertook an independent investigation of the epidemic.

By 1849, about 53,000 cholera deaths were registered for England and Wales. Snow was skeptical of the predominant Miasma Theory, and theorized that the cause of cholera was due to contaminated water as the main form of transmission. In 1854, a cholera epidemic broke out, affecting resident families of tailors and clerks from the shops of nearby Regent Street. The epidemic caused violent diarrhea and very high mortality, with some 600 deaths in one week during September 1854.

The prevailing Miasma Theory was that cholera was caused by airborne transmission of poisonous vapors from foul smells due to poor sanitation. At the same time, the competing Germ Theory that inspired Snow was still an unproven minority opinion in medical circles. Eventually, the foul smells, popularly known at the time as "The Great Stink" from the Thames River flowing past the Houses of Parliament were so severe that the MPs decided to take action. Finally, in 1864 with the plan of Sir Joseph Bazalgette, two enormous sewers were laid along the Thames, diverting the sewage downstream with development of sewage farms to manage the effluent. The system is still in use, but becoming too small to cope with the demands being placed on it as a result of increasing population and land development.

The Report of the Committee on Scientific Inquiries in Relation to the Cholera Epidemic of 1854 concluded that:

"Either in air or water it seems probable that the infection can grow. Often it is not easy to say which of these media may have been the chief scene of poisonous fermentation; for the impurity of one commonly implies the impurity of both; and in considerable parts of the metropolis (where the cholera has severely raged) there is rivalry of foulness between the two."

When the next cholera epidemic struck London from August to September, 1854, primarily in the Soho area adjacent to Broad Street, Snow investigated it and traced some 600 cholera deaths occurring in a 10-day period. He was struck by the observation that the cases either lived close to or were using the Broad Street pump for drinking water. He also determined that brewery workers and poorhouse residents in the area, both of whom relied on local wells, escaped the epidemic. Snow concluded that access to uncontaminated water prevented them from cholera infection, while users of the Broad Street pump became infected. He persuaded the doubtful civic authorities to remove the handle from the Broad Street pump, and the already subsiding epidemic disappeared within a few days.

As noted in Snow's report on cholera:

"The most terrible outbreak of cholera ... took place (in London) in Broad Street, Golden Square, and the adjoining streets, a few weeks ago ... there were upwards of five hundred fatal attacks of cholera in ten days. The mortality ... probably equals any that was ever caused in this country, even by the plague; and it was much more sudden, ... The mortality would undoubtedly have been much greater had it not been for the flight of the population ... in less than six days ... the most afflicted streets were deserted by more than three-quarters of their inhabitants."

"There were a few cases of cholera in the neighborhood of Broad Street, Golden Square, in the latter part of August; and the so-called outbreak which commenced in the night of 31 August and the 1st September, was, in all similar instances only a violent increase of the malady. I suspected some contamination of the water of the much-frequented pump in Broad Street ... but on examining the water, I found so little impurity in it of an organic nature ... I requested ... to take a list, at the General Registrar's Office, of the deaths of cholera, registered during the week ending 2nd September ... Eighty-nine deaths from cholera were registered during the week, in the three subdistricts."

"I found that nearly all the deaths had taken place within a short distance of the pump ... With regard to the deaths ... there were sixty-one instances in which I was informed that the deceased persons used to drink the water from Broad Street, either constantly or occasionally..."

"The Workhouse in Poland Street is more than three-quarters surrounded by houses in which deaths from cholera occurred, yet out of five hundred and thirty five inmates, only five died of cholera ... The Workhouse has a pump-well on the premises, in addition to the supply from the Grand Junction Waterworks, and the inmates never sent to the Broad Street for water. If the mortality in the Workhouse has been equal to that in the streets immediately surrounding it ... upward of one hundred persons would have died."

"There is a brewery in Broad Street, near the pump, and ... no brewer's men were registered as having died of cholera, ... above seventy workmen

employed in the brewery, none of them had suffered from cholera ... at the time the disease prevailed. The men ... do not drink water at all .... There is a deep well in the brewery, in addition to the New River water."

"The result of the inquiry then was that there has been no particular outbreak or increase of cholera, in this part of London, except among the persons who were in the habit of drinking water of the above-mentioned pump-well. I had an interview with the Board of Guardians of St. James parish, ... the handle of the pump was removed the following day."

The cholera epidemic, which was already declining, fell off and disappeared once the pump usage stopped. As a result of this episode, Benjamin Disraeli, together with other members of Parliament, adopted the plan of the Thames Authority and passed legislation forcing the overhaul of London's water and sewage systems, which after completion, contributed to the nonreturn of cholera.

In the next London cholera epidemic of September to October 1854, the highest rates of cholera occurred in areas of the city where two companies with overlapping water mains supplied homes. One of these—the Lambeth Company—moved its water intake to a less polluted part upstream of the Thames River, while the Southwark and Vauxhall company left its intake in a part of the Thames heavily polluted with sewage.

Again, suspecting water transmission, Snow's investigation identified cases of mortality from cholera by place of residence and by the two water companies that supplied the homes. During the first four weeks the impure water of Southwark and Vauxhall accounted for fatalities 14 times as great as those of the Lambeth water supply. Snow calculated the cholera rates for a 7-week period in homes supplied by each of the two in possibly the most famous presentation table in epidemiology (Table 5.1).

TABLE 5.1 Deaths From Cholera Epidemic in Districts of London Supplied by Two Water Companies Over 7 Weeks, 1854

Water Supply Company	Number of Houses	Deaths From Cholera	Cholera Deaths per 10,000 Houses
Southwark and Vauxhall	40,046	1,263	315
Lambeth	26,107	98	37
Rest of London	256,423	1,422	59

Source: Snow J. On the mode of transmission of cholera. London: John Churchill, 1855, pp. 55–98. Part 3, Table IX, Reprinted by UCLA Fielding School of Public Health 2001. Available at: http://www.ph.ucla.edu/epi/snow/snowbook3.html (accessed 26 June 2016).

Homes supplied by the Southwark and Vauxhall Water Company were affected by high cholera death rates, whereas adjacent homes supplied by the Lambeth Company had rates lower than throughout the rest of London. This provided overwhelming epidemiologic support for his hypothesis that the source of the cholera epidemic was the contaminated water from the Thames River, distributed to homes in a large area of south London.

Snow's pioneering epidemiologic investigation proved the mode of transmission of a waterborne disease that ravaged many parts of the world in the 19th century and still occurs in the 21st century. The *V. cholera* organism was originally grown in 1854 but was reported in local Italian medical literature and not recognized internationally. International recognition for the definitive identification and growth of the organism during his investigation of an epidemic of cholera in Egypt was given to the eminent German bacteriologist, Robert Koch in 1883. Filipo Pucini was ultimately recognized for the discovery in 1984 when the organism was formally named *Vibrio cholerae pucini 1854*. Robert Koch was the discoverer of anthrax in 1880, and tuberculosis in 1882, and leader in defining criteria for causation of infectious diseases; he was awarded a Nobel Prize in Medicine in 1905 (see Chapter 7).

The Broad Street pump episode demonstrated that cholera was water-borne and thus the means to prevent it had already been identified almost 30 years before. Snow also established the basic methodology of modern public health for infectious disease investigation and contributed to establishing the validity of the Germ Theory, which was still highly controversial at this time.

With the understanding of the causal relation between microorganisms and diseases at the end of the 19th century, the process for reducing large-scale morbidity and mortality via disinfection was initiated. The first use of chlorine as a disinfectant for water facilities was in 1897 in England. The first use of this method for municipal water facilities in the United States was in Jersey City, New Jersey, and Chicago, Illinois, in 1915. Other cities followed and the use of chlorination as standard treatment for water disinfection rapidly grew. During the 20th century, death rates from waterborne diseases decreased significantly, and although other additional factors contributed to the general improvements in health (such as sanitation, improved quality of life, and nutrition), the improvement of water quality was, without doubt, a major reason. The decline in typhoid fever in the United States between 1900 and 1945 as a result of improved water supply systems and use of chlorination is seen in Figure 5.1.

The disinfection of drinking water through both filtration and chlorination processes has been one of the major achievements of public health. Clean water was responsible for nearly half the total mortality reduction in major cities, three-quarters of the infant mortality reduction, and nearly two-thirds of child mortality reduction.

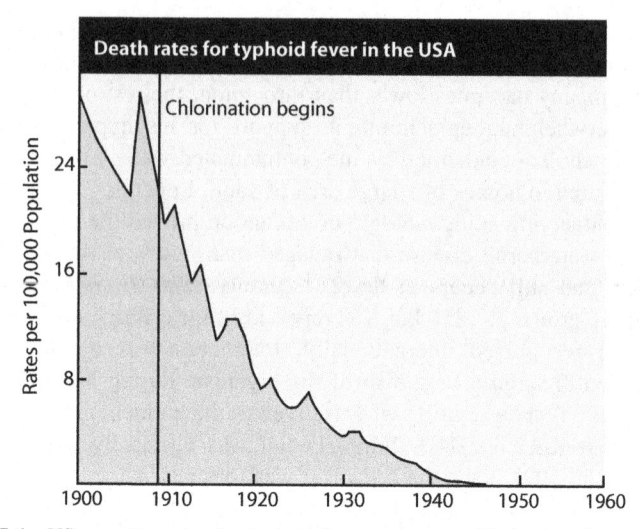

FIGURE 5.1   US mortality rates for typhoid fever and water chlorination. *Source: Chlorine Chemistry Council (C3) and Canadian Chlorine Coordinating Committee (C4). Drinking water chlorination: a review of disinfection practices and issues. Adapted from US Centers for Disease Control and Prevention, Summary of Notifiable Diseases, 1997. Available at: http://www. waterandhealth.org/drinkingwater/wp.html (accessed 16 August 2016).*

CURRENT RELEVANCE

In 2014, an estimated 3—5 million cases of cholera occurred globally with more than 100,000 deaths, mainly in developing countries without safe drinking water treatment and sanitation.

Epidemics of cholera also occur in natural disaster situations, particularly in those areas where sanitation systems break down. A current example of such events is seen in Haiti, where an earthquake in 2010 killed over 200,000 people and displaced over one million persons. This was followed by a massive cholera outbreak 10 months later, with over 665,000 cases and 8,183 deaths. Intensive efforts of the Haitian Ministry of Health together with the Centers for Disease Control (CDC), World Health Organization (WHO), and other international organizations, with massive vaccinations against cholera, prevented thousands of deaths from cholera, but transmission of the disease continued in the following years.

Making matters worse, while Haiti was already struggling with effects of the cholera outbreak since 2010, a major hurricane (Hurricane Matthew) struck in October, 2016. The WHO shipped a million cholera vaccines to Haiti, attempting to minimize the risk of further increases of cases. The UN reports that since the cholera outbreak of 2010 some 780,000 persons have been infected with cholera and 9,145 have died of the disease. Moreover, since the hurricane in 2016, almost 800 new cases arise each week.

The cholera epidemic in Haiti since 2010 has been attributed to importation of the *Vibrio* bacterium by UN peacekeeper forces from Nepal, still a cholera-endemic country. The sewage contamination in UN peacekeeper camps with poor sanitation spread to nearby camps for displaced homeless Haitians following the earthquake.

Cholera can be imported via travelers from areas still endemic with cholera exposure to street, or other contaminated foods. Cholera and other water-borne diseases remain major global public health problems in the 21st century, particularly in areas of poverty. Both the WHO and the United Nations have recently acknowledged that the Haitian epidemic resulted from entry of the organism into poor hygienic camps by UN troops that were sent in to maintain order. Epidemiologists identified that the cholera strain found in Haiti was the same as one that originated in Nepal, where the disease is still endemic. Improving Haiti's water and sanitation infrastructure is critical to achieving large health gains and reducing the opportunity for cholera to spread with responsibility attributed to United Nation peacekeeper soldiers from Nepal.

During the 1970s, in the medical and public health professions public health community there was a widespread idea that infectious diseases were gradually going to disappear under the combined influence of hygiene, antibiotics, and vaccines. This false sense of security was shattered with the advent of AIDS in the 1980s, and the subsequent return of diseases previously thought to be under control, such as tuberculosis, malaria, dengue, and plague. The complacency was replaced by a high degree of concern as new infectious diseases continued to arrive, such as HIV in the 1980s, bovine spongiform encephalopathy (BSE) in the 1990s, severe acute respiratory syndrome (SARS) in 2003, Ebola in 2015 and Zika virus in 2016 is now seen as a global public health crisis with few new antibiotics in the pipeline of development, testing, licensure and production. Growing resistance of many organisms to currently available antibiotics and health care associated infections, as well as spread of diseases from tropical areas to temperate zone countries in North America, Europe and other regions such as West Nile Fever, Chikungunya, and Zika. A further concern was the return of old diseases thought to be controlled such as the sexually transmitted diseases, as well as diphtheria and pertussis.

In the early 21st century, the spread of infectious diseases as weapons of terror and even war, including anthrax, came to grip the public and created a whole new spectrum of terrorism. In 2004, another concern came to the fore, with the lack of an influenza vaccine to protect vulnerable people in the population, due to difficulties with production and regulation. In particular, this placed caregivers at high risk of infecting patients or bringing the disease home from the hospital setting.

Today, waterborne disease is given less recognition, as standards of water and sewage treatment are assumed to be part of modern living. However, waterborne enteric disease continues to be among the major killers in many parts of the world, especially among children. Waterborne disease may be so common that it escapes detection in many countries, especially those where hepatitis (especially A and E) is endemic and where incidence of gastroenteritis from *shigella*, *Escherichia coli*, rotavirus, and many other enteric infectious agents remains high. Another example is *Helicobacter pylori*, the cause of chronic peptic ulcer disease and the recognized cause for gastric cancer. Helicobacter, which affects nearly half of the world's population and is related to poverty and poor hygiene is also waterborne.

In Western industrialized countries, waterborne disease outbreaks have become relatively uncommon due to high levels of water management. Water contamination and enteric disease can also occur from organisms for which routine testing is not currently practiced. For example, testing for rotaviruses (which cause enteric disease) and organisms such as *campylobacter* and *giardia* is not routinely done, but water is tested if there is a suspicion of contamination.

In 1999, the CDC reported on achievements of public health during the 20th century in the United States addressing the problem of waterborne disease as follows:

By 1900, however, the incidence of many of these diseases had begun to decline because of public health improvements, implementation of which continued into the 20th century. Local, state, and federal efforts to improve sanitation and hygiene reinforced the concept of collective "public health" action (e.g., to prevent infection by providing clean drinking water). By 1900, 40 of the 45 states had established health departments. The first county health departments were established in 1908. From the 1930s through the 1950s, state and local health departments made substantial progress in disease prevention activities, including sewage disposal, water treatment, food safety, organized solid waste disposal, and public education about hygienic practices (e.g., food-handling and handwashing). Chlorination and other treatments of drinking water began in the early 1900s and became widespread public health practices, further decreasing the incidence of waterborne diseases.

In 2003, bacterial contamination of the municipal water system in Walkerton, Ontario, Canada resulted in a public health disaster with 7 deaths and 2,300 persons ill. A public inquiry revealed that improper practices and systemic fraudulence by the public utility operators, privatization of municipal water testing, absence of mandatory criteria governing quality of testing, and the lack of provisions for notification of results to multiple authorities all contributed to the crisis. Warnings of significant concerns two years before the outbreak were ineffective as budgetary cuts destroyed the checks and balances needed to ensure municipal water safety.

Safe water also includes ensuring chemical safety through measures such as prevention of lead poisoning from deterioration in distribution systems, such as occurred in Flint, Michigan, in the United States, in 2015. Safe water supply requires exacting physical treatment as well as disinfection, especially of all surface water sources. Effective water management can reduce the burden of gastroenteric disease even in a relatively well-developed country.

Water treatment is one of the fundamentals of preserving public health not only at the sources. Residual chlorine throughout the distribution system prevents secondary contamination from faults in the pipes and leakage of sewage into the system. Many steps are essential for assurance of safe water supplies, including well-organized sanitary and laboratory monitoring by the public health authorities and not only the supplier. Yet waterborne diseases can occur and spread due to error, negligence or as in the case of Haiti unintended consequences of well meant interventions.

Cholera, typhoid fever, dysentery, and hepatitis A and E, and many other bacterial, viral, and parasitic diseases are waterborne diseases, i.e., caused by pathogens transmitted via water supplies. An immensely important public health challenge at the beginning of the 20th century was therefore the improvement and safety of drinking water quality, aiming to significantly reduce illness and death caused by contaminated drinking water.

In 1991, *V. cholera* O1 apparently arrived in a cargo ship from China whose sewage was spread into the harbor of Lima, Peru. It contaminated shellfish, popular among the local population, and therewith created a local epidemic that continued to spread in Central and South America between 1991 and 1994. The Pan American Health Organization (PAHO) reported a total of over one million cases and almost 10,000 deaths (case-fatality rate: 0.9%) from countries in the western hemisphere in this period. In southern Asia, an epidemic caused by a newly recognized strain of *V. cholera*, which began in late 1992, then spread to several areas of Central America, Brazil, and Argentina. In 2011, 58 countries from all continents reported a cumulative total of 589,854 cholera cases, representing an increase of 85 percent from 2010, with the greatest proportion of cases in Haiti and the African continent. In 2014, 55 percent of all reported cholera cases were from Africa and 15% from the Americas, the latter clearly resulting from the Haiti outbreak that started in 2010. The case fatality rate for cholera increased by 47 percent from 2013 compared to 2014. In 2014, a case fatality rate of 1.17 percent represented 190,549 cases and 2,231 deaths, mainly in Afghanistan, Democratic Republic of Congo (DRC), Ghana, Haiti, and Nigeria.

Waterborne disease outbreaks reported in the United States between 1920 and 2002, included at least 1,870 events associated with drinking water, an average of 22.5 per year, with 883,806 illnesses, for an average of 10,648 cases per year. Of more recent cases, just over half of the outbreaks had no organisms that were specifically identified but were epidemiologically identified as viral in origin. In addition to the disease outbreaks, these waterborne organisms constitute a special risk of death for persons with compromised immune systems, including cancer patients being treated with chemotherapy,

HIV-positive persons, and patients being treated with immunosuppressants. Outbreaks of waterborne giardia and cryptosporidium in the United States raised concerns, because these organisms are not efficiently eliminated by standard water treatment.

ETHICAL ISSUES

The principal ethical issue is implementation of existing technology of public health globally to save human lives now being lost to waterborne and other diarrheal diseases. Diarrheal disease caused by contaminated water, food, or transmission from person to person can be caused by many bacteria, viruses, and parasites. Together, these are the second leading cause of death in children under 5 years of age, killing some 760,000 children every year. The most serious complication of severe diarrheal disease in young children results from dehydration due to the loss of fluids and salts necessary for survival. Dehydration is mostly treatable with oral rehydration solutions (ORS), one of the great public health innovations of the past half century, now used globally. Children most at risk are those that have been previously malnourished or with impaired immunity. Prevention includes access to safe drinking water; improved sanitation; handwashing with soap; exclusive breastfeeding for the first six months of life; good personal and food hygiene; health education about how infections spread; and rotavirus vaccination.

Clearly, the issues related to control of infectious diseases are not gone, nor are they likely to be without major new breakthroughs in vaccine production and new modes of treatment. But control of waterborne enteric diseases continues to depend on well-tested and effective traditional means of infectious disease control. Public health organizations require strong emphasis on monitoring of water security, adequate waste disposal systems, disease reporting systems, training of health workers and the public, and strong laboratory capacity and support.

Other causes of diarrheal disease morbidity are no less important. Rotavirus is a major cause of disease and death among children up to age five years, even in high- and medium-income countries. But the burden is mainly on low-income populations especially in low-income countries led by India, Nigeria, Pakistan, and sub-Saharan African countries. Oral rotavirus vaccines introduced in the industrialized world in 2006 have had a great impact in the United States, reducing hospitalizations for severe rotavirus by as much as 80 percent. Rotavirus globally is estimated by the WHO to cause annually approximately 111 million episodes of gastroenteritis, 25 million clinic visits, two million hospitalizations, and 352,000−592,000 deaths (median 440,000 deaths) in children up to five years of age.

Rotavirus causes severe acute gastroenteritis with diarrhea and vomiting, primarily in infants and young children. The oral vaccine has been introduced in 90 countries by the end of 2016, with global child coverage estimated at 25 percent, having been adopted in most high- and many medium-income countries and gradually introduced in low-income countries. Adoption of rotavirus vaccine in routine national immunization programs resulted in reduction of over 85 percent of rotavirus hospitalizations in Belgium, and similar reductions in hospitalizations for rotavirus-induced diarrheal conditions showed the high effectiveness of the rotavirus vaccines (over 85%). In many countries, the vaccine is only partially reimbursed on a per-prescription basis. A systematic review of ecological studies from eight countries reported a 49−89 percent decline in laboratory-confirmed rotavirus hospital admissions in children less than five years old within two years of vaccine introduction. Increasing the use of rotavirus vaccine with proven efficacy and cost effectiveness, along with efforts to improve access to safe water supplies, improved food and sewage management, and personal hygiene will continue to reduce the burden of disease and death in the vulnerable child population where sanitation is still poor. Clean sanitary facilities in homes supported by safe public sewage collection and treatment systems are essential for prevention of enteric infections. A World Bank data base review of percentage of homes with access to improved sanitary faclities with change between 1990 and 2015 showed high income countries such as the US, Canada, UK, Netherlands and Australia with 99−100% in both years. China increased from 48 to 77 percent, and India from 17 to 40 percent. Global coverage increased from 53 to 67 percent.

Meeting the goal of clean, safe drinking/potable water requires implementing a multibarrier approach that includes: protecting source water from contamination, appropriately treating raw source water, especially surface water, and ensuring safe distribution of treated water to the consumers. While chlorination is a mainstay in protecting water supplies, filtration and coagulation are equally important. Filtration, coagulation, and disinfection of water are the optimal combination known to date, where chlorination kills or inactivates bacteria and viruses and filtration completes the action of eliminating pathogens in particles and eliminating parasitic protozoa.

Wastewater includes water with human waste, food scraps, oils, soaps, and chemicals from homes, from industry, and from storm runoff. Untreated wastewater discharged to nature can damage the environment and groundwater, making treatment essential. Nature copes well with small amounts, but can be overwhelmed by large amounts of untreated wastewater and sewage. Treatment plants reduce pollutants in wastewater to a level nature can handle. Government regulation of business, industry, and local authorities is a vital part of modern public health. Business and industry are legally accountable, but not well enforced, for ensuring their wastewater runoff is within accepted standards. Use of wastewater for irrigation after extensive treatment for irrigation is part of modern water economies and within supervised standards for field and orchard crops and even in vegetables and other ground crops, including for newly emerging pathogens and chemicals.

Chemical disinfectants in water treatment and sewage usually can result in the formation of chemical byproducts. However, the risks to health from these byproducts are extremely small in comparison to the risks associated with inadequate disinfection. Disinfection efficacy should not be compromised in attempting to control such byproducts. The main advantage of chlorine-based water disinfection over other methods (such as ozone and UV radiation) is its long-lasting effect; its presence also prevents the regrowth of microorganisms, thereby protecting clean water throughout the distribution system. Chlorine as a disinfectant is also easily monitored and controlled as a drinking water disinfectant, and frequent monitoring is recommended wherever chlorination is practiced.

Private water supplies, such as wells, used by millions of people even in high-income countries are not government regulated or well protected. Contamination by animal excretions and agricultural runoff are of serious concern. These sources of water can be made safe by fencing and hard surrounding platform along with regular use of household chlorine (5.25%) bleach. Potential contaminants include microorganisms of human and animal waste products. Chemical contaminants from natural and man-made sources can be equally hazardous.

Cholera continues to spread across many countries with dramatic consequences, overwhelming stretched health systems and diverting resources from other crucial prevention-oriented programs. Global priority for increasing safe water supply as part of the MDGs did achieve its targets of increasing access to safe water, but cholera itself has not been a topic of major priority in global health.

The UN report on MDGs indicates that the global target of halving the proportion of people without access to improved sources of water was met five years ahead of schedule. Between 1990 and 2015, 2.6 billion people gained access to improved drinking water sources. Worldwide 2.1 billion people have gained access to improved sanitation. Despite progress, 2.4 billion are still using unimproved sanitation facilities, including 946 million people still practicing open defecation.

However, WHO reestablished a Global Task Force on Cholera Control in 2012 to increase the visibility of cholera as an important global public health challenge. This emphasizes disseminating information about cholera prevention and control and conducting advocacy and resource mobilization activities to support cholera prevention and control at national, regional, and global levels with participation by the international community of donors and public health professionals.

Cholera can appear in disaster situations such as in severe floods, and other natural calamities including earthquakes, tsunamis, and floods, as well as manmade catastrophes including civil wars and refugee situations as well.

In the second decade of the 21st century, major epidemics of cholera are wreaking havoc in man-made and natural disaster settings. In post-hurricane Haiti as a result of imported vibrio by UN peacekeeper forces and recklessly poor sanitation, contamination of water used by a displaced persons' camp in 2010 resulted in a devastating cholera epidemic persisting for years. This has killed more than 11,000 people and left more than 880,000 infected by June 2017. A deadly cholera epidemic is raging in war torn Yemen with over 200,000 cases and 1,500 deaths reported by WHO. Cholera is also rampant in strife-torn East Africa with Red Cross reports of 51,000 cholera cases in Somalia and nearly 5,000 in South Sudan associated with famine, poor supply of food aid in a vicious tragedy mainly of man-made causes.

ECONOMIC ISSUES

In 1993 in the United States contamination of water sources with the parasite *cryptosporidium* caused major waterborne disease outbreaks in Milwaukee, Wisconsin and elsewhere. The Milwaukee outbreak was the largest reported waterborne disease outbreak in US history, with approximately 403,000 ill persons with 4,400 hospitalizations. Attack rates were as high as 50 percent in some parts of the city. *Cryptosporidium* is transmitted from person to person and from animals to humans, but can also be transmitted in swimming pools and community waters. *Cryptosporidium* was reportedly present in 65−87 percent of surface water samples tested in the United States. The total cost of illness in this outbreak was calculated at $96.3 million: $31.7 million in medical costs and $64.6 million in productivity losses.

Giardia lamblia is another parasite that can be transmitted in inadequately filtered surface water and for which chlorination is inadequate to disinfect. In the period 2011−12, in the United States 32 drinking water-associated outbreaks were reported, with at least 431 cases of illness, 102 hospitalizations, and 14 deaths. *Legionella* was responsible for 66 percent of these outbreaks and 26 percent of illnesses; other bacteria and viruses accounted for 16 percent of outbreaks and 53 percent of illnesses.

Helicobacter pylori as the major cause of acute and chronic peptic ulcer disease (PUD) and gastric cancer is known to be related to hygienic conditions including water safety, and is thought to be prevalent in more than half the world population with a high economic impact on health systems. One of the important measures for its control is water security, especially for low- and medium-income countries (see Chapter 22).

Prevention of waterborne diseases requires high standards for community, food, and personal hygiene, sanitation including garbage disposal, supply and treatment of safe drinking water, and prohibiting the use of raw or partially treated sewage for irrigation of crops. Sanitation, particularly the filtration and chlorination of drinking water, prohibiting the use of raw or partially treated sewage for the irrigation of ground crops. Crucial treatment for diarrhea is prompt fluid therapy with sugar electrolytes in large volumes to replace all fluid loss with oral rehydration therapy (ORT). Using this form of treatment can successfully treat up to 80 percent of cholera cases.

Tetracycline shortens the duration of the disease, and chemoprophylaxis for contacts following stool samples may help in reducing its spread. A vaccine is also available, which can help to control outbreaks. Rehydration is a cornerstone of treatment and can reduce the fatality rate to less than one percent.

Cholera and its burden on a country serve as indicators of poverty and inadequate social infrastructure and development. It persists as a major public health challenge in developing countries that lack fundamental sanitary infrastructure, with effective public health systems capable of providing clean, safe water. Due to unsanitary living conditions, these populations and communities are at high risk of major cholera outbreaks as well as other diarrheal diseases.

Cholera infection still endemic in more than 50 countries is caused by *V. cholera* O1 (99% of cases worldwide), which produces a toxin causing severe watery diarrhea that can be rapidly fatal without treatment of dehydration. Globally, gastroenteric infections kill some three million children per year and must remain one of the high priority issues in international aid for the coming decades. Even industrialized countries with proper sanitation and water supply systems face the risks of waterborne disease outbreaks, since these can occur due to malfunctions and human error in monitoring water supply and safety, as the examples of Milwaukee and Walkerton, Canada, in 2003 showed.

The United Nations 1966 International Covenant on Economic, Social and Cultural Rights (ICESCR) confirmed the right to water in international law, noting that such a right is "indispensable for leading a life in human dignity" and "a prerequisite for the realization of other human rights." This international commitment was reaffirmed in 2002 that: The "human right to water entitles everyone to sufficient, safe, acceptable, physically accessible and affordable water for personal and domestic uses" (see Box 5.1). This right is implicit in the rights to health, housing, food, life, and

---

BOX 5.1 United Nations: Human Rights to Water and Sanitation

Sufficient and continuous water supply for personal and domestic uses; the WHO estimates this should be 50–100 liters per person daily.

Safe, i.e., free from microorganisms, chemical substances, and radiological hazards that threaten health.

Acceptable in color, taste, and odor.

Physically accessible, i.e., within 1,000 meters of the home and collection time not to exceed 30 minutes, and safe for gender privacy.

Affordable for all and costs should not exceed three percent of household income.

Source: United Nations. Available at: http://www.un.org/waterforlifedecade/ human_right_to_water.shtml (accessed 14 November 2016).

dignity enshrined in other international conventions, such as the International Bill of Human Rights and the Convention on the Rights of the Child. The focus is explicitly on the responsibilities of governments for delivering clean water and adequate sanitation services to all.

The global initiative of the Millennium Development Goals (MDGs) from 2001 to 2015 was a consensus-combined effort of 140 countries to achieve reduced poverty, improved education and health of women and children, and improved access to sanitation, as well as control of diseases such as malaria, HIV, and TB. The MDGs included a specific goal to increase access to safe water supplies. Since 2011, the WHO Global Task Force on Cholera Control has also worked to support the design and implementation of global strategies to contribute to capacity development for cholera prevention and control.

Between 1990 and 2015, progress was made so that 1.9 billion people gained access to piped drinking water and 2.1 billion people gained access to improved sanitation. After the MDGs the UN created Sustainable Development Goals (SDGs), which incorporate many of the MDG goals and an agenda for global sustainable development until 2030. Among the 17 goals, number six is on "clean water and sanitation," and other goals are likely to seek to contribute to prevention and control of waterborne diseases (e.g., Goal 3: Good Health and Well-being).

CONCLUSION

Policy initiatives are essential to support the development and implementation of global strategies for policy and capacity development for cholera prevention locally, nationally, and globally. This is meant to promote donor support, technical exchange, coordination, and cooperation on cholera-related activities; to strengthen countries' policies and capacity to prevent and control cholera; to disseminate technical guidelines and operational manuals; and to support development of a research agenda with emphasis on evaluating innovative approaches to cholera prevention and control in affected countries.

Snow's brilliant, game-changing studies of cholera in 1854 earned him the title "the father of modern epidemiology." His work led directly to steps taken to improve water safety in London, setting new standards for other urban centers across the industrialized world, resulting in cholera, typhoid, and other enteric infectious diseases largely disappearing in many countries and saving of millions of lives over the years. Yet cholera, along with many other waterborne diseases, remains a serious challenge to public health with severe health, economic, and social effects globally particularly on the poorest populations, especially those in developing countries or in disaster situations in the 21st century.

The potential to relieve suffering and death from cholera, and other gastroenteric infections from contaminated water (and food) resulting from John Snow's work, is still far from being fully achieved. But his contribution has saved millions of lives. Improving sanitation and reducing poverty are still closely linked issues in public health today in both industrialized and developing countries. The WHO has called for recognition of cholera as a Neglected Tropical Disease and promotes its prevention and control globally. But clearly cholera and its many brother waterborne diseases are real and present dangers in a globalized world with millions traveling for business, tourism, and migration. John Snow pointed the way, and the modern world needs to apply lessons learned from this case.

The WHO Global Task Force on Cholera Control, and WHO work to:

1. Support the design and implementation of global strategies to contribute to capacity development for cholera prevention and control globally;
2. Provide a forum for technical exchange, coordination, and cooperation on cholera-related activities to strengthen countries' capacity to prevent and control cholera;
3. Support countries for the implementation of effective cholera control strategies and monitoring of progress;
4. Disseminate technical guidelines and operational manuals;
5. Support the development of a research agenda with emphasis on evaluating innovative approaches to cholera prevention and control in affected countries;
6. Increase the visibility of cholera as an important global public health problem through the dissemination of information about cholera prevention and control, and
7. Conduct advocacy and resource mobilization activities to support cholera prevention and control at national, regional, and global levels.

RECOMMENDATIONS

The following recommendations represent key lines of action highlighting the Millennium Development Goals and the follow-up Sustainable Development Goals recommended actions for increased access to safe water supplies and preventive care for diarrheal disease which despite progress with MDGs are still one of the leading causes of death under age 5 globally.

1. Continued global health efforts of the WHO and UN and other international agencies should expand efforts to improve safe water, improved sanitary home facilities and safe community sewage management in low- and medium-income countries.
2. Control and elimination of cholera and other microbiological causes of severe diarrheal disease must be given high priority on the global health agenda with training and improved safety of water sources and distribution systems.
3. Research to develop effective vaccines that can be introduced to routine vaccination programs such as has successfully occurred with rotavirus

vaccine should be of high priority of public private partnerships working to advance global health.

4. Funding assistance to low-income countries and poor regions of middle- and high-income countries and donors should include resources for the essential water infrastructure and monitoring systems and training of monitoring and laboratory personnel.

5. Education for public health workers, political leaders, and the general public should stress the multiple interventions needed to ensure the quality and quality of safe drinking water, improved home sanitary facilities and community sewage systems, as fundamental to public health especially for preparation in disaster situations.

STUDENT REVIEW QUESTIONS

1. How did the emptying of raw sewage into the Thames River contribute to the cholera epidemics of the 1850s?

2. What were the alternative explanations for the London cholera epidemics at the time of the mid-19th century epidemics?

3. What were the characteristics of the cholera epidemics discovered by Snow in his investigation that led to him identify water as the vehicle for transmission of the disease?

4. What is the state of waterborne gastroenteric disease in the total burden of disease globally at the present time?

5. How did cholera become established in Haiti following the earthquake and hurricane in 2004 and 2016? What happened as a result of the presence of United Nations troops contaminating local sewage near a refugee camp?

6. What are the key prevention measures of waterborne diseases crucial to public health?

7. What are the key components for assuring safety of community water supplies?

8. How are *cryptosporidium*, *shigellosis*, *rotavirus*, and *Helicobacter pylori* related to cholera?

9. What are the differences between proof of *association* and proof of *causation* in epidemiology? Explain which applied to John Snow's studies?

10. What are the advantages and disadvantages of chlorine disinfection of community and household water supplies?

RECOMMENDED READINGS

1. Anderson C. Cholera epidemic traced to risk miscalculation. Nature. 1991;354:255.

2. Albert MJ, Neira M. The role of food in the epidemiology of cholera. World Health Stat Q. 1997;50(1−2):111−118. Abstract available at: http://www.ncbi.nlm.nih.gov/pubmed/9282393 (accessed 29 June 2016).

3. Ali M, Nelson AR, Lopez AL, Sack DA. Updated global burden of cholera in endemic countries. PLoS Negl Trop Dis. 2015;9(6):e0003832. Available at: http://www.ncbi.nlm. nih.gov/pmc/articles/PMC4455997/pdf/pntd.0003832.pdf (accessed 20 August 2016).

4. Benedict KM, Reses H, Vigar M, Roth DM, Roberts VA, Mattioli M, et al. Surveillance for waterborne disease outbreaks associated with drinking water — United States, 2013–2014. MMWR Morb Mortal Wkly Rep. 2017;66:1216–1221. doi:https://doi.org/ 10.15585/mmwr.mm6644a3. Available at: https://www.cdc.gov/mmwr/volumes/66/wr/ mm6644a3.htm?s_cid = mm6644a3_e (accessed 9 November 2017).

5. Beer KD, Gargano JW, Roberts VA, Hill VA, Garrison LE, Kutty PK, et al. Surveillance for waterborne disease outbreaks associated with drinking water—United States, 2011–2012. Morb Mortal Wkly Rep. 2015;64(31):842–848. Available at: http://www.cdc. gov/mmwr/preview/mmwrhtml/mm6431a2.htm (accessed 26 June 2016).

6. Centers for Disease Control and Prevention. Update: *Vibrio cholerae* 01—Western Hemisphere, 1991–1994, and *V. cholerae* 0139—Asia, 1994. Morb Mortal Wkly Rep. 1995;44(11):215–219. Available at: https://www.cdc.gov/mmwr/preview/mmwrhtml/ 00036609.htm (accessed 4 July 2016).

7. Centers for Disease Control and Prevention. Achievements in public health, 1900–1999: control of infectious diseases. Morb Mortal Wkly Rep. 1999;48(29):621–629. Available at: http://www.cdc.gov/mmwr/pdf/wk/mm4829.pdf (accessed 29 June 2016).

8. Centers for Disease Control and Prevention. A century of U.S. water chlorination and treatment: one of the ten greatest public health achievements of the 20th century. Morb Mortal Wkly Rep. 1999;48(29):621–629. Available at: http://www.cdc.gov/healthywater/drinking/ history.html (accessed 17 August 2016).

9. Centers for Disease Control and Prevention. Cholera epidemic associated with raw vegetables— Lusaka, Zambia, 2003–2004. Morb Mortal Wkly Rep. 2004;53(34):783–786. Available at: http://www.cdc.gov/mmwr/preview/mmwrhtml/mm5334a2.htm (accessed 29 June 2016).

10. Centers for Disease Control and Prevention. 150th anniversary of John Snow and the pump handle. Morb Mortal Wkly Rep. 2004;53(34):783. Available at: https://www.cdc.gov/ mmwr/preview/mmwrhtml/mm5334a1.htm (accessed 4 July 2017).

11. Centers for Disease Control and Prevention. Haiti cholera outbreak: cholera in Haiti one year later, 2011. Available at: https://www.cdc.gov/cholera/haiti/haiti-one-year-later.html (accessed 26 June 2016).

12. Centers for Disease Control and Prevention. Cholera in Haiti, 2014. Available at: http:// www.cdc.gov/cholera/haiti/index.html (accessed 26 June 2016).

13. Centers for Disease Control and Prevention. Water treatment, community water treatment, 2015. Available at: http://www.cdc.gov/healthywater/drinking/public/water_treatment.html (accessed 26 June 2016).

14. Chin CS, Sorenson J, Harris JB, Robins WP, Charles RC, Jean-Charles RR, et al. The origin of the Haitian cholera outbreak strain. N Engl J Med. 2011;364(1):33–42. Available at: http://www.nejm.org/doi/full/10.1056/NEJMoa1012928 (accessed 15 August 2016).

15. Chlorine Chemistry Council and Canadian Chlorine Coordinating Committee. Water quality and health. Drinking water chlorination, a review of disinfection practices and issues. Available at: http://www.waterandhealth.org/drinkingwater/wp.html (accessed 16 August 2016).

16. Corso PS, Kramer MH, Blair KA, Addin DG, Davis JP, Haddix AC. Cost of illness in the 1993 waterborne *Cryptosporidium* outbreak, Milwaukee, Wisconsin. Emerg Infect Dis. 2003;9(4):426–431. Available at: http://wwwnc.cdc.gov/eid/article/9/4/02-0417_article (accessed 26 June 2016).

17. Craun MF, Craun GF, Calderon RL, Beach MJ. Waterborne outbreaks reported in the United States. J. Water Health. 2006;4(Suppl. 2):19−30. Abstract available at: http://www. ncbi.nlm.nih.gov/pubmed/16895084 (accessed 26 June 2016).

18. Crockett CS. The role of wastewater treatment in protecting water supplies against emerging pathogens. Water Environ Res. 2007;79(3):221−232. Abstract available at: http://www. ncbi.nlm.nih.gov/pubmed/17469654 (accessed 20 August 2016).

19. Crump JA, Mintz ED. Global trends in typhoid and paratyphoid fever. Clin Infect Dis. 2010;50(2):241−246. Available at: http://cid.oxfordjournals.org/content/50/2/241.long (accessed 17 August 2016).

20. Cutler D, Miller G. The role of public health improvements in health advances: the twentieth-century United States. Demography. 2005;42(1):1−22. Available at: http://www. ncbi.nlm.nih.gov/pubmed/15782893.

21. Department of Epidemiology, Fielding School of Public Health, University of California at Los Angeles (UCLA). John Snow. Available at: http://www.ph.ucla.edu/epi/snow.html (accessed 5 July 2017).

22. Esrey SA, Potash JB, Roberts L, Shiff C. Effects of improved water supply on ascariasis, diarrhoea, dracunculiasis, hookworm infection, schistosomiasis, and trachoma. Bull World Health Organ. 1991;69:609−621. Available at: http://apps.who.int/iris/bitstream/10665/ 48164/1/bulletin_1991_69%285%29_609-621.pdf (accessed 12 November 2016).

23. Frerichs RR, Keim PS, Barrais R, Piarroux R. Nepalese origin of cholera epidemic in Haiti. Clin Microbiol Infect. 2012;18(6):E158−E163. Available at: http://www.sciencedirect.com/science/article/pii/S1198743X14641343 (accessed 14 November 2016).

24. George G, Rotich J, Kigen H, Catherine K, Waweru B, Boru W, et al. Notes from the field: ongoing cholera outbreak—Kenya, 2014−2016. Morb Mortal Wkly Rep. 2016;65:68−69. Available at: http://dx.doi.org/10.15585/mmwr.mm6503a7 (accessed 17 August 2016).

25. Harris JB, LaRocque RC, Qadri F, Ryan ET, Calderwood SB. Cholera. Lancet. 2012;379 (9835):2466−2476. doi:10.1016/S0140-6736(12)60436-X.V. Available at: http:// europepmc.org/backend/ptpmcrender.fcgi?accid=PMC3761070&blobtype=pdf (accessed 14 June 2016).

26. History of the Thames 1999−2016. Available at: http://www.riverthames.co.uk/history.htm (accessed 15 July 2016).

27. Hrudey SE, Payment P, Huck PM, Gillam RW, Hrudey EJ. A fatal waterborne disease epidemic in Walkerton, Ontario: comparison with other waterborne outbreaks in the developed world. Water Sci Technol. 2003;47(3):7−14. Available at: http://www.ncbi.nlm.nih.gov/ pubmed/12638998 (accessed 26 June 2016).

28. Hurst CJ. Presence of enteric viruses in freshwater and their removal by the conventional drinking water treatment process. Bull World Health Organ. 1991;69:113−119. Available at: http://www.ncbi.nlm.nih.gov/pmc/articles/PMC2393205/pdf/bullwho00046-0120.pdf (accessed 26 June 2016).

29. Katz JM. UN admits role in Cholera epidemic in Haiti. Available at: https://www.nytimes.com/ 2016/08/18/world/americas/united-nations-haiti-cholera.html?_r=1 (accessed 19 August 2016).

30. MacKenzie WR, Hoxie NJ, Proctor ME, Gradus MS, Blair KA, Peterson DE, et al. A massive outbreak in Milwaukee of cryptosporidium infection transmitted through the public water supply system. N Engl J Med. 1994;331:161−167. Available at: http://www.nejm. org/doi/pdf/10.1056/NEJM199407213310304 (accessed 25 June 2016).

31. Morris JG. Cholera—modern pandemic disease of ancient lineage. Emerg Infect Dis. 2011;17:2099−2104. Available at: http://www.ncbi.nlm.nih.gov/pmc/articles/PMC3310593/ (accessed 16 August 2012).

32. Paneth N, Vinten-Johansen P, Brody H, Rip M. A rivalry of foulness: official and unofficial investigations of the London cholera epidemic of 1854. Am J Public Health. 1998;88:1545−1553. Available at: http://www.ncbi.nlm.nih.gov/pmc/articles/PMC1508470/pdf/amjph00022-0105.pdf (accessed 4 July 2016).

33. Piarroux R, Barrais R, Faucher B, Haus R, Piarroux M, Gaudart J, et al. Understanding the cholera epidemic, Haiti. Emerg Infect Dis. 2011;17(7):1161−1168. Available at: http://wwwnc.cdc.gov/eid/article/17/7/11-0059_article#r32 (accessed 26 June 2016).

34. Reuters Health News. U.N. remarks on Haiti cholera a "groundbreaking" step to justice, say lawyers, August 18, 2016. Available at: http://www.reuters.com/article/us-haiti-cholera-idUSKCN10T209 (accessed 13 November 2016).

35. Rosen G. A history of public health. Expanded edition. Baltimore, MD: The Johns Hopkins University Press, 1993.

36. Sabbe M, Berger N, Blommaert A, Ogunjimi B, Grammens B, Callens M, et al. Sustained low rotavirus activity and hospitalisation rates in the post-vaccination era in Belgium, 2007 to 2014. Euro Surveill. 2016;21(27):pii=30273. Available at: http://www.eurosurveillance.org/ViewArticle.aspx?ArticleId=22518 (accessed 8 July 2016).

37. Salvadori MI, Sontroop J, Garg AX, Moist LM, Suri RS, Clark WF. Factors that led to the Walkerton tragedy. Kidney Int Suppl. 2009;112:S33−S34. Available at: http://www.kidney-international.org/article/S0085-2538(15)53612-0/pdf (accessed 16 August 2016).

38. Schoenen D. Role of disinfection in suppressing the spread of pathogens with drinking water: possibilities and limitations. Water Res. 2002;36(15):3874−3888. Abstract available at: http://www.ncbi.nlm.nih.gov/pubmed/12369533 (accessed 29 June 2016).

39. Snow J. On the mode of transmission of cholera, 1855. Snow on cholera. New York: The Commonwealth Fund, 1936. Reprinted by UCLA Fielding School of Public Health 2001. Available at: http://www.ph.ucla.edu/epi/snow/snowbook2.html (accessed 4 July 2016).

40. Tappero JW, Tauxe RV. Lessons learned during public health response to cholera epidemic in Haiti and the Dominican Republic. Emerg Infect Dis. 2011;17(11):2087−2093. Available at: http://www.medscape.com/viewarticle/754871_7 (accessed 13 November 2016).

41. Tulchinsky TH, Burla E, Clayman M, Sadik C, Brown A, Goldberger S. Safety of community drinking-water and outbreaks of waterborne enteric disease outbreak: Israel, 1976−97. Bull World Health Organ. 2001;78:1466−1473. Abstract available at: http://www.ncbi.nlm.nih.gov/pmc/articles/PMC2560668/pdf/11196499.pdf (accessed 29 June 2016).

42. United Nations, Department of Economic and Social Affairs (UNDESA), International decade for action: water for life, 2005−2015, Available at: http://www.un.org/waterforlifedecade/scarcity.shtml (accessed 16 August 2016).

43. United Nations Development Programme. Water governance for poverty reduction, 2004. New York: United Nation, 2004. Available at: http://www.undp.org/content/dam/aplaws/publication/en/publications/environment-energy/www-ee-library/water-governance/water-governance-for-poverty-reduction/UNDP_Water%20Governance%20for%20Poverty%20Reduction.pdf (accessed 14 November 2016).

44. United Nations. The Millennium Development Goals report 2015. Available at: http://www.un.org/millenniumgoals/2015_MDG_Report/pdf/MDG%202015%20rev%20(July%201).pdf (accessed 28 June 2016).

45. United Nations. Report of the Special Rapporteur on extreme poverty and human rights. General Assembly, August, 2016. New York: United Nations, 2016. Available at: http://chrgj.org/wp-content/uploads/2016/08/G-A7140823.pdf (accessed 12 November 2016).

46. Vachon D. Father of modern epidemiology: John Snow. Los Angeles, CA: University of California, Los Angeles (UCLA), 2005. Available at: http://www.ph.ucla.edu/epi/snow/fatherofepidemiology.html (accessed 25 June 2016).

47. Vinten-Johansen P, Brody H, Paneth N, Rachman S, Rip M. Cholera, chloroform, and the science of medicine: a life of John Snow. New York: Oxford University Press, 2003. Book review in: NEJM. 2004;350:90−91. Available at: http://www.nejm.org/doi/full/10.1056/NEJM200401013500122 (accessed 26 June 2016).

48. World Health Organization. Cholera 2015. Wkly Epidemiol Rec. 2016;91(40):433−440. Available at: http://apps.who.int/iris/bitstream/10665/250142/1/WER9138.pdf (accessed 15 November 2016).

49. World Health Organization. Guidelines for drinking-water quality. 4th edition. Geneva, Switzerland: WHO, 2011. Available at: http://apps.who.int/iris/bitstream/10665/44584/1/9789241548151_eng.pdf http://www.who.int/water_sanitation_health/publications/2011/dwq_guidelines/en/ (accessed 29 June 2016).

50. World Health Organization. Epidemic focus cholera: the genie that escaped. Wkly Epidemiol Rec. 2016;91(23):297−304. Available at: http://www.who.int/wer/2016/wer9123.pdf?ua = 1 (accessed 4 July 2016).

51. World Health Organization. Diarrhoeal disease: fact sheet updated May 2017. Available at: http://www.who.int/mediacentre/factsheets/fs330/en/ (accessed 26 June 2016).

52. World Health Organization. Cholera: fact sheet, updated October 2016. Available at: http://www.who.int/mediacentre/factsheets/fs107/en/ (accessed 14 November 2016).

53. World Health Organization. Rotavirus, June 3, 2016. Available at: http://www.who.int/immunization/diseases/rotavirus/en/ (accessed 26 June 2016).

54. World Health Organization. Estimated rotavirus deaths for children under 5 years of age: 2013, 215,000. Available at: http://www.who.int/immunization/monitoring_surveillance/burden/estimates/rotavirus/en/ (accessed 26 June 2016).

55. World Health Organization. The Global Task Force on Cholera Control. Available at: http://www.who.int/cholera/task_force/en/ (accessed 21 August 2016).

56. World Health Organization. Number of reported cholera cases. Available at: http://www.who.int/gho/epidemic_diseases/cholera/cases_text/en/ (accessed 15 October 2016).

57. Yen C, Tate JE, Patel MM, Parahar UD. Rotavirus vaccines: update on global impact and future priorities. Hum Vaccin. 2011;7(12):1282−1290. Available at: https://www.ncbi.nlm.nih.gov/pmc/articles/PMC3338930/ (accessed 5 July 2016).

58. Zeng M, Mao XH, Li JX, Tong WD, Wang B, Zhang YJ, et al. Efficacy, safety, and immunogenicity of an oral recombinant *Helicobacter pylori* vaccine in children in China: a randomised, double-blind, placebo-controlled, phase 3 trial. Lancet. 2015;386 (10002):1457−1464. doi:10.1016/S0140-6736(15)60310-5. Abstract available at: http://www.thelancet.com/journals/lancet/article/PIIS0140-6736(15)60310-5/abstract (accessed 26 June 2016).

Chapter 6

Pasteur on Microbes and Infectious Diseases

ABSTRACT

Louis Pasteur became a dominant figure in European science as a young man demonstrating conclusive evidence of the Germ Theory and applying it for industrial use in the wine, beer, and milk industries inventing "pasteurization," a term in common use worldwide. Pasteur's brilliant laboratory work demonstrated that microbes were the cause of contamination. He developed key veterinary vaccines for anthrax and chicken cholera, and subsequently human vaccine against rabies. His proof of the concept of attenuation or weakening of live disease-causing organisms enabled development of antibodies to protect against later exposure to the natural organisms for many diseases by follow-up scientists. He strongly advocated the work of Semmelweis in Vienna promoting handwashing by obstetricians and boiling instruments for preventing high rates of mortality from childbirth fever and for hygiene in surgery as advocated by Lister in England. Pasteur is recognized as one of the all-time giants of science and his contributions to public health were essential for the evolution of modern society.

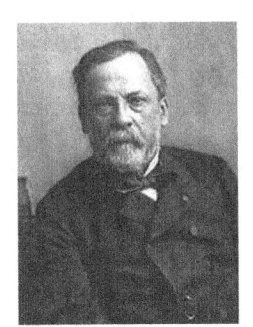

Louis Pasteur (1822–1895) is world renowned as the founder of microbiology for his proof of the principles microbial growth, of pasteurization and for vaccination. *Photo courtesy of Pasteur Foundation Museum, Paris at: http://www.pasteurfoundation.org/contact (photograph by Nadar).*

Case Studies in Public Health. DOI: http://dx.doi.org/10.1016/B978-0-12-804571-8.00008-1

Science knows no country, because knowledge belongs to humanity, and is the torch which illuminates the world.

Source: http://www.brainyquote.com/quotes/quotes/l/louispaste468082.html.

BACKGROUND

Louis Pasteur was born in 1822 in the village of Dole located in the mountainous Jura region of eastern France, the son of a poor tanner and former soldier in the Napoleonic wars. At age nine, he observed an outbreak of rabies spread by rabid dog bites in Arbois, France. Despite modest performance at school, he completed a bachelor's degree in science in 1842, and earned a master's degree in chemistry in 1845 at the *Ecole Normale Superieure* in Paris. He received his PhD in chemistry and physics in 1847 demonstrating that two forms of the crystals of tartaric acid reflect polarized light in opposite directions, establishing the field of stereochemistry.

At age 27, he was appointed professor of physics at Dijon University, and subsequently professor of chemistry at Strasbourg University (1849) and chairman of the department in 1852. He went on to become a world famous iconic figure for pioneering investigations leading to development of bacteriology and immunology with monumental advances for public health.

Between 1857 and 1863 Pasteur's experiments demonstrated that "spontaneous generation" of living matter (microorganisms) from nonliving matter did not occur, which despite continuing controversy, paved the way for the sciences of microbiology and later immunology. In 1862, Pasteur's findings were presented to the French Academy of Science winning the prize for the challenge to "to shed light on the concept of spontaneous generation" and the then widely accepted concept that spontaneous generation of life can arise from nonliving materials, such as mud or water.

Appointed Director of Scientific Studies at the *École Normale Supérieure*, a prestigious higher education institution in Paris, Pasteur continued his studies of fermentation demonstrating that it was a biological process of tiny organisms in both anaerobic and aerobic processes. He showed that the organisms could be eliminated from solutions by heating or by filtering (1857–63), greatly strengthening the foundations of proof of the Germ Theory of disease. This knowledge was later applied to prevention of spoilage of agricultural products, as well as to the health of animals and subsequently to human diseases. Appointed professor of chemistry at the Sorbonne (1867–89), and later founding director of the Pasteur Institute (1889–95) in Paris, with public funds to treat rabies, he surrounded himself with gifted researchers on a multidisciplinary basis—chemistry, physics, medicine, and others—which in essence became a center of research focused on unity of research and application. Pasteur became recognized as France's leading scientist and national hero, as well as an iconic international figure in science to the present time.

Pasteur was asked by representatives of the wine and beer industries to investigate spoilage in their products. Between 1863 and 1871, he demonstrated that spoilage of beer and wine occurred during storage or transportation causing heavy financial losses to these industries, which were of vital importance to the French economy. He identified yeasts crucial to the fermentation process and experimentally showed that heating of the beer and wine to 55°C protected them from souring by killing contaminant organisms. This process was later applied to destroying harmful organisms such as *Escherichia coli (E.coli)*, listeria, and tuberculosis (TB) transmission by contaminated milk interrupted by the process of pasteurization. This immediately resulted in great economic and health benefits to these French industries and people, and subsequently to the whole world since "pasteurization" became the global standard for food, and especially for milk production.

Recognition of this achievement brought a new challenge to Pasteur when he was approached to resolve a crisis in the silkworm industry, one of the principal industries in rural France. Aided by his capable wife Marie, he devoted five years to studying this problem and by 1870 he had devised methods to identify, isolate and destroy sick moths and silkworms, leading to elimination of the epidemic that had previously endangered the entire industry. He proved that independent mobile corpuscles, which caused the silk plague, were present in all the cyclical alterations of the insect's life. He showed that they could be readily detected only in the moth, suggesting the selection of healthy moths, which proved to be effective in restoring the silk industry of France.

In 1878, Pasteur was asked to investigate an economic problem associated with chicken cholera. He found that using an aged culture of weakened (attenuated) organisms did not cause the disease but helped the chicks develop immunity against fresh (virulent) strains of the bacterium. This resulted in protection of the chicks from subsequent inoculation with fresh virulent organisms. Realizing the importance of this crucial scientific finding, Pasteur went on to carry out a series of momentous investigations showing that exposure of a host to a weakened organism could cause the production of defenses or "immunity" to fully virulent cultures of the same organism. In other words, he discovered how to produce antibacterial vaccines.

Despite suffering a stroke in 1868 at age 46 with partial paralysis of his left side, Pasteur began to work on another agricultural economic problem of widespread prevalence of anthrax among sheep and other domestic animals in France. Anthrax was devastating to French agriculture, and widely thought to be due to toxic plants, biting insects, the sun, or hot weather as the cause of this highly fatal animal disease. Pasteur confirmed the work of his German rival Robert Koch who in 1876 (see Chapter 7) had identified and grown the anthrax bacillus organism and proved that it was the causative agent of clinical anthrax. Using trial-and-error experimentation, Pasteur showed that age-attenuated anthrax cultures were too weak to cause the disease in a host animal, but were sufficient to induce protective immunity in the inoculated host later exposed to highly pathogenic anthrax organisms.

Pasteur was by then both a national and international hero, besieged by stock raisers begging for his anthrax vaccine. However, problems in standardizing safety and efficacy in production of attenuated organisms for a vaccine kept the issue controversial for some years. The debate was especially heated between the two scientific giants of the field, the egotistical and quick-tempered Pasteur, and his bitter rival, Germany's leading bacteriologist, Robert Koch, the discoverer of the anthrax organism.

In 1881, Pasteur was invited to conduct a highly publicized field experiment as a clinical trial of his anthrax vaccine. Some 200 observers from agriculture, veterinary, military, and the general press attended the clinical trial events. The trial involved 60 sheep; 25 given the vaccine, 25 given no vaccine, and 10 given no vaccine and no infected material. After several weeks, the 25 vaccinated and the 25 nonvaccinated sheep were given injections of live culture of virulent anthrax bacteria. All the vaccinated test group given the culture survived; the control group of sheep without the vaccine died of anthrax; the 10 given nothing survived. The results of this experiment attracted national and international publicity and were accepted by the medical community as well. Earlier work by Toussaint, a French veterinary had produced a killed vaccine which in small studies had proven effective. Controversy arose in recent years as to whether Pasteur's vaccine was live attenuated or killed as per Toussaint's method (Smith, 2005). Despite recent controversy this clinical trial was seen as and remains a dramatic event in public health history inaugurating a laboratory vaccine prepared by attenuation of the living agent of the disease, a widely used method in the 20th century.

In 1882, at age 60, Pasteur took up the issue of rabies, then a universally fatal disease of persons and animals after being bitten by a rabid animal. He reasoned that the disease was transmitted by an as yet unidentified microorganism that attacked the central nervous system via the peripheral nerves. He devised methods of inoculating dogs with extracts of spinal cords of infected animals and methods of weakening the virus by attenuation. This was achieved by passing the virus from one animal to subsequent animals on 13 succeeding days to increase attenuation of the virus.

By 1885, when faced with the challenge of a nine-year-old boy, Joseph Meister, who had been severely bitten by a rabid dog, Pasteur was confident of the treatment efficacy of his two-week vaccination method. Attending physicians urged Pasteur, who was not a physician, to try the vaccine, which saved the boy's life by developing antibodies before the viral infection could overcome the child. Almost immediately, this method was confirmed when the Czar of Russia sent 19 peasants who had been bitten by rabid wolves to Paris for this new treatment. Pasteur's immunization saved 16 of them, thus gaining international scientific and worldwide popular acclaim. This led to launching of the famous Pasteur Institute in Paris. Originally the rabies vaccine was prepared from animal nerve tissue, later in eggs, and since around 1960 the rabies virus has been grown in human diploid cells.

Pasteur is recognized as the father of the study of microorganisms, and the triumph of the Germ Theory over its many hostile opponents and sincere doubters. He was acclaimed as founder of the rapidly growing fields of study of microorganisms and their role in human and animal disease. His many accomplishments of lasting importance to bacteriology, immunology, public health, veterinary public health, and the manufacturing industries include:

- proof of the germ theory and rejection of spontaneous generation of disease-causing organisms;
- pasteurization to destroy harmful bacteria that spoiled milk, beer, and wine, protecting countless humans from exposure to serious diseases caused by *E. coli*, listeria, TB, and other dangerous microorganisms;
- development of the concept of attenuation of pathogenic organisms to produce a vaccine for protection of animals from anthrax; and
- development of an effective rabies immunization vaccine to protect humans at risk for the disease by exposure to infected domestic or wild animals.

Pasteur died in 1895 before the first Nobel Prize awarded in 1901, but he was highly honored, including by the French Academy of Science, the Leeuwenhoek medal, microbiology's highest honor, in 1895, and the Grand Croix of the Legion of Honor, one of only 75 in all of France at that time. His name was known widely and made more famous by a 1936 Hollywood Academy Award winning motion picture starring Paul Muni.

The 20th century has seen a blossoming of the fields of microbiology, and immunology with great achievements in vaccinology (see Chapters 16 and 19). Pasteur's concept of live attenuated vaccines is alive and well including smallpox, oral poliomyelitis (Sabin) vaccines as well as many others such as measles, mumps, rubella, rotavirus, influenza (nasal), varicella, yellow fever, and influenza. At the same time important killed vaccines for both bacterial and viral organisms have been developed for many diseases including pertussis, hepatitis A, poliomyelitis (Salk), influenza, cholera, typhoid, and plague. A recombinant vaccine is developed with a part of the disease causing organism as an antigen (e.g., part of surface protein), such as hepatitis B vaccine now used worldwide.

In the early and middle 19th century, the causation of disease was hotly debated. The Miasma Theory, holding that disease was the result of environmental emanations or miasmas, went back to Greek and Roman medicine, and the Hippocrates treatise (*Air, Water, and Places*). Miasmists believed that disease was caused by infectious mists or noxious vapors emanating from filth in the towns and that the method of prevention of infectious diseases was to clean the streets of garbage, sewage, animal carcasses, and wastes that were features of urban living. This view did stimulate the growth of the "Sanitary Movement" and greatly improved adverse health conditions. The Miasma Theory had strong proponents well into the latter part of the 19th century.

The "Miasma Theory" was the predominant view of the medical profession and many leading figures of the day including Rudolph Virchow in Germany and Florence Nightingale in Britain. The scientific importance of Pasteur's work was in laying the scientific basis for the triumph of the "Germ Theory" of disease as opposed to the then more widely accepted theory of "spontaneous generation" by "putrefaction from within." His experiments showed that microbes would not occur spontaneously if not exposed to, and contaminated by microbial entry from outside air.

Pasteur's ideas were based on a small but growing acceptance of the contagion or germ theory, which gained ground, despite the lack of scientific proof. Isolation of lepers and quarantine of other infectious conditions during the Biblical and Middle Ages contributed to persistence of the contagion theories. In 1546, Girolamo Fracastoro published *De Contagione*, a treatise on microbiological organisms as the case of specific diseases. The Germ Theory was strengthened by the work of Anton van Leeuwenhoek, who developed the microscope in 1676, a watershed in the history of science. Van Leeuwenhoek's intense and well-documented research showed the existence of minute single-celled microorganisms. He was also the first microbiologist to study muscle fibers, bacteria, moulds, sperm, bees, and blood flow in capillaries. His work led to his recognition as a Fellow of the Royal Society of London in 1680. The germ theorists belief was strengthened that microbes, such as those described by van Leeuwenhoek, were the cause of diseases and were transmitted from person to person or by contact with sewage or contaminated water.

Major contributions to resolving this issue came from the epidemiologic studies of Peter Panum on measles, John Snow, and William Budd in the 1850s, proving waterborne transmission of cholera and typhoid. The classic study of a measles epidemic in the remote Faroe Islands by Peter Panum in 1846 clearly showed person-to-person transmission of this disease, its incubation period, and the lifelong natural immunity that previous exposure gives. The Germ Theory was gaining ground (see Chapters 3, 4, 6, and 7).

Pasteur succeeded in producing vaccines through attenuation, or weakening an organism's strength aging of the organism in the culture media, as for chicken cholera vaccine, or by passing it successively through animals, recovering it, and retransmitting it to other animals. He postulated that if a vaccine can prevent smallpox, then one can be created for all diseases. In collaboration with a physician, he inoculated chickens with chicken cholera germs taken from an old culture. The dispute continued, however, with "germ theorists," "miasmists," or "sanitationists" arguing with equal vehemence.

When Pasteur published the concept that the very microorganisms that contaminated the liquids also floated in the air, it was met with ridicule and rejected by the medical establishment. Pasteur's monumental proof of the Germ Theory, over time drastically influenced the way in which public health evolved. He proved the existence of germs and their role in disease causation, confirming previous discoveries and promoting new scientific development in microbiology and immunology.

While the Germ versus Miasma issue was debated until the end of the 19th century, the practical application of sanitary reform was promoted by both theories. Increasing attention to sewage, water safety, and removal of waste products by organized municipal activities was adopted in European and North American cities. The Sanitary Revolution proceeded while the debates raged and solid scientific proof of the Germ Theory accumulated, primarily in the 1880s. Fear of cholera stimulated New York City to establish a Board of Health in 1866. In the city of Hamburg, Germany, a Board of Health was established in 1892 only after a cholera epidemic attacked the city, while the neighboring town remained cholera-free because it had established a water-filtration plant.

The specific causation of disease (Germ Theory) has been a vital part of the development of public health. The bacteriologic revolution led by the work of Louis Pasteur and his rival Robert Koch provided enormous benefit to medicine and public health. But those who argued that disease is environmental in origin (the Miasma Theory) also contributed to public health because of their recognition of the importance of social or other environmental factors, such as poor sanitation and housing conditions or nutritional status, all of which increase susceptibility to specific agents of disease, or the severity of disease.

Pasteur moved on to experimental trials, demonstrating that microbes were the reason behind the decay of meat. He was confident that this concept explained the development of disease, arguing that the multiplication of germs leads to a specific disease. This was a very significant realization, as it meant that microbes not only affected beer, milk, and various foods, but also affected humans and animals as well.

His experiment illustrated the principles of attenuation of disease-causing organisms to produce immunity through vaccination. Pasteur showed that weakening the virulence of germs by passing them through successive generations of animals led to a vaccine which produced a defense and establishing protection to fight the stronger, more potent germs later presented in the fresh sample. In 1883, he produced a similar protective vaccine for swine erysipelas, and then in 1884–85 a vaccine for rabies.

Pasteur was a determined and brilliant scientific pioneer with many outstanding achievements that greatly contributed to the advance of medical sciences and public health. His demonstration of effective vaccines for anthrax and rabies showed many scientists and the general public that vaccination could protect against many infectious diseases with enormous benefit to human society.

His work showing heat kills microbes in wine, beer, and milk led to enormous gains in public health. Pasteurization of milk led to adoption of practices in food and preventing transmission of many infectious diseases such as TB, *E. coli*, brucellosis, diphtheria, and others, which had been causes of high morbidity and mortality especially among children and the elderly. The savings in costs of hospitalization and family and work disruption and greater control of environmental hazards were vital to the increasing urbanized societies developing as a result of the industrial revolution.

Because he was a chemist and nonphysician, Pasteur met with opposition to his work with human vaccines from the medical community despite successes and acceptance of the veterinary, agricultural, and business communities as well the general public to whom he became a folk hero. But his fame and scientific reputation promoted the idea that science is a crucial source of human progress and its international role of betterment of humanity.

Pasteur was powerfully influenced by the work of Ignaz Semmelweis, a Hungarian doctor in Vienna in the 1860s where maternal mortality rates were extremely high and doctors and medical students did the deliveries and autopsies. Semmelweis showed that washing hands of doctors (*accoucheurs*) and midwives between delivering babies especially after autopsies on maternal deaths reduced the high mortality rates of mothers from childbed fever. Pasteur vigorously promoted Semmelweis'ideas of hand hygiene for doctors convinced that microbes were transmitted on contaminated hands transferred the disease from the autopsies of the dead to living women in labor (see Chapter 4).

Pasteur, like Semmelweis, was seen as a challenge to the mainstream medical profession which worked to discredit the "Germ Theory" and attack its proponents. Pasteur's work proved that microbes existed and transmitted specific diseases advancing medicine and public health a giant step forward. Pasteur also inspired and benefitted from support of the highly prestigious British surgeon Joseph Lister who read Pasteur's work on microorganisms. Lister experimented using one of Pasteur's proposed techniques of using dressings soaked with carbolic acid. Lister thus adopted and promoted antiseptic practices in surgery, which reduced wound infections and deaths.

A 1936 Hollywood movie *The Life of Louis Pasteur* (starring Paul Muni who won an Oscar for his performance) portrayed Pasteur's life brilliantly. His struggles against medical dogma to establish proof of the microorganisms that cause diseases of animals and humans are dramatized in the movie and helped to ensure his fame in the popular culture of human progress. Semmelweis's life was also made into a documentary movie *That Mothers Might Live*.

CURRENT RELEVANCE

Anthrax is primarily a disease of domestic and wild herbivores caused by *Bacillus anthracis* from ingestion of spores in contaminated soil, plants, or water where animals have had anthrax in the past. Humans in contact with infected animals or their products, directly or indirectly can acquire the disease. Routine vaccination helps prevent outbreaks. Anthrax spores can be found in nature on all continents and when inhaled or ingested can cause disease in unvaccinated affected domestic or wild animals, and in people contaminated while working with affected animals exposed to the live organism, especially in developing countries such as Central and South America, sub-Saharan Africa, central and southwestern Asia, southern and Eastern Europe, and the Caribbean.

Annual vaccination of livestock is recommended in areas where animals have had anthrax in the past. Human disease has become rare in developed countries where veterinary services and animal immunization are well developed or where exposure occurs inadvertently or deliberately. Anthrax was used as a biological warfare weapon during World War I and developed further during the Cold War (1947 − 1991). In 2001 anthrax was used as a terrorist biological weapon and raised widespread public and governmental concern; and remains a major terrorist threat along with chemical weapons and many other forms of violence. Anthrax outbreaks still occur with incidents in the United States with exposure of CDC laboratory workers to live anthrax, and outbreaks of the disease in Canada, Bulgaria, Peru, China, Zimbabwe, and many other countries in the 21st century. Anthrax remains a global health problem among domestic and wild animals despite many new vaccines developed in the past century, as well as availability of veterinary antibiotics. Vaccines for humans were developed by the Soviet Union in the late 1930s and in the United States and United Kingdom in the 1950s. Recombinant vaccines in the 1960s are safer and approved by the US Food and Drug Administration (FDA). These were developed for protection of people who work with animals and their products but mainly for defense purposes especially for threats of terrorists.

Rabies continues to be a global public health issue. Although domestic animals are required to be vaccinated against rabies, the disease occurs in nature in wild animals with periodic transmission to humans directly or via unvaccinated cats, dogs, and other pets. Rabies still exists in bats, the most common source of human rabies infection in the United States. Skunks, raccoons, coyotes, foxes, and other mammals can also transmit the disease. Rabies vaccine is now made with killed rabies virus, and is given to people at high risk of rabies to protect them if they are exposed. It can also prevent the disease if given to a person after they have been exposed.

But the importance of Pasteur's opening the era of created vaccines goes far beyond these specific diseases. His work and support for the ideas of Semmelweis in handwashing in hospitals is a current issue in prevention of hospital acquired infections, and in the work of sterility in surgery pioneered by Lister. Pasteur's work has been one of the greatest scientific achievements with profound effects for public health through vaccine and food safety developments with human life and well-being vastly improved through control of communicable diseases including some which cause cancers and other chronic diseases.

Pasteur's legacy continues through the Pasteur Institute in 32 countries on five continents with major public health organizations and health ministries. The Paris Institute includes some nine research departments, 70 units in fundamental research fields resulting more than 500 researchers, and over 600 trainees. Box 6.1 shows the notable discoveries of the Pasteur Institute.

Among the Pasteur Institute staff are 10 Nobel Prize recipients since 1900 including:

- 1907: Charles Louis Alphonse Laveran for discovery of the malaria protozoa
- 1908: Ilya Metchnikoff for his work on cellular immunity
- 1919: Jules Bordet for discoveries related to immunity

BOX 6.1 Pasteur Foundation: Notable Discoveries

19th Century
- First vaccine against rabies (1885)
- Serotherapy treatments of diphtheria (1894)
- Identification of bubonic plague bacillus (1894)

20th Century
- Development of vaccines for diphtheria and tetanus (1920s)
- Vaccine against yellow fever (1920s)
- Discovery of the anti-infectious power of sulfa drugs (1960)
- First to isolate HIV, the virus that causes AIDS (1983)
- Development of the AIDS blood test (1984)
- Isolation of the second AIDs virus, HIV-2 (1985)
- Genetically engineered vaccine against hepatitis B (1989)
- First probe to detect listeria in food (1990)
- Rapid diagnostic tests for Helicobacter pylori bacterium (stomach ulcers) (1990)
- Rapid tests to detect multidrug-resistant tuberculosis (1993)

21st Century
- Vaccine against *Helicobacter pylori* (2000s)
- Early detection test for colon cancer (2000s)
- Identification of the role nicotine plays in sudden infant death syndrome (SIDS)
- Identification of new susceptibility genes for autism (2000s)
- First identification of the genes involved in deafness (2000s)

Courtesy, Pasteur Institute. Notable discoveries. Available at: http://www.pasteurfoundation.org/discovery/notable-discoveries (accessed 11 September 2017).

- 1928: Charles Jules Henri Nicolle for discoveries related to typhus
- 1957: Daniel Bovet for discoveries in chemical pharmacology elated to neuromuscular transmission in the autonomous nervous system
- 1965: François Jacob, André Lwoff, and Jacques Monod for genetic control of enzyme and virus synthesis
- 2008: Françoise Barré–Sinoussi and Luc Montagnier for their discovery of HIV

ETHICAL ISSUES

Pasteur was a brilliant scientific pioneer, with many outstanding achievements, who greatly contributed to the advance of medical sciences and public health with the belief that "Science belongs to no country; science belongs to humanity." He was talented in art since his boyhood with and in adult life friends with French and other artists. He believed art enriched his life and his science in the name of all humanity. He elevated the application of science. He is famously quoted as saying, "chance favors the prepared mind," and "do not let yourself be tainted with a barren skepticism," thus helping promote science for all of humanity.

He was dedicated to science to improve the world. His steadfast commitment to science and experimentation and his support of hospital hygiene was drawn from his ethical commitment to science in the service of humanity.

He faced opposition. The medical profession did not accept his work to disprove the Miasma Theory that spontaneous generation of disease was due to foul odors. Their opposition included his demonstration of effective anthrax and rabies vaccine, but finally late in his life recognized his momentous contributions to medicine and to humanity. This serves as a reminder for the ethics of scientific research to the present time. His work and scientists that followed have saved countless lives. The threat of biological warfare by terrorists or rogue state us anthrax, or other organisms, as a biological weapon.

Ethics in science were seriously compromised in the 20th century by the Eugenics movement descending into justification for forced sterilization and mass murder of mentally ill and handicapped children in Nazi Germany with full support of professional and scientific communities of Germany. This led to the Holocaust of European Jewry including, unethical pseudo-scientific experimentation. The postwar Nuremberg Trials and the Helsinki Declaration of ethical standards for scientific experimentation (see Chapter 13).

The corruption of science constitutes not only serious ethical travesty, but also potential for terrorist or rogue state catastrophic use of anthrax as a biological weapon for mass murder.

While Pasteur may not have foreseen such possibilities, he understood that developing the means of preventing serious infectious diseases was a vital task of the scientific community. He did not hesitate to undertake, successfully, to treat Russian peasants stricken with rabies exposure as a human and scientific responsibility when called upon to do so.

Science in the 21st century is moving rapidly into use of genetic methods to alter microorganisms to produce new, less costly and safer vaccines, as well as for therapy to prevent birth defects and improve the life of those born with defects such as cystic fibrosis. The science of the 21st century has enormous potential, as predicted by Pasteur, to improve the world as he dreamed of doing.

Pasteur also showed the importance of advocacy as part of the role of science and implicitly as an ethical responsibility of public health.

ECONOMIC ISSUES

Pasteur's achievements were seminal in the development of bacteriology and immunology, applying basic science to agricultural and industrial problems, such as the silkworm and beer and wine industries in the late 19th century France. One of the most significant contributions was the safe preservation of foods for human consumption through thermal methods such as pasteurization of milk, which has had enormous implications on the practice of food safety for control of preventable infections and the proper use of health facilities.

Pasteur developed the basis for experimental bacteriology and immunology with monumental successes of vaccination in the 20th century contributing to human betterment and economic growth. His scientific leadership increased the possibilities to prevent disease and speed treatment with huge implications for human longevity, productivity, healthcare costs, and the use of healthcare facilities and programs.

The 20th century has seen a dynamic period of development of microbiology and immunology leading directly to the saving of millions of lives. The advances based on the work of Pasteur, Koch, and many others created a revolution in population health. Pasteur's method of attenuation of live infectious organisms brought forth a host of vaccines used world-wide today including poliomyelitis (Sabin), measles, mumps, rubella, varicella, rotavirus, and many others. The method of developing vaccines based on inactivated organisms by heat or chemical processes has also been highly productive with examples of poliomyelitis (Salk), rabies, and hepatitis A virus vaccine. Subunit (conjugate) vaccines based on a portion of the cell wall to a protein with strong immunogenic properties has also come to the fore in vaccinology with the hepatitis B vaccine, influenza (injection), hemophilus influenza b, human papilloma virus (HPV), pertussis, pneumococcal pneumonia, meningitis now used world-wide.

CONCLUSION

Pasteur's work remains unfinished with long known and newly emerging infectious diseases still vitally important in public health alongside non-communicable diseases, some of which originate in infectious organisms. Rabies and anthrax are still public health challenges, and new knowledge is showing that infectious agents are causes of chronic disease such as cancer of the liver, cervix, and others.

Pasteur was a powerful advocate and developed the basis for the Germ Theory through his experimental bacteriology and immunology. He showed that reducing virulence of microorganisms could produce vaccines to prevent microorganisms from causing specific disease in the vaccinated person. This led to the monumental successes of vaccination in the 20th century, saving millions of lives. While there is still some controversy regarding the anthrax vaccine used in his famous sheep experiment, Pasteur demonstrated the efficacy of vaccination and inaugurated laboratory attenuated vaccine as the follow-up to smallpox vaccine. Many of the modern vaccines are based on live attenuated organisms, such as measles, mumps, rubella, and many others.

Pasteur trained and inspired a whole generation of pioneers in this field, making science and scientists popular heroes of the late 19th and early 20th centuries. He demonstrated beyond all reasonable doubt experimental methods and the benefits of science for the health and well-being of a nation and humanity as a whole. The *Institut Pasteur* established by Pasteur is recognized as the origin of microbiology, immunology, and molecular biology and with a global network of more than 30 Institutes.

Despite his contributions and those of his rivals and followers and societal acceptance of his ideas and benefits, tax-based funding for research and training of researchers remains a struggle with long delays in development of feasible applicable science, such as in vaccine development for microbial and parasitic diseases still costing millions of lives annually. This remains an important issue for forward-looking organizations, decision-makers, and donors when skepticism is widespread regarding the ethics and merits of science and the need to use tax-based public monies to promote such work.

Pasteur's name is part of not only science but of modern human culture. Despite opposition and even vilification he proved the scientific method of experimentation, the validity of the Germ Theory, and contributed to industrial, animal and human health, saving countless lives through food safety and vaccination. His contribution to society is recognized by public awareness of his name along with other giants of science such as those of Newton, Darwin, and Einstein.

RECOMMENDATIONS

1. Research in microbiology and vaccinology should be strongly supported by governments and donor organizations as essential to improve health protection globally.

2. Education systems (primary, secondary, and post secondary) should include history of public health and its innovators such as Pasteur as part of general civilization studies.
3. Medical educators and curricula should include consideration of alternative theories with evidence developed scientifically for causation, prevention and management of disease.
4. Infectious organisms causing chronic diseases should be aggressively researched along with environmental and nutritional causes.
5. Causes of disease of single micro-organisms, along with multiple risk factor causation, individual behavior and the societal causation of diseases should all be integral to education and research in health at all levels of academic awareness.

STUDENT REVIEW QUESTIONS

1. What was the controversy between the Germ and Miasma theories?
2. What was the influence of the prevention of childbed fever by Semmelweis in Vienna on Pasteur's search and proof of existence of disease-causing microbes?
3. What was the importance of Pasteur's experiment showing spoilage of fluids open to airborne contamination versus the same fluids protected against that contamination?
4. As a chemist how was his contribution to medicine and public health received by the medical profession and by posterity?
5. What was the importance of Pasteur's scientific investigations for agriculture and the wine, beer, silkworm and milk industries?
6. How did Pasteur's work save the French sheep industry from anthrax, a lethal disease for animals and human contacts?
7. What were Pasteur's contributions in development of experimental microbiological methods and the science of immunology?
8. Why is the term pasteurization known world-wide in multiple languages and a part of modern society and culture?
9. Explain live/attenuated, killed/inactivated, subunit/conjugate vaccines with examples.
10. Name and discuss "new" infectious diseases that do not have proven vaccines that have caused global public health threats in the 21st century.

RECOMMENDED READINGS

1. Brachman PS. Bioterrorism: an update with a focus on anthrax. Am J Epidemiol. 2002;155(11):981−987. Available at: https://academic.oup.com/aje/article/155/11/981/57382/Bioterrorism-An-Update-with-a-Focus-on-Anthra (accessed 6 September 2017).
2. British Broadcasting Corporation. Louis Pasteur: the man who led the fight against germs. Available at: http://www.bbc.co.uk/timelines/z9kj2hv#z3r7xnb (accessed 12 September 2017).

3. Centers for Disease Control and Prevention. Rabies vaccination information statement, June 13, 2014. Available at: http://www.cdc.gov/vaccines/hcp/vis/vis-statements/rabies. html (accessed 21 September 2017).

4. Centers for Disease Control and Prevention. A history of anthrax, last updated 15 August 2016. Available at: http://www.cdc.gov/anthrax/resources/history/index.html (accessed 21 September 2017).

5. College of Physicians of Philadelphia. The history of vaccines. Available at: http://www. historyofvaccines.org/content/timelines/pasteur (accessed 12 September 2017).

6. Encyclopedia Brittanica. Louis Pasteur: French chemist and microbiologist. Available at: http://www.britannica.com/biography/Louis-Pasteur (accessed 7 September 2017).

7. Friedman M, Friedland GW. Medicine's 10 greatest discoveries. New Haven, CT: Yale University Press, 1998.

8. Garrison FH. An introduction to the history of medicine, with medical chronology, suggestions for study and bibliographical data. 4th edition. Philadelphia, PA: WB Saunders, 1929reprinted 1966. Book digitized by Google from the library of Harvard University and uploaded to the Internet Archive at: https://archive.org/details/anintroductiont04garrgoog (accessed 7 September 2017).

9. Hammill HA. Puerperal fever from Hippocrates to Pasteur. Houston history of medicine lectures 9. Houston, TX: Texas Medical Center, 2012. Available at: http://digitalcommons. library.tmc.edu/homl/9 (accessed 20 September 2017).

10. Hansen B, Weisberg RE. Louis Pasteur's three artist compatriots-Henner, Pointelin, and Perraud: a story of friendship, science, and art in the 1870s and 1880s. J Med Biogr. 2017;25(1):18−27. doi:10.1177/0967772015575887. Abstract available at: https://www. ncbi.nlm.nih.gov/pubmed/26025839 (accessed 13 September 2017).

11. Hugh-Jones ME. Overview of anthrax. Merck MSD Veterinary Manual, 2016. Available at: http://www.msdvetmanual.com/generalized-conditions/anthrax/overview-of-anthrax (accessed 11 September 2017).

12. Institut Pasteur. Louis Pasteur. Available at: http://www.pasteur.fr/en/institut-pasteur/history/louis-pasteur (accessed 11 September 2017).

13. Lister J. On the antiseptic principle in the practice of surgery. BMJ. 1867;2(351):246−248. Available at: https://www.ncbi.nlm.nih.gov/pmc/articles/PMC2310614/pdf/brmedj05631-0002.pdf (accessed 11 September 2017).

14. Louis Pasteur (1822−1895). London: brought to life science museum. Available at: http:// www.sciencemuseum.org.uk/broughttolife/people/louispasteur.aspx (accessed 19 June 2017).

15. Louis Pasteur, United Kingdom: history learning site, updated 2012. Available at: http:// www.historylearningsite.co.uk/louis_pasteur.htm (accessed 19 June 2017).

16. Moorhead R. William Budd and typhoid fever. J Royal Soc Med. 2002;95(11):561−564. Available at: https://www.ncbi.nlm.nih.gov/pmc/articles/PMC1279260/pdf/0950561.pdf (accessed 13 September 2017).

17. Nobel Prize Organization. List of Nobel prizes and laureates: the Pasteur Institute. Available at: http://www.nobelprize.org/nobel_prizes/themes/medicine/jacob/ (accessed 25 September 2017).

18. Pasteur Brewing Articles. Louis Pasteur is dead: inspiring career of a great and modest man of science. *New York Times*, Monday, April 6, 2009. Available at: http://www.pasteur-brewing.com/articles/life-of-pasteur/louis-pasteur-is-dead.html (accessed 7 September 2017).

19. Pasteur Foundation. Notable discoveries. Available at: http://pasteurfoundation.redfinsolutions.net/discovery/notable-discoveries (accessed 25 September 2017).

20. Rosen G. A history of public health, paperback revised. Expanded edition. Baltimore, MA: Johns Hopkins University Press, 1993.

21. Science Museum. Joseph Lister (1827–1912). Available at: http://www.sciencemuseum. org.uk/broughttolife/people/josephlister.aspx (accessed 12 September 2017).

22. Schlipköter U, Flahault A. Communicable diseases: achievements and challenges for public health. Public Health Rev. 2010;32:90–119. Available at: https://www.biomedcentral.com/ search?query=flahault+&searchType=publisherSearch (accessed 12 September 2017).

23. Semmelweis I. The etiology, concept, and prophylaxis of childbed fever. In: Buck C, Llopis A, Najera E, Terris M, editors. The challenge of epidemiology: issues and selected readings. Washington, DC: World Health Organization, 198846–59. Available at: http:// graphics8.nytimes.com/images/blogs/freakonomics/pdf/the%20etiology,%20concept%20and %20prophylaxis%20of%20childbed%20fever.pdf (accessed 29 September 201715).

24. Stone SP. Hand hygiene—the case for evidence-based education. J R Soc Med. 2001;94 (6):278–281. Available at: http://www.ncbi.nlm.nih.gov/pmc/articles/PMC1281522/ (accessed 21 September 2017).

25. Smith KA. Wanted, an anthrax vaccine: dead or alive? Med Immunol. 2005;4:5. doi:10.1186/1476-9433-4-5. Available at: https://www.ncbi.nlm.nih.gov/pmc/articles/ PMC1087873/pdf/1476-9433-4-5.pdf (accessed 11 September 2017).

26. TCM Movie Database. The story of Louis Pasteur. This 1936 classic Warner Brothers movie starred Paul Muni, who was awarded an Academy Award for Best Actor, while writers Collings and Gibney won for Best Screenplay and Best Story. Available at: http:// www.imdb.com/title/tt0028313/ (accessed 10 August 2017).

27. That Mothers Might Live. USA 1938. MGM (Director: Fred Zinnemann) won the Academy Award Oscar for the best short film. Available at: http://www.tcm.com/this-month/article.html?isPreview=&id=142631%7C143139&name=Fred-Zinnemann-Shorts; http://www.imdb.com/title/tt0030855/ (accessed 29 September 2017).

28. Tulchinsky TH, Varavikova EA. The new public health. 3rd edition. Amsterdam: Elsevier/ Academic Press, 2014. Chapter 1.

29. Weisberg RE, Hansen B. Collaboration of art and science in Albert Edelfelt's portrait of Louis Pasteur: the making of an enduring medical icon. Bull Hist Med. 2015;89(1):59–91. Avaialble at: https://www.ncbi.nlm.nih.gov/pubmed/25913463 (accessed 13 September 2017).

30. World Health Organization. Anthrax in humans and animals. In cooperation with the Food and Agriculture Organization and the World Organization for Animal Health. fourth edition. Geneva: World Health Organization, 2008. Available at: http://www.who.int/csr/ resources/publications/anthrax_web.pdf (accessed 4 September 2017).

31. World Health Organization. WHO expert consultation on rabies. Second report, 2013. Available at: http://apps.who.int/iris/bitstream/10665/85346/1/9789240690943_eng.pdf? ua=1 (accessed 6 September 2017)ADD REFWorld Health Organization. Emergency preparedness and response: Anthrax. Available at: http://www.who.int/csr/disease/Anthrax/en/ (accessed 4 September 2017).

32. World Health Organization. Emergency preparedness and response: Anthrax. Available at: http://www.who.int/csr/disease/Anthrax/en/ (accessed 4 September 2017).

33. World Health Organization. Rabies: a neglected zoonotic disease, 2014. Available at: http://www.who.int/rabies/about/en/ (accessed 6 September 2017).

34. World Health Organization. Neglected tropical diseases: WHO expert consultation on rabies re-evaluates the burden and methods of treatment. Available at: http://www.who.int/ neglected_diseases/support_to_rabies_elimination_2013/en/ (accessed 6 September 2017).

Chapter 7

Robert Koch and Paul Ehrlich: Criteria of Causation of Disease and Chemotherapy as "Magic Bullets"

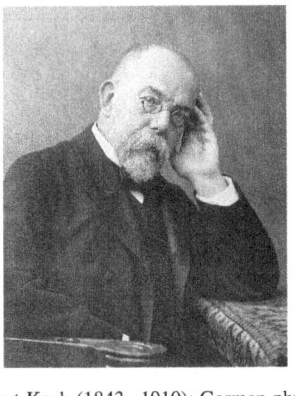

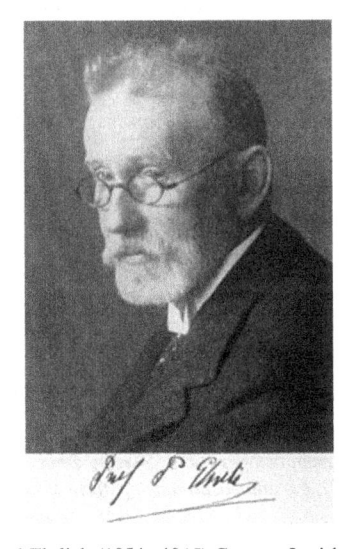

Robert Koch (1843–1910); German physician and a key founder of bacteriology and microbiology; discovered the organism of anthrax in 1876, of tuberculosis in 1882, and cholera in 1883; formulated Koch's postulates of disease causation; awarded the 1905 Nobel Prize in Physiology for Medicine. *Source: https://commons.wikimedia.org/wiki/Robert_Koch.*

Paul Ehrlich (1854 –1915) German-Jewish physician and scientist; pioneer in hematology, immunology, and antimicrobial chemotherapy; awarded Noble Prize in 1908 with Ilya Mechnikov for their work on immunity; discoverer of Salvarsan in 1909, the first effective treatment for syphilis, dubbed "the Magic Bullet". *Wikimedia Commons Available at: https://upload.wikimedia.org/wikipedia/commons/thumb/0/05/Paul_Ehrlich_1915.jpg/800px-Paul_Ehrlich_1915.jpg (accessed 12 November 2017).*

Case Studies in Public Health. DOI: http://dx.doi.org/10.1016/B978-0-12-804571-8.00016-0

ABSTRACT

The biological foundations of infectious disease were developed in the 19th century, building on the work of Louis Pasteur. The methodologies of microbiology were greatly advanced by Robert Koch, in Germany, discoverer of tuberculosis , anthrax and cholera organisms and establishing criteria of proof for the "Germ Theory" causation of disease by microbial agents. Paul Ehrlich later developed the "magic bullet" of Salvarsan chemotherapy for treating syphilis. The pioneering work and findings of Koch and Ehrlich were recognized by Nobel Prizes, awarded to Koch in 1905 and to Ehrlich in 1908, respectively. These scientific pioneers provided the foundation for development of microbiology and immunology as well as the search for magic bullets to cure not only infectious diseases but others as well such as cancers. Current research is working to develop specific treatments based on genetic studies of the patient for "personalized magic bullets" now being developed as "precision medicine" to treat cancer and improve survival. The biomedical model is still a cornerstone of public health and overlaps with health protection and health promotion aspects as well as priority setting and good management of limited health resources.

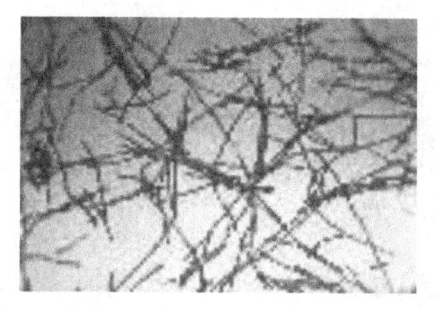

Photomicrograph of Bacillus anthracis bacteria using Gram's stain technique; ultrastructural morphology of numerous rod-shaped, Bacillus anthracis bacteria, many of which had formed long chain configurations. *Source: Centers for Disease Control and Prevention. Anthrax Photos ID# 2226 Available at:https://phil.cdc.gov/ImageIDSearch.aspx?key = true.*

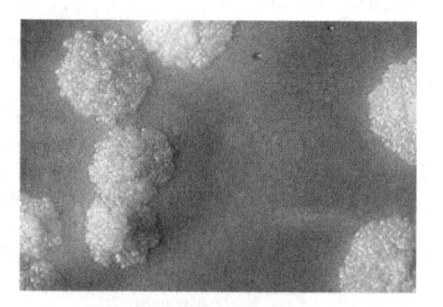

Close-up of a Mycobacterium tuberculosis culture revealing this organism's colonial morphology. *Source: Centers for Disease Control and Prevention, Public Health Image Library (PHIL), ID no. #4428 Available at: https://phil.cdc.gov/Details.aspx?pid = 4428 (accessed 14 November 2017).*

BACKGROUND

Robert Koch

Robert Koch (1843–1910) was born in Clausthal, Germany, in the Upper Harz Mountains of Germany, the son of a mining engineer. He was an outstanding student at the local high school and showed an interest in biology. In 1862 Koch studied medicine at the University of Göttingen, Germany, where Professor, Jacob Henle, influenced him of his view, published in 1840, that infectious diseases were caused by living micro-organisms. Graduating in 1866, Koch absorbed the concept that infectious diseases were caused by specific living organisms or microbes as advanced by Louis Pasteur. Following graduation, he served as a volunteer military surgeon in the Franco-Prussian war of 1870–72. He then became a rural family physician and district medical officer working to pioneer in the field of bacteriology. His innovations in techniques of experimentation advanced the work of Pasteur, Cohn, Ehrlich, and others to open important basic scientific aspects of public health and going on to be widely recognized as "a founding father of modern bacteriology."

Working independently with very limited facilities Koch demonstrated in 1876 recovery of anthrax from dead animals, isolating the organism, growing it in culture media he developed, and then transmitting the live bacteria to mice. He grew the organism in his own improvised culture media and developed staining techniques for visual microscopic identification of the bacteria. He used the blood of cattle that died of anthrax and inoculated successive generations of mice which died of anthrax, then retrieved, grew, and identified the anthrax organism. The mice inoculated with blood of healthy cattle did not develop the disease. Thus he proved the transmission of specific disease by specific microorganisms and established criteria for causation of disease.

In 1878 Koch was appointed assistant at the Berlin Medical Clinic with facilities to work with dyes for staining of tissues. He showed how dyes could be classified as basic, acid, or neutral, and his work on the staining of granules in blood cells laid the foundations of future work on hematology and the staining of tissues.

Cholera was a recurring epidemic in many cities of Europe in the mid-19th century. Following years of study of recurrent cholera epidemics in London, John Snow documented the 1854 cholera epidemic in London demonstrating higher rates of cholera among users of the Broad Street pump in Soho and cessation of the epidemic following removal of the pump handle. Separating drinking water from sewage-contaminated water was effectively demonstrated by stopping cholera. Removing the pump handle was quickly followed by the cholera epidemic subsiding (see Chapter 5).

In 1882, as an advisor with the Imperial Department of Health in Berlin, Koch undertook research on tuberculosis. Tuberculosis was then generally considered to be an inherited disease, but Koch was able to culture the tubercle bacillus and demonstrate that it was an infectious disease.

Koch was appointed head of the German Cholera Commission to investigate continuing epidemics in Egypt and India in 1883, isolating and identifying *Vibrio cholerae*. He demonstrated the efficacy of filtrating water in order to prevent of transmission of enteric diseases including cholera. His methods of investigation in isolating the organism and demonstrating onward transmission of the disease led to the formulation of criteria of causation of diseases. In 1883, Koch adapted the clinician-pathologist Jacob Henle's postulates on causation of disease. He established criteria for attribution of causation of a disease to a particular organism or agent. These were fundamental to establishing the science of bacteriology and the relationship of microorganisms to disease causation.

The Koch–Henle postulates in their pure form were too rigid, and would limit identification of the causes of many diseases. But they were important to establish the Germ Theory and the scientific basis of bacteriology, competing with many other theories of disease that were still widespread in the late 19th century, specifically the Miasma Theory, which was predominant in medical thinking, and the sociopolitical theory of Rudolph Virchow.

The Miasma Theory contributed to the Sanitary Movement goal of reducing exposure to sewage. The societal factor in disease prevalence and prevention foretold by Virchow and others in the mid-19th century became part of public health practice in the 20th century when universal education and rising standards of living in industrial nations led to improved nutrition, and municipal sanitation of community water supplies and sewage drainage. As chronic diseases became the major health issues, a more complex approach than the single causation biomedical model became vital. These criteria of causation of noncommunicable diseases have evolved to take into account multiple risk factors as opposed to the single causative concept of the "Germ Theory" and its pioneers including Koch and his successors.

The Koch–Henle postulates needed adaptation with more complex postulates to include other causes of infection and for noninfectious disease-causing agents such as smoking, nutrition, cholesterol, hypertension, genetics, exercise, and other risk factors in causation of many noncommunicable diseases that began to dominate epidemiology and public health practice by the middle of the 20th century. In the 21st century, the predominant causes of disease and death are noncommunicable diseases associated with lifestyle, genetics, health care, poverty, injury, and social conditions (see Chapter 21), but infectious diseases emerge as new challenges and old diseases reemerge as renewed public health issues.

Robert Koch discovered the anthrax bacillus and investigated the anthrax disease cycle in 1876. He discovered the bacteria of tuberculosis in 1882 and cholera in 1883. Robert Koch's contributions were acknowledged with the Nobel Prize for Medicine in 1905. Medicine and epidemiology still rely on the Koch principles of affirming the causes of infectious diseases. Koch died in 1910 at age 66. He advanced the field of medical bacteriology opening a "golden age" of scientific work with profound influence on public health and human civilization.

Paul Ehrlich and "Magic Bullets"

Paul Ehrlich (1854–1910) was born to a Jewish family in Strehlen in Upper Silesia, Germany. He was educated at the Gymnasium at Breslau and subsequently at the universities of Breslau, Strasburg, Freiburg, and Leipzig. He graduated as a doctor of medicine in 1878 with a dissertation on the theory and practice of staining animal tissues.

Ehrlich was appointed in 1878 to the Berlin Medical Clinic as an assistant with access to laboratory facilities, where he continued his work with dyes for staining of tissues. He classified dyes as basic, acidic, or neutral to work on staining microorganisms and blood cells laying the foundation of future work on hematology and the pathologic staining of tissues. In 1882 Ehrlich published his method of staining the tubercle bacillus, newly discovered by Robert Koch, and his methods with later modifications are still used today. His method also led to the Gram method of staining and classifying bacteria used by modern bacteriologists.

In 1887 Ehrlich became an unpaid instructor based on his thesis and later appointed Associate Professor in the Faculty of Medicine at the University of Berlin and Senior House Physician at the Charité Hospital in Berlin. In 1890 he was appointed assistant to Robert Koch, Director of the Institute for Infectious Diseases, and began his reputation for immunological studies. At the end of 1896 he was appointed director of a newly established Institute for the control of therapeutic sera in Berlin. His work on immunology focused on the chemical toxin-antitoxin necessary to establish standards of measuring antitoxin content. He used antidiphtheritic serum to standardize units of serum, providing a method for future standardization of sera and the theory of immunity. In 1897 Ehrlich was appointed Public Health Officer in Frankfurt and in 1899 Director of the new Royal Institute of Experimental Therapy established at Frankfurt. He applied his ideas from his doctorate thesis to chemotherapy, studying the chemical constitution of drugs in relation to their affinity for the disease-causing organism.

Ehrlich and his team worked to find chemical substances with special affinities for pathogenic bacterial organisms. They sought what he called "magic bullets" or chemicals that would attach directly to the organisms at which they were aimed and destroy them. Ehrlich and his assistants tested hundreds of selected chemical substances. Among other subjects, they sought chemicals for treatment of trypanosomiasis and other protozoal diseases.

Ehrlich decided to seek a drug (the "Magic Bullet") that would be effective against the *Treponema pallidum* bacteria causing syphilis, then a common and serious disease and a major public health threat in Europe. His team conducted hundreds of experiments eventually showing that the 606th compound tested, called Salvarsan, was found active in rabbits and then in humans repeatedly proving its efficacy against syphilis. The first clinical trial of 50 patients with late-stage syphilis using Salvarsan conducted in 1909 ended with an impressive positive outcome. However, as Salvarsan became more widely used, side effects were frequently reported, and Ehrlich was highly criticized. He launched further studies of chemical modification of Salvarsan to produce a water-soluble analogue that was stable and retained its high therapeutic activity. After another 300 derivatives of Salvarsan were tested, in 1912 Neosalvarsan (compound 914) was shown to be safe, with curative effects but more easily manufactured and administered. There was much opposition in the medical community until Salvarsan or Neosalvarsan were proven based on practical application and were accepted for treatment of human syphilis. Wide use of Neosalvarsan led to a decline of syphilis as a public health problem by the 1920s, and syphilis continued to decline as effective sulfa drugs replaced arsenicals in the 1930s and antibiotics such as penicillin when they became available in the 1940s.

Ehrlich became famous as one of the key founders of chemotherapy and experimental work on immune therapies for cancers. He had a "combination of intuition and deduction that marked him as a genius," and became recognized as the "father of hematology, a revolutionary immunologist, and the creator of the field of chemotherapy.

CURRENT RELEVANCE

The Koch–Henle postulates on microorganisms as the cause of disease provided a model for proof of causation of infectious diseases. The postulates included:

1. The organism (agent) must be shown to be present in every case of the disease by isolation in pure culture.
2. The agent should not be found in cases of any other disease.
3. Once isolated, the agent should be grown in a series of cultures, and then must be capable of reproducing the disease in experimental animals.
4. The agent must then be recovered from the disease produced in experimental animals.

The Koch–Henle postulates serve as guidelines that in their pure form are important to developing the field of infectious disease-related sciences, dispelling the many other theories of disease that were widespread in the late 19th century. These postulates, developed based on experience with anthrax and tuberculosis, served to provide a rational scientific framework for evidence of causation in the study of infectious diseases for their prevention and treatment. Koch realized these criteria were not fulfilled in the case of cholera where the organism may be present in humans without causing the disease, and this was later seen as even more of a problem for viral diseases. Later, they were seen as too rigid, limiting identification of the multiple factors that together cause many diseases especially noncommunicable diseases. But even for infectious diseases there are multiple factors as well as the "causative organisms" such as poverty, poor nutrition, lack of access to health care, and other social inequalities not only in the incidence of disease but even more so in the severity of an infectious disease.

Later definitions of association and causation required more complex criteria especially in regard to noncommunicable diseases with multiple risk factors. The criteria of evidence of association/causation as proposed by Bradford Hill in the 1950s for smoking and lung cancer were based on evidence of strength of association; consistency; specificity; temporality; biological gradient; plausibility; coherence, experiment, and analogy; and even more so on complex social and environmental factors in origins of disease in populations.

However, the Koch–Henle postulates continue to be basic tools for providing evidence of causation of disease as in the identification of *Helicobacter pylori* as the major cause of chronic peptic ulcer disease in the early 1980s by Robin Warren and Barry Marshall (see Chapter 22). The finding of the causative bacteria *H. pylori* led to simple and inexpensive diagnostic and curative treatment. Since the early 1980s this development has resulted in emptying surgical wards of gastrectomy and vagotomy cases as well as medical wards of many patients suffering from peptic ulcers. *Helicobacter pylori* is considered to be present in half the world's population and a cause of gastric cancer. As sanitation and living conditions improved in the 20th century, gastric cancer incidence gradually declined in many countries. The simple diagnosis for *H. pylori*, which produces urease, a chemical that protects the organism from the acidity of the stomach and that is detectible by breath tests has opened a whole new field of medical screening diagnostics.

Ehrlich's achievement over a century ago of developing arsenic-based drugs to treat syphilis with Salvarsan initiated effective treatment for an important clinical and public health issue. Within 5 years, the incidence of syphilis in several European countries decreased by 50 percent. Ehrlich was awarded the Nobel Prize in Physiology of Medicine in 1908. In subsequent decades new antibacterial drugs were discovered: sulfa (Gerhard Domagk), penicillin (Sir Alexander Fleming, curative against syphilis and other bacterial infections), streptomycin (Selman Waksman, the first antibiotic effective against tuberculosis), and many new generations of antibiotics and later antiviral drugs that have revolutionized medicine. But clinical antibiotic overuse and widespread use of antibiotics routinely in animal husbandry and spread of infections in health care facilities have led to resistant organisms with potential loss of successful control of many infectious diseases until new generations or parallel methods are developed. This issue is now apparent for many infectious diseases including tuberculosis, malaria, and syphilis.

ETHICAL ISSUES

The ethical issue that drove Ehrlich, was to advance science and finding a cure for syphilis, a devastating and common, but socially reprehensible, disease in his time. The decline in syphilis infection by the end of the 20th century was related to effects on behaviors associated with the AIDS epidemic and raised hopes that the disease could be eradicated in the United States with public health efforts focused on high-incidence population groups. But the reality of return of syphilis disease led the US CDC to terminate the program for near-term eradication of syphilis as rates of new cases have increased since 2000 and focus has again shifted to prevention of maternal-infant transmission. Despite the breakthroughs of Ehrlich and his co-workers over a century ago, syphilis is returning as a major public health challenge and control will require new tools and more emphasis on targeted screening, health promotion, and hope for a new breakthrough in patient-specific "precision medicine" management tools. At the same time advances in medicine and medical technology are improving early diagnosis by prevention, screening and early treatment of life-threatening diseases such as cervix, colorectal, and lung cancers.

The search for "Magic Bullets" such as anti-viral agents and increasingly resistant dangerous bacterial organisms for important infectious diseases and new treatments is now growing in genetic determinations of cancers in individual patients and is leading to anticancer-targeted medications specific to the genetic makeup of the malignancy in a patient. New screening tests for early diagnosis of cancer of the lung and other malignancies can facilitate early therapy with better life expectancy and quality.

The biomedical scientific methods pioneered by Koch, Ehrlich, and their many followers were the foundation of one of the most dynamic and productive aspects of even the social model public health in the context of health protection including sanitation, food and water safety, work and road safety, and many others. In addition for the 30 years since the Ottawa Charter, health promotion has become an increasingly crucial element of public health in risk factors for noncommunicable diseases such as cancer and cardiovascular diseases by promoting healthy lifestyle and reduction of risk factors such as smoking. Health promotion also plays a vital role in control or elimination of infectious diseases where human behavior is critical in acceptance of effective vaccines and in safe-sex behavior. Comprehensive and community-oriented elements of public health, recognizing and addressing social inequalities, have major potential for reducing health inequities between countries as well as with high-, medium-, and low-income countries.

ECONOMIC ISSUES

The dominance of infectious diseases in the health burden in the 19th century and early 20th century was a major factor in low life expectancy and economic hardship for most of the populations of even the most advanced countries. The research and innovations pioneered by Pasteur and followers with crucial steps forward by Koch and Ehrlich provided the conceptual and methodological basis for reducing the heavy social and economic burden of infectious disease. The results provided crucial tools for population health advances in the 20th century (see Chapter 21).

Elimination and/or eradication of infectious and even some noncommunicable conditions could be achieved based on the work of these pioneering microbiologists and their successors. Smallpox was eradicated by 1977 some 180 years after discovery of vaccination. Polio eradication is on the horizon with a target by 2020. Measles, thought to have been eliminated in the Americas and Europe with potential for eradication by 2025, returned with epidemics in Europe that spread to the United States and other parts of the world (see Chapter 3). Important tropical diseases are being controlled and locally eliminated with hopes of gradual elimination, including tropical diseases such as onchocerciasis and dracunculiasis.

Simultaneously, advances in molecular biology and genetic research have expedited cancer drug development with an emphasis on "personalized and tailored drugs" that precisely target the specific molecular defects of a cancer patient. This is based on the intellectual and scientific foundations of Paul Ehrlich, the founder of chemotherapy over 100 years ago. His work included three creative periods: he developed histological staining; he carried out ground-breaking work in immunology; he invented chemotherapy. His vision and success in creating the "Magic Bullet" of a successful chemotherapy for syphilis, now enriched by enormous progress in molecular biology and genetics, provide new tools and inspiration for new generations of scientists to develop individualized precision cancer treatments or new Magic Bullets molecular cancer therapeutics.

CONCLUSION

Koch and Ehrlich followed the work of Pasteur, Lister, and others who opened the fields of application of the Germ Theory to scientific bacteriology and immunology later becoming fundamental aspects of medicine and public health. Establishing accepted criteria for proof of causation helped scientists and epidemiologists everywhere to focus on research design and acceptable proof of their investigations.

Diseases once thought to be controlled have come back because of failures in achieving complete "herd immunity" of vaccines such as measles, or the development of resistance in organisms to current antibiotics largely due to overuse of antibiotics in animal husbandry and in medical practice, so that resistant strains of antibiotics develop faster than new antibiotics are developed. Antimicrobial resistance is a global challenge to successful management of infectious diseases, and is undermining many other advances in health and medicine. In 2015 the World Health Assembly endorsed a global action plan to tackle antimicrobial resistance—including antibiotic resistance, the most urgent drug resistance trend. The plan focuses on continuity of surveillance and prevention and successful treatment of infectious diseases with effective and safe methods, promoting research for new methods and high-quality antibiotics used responsibly. Complacency and reckless human behavior promote recurrence of diseases transferred by unsafe sex such as syphilis or HIV, or by parental refusal of immunizations for their children.

The Pasteur—Koch—Ehrlich biomedical model that contributed so much to development of public health is also greatly augmented by the social model of Virchow and others in the 19th century now highlighting social inequalities in health in the 21st century. The health-promotion model of reducing risk factors for chronic disease by regulatory and health promotion and political socioeconomic measures to address diseases and the sociopolitical contexts has become a strong element of a New Public Health, addressing the biomedical, socio economic, health promotion and social inequities still prevalent in health in some degree in all countries.

The work of these pioneers and their followers has resulted in preventing millions of deaths worldwide, and in reductions in the need for costly treatment interventions such as hospitalization. New methods of precise targeting the pathogens and limiting indiscriminate use of antimicrobials are essential to prevent emergence of resistance mechanisms. Research on antibiotic resistance and dissemination is vital to early warning and preventive measures to preserve efficacy of antimicrobials and chemotherapy.

Ehrlich's success in developing his "Magic Bullet" concept for synthesis of antibacterials introduced concepts such as chemoreceptors and chemotherapy, linking the chemical structure of compounds to their pharmacological activity. This established the transition from experimental pharmacology to therapeutic pharmacology. Current research is showing promising achievements to provide new "Magic Bullet" of greater precision and wider coverage for early diagnosis, prevention, and treatment of new and reemerging infectious diseases, cancers, genetic disorders, noncommunicable diseases, and other threats to human health.

Epidemiology and public health practice move forward incorporating programs to address social determinants which are major factors in health in countries at all levels of development. The double burden of infectious and noncommunicable disease, and their overlap, provides a new challenge for a comprehensive linkage of these themes. Emerging economies are facing major health threats of chronic diseases that will demand more national and external financial and policy assistance. Ethical policies in health will require greater self-reliance and adoption of health promotion and disease prevention strategies. The Koch and Ehrlich pioneering is still vitally relevant but in the context of a wider world view for health in the 21st century.

RECOMMENDATIONS

1. Research priorities should place major emphasis on immunology related to infectious and chronic diseases and their interaction such as has successfully occurred with human papilloma virus and cervical cancer with a successful vaccine already reducing this important cancer in low-income countries particularly.
2. Policy development in population health should promote translation of current scientific and sociological knowledge to improve population health with attention to reducing inequalities in health status in and between countries.
3. Promotion of biomedical and socio-political public health in educational programs to foster understanding and recruitment of talented candidates to engage in professional careers in related fields.
4. Policy forums should include multidisciplinary participation to promote transparency and commonality of purpose in addressing population health issues.
5. Epidemiological/public health studies should recognize that poverty-related health inequalities are causal factors in major health threats for both infectious and noncommunicable diseases, seeking methodologies to address social determinants of health in poverty populations in high-, medium- and particularly in low-income countries.

STUDENT REVIEW QUESTIONS

1. How do the germ theory and the miasma theory interact in applied public health?
2. How do the social medicine theories of Virchow in the 19th century and Marmot in the 21st century interact with regard to control of infectious diseases?
3. Why was the definition of proof of causation important for public health?

4. How do the Koch postulates apply to chronic diseases?

5. How do the Koch postulates apply to infections causing chronic disease? Give examples.

6. What is a "Magic Bullet" in health? Give examples.

7. What applications in medicine and public health followed the basic idea that Ehrlich pioneered?

8. Why do diseases that are preventable or treatable come back to haunt us?

9. How does the idea of "Magic Bullet" affect new research with genetic aspects of cancer?

10. What "Magic Bullet" in health promotion can contribute to infectious disease control?

RECOMMENDED READINGS

1. Aminov RI. A brief history of the antibiotic era: lessons learned and challenges for the future. Front Microbiol. 2010;1:134. Available at: https://www.ncbi.nlm.nih.gov/pmc/articles/PMC3109405/ (accessed 23 July 2017).

2. Bosch F, Rosich L. The contributions of Paul Ehrlich to pharmacology: a tribute on the occasion of the centenary of his Nobel Prize. Pharmacology. 2008;82(3):171–179. doi:10.1159/000149583. Available at: http://www.ncbi.nlm.nih.gov/pmc/articles/PMC2790789/ (accessed 10 July 2017).

3. Blevins SM, Bronze S. Robert Koch and the "golden age" of bacteriology. Int J Inf Dis. 2010;14(9):e744–e751. Available at: http://www.sciencedirect.com/science/article/pii/S1201971210023143 (accessed 10 July 2017).

4. Clement ME, Hicks CB. Syphilis on the rise: what went wrong? JAMA. 2016;315 (21):2281–2283. doi:10.1001/jama.2016.7073. Available at: https://jama.jamanetwork.com/article.aspx?articleid = 2526614 (accessed 12 June 2017).

5. Centers for Disease Control and Prevention. Cholera: *Vibrio cholerae* infection, 2014. Available at: http://www.sciencedirect.com/science/article/pii/S1201971210023143t: http://www.cdc.gov/cholera/index.html (accessed 2 July 2017).

6. Centers for Disease Control and Prevention. Sexually transmitted diseases: CDC factsheet (detailed), May 2016. Available at: http://www.cdc.gov/std/syphilis/stdfact-syphilis-detailed.htm (accessed 2 July 2017).

7. Chemica Heria Foundation. Paul Ehrlich. Available at: http://www.chemheritage.org/discover/online-resources/chemistry-in-history/themes/pharmaceuticals/preventing-and-treating-infectious-diseases/ehrlich.aspx (accessed 10 July 2017).

8. Cleveland Clinic. Breath tests for helicobacter, 2016. Available at: http://my.clevelandclinic.org/health/diagnostics/hic_Breat_Test_for_H_Pylori (accessed 8 June 2017).

9. College of Physicians of Philadelphia. Vaccines: vaccine development and licensing events. Available at: http://www.historyofvaccines.org/content/articles/vaccine-development-licensing-events (accessed 15 June 2017).

10. DeWalt DA, Pincus T. The legacies of Rudolf Virchow: cellular medicine in the 20th century and social medicine in the 21st century. Isr Med Assoc J. 2003;5:395–397. Available at: https://www.ima.org.il/FilesUpload/IMAJ/0/53/26937.pdf (accessed 3 July 2017).

11. Doll R. Proof of causality: deduction for epidemiologic observation. Perspect Biol Med. 2002;45(SU01):499–515. Available at: http://muse.jhu.edu/article/26159 (accessed 3 May 2017).

12. Evans AF. Causation and disease: the Henle-Koch postulates revisited. Yale J Biol Med. 1976;49:175–195. Available at: https://www.ncbi.nlm.nih.gov/pmc/articles/PMC2595276/ (accessed 4 November 2017).

13. Ferri M, Ranucci E, Romagnoli P, Giaccone V. Antimicrobial resistance: a global emerging threat to public health systems. Crit Rev Food Sci Nutr. 2015;0. Abstract available at: http://www.tandfonline.com/doi/full/10.1080/10408398.2015.1077192 (accessed 6 July 2017).

14. Frederichs DN, Relman DA. Sequence-based identification of microbial pathogens: a reconsideration of Koch's postulates. Clin Microbiol Rev. 1996;9:18–33. Available at: https://www.ncbi.nlm.nih.gov/pmc/articles/PMC172879/pdf/090018.pdf (accessed 5 July 2017).

15. Gensini GF, Conti AA, Lippi D. The contributions of Paul Ehrlich to infectious disease. J Infect. 2007;54(3):221–224. Epub 2006 Mar 29. Abstract available at: https://www.ncbi.nlm.nih.gov/pubmed/16567000 (accessed 6 November 2017).

16. Greenberg H. The epidemiological challenge of traditional chronic disease risk factors in emerging economies. Int J Epidemiol. 2017;4(5):1351–1353. Available at: https://doi.org/10.1093/ije/dyx214. Abstract available at: https://academic.oup.com/ije/article-abstract/46/5/1351/4360949?redirectedFrom = fulltext (accessed 12 November 2017).

17. Hebar A, Valent P, Selzer E. The impact of molecular targets in cancer drug development: major hurdles and future strategies. Expert Rev Clin Pharmacol. 2013;6(1):23–34. doi:10.1586/ecp.12.71. Available at: http://www.tandfonline.com/doi/full/10.1586/ecp.12.71 (accessed 6 July 2017).

18. Henderson DA. Eradication: lessons from the past. Morb Mort Wkly Rep. 1999;48 (SU01):16–22. Available at: http://www.cdc.gov/mmwr/preview/mmwrhtml/su48a6.htm (accessed 18 October 2017).

19. Hughes MF, Beck BD, Chen Y, Lewis AS, Thomas DJ. Arsenic exposure and toxicology: a historical perspective. Toxicol Sci. 2011;123(2):305–332. Abstract available at: http://toxsci.oxfordjournals.org/content/123/2/305.full (accessed 1 July 2017).

20. Kasten FH. Paul Ehrlich: pathfinder in cell biology. 1. Chronicle of his life and accomplishments in immunology, cancer research, and chemotherapy. Biotech. Histochem. 1996;71(1):2–37. Available at: https://www.ncbi.nlm.nih.gov/pubmed/9138526 (accessed 5 November 2017).

21. Kaufmann SHE. Paul Ehrlich: founder of chemotherapy. Nat Rev Drug Discov. 2008;7:373. doi:10.1038/nrd2582. Available at: http://www.nature.com/nrd/journal/v7/n5/full/nrd2582.html (accessed 11 July 2017).

22. Last JM. A dictionary of public health. Oxford: Oxford University Press, 2006.

23. Lucas RM, Mc Michael AJ. Association or causation: evaluating links between environment and disease. Bull World Health Org. 2005;83(10):792–795. Available at: http://www.who.int/bulletin/volumes/83/10/792.pdf (accessed 3 May 2017).

24. Marmot M. Social determinants of health inequalities. Lancet. 2005;365:1099–1104. Available at: http://www.who.int/social_determinants/strategy/en/Marmot-Social%20determinants%20of%20health%20inqualities.pdf (accessed 11 July 2017).

25. MedicineNet. Definition of Koch's postulates. New York: MedicineNet, updated 10 October 1998. Available at: https://www.medicinenet.com/script/main/art.asp?articlekey = 7105 (accessed 6 July 2017).

26. New York School of Medicine. Dr. Ehrlich's magic bullet, 1940. Warner Brothers, Biographical Film, Nominated for Academy Award 1940. Available at: http://medhum.med.nyu.edu/view/10059 (accessed 10 July 2017).

27. Nobelprize.org. Robert Koch biography. Available at: http://www.nobelprize.org/nobel_prizes/medicine/laureates/1905/koch-bio.html (accessed 1 July 2017).
28. Nobel Media AB. Paul Ehrlich-Biographical. Nobelprize.org, 2014. Web. June 11, 2016. Available at: http://www.nobelprize.org/nobel_prizes/medicine/laureates/1908/ehrlich-bio.html (accessed 12 June 2017).
29. Patlak M, Shastri N. Vaccines: essential weapons in the fight against disease. Breakthroughs in bioscience. Bethesda, MD: Federation of American Societies for Experimental biology, 2014. Available at: https://www.faseb.org/Portals/2/PDFs/opa/2015/10.23.15%20FASEB-BreakthroughsInBioscience-Vaccines%20-WEB.pdf (accessed 10 July 2017).
30. Racaniello V. Koch's postulates in the 21st century. Virology blog, 2015. Available at: http://www.virology.ws/2010/01/22/kochs-postulates-in-the-21st-century/ (accessed 10 July 2017).
31. Rosen G. A history of public health. Expanded edition. Baltimore MD: The Johns Hopkins University Press, 1993.
32. Rubin RP. A brief history of great discoveries in pharmacology: in celebration of the centennial anniversary of the founding of the American Society of Pharmacology and Experimental Therapeutics. Pharmacol Rev. 2007;59(4):289−359. Available at: http://pharmrev.aspetjournals.org/content/59/4/289.full#title16 (accessed 8 July 2017).
33. Schwartz RS. Paul Ehrlich's magic bullets. N Engl J Med. 2004;350:1079−1080. Abstract available at: http://www.nejm.org/doi/full/10.1056/NEJMp048021 (accessed 1 July 2017).
34. Strebhardt K, Ullrich A. Paul Ehrlich's magic bullet concept: 100 years of progress. Nat Rev Cancer. 2008;8:473−480. doi:10.1038/nrc2394. Abstract available at: http://www.ncbi.nlm.nih.gov/pubmed/18469827 (accessed 12 June 2017).
35. Tulchinsky TH, Varavikova EA. What is the "New Public Health"? Public Health Rev. 2010;32:25−53. Available at: https://publichealthreviews.biomedcentral.com/articles/10.1007/BF03391592 (accessed 23 July 2017).
36. Warren JR. Reminiscences on *Helicobacter pylori*. Public Health Rev. 2010;32:10−14. Available at: https://publichealthreviews.biomedcentral.com/articles/10.1007/BF03391589 (accessed 23 July 2017).
37. World Health Organization. Drug resistance: global action plan on microbial resistance. Available at: http://www.who.int/drugresistance/global_action_plan/en/ (accessed 2 July 2017).

Chapter 8

Bismarck and the Long Road to Universal Health Coverage

ABSTRACT

The 2015 Sustainable Development Goals (SDGs) state that All United Nations Member States have agreed to try to achieve Universal Health Coverage by 2030. This includes financial risk protection, access to quality essential health care services and access to safe, effective, quality and affordable essential medicines and vaccines for all. Universal health coverage (UHC) means inclusion and empowerment for all people to access medical care, including treatment and prevention services. UHC exists in all the industrial nations except the US, which has a mixed public-private system and struggles with closing the gap between the insured and the uninsured population. Middle- and low-income countries face many challenges for UHC achievement, including low levels of funding, lack of personnel, weak health management, and issues of availability of services favoring middle- and upper-class communities. Community health services for preventive and curative health services for needs in populations at risk for poor health in low-income countries must be addressed with proactive health promotion initiatives for the double burden of infectious and noncommunicable diseases. Each nation will develop its own unique approach to national health systems, but there are models used by a number of countries based on principles of national responsibility for health, social solidarity for providing funding, and for effective ways of providing care with comprehensiveness, efficiency, quality, and cost containment. Universal access does not eliminate social inequalities in health by itself, including a wide context of reducing social inequities. Understanding national health systems requires examining representative models of different systems.

Health reform is necessarily a continuing process as all countries must adapt to face challenges of cost constraints, inequalities in access to care, aging populations, emergence of new disease conditions and advancing technology including the growing capacity of medicine, public health and health promotion. The growing stress of increasing obesity, diabetes, and other chronic diseases, requires nations to modify their health care systems. Learning from the systems developed in different countries helps to learn from the processes of change in other countries.

Case Studies in Public Health. DOI: http://dx.doi.org/10.1016/B978-0-12-804571-8.00031-7
131

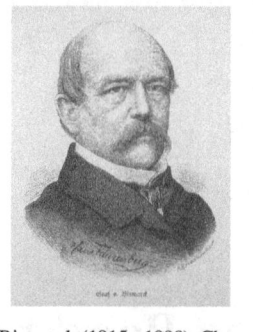

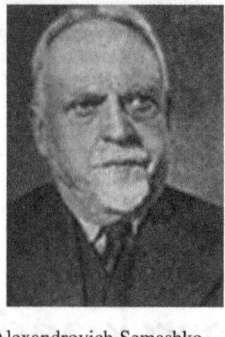

Otto von Bismarck (1815–1898), Chancellor of Germany, Founder of the Social Security health insurance model in 1883. *Source: https://commons.wikimedia.org/wiki/File:Graf_v._Bismarck. JPG (accessed 6 October 2017).*

Nikolai Alexandrovich Semashko (1874–1949), founder of the Soviet health system 1917. *Source: Marxists Internet Archive Available at: https://www.marxists. org/archive/semashko/1923/06/health.htm (accessed 6 October 2017).*

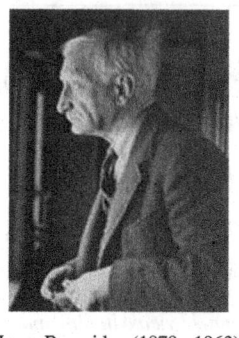

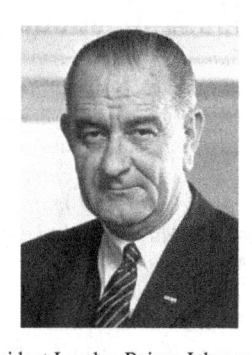

William Henry Beveridge (1879–1963); circa 1947; Baron Beveridge; economist, London School of Economics; author of the Social Insurance and Allied Services ("Beveridge Report" on the Welfare State) in the United Kingdom 1942; visionary of the UK National Health Service 1948. *Source: London School of Economics LSE ref no. IMAGELIBRARY/1290. Available at: https://archives.lse.ac.uk/Record. aspx?src=CalmView.Catalog&id=IMAGELIBR ARY%2f1290 (accessed 2 Oct 2017).*

US President Lyndon Baines Johnson (1908–1973); president (1963-1969) introduced Medicare (1965), Medicaid (1965). *Source: US government official portrait courtesy LB Johnson Library credit Frank Muto, Available at: http://www.lbjlibrary.net/ collections/quick-facts/ (accessed 6 October 2017).*

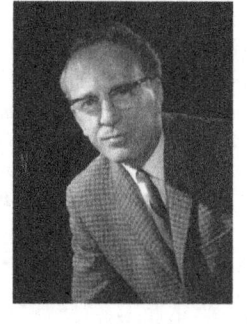

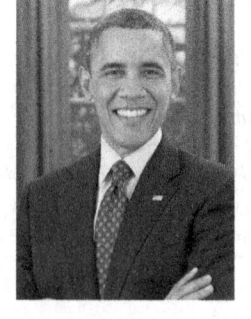

Thomas Clement (Tommy) Douglas (1904–1986); Father of the Canadian Medicare universal health plan (1946–1971); Premier of Saskatchewan; a national survey, voted Tommy "The Greatest Canadian" 2014. *Courtesy of Joan Dianne Douglas on behalf of the Douglas family (accessed 10 October 2017).*

US President Barack Obama (1961) 44th president 2009-2017. *Source: US government official photograph in the Oval Office, December 2012, available at: https://commons. wikimedia.org/wiki/File:President_Barack_ Obama.jpg (accessed 8 October 2017).*

BACKGROUND

In almost all high- and many medium-income countries, the State has assumed the responsibilities for social security and health care for all their citizens. The "welfare state" took on measures such as workers compensation, unemployment and disability insurance, and special disability benefits for the blind, widows, orphans, and the elderly through pensions. Some states instituted child benefits to raise levels of child care and nutrition through child allowances provided from taxation and other government revenues. The main models of *state-operated health services* are the German "Bismarckian system", the Soviet "Semashko system", the British National Health Service "Beveridge system: and the Canadian National Health Insurance system". Although there are many national variations, the classical national health insurance models are the Bismarckian Social Security system, and the Canadian National Health Insurance system operated by the provinces with federal standards and cost sharing. Other nations, such as the United States, have mixed public-private systems of prepaid and self paid health care.

Medium- and low-income countries aspiring to universal access for the total population must face the need to allocate at least 5–6 percent of gross domestic product (GDP) for health, to define health targets and give priority to programs that address those targets, along the lines of the Sustainable Development Goals (SDGs). Other requirements include the need to train people at different levels to plan, manage, administer and deliver services; to develop the capacity to monitor the epidemiology of population health; and, to give strong political support to health and related issues of social support, education, community infrastructure, especially emphasizing the values of prevention and health promotion.

Assuring access to quality health care for all is accepted as a basic principle of public health and human rights. This includes medical and hospital care, but these alone, while vital, are not sufficient to produce a high standard of population health for all. There are many self care, genetic, socioeconomic, and community factors that affect health status, with medical care being one of the vital aspects of the broad spectrum of health needs (see Chapter 21). In order to promote optimal health, effective population-level prevention, availability, and access to care must be seen in the wider context of the individual- and of societal conditions which increased risk of disease, and application of appropriate measures to reduce those risks to prevent disease and promote health. Some interventions are provided by medical care including its preventive role, while others are social, sanitary, environmental, nutritional, legal, economic, and educational, among other factors. This interrelates with human resources for health, financing and economics, organization, technology, law, ethics, and globalized health.

The World Health Organization (WHO) defines a health system as: *"The people, institutions and resources, arranged together in accordance with established policies, to improve the health of the population they serve, while responding to people's legitimate expectations and protecting them against the cost of ill-health through a variety of activities whose primary intent is to improve health. It is a set of elements and their relationship in a complex whole, designed to serve the health needs of the population. Health systems fulfill three main functions: Health care delivery, fair treatment to all, and meeting health expectations of the population."*

WHO's World Health Reports (2000, 2006, 2013) focused on health systems financing and management in the search for universal health coverage. Under the globally endorsed SDGs, universal health coverage (UHC) is designated Goal 3 (Health and Wellbeing), target 3.8: *"Achieve universal health coverage (UHC), including financial risk protection, access to quality essential health care services, and access to safe, effective, quality, and affordable essential medicines and vaccines for all"*. Box 8.1 outlines WHO building blocks for UHC.

Universal access is a means of assuring that the economic barrier to health care is mostly if not completely removed for the total population and may lead to increased access to medical and hospital services for those previously excluded. While UHC increases access to medical care and health indices, it does not, of itself, guarantee achievement of many important health targets. Allocation of resources is an even more fundamental problem to address the needs of those with the highest risk of early disability or avoidable premature death. A system of national health must be able to allocate resources to meet those needs and must not simply be a payment system for doctors and hospitals. Changing demographics, medical advances and epidemiological challenges including social and health inequalities also be addressed with high priority.

BOX 8.1 "Building Blocks" for Universal National Health Coverage

- Adequate financing with pooling of risk.
- A well-trained and adequately remunerated workforce.
- Information on which to base policy and management decisions.
- Logistics that get medicine, vaccines, and technologies to where they are needed.
- Well-maintained facilities organized as part of a service delivery and referral network.
- Leadership that sets and enforces the rules of the game, provides clear direction, and harnesses the energies of all stakeholders including communities and other sectors.

Source: World Health Organization. Strategic vision: Better health outcomes depend on better health systems. Available at: http://www.who.int/nationalpolicies/vision/en/ (accessed 14 May 2017).

This case study provides the background and experience of the development of UHC over the past century and a half, with lessons learned for consideration in how—and what—is done to achieve this goal. Most industrialized countries have implemented national health programs such as health insurance systems or national health services. Each system developed in the political, social, and historical context of the country—and continues to evolve. Medium- and low-income countries are also struggling to achieve universal access to care and health for all by expanding primary health care and social security plans which provide benefits to workers and for certain vulnerable populations—primarily mothers and children. As they move up the scale of economic development, developing countries must also address the problem of how to decrease morbidity and mortality, achieve equity in access to health care, and expand the funding basis for health care through national health insurance. Some countries experience rapid economic development, but lag behind in directing increased national wealth towards improving health status. This is often due to a lack of focused political commitment, trained policy analysts, and cultural adaptation to the crucial importance of public health.

Each national health system has its own characteristics and challenges. Systems management requires continuous evaluation based on well-developed information systems, trained health management personnel, societal involvement through all levels of government, as well as the private sector, professional organizations and advocacy groups. There is no defined "gold standard" plan for providing universal access to health care that is suitable for all countries. Each country develops and modifies a program of national health appropriate to its own political and cultural needs and available resources. However, there are evolving patterns in health care organization, so that networking within and between countries ensures that they can—and do—learn from one another (Box 8.2).

Barriers to necessary health care can be geographic, ethnic, cultural, social, lack of information and awareness, psychological, financial, and poverty. Removing financial barriers to care is necessary and constructive, but not sufficient to address the health problems of individuals and of a society. Equity in financial access with universal coverage is vital to population and individual health since anyone can have serious illness at any time. But equally important, long-term preventive care and health promotion are essential to good population and individual health standards. Inequities exist in all societies, but many countries have successfully reduced these by poverty alleviation, job creation, education, and other programs that reduce interregional, socioeconomic, and demographic differences in health. Special attention to high-risk groups in a population is essential. Groups at-risk may be based on age, gender, ethnicity, genetic legacy, occupation, risky lifestyle, location of residence, religion, sexual orientation, economic status, or other factors that increase susceptibility to disease, premature death, or disability. Services must be based on need and not only demand, which can escalate costs by

BOX 8.2 Key Elements of National Health Systems

1. A tradition of government and nongovernmental initiatives to improve health of the population.
2. Public administration and regulation; public-private partnerships.
3. Intersectoral cooperation with education, social services and the private sector.
4. Demographic, economic, and epidemiologic monitoring.
5. Health targets monitored with accessible data systems.
6. Public health programs, including strong elements of health promotion.
7. Universal coverage by public insurance or service system.
8. Access to a broad range of health services.
9. Strategic planning for health and social policies.
10. Monitoring health status indicators.
11. Recognition of special needs of high-risk groups and related issues.
12. Portability and accessibility of benefits when changing employer or residence.
13. Efforts to reduce inequity in regional and socio-demographic accessibility and quality of care.
14. Adequacy of financing.
15. Cost containment.
16. Efficient use of resources for a well-balanced health system.
17. Consumer satisfaction and choice of primary care provider.
18. Provider satisfaction and choice of referral services.
19. Promotion of high-quality service.
20. Promote patient and staff safety.
21. Comprehensive public health and health promotion programs.
22. Comprehensive primary, secondary, and tertiary levels of medical care.
23. Well-developed information and monitoring systems.
24. Continual policy and management review.
25. Promotion of standards and accreditation of services, professional education, training, research.
26. Governmental and private provision of services.
27. Decentralized management and community participation.
28. Assurance of ethical standards of care for all.
29. Conduct epidemiological, basic sciences and health systems research.
30. Preparation for mass casualties from disasters and terrorism.

Source: Adapted from Tulchinsky TH, Varavikova EA. The New Public Health, Third Edition, chapter 13, Box 13.3, page 644. San Diego, CA; Academic Press/Elsevier, 2014.

over-servicing. Health systems planning needs to promote access to patient care, but also those services that reach the entire population, especially people at high risk who are often least able to seek and access appropriate care.

A program that provides equal access for all may not achieve the objective of better health for the population unless accompanied by other important governmental, community and personal self-care activities. These include enactment and enforcement of environmental and occupational health laws, food safety, nutrition standards, clean water, improved rural care, higher educational levels, and provision of health information to the public. Additional national programs are needed to promote health generally and to reduce specific risk factors for morbidity and mortality. Responsibility for health lies not only with medical and other health professionals, but also with governmental and voluntary organizations, the community, the family, and the individual.

Individual access to an essential "basket of services" as a prepaid insured benefit is fundamental to a successful national health program. Each country addresses this issue according to its means and traditions, but cost-effective evidence-based methods of meeting a country's epidemiologic and demographic needs should be prioritized. Coverage and payments for heart transplantation, for example, may be beyond the means of a health system, but early and aggressive management of hypertension, smoking, poor diet, physical inactivity, and rapid care for acute myocardial infarction are effective in saving lives at modest cost and containing the need for more intrusive health care interventions. Prevention is cost-effective and should be integral to the development of service priorities within the insured benefits with incentives included in the "basket of services".

Globalization affects health systems around the world not only in the ease of spread of infectious diseases, but in increased access to modern preventive, diagnostic, treatment modalities. Access to antiretroviral drugs has dramatically changed the face of HIV/AIDS globally, including in low-income countries with support of international and bilateral donors. The same is true for vaccines, including the MMR (measles, mumps, rubella, 2 doses), Hib (Hemophilus influenza b), rotavirus, pneumococcal pneumonia and HPV (Human papillomavirus) vaccines, which will save millions of children's lives and foster well being in the coming decade. Information technology, migration of medical professionals, and internalization of educational standards are all global health issues affecting national health systems.

Health systems in all countries are facing common problems in population health, with rising population age, hypertension, obesity and diabetes prevalence, and rising health care costs. Health systems research capacity is important in each country as it attempts to cope with rapid changes in population health and individual health needs with limited resources. Development of research capacity enables improved capacity of decision-makers for informed, cost-effective decisions. In developing countries, low levels of funding for health in general—including research—impede evidence-based health system development and training of the new health workforce. Strengthening reporting systems of data aggregation, as well as economic and epidemiologic analysis, are vital for health policy and management.

National Health Systems

National health systems from Germany, UK, Canada, US and Russia are presented here as representing major models of organization. These organizational models influence health care system formulation in both developing and developed countries, as well as for countries restructuring their health services. Health care systems and financing are under pressure everywhere, not only to assure access to health for all citizens, but also to keep up with advancing medical technology, and contain the cost increase at sustainable levels. Because a health system is judged by more than its cost and measure of medical services, indicators of health status of the population, as well as morbidity and mortality are vital and should be available for the public through community organizations and the media. This topic has developed a complex terminology of its own. The World Health Organization (WHO) helps development of national health systems as shown in Box 8.3.

BOX 8.3 WHO Definition, Rationale and Content of Health Systems

Universal health coverage is defined as ensuring that all people have access to needed health promotion, preventive, curative and rehabilitative health services, of sufficient quality to be effective, while also ensuring that people do not suffer financial hardship when paying for these services.

- Good health is essential to sustained economic and social development and poverty reduction.
- Access to needed health services is crucial for maintaining and improving health.
- At the same time, people need to be protected from being forced into poverty because of the cost of health care.
- A well-functioning health system working in harmony is built on having:
  Trained and motivated health workers;
  A well-maintained infrastructure;
  A reliable supply of medicine and technologies;
  Backed by adequate funding;
  Strong health plans;
  Evidence-based policies.

WHO assists in creating resilient health systems by supporting countries to:
- *"Develop, implement, and monitor solid national health policies, strategies and plans.*
- *Assure the availability of equitable integrated people-centered health services at an affordable price.*
- *Facilitate access to affordable, safe, and effective medicine and health technologies.*
- *Strengthen their health information systems and evidence-based policy-making, and to provide information and evidence on health-related matters."*

Source: World Health Organization. Health systems. Available at: http://www.who.int/healthsystems/about/en/ (accessed 2 May 2017).

TABLE 8.1 Life Expectancy at Birth, Selected Countries, 1960–2015

	1960	2015
Canada	71	82
China	43	76
France	70	83
Germany	60	81
India	41	68
Nigeria	37	53
UK	71	82
USA	70	79
World	52	72

Source: Derived from World Bank. Life expectancy at birth, total (years). Available at http://data.worldbank.org/indicator/SP.DYN.LE00.IN (accessed 15 October 2017).

Health systems are meant to improve health and quality of life, as measured by quantitative and qualitative methods. The Human Development Index (HDI) provides a standard method of comparison which combines many health and social indices into a summary figure for social development of countries. These include life expectancy at birth, gross domestic product (GDP) per capita, child mortality, education and others. Table 8.1 shows life expectancy, still a valued health status indicator, for some industrialized, mid-level, and developing countries. Comparisons between countries health indicators are useful to portray relative international health status among nations.

The foundations of public responsibility for health care systems go back to ancient Greece and Rome where city states employed municipal doctors to service the poor and slaves. In the Medieval and Renaissance periods, monasteries and nunneries provided charitable care to the poor while professional guilds provided prepaid medical care and other social benefits to members and their families. These later evolved into the Friendly (benevolent) Societies, as mutual benefit programs that provided for burials, pensions, and payment for health services for members. In the twentieth century, these developed through collective bargaining into health insurance plans through private or professionally sponsored insurers, and labor union–sponsored health plans. Governmental responsibility for health systems evolved in public health and health protection systems in the nineteenth and twentieth centuries and continues to evolve to face new challenges as well as preventive and treatment capacities.

The health systems described highlight the unique and common features of national health systems in the search for "health for all", and policies for making health a priority in resource allocation, policy priority for human rights, and for socioeconomic development. Figure 8.1 indicates the 1995–2014 trends in total health expenditures as percent of Gross Domestic Products of selected countries in the European Region of WHO. German and Swedish expenditures rose to between 11% and 12%, in the United Kingdom to over 9% while Israel is relatively stable under 8% and the Russian Federation expenditures rose to 7% of GDP.

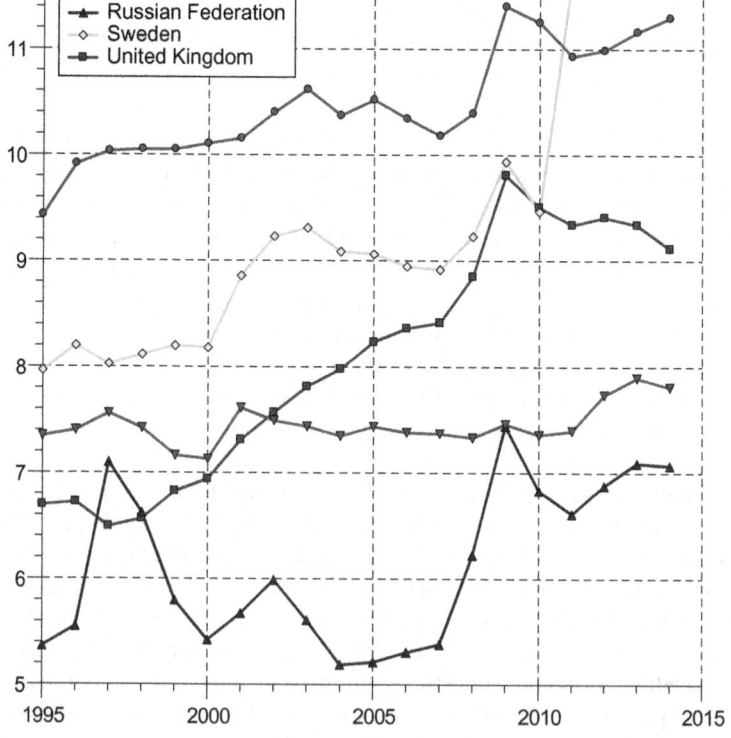

FIGURE 8.1 Total health expenditures as percent of Gross Domestic Product, WHO estimates, selected countries European region, 1995–2014. *Source: World Health Organization European Region, Health for All Data Base, 2016. Available at: http://data.euro.who.int/hfadb/ (accessed 12 November 2017).*

Germany: The Bismarckian System

Otto von Bismark was born in Schönhausen, Pomerania to a noble landowning family. He studied law at Göttingen and Berlin and entered the civil service. Following failure of the 1848 revolution he entered political life as a conservative. He became a prominent hero in the Franco-Prussian War of 1870 and unified the German Confederation becoming Chancellor from 1871 to 1890. Despite his aristocratic roots and deep political conservatism, Bismarck created Europe's first modern welfare state in the 1880s, establishing national health insurance for workers and their families (1883), accident insurance (1884) and old age pensions (1889). While his motivation may have been political—to stem the rising popularity of socialist parties—it also served nationalistic purposes to develop healthier children as future workers and soldiers. His legacy of employment-based social insurance for the health of workers and their families is widely emulated and remembered to this day as the "Bismarckian model" of national health insurance built on the principles of solidarity, self-governance and competition. The Bismarckian model established state social insurance with prepayment by workers and their employers. It utilized Sick Funds (*Krankenkassen*) as insurers to provide payment to the physician, hospital, or other provider.

Germany's health care system today is characterized by participation as well as sharing of decision-making powers between the states (*Länder*), the federal government and civil society organizations. Since 2009, Statutory Health Insurance (SHI) has been mandatory for all citizens and permanent residents pay a uniform contribution of 15.5 percent of their income (*Gesetzliche Krankenversicherung*) with 118 sickness funds (*Krankenkassen, January 2016*). SHI covers 85 percent of the population, who have the right to choose their preferred sickness fund for a comprehensive range of services. The sickness funds are linked to associations of physicians accredited to treat patients covered by SHI. Private health insurance (PHI) covers 11 percent of the population for designated groups such as civil servants. Others (4%) such as the military are included in other specific governmental programs. Since the 1990s financial incentives are being introduced to improve quality and efficiency of care along with beneficiaries right to choose between sickness funds increasing competition and a market orientation. Hospitals are paid by diagnosis related groups (DRGs)—i.e., payment by diagnostic category rather than hospital length of stay, adopted from US experience. Physicians are paid by a capitation system—i.e., a fixed payment for each person registered for care with a doctor for a fixed period of time (as opposed to fee-for-service) in the doctor's medical associations. Long-term care is covered by a federal mandatory program. Germany expends 11.3 percent of GDP (2015) on health, one of the highest levels among EU members, with 73 percent from public sources and 27 percent privately sourced. In 2014, Germany had 6.2 acute care beds per 1,000 beds per 1000 population, nearly 40 percent above the rate for the original EU countries (3.8 per 1,000). Of these, 48 percent of beds were in publicly owned, 34 percent in private nonprofit, and 18 percent in private for-profit hospitals. Busse et al. (2017) describes reforms since its founding in 1883 gradually achieving universal coverage. The system is also seeking greater cost effectiveness as compared to neighboring countries.

In Europe, many countries developed taxation or social security models based on the Bismarckian approach, with compulsory contributions by workers and their employers to a national social security system. This then financed approved services usually paid through private medical practice with fee-for-service payment. Many European countries and Japan gradually developed similar forms of compulsory health insurance for workers and their families following World War I, or later after World War II, expanding to universal coverage health insurance systems. This model is used in France, Belgium, the Netherlands, Japan, Switzerland, and Latin America as well as post-Soviet health reforms and countries of Eastern Europe (CEE).

The Israeli system, adopted in 1995, based on the Bismarckian model is mandatory national health insurance in which everyone must choose one of four long-standing Sick Funds now called Health Organizations. They compete for members, and are paid a per capita sum for which they are obliged to provide comprehensive services including hospital, primary care, and preventive services. The services improved vastly under national health insurance, with services kept up to date with annual additions to the statutory "basket of services." Health statistics show Israel as among the top countries for life expectancy, with rapidly falling mortality from strokes, coronary heart diseases, and cancers. Consumer satisfaction is high, maternal and child health are stressed, a low hospital bed to population ratio, while health expenditures are relatively modest and a stable per capita health expenditure just under eight percent of GDP (Lancet 2017).

The United Kingdom: The Beveridge System

William Beveridge was born in 1879 in Bengal, India, where his father was a judge in the Indian Civil Service. He trained as a lawyer coming to prominence in the British Liberal government of 1906–14 when he advised David Lloyd George (Chancellor of the Exchequer from 1908 to 1915, Prime Minister from 1916 to 1922) on old age pensions and national insurance. In 1911, initiated by Lloyd-George, influenced by the German compulsory health insurance scheme, the Liberal government of Great Britain introduced the National Health Insurance Act. It was compulsory for all wage earners between 16 and 70 years of age. This was a two-part plan based on a worker and employer contributory system for both unemployment insurance and for medical care for workers and their families. Administration was through approved mutual benefit societies (the Friendly Societies), some based on insurance companies, and others by professional associations and trade unions. General practitioner services were paid on a capitation basis rather than a salary, preserving their status as self-employed professionals. Initially this plan covered one-third of the population increasing to half by 1940, however there was disruption due to mass unemployment during the Great Depression starting in 1929 and continuing to the late 1930s.

In the early days of World War II, the British government established a National Emergency Medical Service for hospitals in preparation for the anticipated large-scale civilian casualties that were expected during the Blitz bombing by Nazi Germany. This established national health planning and rescued many hospitals from near bankruptcy due to the effects of the Great Depression in the United Kingdom (UK). During World War II, at the behest of Prime Minister Winston Churchill, Beveridge developed a postwar social reconstruction program. The Beveridge Report of 1942, *Social Insurance and Health Services*, outlined the concept of a future welfare state including a national health service, placing medical care in the context of general social policy for the total population. The wartime government coalition approved the principle of a national health service, which had wide public support, despite opposition from the medical association.

In 1945, the newly elected Labour government of Clement Attlee took up the recommendations of Beveridge to introduce the National Insurance Act (1946) as a comprehensive system of unemployment, sickness, maternity, and pension benefits funded by employers, employees and the government. The National Health Service (NHS) Act was instituted in 1948 under the leadership of Aneurin Bevan, against continued opposition from medical organizations, as a universal state health service in Britain. The NHS provides a nationally tax-based financed, universal coverage system providing free care by general practitioners, specialists, hospitals, and public health services. This includes diagnosis and treatment of illnesses at home or in hospital, including dental and optometric care. The original NHS structure was divided into three separate services: hospital, general practitioner, and community health services. The hospital and specialist services were under the authority of 14 regional boards. General practitioners worked under national contracts, and community health services, such as public health, home nursing and health visitors, midwives, maternal- and child care, came under the control of the county and city local authorities. All units reported to the minister of health and his staff. The hospital bed supply in the UK in 2014 was just under half the rate in France and one third of the rate of beds in Germany per 1,000 population. Hospital based specialists are salaried but highly independent; general practitioners ran their own practices and provided the foundation of the NHS system. Over time, this tripartite structure evolved to some degree of integration of GP and community health services, along with hospitals under Hospital Trusts reporting to Regional Health Authorities. The NHS, with periodic reforms, is still in place in the UK and well accepted by the population and—over time—even by conservative governments and by the medical profession.

There are differences between the NHS systems of the UK: England, Scotland, Wales and Northern Ireland each operate their own NHS, albeit with funding and structure of the central NHS. Regional disparities in health indicators still exist despite changes in funding giving greater resources within regions (north-south divide) of England; each of the four has their own, policy directions. Social class and geographic inequities in health within the NHS have been recognized since the 1970s with a series of reports and analyses showing large gaps in life expectancy, avoidable (i.e., preventable) mortality between the south and north of England and even more so with Scotland and significantly poorer health indicators. The Marmot Report on inequalities from 2010 indicated the scope of the problem: *"People living in the most deprived neighborhoods will on average die seven years earlier than people living in the richest neighborhoods. Even more disturbing, people living in poorer areas not only die sooner, but spend more of their lives with disability—an average total difference of 17 years. The review has estimated the cost of health inequalities in England: productivity losses of £31—33 billion every year; lost taxes and higher welfare payments in the range of £20—32 billion per year; and additional NHS healthcare costs well in excess of £5.5 billion per year."*

The "Beveridge model" is a term used for the National Health Service model, which has since been adopted by many European countries and should be regarded as a strong model for countries reforming their universal health care systems, such as Spain and Italy. The Scottish NHS diverges from the central English NHS in addressing inequalities by a focus on the health sector as the sole responsibility for reduction of inequalities. The English NHS and other government agencies see the problem more broadly and adopted poverty-fighting measures with some success in improving mortality and morbidity social and health disparities since 2000. The NHS system remains generally popular in providing health security for all, and reaching good outcome measures despite regional inequities. No change of governing political party has led to dismantling the NHS for a privatized health system over the seven decades since its inception.

Canada: National Health Insurance

TC (Tommy) Douglas was born in Falkirk, Scotland and immigrated at the age of 10 with his working class family to Winnipeg, Manitoba, Canada. He developed osteoarthritis and the doctors were going to amputate his leg as the family lacked funds for long-term medical care. His leg was saved by a senior surgeon who refused the amputation. This made Tommy a lifelong advocate and fighter for publicly administered, universal health care for all. He became a Baptist minister and entered politics winning the Saskatchewan general election of 1944 for the CCF party in a massive victory. It was the first democratic socialist government elected in North America. He held the office for 17 years, during which time he pioneered many major social and economic reforms.

Canada (population 35.5 million) is a federal state and a constitutional monarchy with parliamentary systems at national and provincial/territorial levels. Health is primarily a provincial responsibility, but federal funding and standards play an important role in the Canadian health system. Local authorities also carry out many primary public health services including sanitation, water safety, and supervision of food safety, among other responsibilities. The Provinces/Territories are responsible for the funding of hospital, community, home and long-term care, as well as mental and public health services. Starting in the 1930s, federal grants-in-aid were given to the Provinces/ Territories for categorical health programs, such as cancer and public health services programs. Since the SARS (severe acute respiratory syndrome) epidemic in 2003, the Canadian federal government has increased its capacity in public health with a new federal department of public health, regional laboratories and encouragement of many schools of public health across the country.

Canada's national health program evolved as a system of provincial health insurance with federal government financial support and standards. Initiatives for national health insurance in Canada go back to the 1920s, but definitive action occurred only after World War II. The federal government regulates drug and medical device safety, funds research and provides services to the Native indigenous population groups, the military, RCMP (Royal Canadian Mounted Police) and federal prison inmates. Services for veterans were later transferred to provincial Medicare programs.

The development of national health insurance was largely due to the bitter experience of the Great Depression of the 1930s, a strong agrarian cooperative movement, and the collective wish for a better society following World War II. In 1946, the social democratic Cooperative Commonwealth Federation (CCF) party under the leadership of Tommy Douglas formed the government of Saskatchewan, a large wheat-growing province of one million people on the western prairies. The national universal health insurance program evolved from the provincial initiatives led by Tommy Douglas, now considered "the Father of Canada's universal Medicare plan." Douglas established the Saskatchewan Hospital Insurance and Diagnostic Services Act in 1946 under provincial public administration. In 1956 a federal cost-sharing formula began providing approximately 50 percent cost-sharing with greater levels of funding going to the poorer provinces. By 1961, all 10 Provinces and two Territories had implemented hospital insurance plans, in a two-tiered national health insurance plan—i.e., universal provincial/territorial health plans with federal standards and cost-sharing. In 1962, again in Saskatchewan, the medical care insurance plan (Medicare) was implemented after a bitter doctors' strike. In 1961, the federal government appointed a

Royal Commission on Health Services (the Hall Commission) which in 1964 recommended adoption of the Saskatchewan model across the country with federal support and standards. The Saskatchewan plan was rapidly followed by similar plans in other provinces encouraged by generous federal cost-sharing.

The Federal government cost-shares provincial and territorial programs. Provinces/Territories must adhere to the standards of the Canada Health Act (1984), which defines services to be covered for hospital, diagnostic, and physician services. There is federal funding support for provincial/territorial public health, long-term care, home care and community mental health services. This federal legislation was expanded to provide co-funding for provincial/territorial Medicare plans, which over a short period brought all Canadians into provincially administered systems of publicly financed health care, while retaining the private practice model of medical care. Hospital care is provided mostly through non-profit, non-governmental hospitals.

Developed over the period 1946–71, the provincial/territorial health insurance plans were promoted by federal governmental cost-sharing, political support, and national standards. The plans were initially financed by taxation and premiums, but later solely by general tax revenues with federal support under the Canada Health Act of 1984. Federal standards required the provincial plans to be: publicly administered; comprehensive in coverage of health services; universal; portable across provinces; and, accessible without user fees. Federal reimbursement to the provinces/territories initially covered 25 percent of national average medical care expenditures per capita and 25 percent of the actual expenditures by each individual province. This provided higher-than-national-average rates of support to poorer provinces as well as portability between provinces/territories. By 1971, all provinces had implemented such plans, and a high degree of health services equity was achieved across the country.

Care is provided by private medical practitioners on a fee-for-service basis under negotiated medical fee schedules with no extra billing allowed. Hospitals are operated by nonprofit voluntary, religious organizations or municipal authorities, with payment by block budgets. Per capita spending on health in Canada is relatively modest in comparison with that of the US, but above OECD averages. Public spending as a percent of total health expenditures is close to the OECD average (see Box 8.4). This Medicare-type plan was later adopted in a number of other countries including Australia. Medicare is still popular in Canada, with support from all political parties and by most medical professionals. Medicare and federal cost-sharing weighed in favor of the poorer provinces, allowing these to catch up in health care services and standards with the richer provinces.

The Canadian health program differs substantively from those of the United Kingdom and the United States. Health systems are important in the political and cultural life of a country. Each within its own tradition is

BOX 8.4 Health Indicators, Canada, OECD, 2015

- Population: 35.5 million.
- GDP per capita: USD $44,201.
- Hospital bed supply: 2.7/1000 population.
- Average acute care hospital length of stay 7.5 days.
- Life expectancy: 82.2 years.
- Human Development Index: 0.920, ranked 9th country.
- Health spending growth: Growth rate spending per capita in health was fairly strong up to 2010, but slowed markedly in recent years, being close to zero in real terms over the past four years.
- Share of GDP for health spending (excluding capital expenditure): 10.2 percent in 2013, compared with an OECD average of 8.9 percent, and much lower than in the US (16.4%).
- Per capita health spending in Canada: equivalent of USD $4,351 per person in 2013, compared to the OECD average of USD $3,453, but only half of the US (USD $8,713).
- Public sources accounted for 71 percent of overall health spending, slightly less than the OECD average (73%).

Source: OECD. OECD Health Statistics 2015. How does health spending in Canada Compare? Available at: https://www.oecd.org/els/health-systems/Country-Note-CANADA-OECD-Health-Statistics-2015.pdf (accessed 8 May 2017).

attempting to ensure population health through public or private means, to constrain the rate of cost increases. Comparisons using various health indicators can be controversial, but the Canadian universal health service or insurance coverage seems to have improved the health status of the population more rapidly than similar indicators for the total US population, but not necessarily for all segments of the population. After decades of focus on developing national health insurance, Canada became a leading innovator in health promotion prevention (see Chapter 21).

Reform Pressures and Initiatives

The Canadian health program established universal coverage for a comprehensive set of health benefits without changing the basic practice of medicine from individual medical practice on a fee-for-service basis. Poorer provinces were able to use the federal cost-sharing mechanism to raise standards of health services, and a high degree of health services equity was achieved across the country.

Rapid increases in health care costs led to a review of health policies in 1969 (the Federal–Provincial Committee on the Costs of Health Services). The resulting report stressed the need to reduce hospital beds and develop lower-cost alternatives to hospital care, such as home-based care and long-term care. Federally-led initiatives during this period extended coverage to include home-based care and long-term nursing home care, while restricting federal participation in cost-sharing to the rate of increases in the gross national product (GNP). Since then, many provincial and federal reports have examined the issues in health care and recommended changes in financing, cost-sharing, hospital services, development of primary care, and other community services.

In 1974, a new approach to health was outlined by the Federal Minister of Health, Marc Lalonde, in a landmark public policy document, *A New Perspective on the Health of Canadians*. This report described the Health Field Theory in which health was seen as a result of genetic, lifestyle, and environmental issues, as well as medical care itself. As a result, health promotion became a feature of Canadian public policy, with the objective of changing personal lifestyle habits to decrease cross-cutting risky behaviors such as smoking, obesity, and physical inactivity. The pioneering work in nutrition from the National Nutrition Survey published in 1971 led to the adoption of federal mandatory enrichment regulations for basic foods with essential vitamins and minerals. This and other initiatives in the 1980s led to the Ottawa Charter on Health Promotion (see Chapter 21), which has had a global impact with the foundation of Health Promotion as a crucial new aspect of public health and health system policy.

The Canadian health system being primarily the responsibility of the provinces/territories had a down side. During the SARS pandemic of 2003, the provinces dealt with it and were found to be lacking strong public health institutions adequate to the task. Following high level reviews of the SARS episode the federal government established a CDC-like institution, regional laboratories capable of infectious disease challenges and eight schools of public health across the country to ensure continuing development of a competent public health workforce. Universal health care needed to be supplemented by introduction of Lalonde-initiated health promotion and equally so a strong microbiologic public health component to ensure rapid and competent responses to new emerging health challenges.

How does the Canadian public view the universal public single payer Medicare run by the provinces with federal guidelines and cost-sharing program? Despite complaints, mostly from US sources, the Canadian public appreciates their health protection very much. In 2004, the Canadian Broadcasting Corporation (CBC) television conducted a program over many months called "The Greatest Canadian," with 10 candidates and advocates. This included a call to all people in Canada to nominate their greatest Canadian. Canadians from coast to coast were asked to vote and chose Tommy Douglas, known as the "Father of Medicare" and selected by national polling as "The Greatest Canadian of all time." The Canadian public is proud of their Medicare plan, and appreciates the security and social protection as a great achievement for everyone in the country. Australia,

Taiwan, and South Korea have adopted national health insurance systems similar to the Canadian model.

The United States: Public-Private Health System

The US (population 322 million, GDP per capita USD $56,066 in 2015) has a system of government based on the Federal Constitution, with 50 states each having its own elected government. The Constitution gives primary responsibility for health and welfare to the states, while direct federal services are provided to armed forces, veterans, and indigenous (Native) Americans. The federal government has established a major leadership role in national health by the development of national standards, national regulatory powers, funding, and information systems. The federal level has many governmental structures for regulation of food, drugs, and environment, as well as for research, public health services, training programs and health insurance systems for the elderly and the poor. The US has the world's costliest health care system with over 86 percent health insurance coverage, but universal access remains elusive, and population health indicators are well below many less-wealthy countries. However, the US has through trial and error experimentation made major contributions to the content and organization of public health systems, which are important for strengthening health systems in medium- and low-income countries as well as influencing countries with universal health systems (see Chapter 15). Clearly, the US can learn from other countries as well (see Box 8.5).

In 1798, the federal government established the US Marine Hospital Service to provide hospitals for sick and disabled merchant seamen. This later became the uniformed US Public Health Service Commissioned Corps (USPHS) headed by the Surgeon General (1873). Services were added for Native Americans, military personnel and their families (through the

---

BOX 8.5 Health Indicators, US, OECD, 2015

- Population: 319 million.
- GDP per capita: USD $56,066.
- Hospital bed supply: 2.9/1000 population.
- Average acute care hospital length of stay: 6.1 days (2013).
- Life expectancy: 79.3 years.
- Human Development Index: 0.920, ranked 11th country.
- Health Expenditures per capita USD $8,713.
- Share of GDP for health spending (excluding capital expenditure): 16.4 percent.

Source: OECD. OECD Health Statistics 2015. How does health spending in the US Compare? Available at: https://www.oecd.org/unitedstates/Country-Note-UNITED%20STATES-OECD-Health-Statistics-2015.pdf (accessed 8 May 2017).

Veterans Affairs Department), the Food and Drug Administration (FDA), the National Institutes of Health (NIH), the Centers for Disease Control (CDC) and many other world class federal programs of research, service and teaching. Other departments and legislation were added to promote nutrition and hygiene, establish state, municipal, and county health departments, and regulate drugs and health hazards.

In 1921, the Sheppard-Towner Act established the federal Children's Bureau that administered grants to assist states to operate maternal and child health programs. From the 1920s, labor unions won health insurance benefits through collective bargaining, which became the main basis for prepayment for health care in the United States until today. In 1927, the Committee on the Costs of Medical Care recommended a universal national health program. This initiative was set aside during the Great Depression of 1929–39. The US Social Security Act (SSA) of 1935 was introduced by President Franklin D. Roosevelt as part of the "New Deal" to alleviate the mass suffering of the people during this very traumatic period in the US (and Europe). The SSA was intended to include national health insurance, but this part of the SSA was set aside largely due to strong opposition of the insurance industry and the organized medical profession. The SSA provides financial benefits for widows, orphans, and the disabled, as well as pensions for the elderly, and provided a base for future reform including health insurance.

With the outbreak of World War II, a significant percentage of eligible military recruits were found unfit for compulsory service due to preventable health conditions. This, and the wish to maintain population health, led President Roosevelt to initiate regulations in 1941 for fortification of "enriched" foods reaching a majority of the population including salt with iodine, flour with iron and vitamin B complex, and milk with vitamin D. During World War II (1941–45), governmental health insurance was provided to many millions of Americans serving in the armed forces, along with their families. At the same time, health benefits through voluntary insurance for workers were vastly expanded in place of wage increases and this became the major method of prepayment for health care for a majority of the population. At the end of the war, millions of veterans were eligible for health care through the Veterans Administration (VA), which established a national network of federal hospitals and primary care services.

In 1946, President Truman attempted to bring in national health insurance, but the legislation (the Wagner-Murray-Dingell Bill) failed in the US Congress. One section of the bill was approved, enabling the federal government to initiate a program to upgrade country-wide hospital facilities, while limiting the beds to population ratio, under the Hill-Burton Act (see Chapter 15). Legislation also provided massive federal funding for the newly established National Institutes of Health (NIH) to fund and promote research to strengthen public and private medical schools, teaching hospitals, and research facilities. In 1946, President Truman established the federally-assisted School Lunch program through the Department of Agriculture bringing nutritious meals to many (millions increasing from 7 million in 1946 to 30 million in 2016) of school children throughout the US. In the 1950s, the federal government also established the Centers for Disease Control and Prevention (CDC) and increased assistance for state and local public health activities and encouraged expansion of schools of public health across the country.

US Medicare and Medicaid

In the 1960s, a large percentage of elderly and poor Americans lacked health insurance. In 1965, President Lyndon Johnson introduced Medicare for the aged (over age 65), plus disabled persons, and persons on renal dialysis as an amendment (Title XVII) to the 1935 Social Security Act (SSA). Medicare covers hospitalization, skilled nursing home-based care, medical appliances, and other benefits with copayments. Medicaid, Title XIX of the SSA, also enacted in 1965 by President Johnson, provided federal cost-sharing for acceptable state health plans for the poor, with local authority participation. Medicaid is financed through shared responsibilities primarily of the federal, state and local governments. Medicaid has seen substantial increases in adult and children enrollees through expansions of eligibility, such as the State Children's Health Insurance Program (SCHIP) extending Medicaid to large numbers of children.

Medicare and Medicaid together brought about 25 percent of Americans into public systems of health insurance. Limitations included variable definitions of poverty for Medicaid eligibility in each state, and copayments for Medicare beneficiaries. The population enrolled in Medicare increased from 19 million in 1966 to 55.5 million in 2015, including disabled persons under the age of 65. The Medicaid enrolled population increased from 28.2 million in 1991 to 49.3 million in 2006 and to 65 million in 2017, or about one of every five persons in the United States. This contributed to increasing public sector health expenditures rising from under 25 percent of total health expenditures in 1960 to 47.7 percent in 2009, of concern for both critics and supporters of public health care programs.

The Changing US Health Care Environment

In the US during the 1960s through to the 1990s, rapid health cost increases were attributed to many factors including the lack of a national health insurance mechanism. The plethora of health insurance systems fostered high costs and restrictions on access due to pre-existing conditions. Other factors for rapid cost increases included an increasing elderly population, high levels of morbidity in the poor population, the spread of AIDS, rapid innovation and costly medical technology, specialization, high laboratory and diagnostic imaging costs, and large-scale public investment in medical education, research and health facility construction. The US system includes a mix of public health insurance and service programs (Medicare, Medicaid, Veterans Administration, Indian Health services, and military health coverage) which provide for a significant part—36.5 percent in 2014—of the US population. However, the majority (66%) is covered by the private insurance industry through employer-employee contracts which developed rapidly as the dominant health insurance sector with minimal government regulation. The cost of private health insurance to employers included in labor contracts of their employees and pensioners has become very high. In 2008, General Motors reported to a Senate hearing that the cost of health insurance per car produced was double the direct cost of labor and more than the cost of steel per car. This impinged on competitiveness in price with for example with Japan which has a successful universal governmental health insurance plan with public-private mix of services.

The Affordable Care Act (ACA) introduced by President Barack Obama in 2010 brought some 16 million previously uninsured persons into public and private insurance, increased governmental regulation to ensure fair pricing and payment and, especially, to abolish the past abuses of the "pre-existing condition" exclusions from insurance. Other equally important factors were high levels of preventable hospitalization, institutional orientation of the health system, high administrative costs due to multiple private billing agencies in the private insurance industry, high incomes especially for specialist physicians, and high medical malpractice insurance costs. The pressure for cost constraint came from government, industry, and the private insurance industry. (See Chapter 15).

Private medical practice, with payment by fee-for-service, was the major form of medical care in the US until the 1990s. Most hospitals were operated through a mix of nonprofit agencies, including federal, state, and local governments, and voluntary and religious organizations, but a growing percentage are privately owned, for-profit (from 7.8% of beds in 1975 to 20.6% in 2013). In an effort to contain costs, the diversity of insurance systems promoted experimentation with organizational systems. Health Maintenance Organizations (HMOs) and other forms of managed care systems grew rapidly to become the predominant method of organizing health care in the United States.

Prepaid group practice (PGP) originated from private companies contracting to provide medical care, especially in remote mining camps and construction sites. In the 1940s, New York City sponsored the Health Insurance Plan of Greater New York to provide prepaid medical care for residents of urban renewal and low-income housing areas. This was later extended to include organized union groups such as municipal employees and garment industry workers. PGP became best known in the Kaiser Permanente network developed for workers of Henry J. Kaiser Industries, at the Boulder Dam and Grand Coulee Dam construction sites in the 1930s. Kaiser Permanente health plans now provide care for millions of Americans in many other states. Initially opposed by the organized medical profession and the private insurance industry, PGP gained acceptance by providing high-quality, less-costly health care. This became attractive to employers and unions alike, and later to governments seeking ways to constrain increases in health costs.

Since the 1970s, the generic term *Health Maintenance Organization* (HMO) was promoted by the federal government in the HMO Act by President Richard Nixon in 1973. HMOs, which operate their own clinics and staff (i.e., the staff model), or through contracts with medical groups as Preferred Provider Organizations (PPOs), have become an accepted, if criticized, part of medical care in the United States and an important alternative to fee-for-service, private practice medicine. In 2011, 70.2 million Americans were registered in HMO plans or 22.5 percent of the total US population.

In recent years, the terms *Accountable Care Organizations (ACO)*, *Patient-Centered Medical Home (PCMH)* and *Population Health Management System (PHMS)* have come into wide use to denote organizations that take responsibility for comprehensive care for enrolled patients, with payment based on a form of capitation rather than fee-for-service. ACOs are present in all 50 states, Washington, DC, and Puerto Rico, with the population covered increasing from 2.6 million in 2011 to 23.5 million in 2015. The ACO comes in different models, but many include a hospital base and may be linked to independent practice associations (IPAs), and specialty groups, or hospital medical staff organizations, or in a network of hospitals linked with other providers as an organized delivery system. These are not-for-profit group practices led by doctors who are salaried and subject to rigorous annual professional review. This model may be adaptable on a wider scale to improve quality and cost effective care to improve health of Americans.

In 1983, a prospective payment system, called *diagnosis-related groups* (DRGs), was adopted for Medicare, to encourage more efficient use of hospital care, with payment by categories of diagnosis. The DRG is a classification system, for inpatient stays, categorizing possible diagnoses into more than 20 major body systems and subdivides them into almost 500 groups for the purpose of Medicare reimbursement. This replaced the previous system of paying by the number of hospital days, or *per diem* or by itemized billing which encouraged longer hospital stays. DRGs provided incentives for hospitals to diagnose and treat patients expeditiously and effectively. Payment for Medicare and Medicaid patients shifted to this method placed the public insurance plans in a stronger position for payments to hospitals. In many states this has also become standard for patients with private health insurance as well.

During the late 1980s, the term *Managed Care* was introduced, expanding from HMOs of the Kaiser Permanente type to include both non-profit and for-profit systems. These include Independent Practice Associations (IPAs), which operate with physicians in private practice, and Preferred Provider Organizations (PPOs), which provide insured care by doctors and other providers associated with the plan to the enrolled members or beneficiaries at negotiated prices. The DRG payment system and HMOs or managed care systems reduced hospital utilization. While total costs of health care increased in this period, without reduction of hospital utilization the increase would have been considerably higher.

In 1994, President Clinton tried to introduce a health plan based on feder ally administered compulsory universal health insurance through the place of employment. A state could opt to form its own health insurance program including through its own department of health. Physicians could contract with health insurance plans to provide care on a fixed-fee schedule, or in HMOs, whether based on group or individual practice. The Clinton health plan failed in Congress mainly due to well financed opposition by the insurance industry and the organized medical community. In addition, opposition was also widespread among the majority of the population who already had good insurance benefits under their employment-based health insurance plans or Medicare. Their interest was in keeping the status quo so that the bill was defeated.

Following the failure of the Clinton national health insurance proposal, managed care experienced tremendous growth. Managed care systems have been able to cut costs in health care in ways that the US government could not. In the US as a whole, in addition to the nearly 58 million persons enrolled in HMOs, another 91 million persons are enrolled in PPOs, with 25 percent of Medicaid and 10 percent of Medicare beneficiaries in various "managed care plans". The search for cost containment led to the development of a series of important innovations in health care delivery, payment, and information systems. HMOs demonstrated that good care provision can be operated efficiently with lower hospital admission rates than care provided on a fee-for-service basis. The managed care systems brought about profound changes in health care organization in the United States.

In 2010, President Barack Obama established the Patient Protection and Affordable Care Act/Health Care and Education Reconciliation Act of 2010, widely known as The Affordable Care Act (ACA or Obamacare) bringing health insurance to millions of previously uninsured Americans when it went into effect in 2014 (see Box 8.6). The ACA requires most companies to cover their workers, and mandates that everyone has coverage or pay a fine. ACA also requires insurance companies to accept all newcomers, regardless of any preexisting conditions, and assists people unable to afford insurance. This legislation covers young people under their parents' health insurance plans until the age of 26, covering 2.5 million young Americans. It eliminated other limits on coverage, allowing those who had already reached a lifetime limit to be eligible for coverage. The Affordable Care Act

---

BOX 8.6 Health Insurance Population Coverage in the United States: 2015

- Between 2008 and 2013, the uninsured rate was relatively stable; 42 million Americans (13.4 percent) were uninsured in 2013.
- In 2014-2015, the uninsured rate decreased due to the Affordable Care Act.
- In 2015, 9.1 percent or 29 million were uninsured for the entire calendar year.
- The percent of people with health insurance coverage for all or part of the years increased from 86.7 percent in 2013 to 90.9 percent in 2015.
- In 2015, private health insurance coverage was 67.2 percent; government coverage 37.1 percent.
- Employer-based insurance in 2015 covered the most people (55.7 percent of the population), followed by Medicaid (19.6 percent), Medicare (16.3), and direct purchase (16.3).

Source: Barnett JC, Vornovitsky MS. Current population reports P60-257(RV): health insurance coverage in the United States: 2015. US Government Printing Office: Washington, DC, 2016. Available at: https://www.census.gov/content/dam/Census/library/publications/2016/demo/p60-257.pdf (accessed 8 July 2017).

---

introduced discounts as large as 50 percent for pharmaceuticals for seniors. Health care reform is currently a contentious issue with the Donald Trump government planning to repeal the Obama health care reforms to be replaced with a plan still under development.

US health care spending increased from 13.1 percent of GDP in 1995 to 16.6 percent in 2014, threatening the ultimate insolvency of Medicare and cutbacks in Medicaid in the near future.

Social Inequities

Lack of universal access and the empowerment it potentially brings encourages an alienation or non-engagement with early health care for the socially disadvantaged sector of the population. This promotes inappropriate reliance on emergency department care and hospitalization in response to under-treated health needs. With large numbers of uninsured persons and many others lacking adequate health insurance, access and utilization of preventive care are below the levels needed to achieve social equity in health in the US. This is especially true for maternal- and child-health and for chronic diseases such as diabetes, hypertension, cancer, and heart disease. Infant mortality rates in the United States vary greatly by race and ethnicity. As measured by the infant mortality rate, the rate among non-Hispanic black mothers was 2.4 times higher than the rate for white non-Hispanic mothers. A significantly higher rate of infant mortality exists among Puerto Rican and American Indian populations compared with the national average. CDC reports that maternal mortality rates have increased in the United States between 2000 and 2013 from 14.5 to 17.3 per 100,000 live births possibly due to changes in reporting and increase in chronic illnesses and influenza during pregnancy particularly in the African American population.

In 2000, the Department of Health and Human Services (DHHS) released *Healthy People 2010* with two main goals: "increase the quality and years of healthy life" and "eliminate health disparities." These goals focus on 28 specific areas developed by over 350 national membership organizations and 250 state health, mental health, substance abuse, and environmental agencies. Many states have adopted use of these targets as their own measures of health status and performance. The US Public Health Service, in cooperation with the National Center for Health Statistics, regularly make available a wide set of data for updating health status and process measures relating to these national health goals.

Various preventive health initiatives are in place to try to alleviate health disparities, which successfully improved immunization coverage of US infants to meet national health targets, as well as for lead and other efforts directed toward poor population groups. In 2002, a program called Racial and Ethnic Adult Disparities in Immunization Initiative was introduced in order to improve influenza and pneumococcal vaccinations among minorities aged 65 and over.

The US Department of Agriculture's Women, Infants and Children (WIC) program enables millions of poor Americans to have good nutritional security. The WIC program covers pregnant women, breastfeeding women (up to infant's first birthday), non-breastfeeding postpartum women (up to 6 months after the birth of an infant or after pregnancy ends) and infants and children (up to their fifth birthday). WIC serves 53 percent of all infants born in the United States. The benefits include: Supplemental nutritious foods, nutrition education and counseling at WIC clinics, screening, and referrals to other health, welfare and social services such as completion of immunization and special needs counseling.

School lunch programs are widespread under a federally assisted meal program operating in over 100,000 public and non-profit private schools and residential child care institutions, providing nutritionally balanced, low-cost or free lunches to more than 31 million children each school day in 2012. Nutrition support for pregnant women and children in need, alleviates some of the ill effects of poverty in the United States, but lack of health insurance affects these groups severely especially in chronic disease, trauma, and other diseases of poverty.

Health disparities are a complex problem that goes beyond the issue of uninsured Americans. Low-income and illegal immigrants face challenges to access medical insurance. New immigrants must wait five years before they are eligible for Medicaid. The structure of the medical system plays an important role in an individual's ability to obtain medical care. This includes convenience of making an appointment, office hours, waiting times, and transportation. A lack of health literacy also plays a role in an individual's ability to seek medical attention. Individuals not fluent in English experience communication gaps. In 2003, it was estimated that an excess of USD $58 billion a year is spent on health care in the United States as a result of low health literacy. In certain areas of the country, medical facilities are scarce. Minorities are under-represented in medical professions. Black, Latino, and Native American populations make up approximately six percent of the physician workforce, although these populations represent over 26 percent of the population in the United States.

Health disparities remain an important social and political issue in the United States. The Office of Minority Health (OMH) of the Department of Health and Human Services was established in 1986 to address issues of health disparities among racial and ethnic minorities. Important health disparities exist in America in relation to region of residence, with the southern states having high rates of obesity, stroke, and coronary heart disease mortality, which are thought to be due to customary diets rich in fatty and salty foods. State health departments will need to address these issues in order to reduce gaps in life expectancy due to lifestyle factors which are grounded in tradition and poverty as well as lack of health insurance. One of the main goals of *Healthy People 2020* is to eliminate health disparities.

Health Information

The US has developed extensive information systems of domestic and international importance. The CDC publishes the *MMWR (Morbidity and Mortality Weekly Report)*, which sets high standards in disease reporting and policy analysis. The US National Center for Health Statistics (NCHS), the Health Care Financing Administration (HCFA), the US Public Health Service (USPHS), the Food and Drug Administration (USFDA), the National Institutes of Health (NIH), and many nongovernmental organizations (NGOs) carry out data collection, publication, and health services research activities important for health status monitoring. National nutrition surveillance and other systems of health status monitoring are reported in the professional literature and in publications of the CDC. National monitoring of hospital discharge information facilitates the understanding of patterns of utilization and morbidity. These information systems are vital for epidemiologic surveillance and managing the health care system. US Surgeon General Reports have an important influence on health systems not only in the United States, but also internationally.

The CDC created the National Center for Public Health Informatics (NCPHI) in 2005 to provide leadership and coordination of shared systems and services, to build and support a national network of integrated, standards-based, and interoperable public health information systems. This is meant to strengthen capabilities to monitor, detect, register, confirm, report, and analyze data, as well as provide feedback and alerts on important health events. This will enable partners to communicate evidence that supports decisions that impact health. Electronic medical and personal health records are now widely used. These protect patient privacy and confidentiality, and serve legitimate clinical and public health needs.

Media coverage of health-related topics is extensive, and is important to promote health consciousness in the public. However, the sheer volume of information may make it difficult to discern which information is most relevant, and due to misinformation on internet sites, can also create opposition to public health initiatives such as the refusal to vaccinate children. Public levels of health knowledge grow steadily, but vary widely by social class and educational levels.

US Health Targets

In 1979, the US Surgeon General's Report *Healthy People* set a series of national health targets for a wide variety of public health issues. The program defined 226 objectives in 15 program areas within the three categories of prevention, protection, and promotion. These goals and objectives were formulated based on research and consultation by experts in different fields who participated in a conference by the US Public Health Service. Consensus is based on position papers, studies, and conferences involving the national governmental health agencies, the National Academy of Science Institute of Medicine, and professional organizations such as the American Academy of Pediatrics (AAP), the US Preventive Health Services Task Force, and the American College of Obstetrics and Gynecology (ACOG). Many private individuals and organizations contribute to this effort, including state and local health agencies, representatives of consumer and provider groups, academic centers, and voluntary health associations.

These targets are periodically assessed as performance indicators of the US health system and then updated. Progress made during the 1980s included major reductions in death rates for three of the leading causes of death: heart disease, stroke, and unintentional injuries. Infant mortality decreased, as did the incidence of vaccine-preventable infectious diseases.

The latest iteration, *Healthy People 2020*, identifies national health priorities. It strives to increase public awareness and understanding of the determinants of health, disease, disability, and opportunities for progress. It defines measurable objectives and goals for Federal, State, and local authorities in the areas of health promotion, health protection, preventive services, surveillance and data systems, and age-related and special population groups. The final reviews of *Healthy People 2000* showed significant decreases in mortality from coronary heart disease and cancer. *Healthy People 2020* renews this effort to establish national targets which are adopted by state level governments and strongly influence policy in health insurance systems.

The US has managed to achieve many of the targets set by the 1979 Surgeon General's *Healthy People* report. At the same time, the average annual increases in health care expenditures in the United States slowed markedly from the 1986–90 period with average annual increases of 10.7 percent, falling to under 7 percent annually between 1995 and 2005. This is partly due to lower general inflation rates ($<3\%$), but also cost-containment measures being adopted by government insurance (Medicare and Medicaid) programs, the health insurance industry, the growth of managed care, and rationalizing the hospital sector by downsizing and promoting lower-cost alternative forms of care.

National health insurance was delayed by congressional rejection of the Clinton health plan. President Barack Obama's 2010 Affordable Care Act (ACA) provided millions of previously uninsured Americans health insurance within better regulated private insurance or in state-run Medicaid plans, but in 2017 is facing "repeal and replace" efforts by the President Trump administration and Republican Congress. A number of possibilities exist to extend health insurance coverage: state health insurance initiatives with federal waivers and cost-sharing; a federal single payer universal coverage plan based on the federal Medicare model or a federal-state Medicaid model.

Summary of the US Health System

The US health system is often called a costly and inefficient nonsystem. There are many stakeholders and providers, high costs, and poorer population health results than those achieved in other industrialized countries such as Britain, Germany, and Canada. The health system is diffused with high levels of coverage for diverse insurance plans through employment-based insurance along with publicly financed and administered health insurance (e.g., Medicare, Medicaid, ACA). Inequalities are a significant health challenge in the US along with the uninsured, poverty, aging of the population, rising levels of obesity and diabetes. The principle of universal access through public insurance for all is still a highly politicized issue in the United States, although public acceptance seems to be gradually growing.

The US has a reputation for good to outstanding quality of medical care, but for those without insurance, services are limited to hospital emergency care only. Important ethnic, social, and regional inequities in health status are still present, but not necessarily greater than in countries with universal access health care plans such as the UK NHS. Further, there are many parallel programs in the United States that have important positive public health content, such as universal school lunch programs, nutrition support for poor women, infants, and children (the WIC program); food stamps for the working poor; fortification of basic foods, free care for the uninsured in emergency departments, Medicare for the elderly, Medicaid for the poor, and ACA coverage for the near-poor. Box 8.7 shows the challenges of the US health system.

Despite rapid increases in health care expenditures during the 1970s and 1980s, despite improved health promotion activities and rapidly developing medical technology, the health status of the American population

---

BOX 8.7   US Health System: Challenges and Strengths

Challenges
- Lack of universal health coverage;
- Total per capita cost of US health system is by far the highest in the world;
- Private insurance at place of employment for majority of population or individual purchase;
- Public insurance or service plans for high-risk population groups; elderly, poor, veterans, and military populations cover over one-third of the total population;
- Uninsured for 2015 was 9.1 percent; the insured coverage for all or part of the year was 90.1 percent;
- Mediocre performance in overall life expectancy, infant mortality compared with many other countries;
- Rising obesity, diabetes, and other health risk factors;
- High administrative costs for private insurance;
- Rural and ethnic populations disadvantaged in access to care and avoidable mortality;
- Political deadlock on the way ahead;
- Likely reduction in insured coverage of cancelled or revise ACA;
- Single payer systems with competitive systems of providing care could limit cost increases;
- Universal coverage unlikely in the near term but could evolve state by state, or federally through Medicare

Strengths
- Insurance coverage for some 91 percent of US population; 9% uninsured;
- High standards of medical and related professional care;
- High levels of academic standards in professional training;
- Innovative management systems;
- Public health leadership, research, publication innovative, and high quality medical teaching centers across the country;
- Excellence in medical research performance including vaccine development;
- Preventive programs strong tradition; screening for cancer; smoking reduction; food fortification, school lunch programs; nutrition support for poor pregnant women and children (WIC);
- Hospitals obliged to provide emergency care to all regardless of insurance status, citizenship, legal status or ability to pay

has improved less rapidly than that in other western countries and universal coverage has not been achieved. US performance measures are lower than many middle- and high-income countries with much lower per capita health expenditures, including measures such as infant mortality rates and life expectancy. Infant mortality in the US remains high in comparison to OECD countries and ranks 34th among all countries in 2012 (estimated). Even the rate of infant mortality of the white population of the United States was higher than that of 16 countries that spent much less per person and a lesser percentage of GNP per capita on health care. Life expectancy at birth in the United States in 2014 was below that of 24 countries, just behind Costa Rica, Portugal and Slovenia. In 2014, the US life expectancy at birth was 78.8 years, well below the OECD average of 81.6 years.

Social inequities in these health status indicators are further evidence of failures of the United States health system to reach its full potential, despite its being the costliest system in the world and its high quality for those with access (Commonwealth Fund, 2008). The advent of the ACA (Obamacare) introduced in 2010 brought health insurance to millions of Americans, but is challenged as unaffordable. The US still lacks a universal single payer health plan of Canadian or European tradition, but the ACA is a huge step forward in America where the working poor are in large measure excluded from access to health care except for emergencies. The struggle for universal access and cost containment are still formidable political and societal challenges for the United States.

Russian Federation: The Semashko Model

In 1918, following the Russian revolution, the Soviet Union (USSR) introduced its national health plan for universal coverage within a state-run system of health protection. The Soviet model, designed and implemented by Nikolai Semashko, provided free health care for all as a government-financed and -organized service. It brought free health services to the population, with a system of primary- and secondary-care based on the principles of universal and equitable access to care through district organization of services. It achieved control of epidemic and endemic infectious diseases and expanded services into the most remote areas of the vast under-developed country. This model was also applicable in countries included in the USSR following World War II until the collapse of the USSR.

The model developed in the former Soviet Union in 1917 by Semashko brought free health care with governmental management by republic and regional authorities according to national norms set out by the Ministry of Finance. Since the 1930s health care became available for all with mostly underdeveloped basic infrastructure for health care including human resources.

The Semashko plan provided universal access to preventive and curative care, and control of infectious disease in a uniform plan, with many republics previously having only primitive care available, achieving national standards of services and improved health indicators. Since the 1960s, an "epidemiologic transition" was occurring characterized by declining mortality from infectious diseases and rising death rates from non-infectious diseases. Life expectancy increased since 1995, still remains far below levels in many medium-income developed countries.

The transition in health systems following the collapse of the Soviet Union in 1991 took different paths for the socialist Central and Eastern European countries (CEE) as compared to the core countries of the Soviet Union, called the Commonwealth of Independent States (CIS). The CEE countries moved rapidly to dismantle their Soviet, centrally managed sanitary-epidemiological system (Sanepid) system with decentralization while retaining universal coverage with central funding, but with local authority participation in some cases. Most CEE and CIS countries have introduced health insurance systems, with more out-of-pocket payments (both formal and informal), and efforts to strengthen primary health care, with family medicine delivered by general practitioners. In most cases central authorities also maintained responsibility for epidemiological surveillance and environmental monitoring with some transferring responsibilities for environmental health in other ministries. The CEE and CIS countries maintained similar levels of health expenditures as percent of GDP between six and seven percent over the past decade, while the original European Union (EU) countries reached an average of 10 percent of GDP.

The CIS acute care hospital bed capacity ratio declined to six per 1000 population in 2014 far higher than CEE countries (declined to 4.6 per 1000), which were higher than the western countries, although all country groups were declining (see Chapter 15). The importance of these differences lies in the fact that total resources allocated for health in the Soviet system was relatively low while the allocation allowed hospital care to consume some 70 percent of total expenditures compared with less than 50 percent in western countries. The outcome of this allocation of resources was weakness in development of primary care, prevention and community care in favor of an over-developed hospital bed supply.

The Russian Federation adopted a mandatory health insurance (MHI) plan in 1993 to open up additional funding for health care in the face of severe governmental funding constraints. It remains a highly centralized system and is struggling to provide universal access to basic care. Despite this, death rates from avoidable causes such as stroke and coronary heart disease have declined in the past decade and life expectancy has risen modestly, but remaining far below western as well as former socialist countries of Central and Eastern Europe. Fig 8.2 shows the differences in life expectancy of the three groups of countries with the Countries of Eastern Europe (CEE)

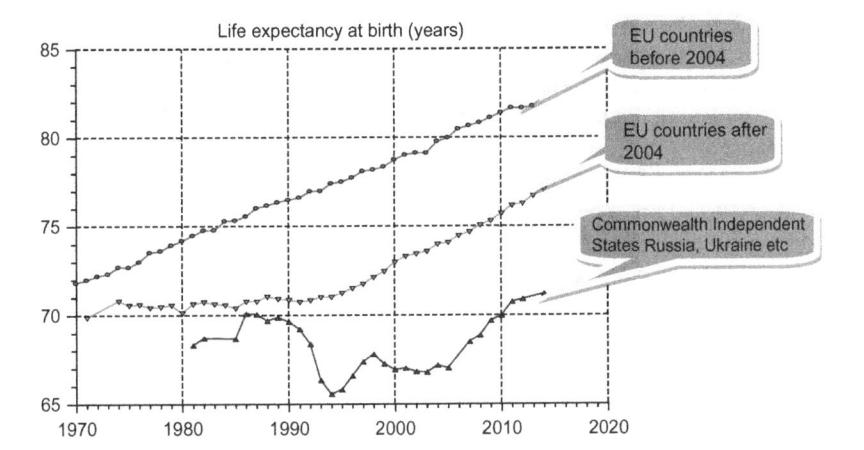

FIGURE 8.2   Life expectancy at birth, EU, EU/EEC and CIS 1970−2013. *Source: Health for All Database. Available at: http://data.euro.who.int/hfadb/ (accessed 5 May 2017).*

(countries which joined the European Union after 2004) improving rapidly since the 1990s.

CURRENT RELEVANCE

Developing national health systems with universal access has been a long process in high-income countries and is an important goal for all countries including medium- and low-income countries to promote improving access to health for the total population. The Commonwealth Fund published an outstanding international profile of selected health care systems in high-income countries (2015) including: Australia, Canada, China, Denmark, England, France, Germany, India, Israel, Italy, Japan, The Netherlands, New Zealand, Norway, Singapore, Sweden, Switzerland, and the United States.

Global spending on health is expected to increase from US$7.83 trillion in 2013 to $18.28 (uncertainty interval 14.42−22.24) trillion in 2040 (in 2010 purchasing power parity−adjusted dollars). We expect per-capita health spending to increase annually by 2.7% (1.9−3.4) in high-income countries, 3.4% (2.4−4.2) in upper middle-income countries, 3.0% (2.3−3.6) in lower middle-income countries, and 2.4% (1.6−3.1) in low-income countries.

Low- and medium-income countries face major difficulties in developing universal health coverage, especially in terms of financial and professional resources. A study of global health care financing (Dielman et al Lancet 2016) reported on health expenditures from 184 countries, including public, donor, and private ("out of pocket") payments between 1995 and 2014. High-income countries spent more, and mostly from public sources, increasing expenditures by an estimated three percent per year. Medium income countries increased their health spending more than three-four percent per year and low-income countries by two percent. Economic development was positively associated with total health spending and a gradual shift away from a reliance on development assistance and out-of-pocket spending towards government spending. In 2014, 59.2 percent of all health spending was financed by the government, although in low-income and lower-middle-income countries, 29 percent and 58 percent of spending was out-of-pocket, 35.7 percent and three percent respectively was with development assistance. Recent growth in development assistance for health has been tepid. Between 2010 and 2016, it grew annually at 1.8 percent, and reached USD $37 · 6 billion in 2016. Nonetheless, there is a great deal of variation revolving around these averages. In 2016 countries spending less than five percent of GDP on health, included many in Asia, the Middle East and sub-Saharan Africa (Institute of Health Metrics and Evaluation, 2016).

While there is wide variation in health spending in low- and lower-middle-income countries and there is overall increased spending in absolute terms, there is still a heavy reliance on out-of-pocket spending and development assistance, which itself is growing very slowly. This indicates that medium- and low-income countries are not providing the financial means to develop universal health access insurance plans. Economic growth also does not translate into adequate funding for universal health care without dramatic changes in policy and decreased dependency on donor aid.

International agencies—such as WHO—are promoting the search for ways to provide universal and equitable care, while controlling costs and improving efficiency in low- and middle-income countries.

ETHICAL ISSUES

The 1948 Universal Declaration of Human Rights, Article 25 states:

"(1) Everyone has the right to a standard of living adequate for the health and well-being of himself and of his family, including food, clothing, housing and medical care and necessary social services, and the right to security in the event of unemployment, sickness, disability, widowhood, old age or other lack of livelihood in circumstances beyond his control.
(2) Motherhood and childhood are entitled to special care and assistance. All children, whether born in or out of wedlock, shall enjoy the same social protection."

The Universal Declaration of Human Rights specific inclusion of access to medical care for all should be seen as a priority in planning universal health insurance (UHI) for promotion of access to health needs for remote rural populations as well as urban poor, and displaced persons. This also applies to conditions of warfare, civil strife, natural disasters as well as incitement to and actual genocide.

As said previously, the global consensus of the MDGs (2000–15) and the SDGs (2015–30) have undertaken to implement key elements of this important declaration. It is easier to be pessimistic than optimistic in the potential for success, but the significant achievements of the MDGs in poverty reduction, educational equity between the genders and in reduction of child and maternal mortality as well as in control of HIV, malaria and tuberculosis are signs of important progress and future possibilities. National governments must take up the financial burdens and management of expanding health systems as well as contributory advances in education, environment and other government sectors toward achieving these goals. Bilateral aid and international donors are vital, but they cannot achieve or sustain all this without national commitments and resources.

National health systems are essential to provide universal access to health care, but must be developed recognizing that restraint in increasing costs, equity in access and quality, as well as efficiency and effectiveness in use of resources are vital to achieve health targets and equity in population health. In the United States, a study of ethnic differences in utilization of services among Medicare beneficiaries who have the same entitlements show significant differences indicating lesser use of preventive services such as mammography and higher rates of lower limb amputation for diabetes indicating poorer management of diabetes. Studies in the United Kingdom also show sharp differences in mortality rates by region of residence that correlate with socioeconomic gradations. Universal access alone does not guarantee equality so that the design of service systems needs to take into account differing needs of groups or regions at higher risk and greater need. Universal access by itself is important, but not sufficient to reduce inequalities, which have more complex needs than medical care alone.

Universal coverage health insurance must be developed with great care to avoid mistakes made in many countries in previous decades of promoting rapid increase in health expenditures to the benefit of the middle class while rural and poor urban populations linger in relatively poor health. A universal health insurance plan without strong incentives for prevention and community health will find itself in a trap of punishing the poor for the benefit of the rich. Population health experience of the past century has shown the power of public health, in all its aspects, to raise life expectancy and quality, yet inequalities still plague all health systems. This provides an ethical challenge in planning, resource allocation and political support.

Beyond financing and resource allocation, there are many "nontariff" barriers to health. Even in highly developed national health systems, social class, place of residence, education level, and ethnicity play significant roles in morbidity and mortality rates. Addressing important health risk factors other than medical or hospital care is vital. The disease-risk factors of diet, smoking, physical fitness, nutrition status including obesity, and untreated hypertension. Such conditions are not necessarily managed even where all residents of a country are insured for health care. Social class, ethnic and regional differences in morbidity and mortality exist due to poverty-associated factors, such as insecurity, lack of control over one's life, lack of financial means or knowledge to purchase healthy foods, as well as fear, loneliness and depression. These are issues that are important and must be addressed in public health policy to reduce inequalities in health and the achievement of national health goals and equity.

ECONOMIC ISSUES

Models of financing of universal health insurance include a variety of methods: general taxation; social security by employee-employer payments through payroll deductions; private insurance under contracts between employee and employer; and private out-of-pocket payments. Taxation financing can be mainly through progressive income tax, resource taxes, surcharges or "sin taxes" (e.g., on cigarettes, alcohol, gasoline) and excise taxes along with local property and business licensing taxation where local authorities have a management role. Funding by general tax revenues at national or state levels or shared between the two levels provides for more local administration while sharing in costs may be the most equitable way of raising funds. Many countries use social security systems based on employer–employee contributions to pay for health services.

The WHO, the World Bank and OECD promote universal health insurance (UHI) for middle-income countries. The advantage will be to reduce the heavy burden of out-of-pocket payments, which are 60 percent of health expenditures in many emerging countries. Universal health insurance provides security for individuals and families against catastrophic health events, for regular medical and hospital care, and for ageing populations with increasing health needs. OECD recommends increasing health expenditures, which improves life expectancy, and to allow UHI implementation. Even a 10 percent increase in national health spending has been shown to reduce child mortality across many countries. Universal health insurance must include promotion of greater efficiency in health care, such as shifting of services from hospital care to outpatient and primary care along with community and home-based care (see Chapter 15). The process requires developing new health care provider roles with emphasis on outreach to groups with greater than average need, promoting public health and preventive care such as for underserved rural or urban communities or groups at special risk for disease such as cardiovascular disease (CVD) and diabetes, making use of epidemiologic and sociologic health data and information systems.

Universal health insurance undoubtedly contributes to improving health indicators such as life expectancy by coverage of the total population, systematizing financing of the health system and providing access to the population. However, without good management of resource allocation, universal health insurance cannot guarantee achievement of important health targets. Allocation of resources is a fundamental problematic aspect of universal health insurance. National health policy governing universal health insurance must invest adequately in health promotion and disease prevention in order to reduce excessive allocation and utilization of hospital care.

Continuous monitoring and evaluation are essential to a health system, but not only for traditional outcome indicators, such as infant, child and maternal mortality rates, and disease-specific mortality rates. These are all valuable indicators of population health, but not sufficient. Input, process and outcome indicators are important and necessary to include, such as supply and distribution of resources e.g., primary care, maternity centers, hospital beds; process measures e.g., immunization rates, incidence of vaccine-preventable diseases, growth patterns and anemia rates in infancy and childhood, food fortification, micronutrient supplements to risk group, prenatal delivery and neonatal care. Outcome measures include prevalence of disabling conditions morbidity and mortality rates. Disability Adjusted Life Years (DALYs) and Quality Adjusted Life Years (QALYs) help change the emphasis from mortality to quality of life measures as part of the evaluation. National health systems require data systems that generate information needed for this continuous process of monitoring. Monitoring of hospitalizations, length of stay, health-care facility acquired (nosocomial) infection, readmission rate by diagnosis and many more indicators, compliance with standards of care such as in infection control, surgical and maternal mortality, including infection and error rates, and other qualitative measures are now part of monitoring and payment systems. High-quality academic centers are needed for training epidemiologic, sociologic, and economic analyses professionals as well as health system managers and to carry out the studies and research vital for health progress.

Health systems are large-scale employers and among the largest economic sectors in their respective countries, with $7-16$ percent of GDP in middle- and high-income countries and, therefore, a major factor in the total national economy. But the gap between countries is very high. Many countries have per capita spending of less than USD $100 per year, so that inadequate resources prevent people from receiving quality health care, without unaffordable out of pocket expenditures. In contrast, in many high-income countries annual health expenditures are above USD $5,000 per capita. Donor aid to low-income countries from bilateral or international agencies or other donors rose rapidly from 2000 with an estimated $10 billion USD to a peak of USD $37 billion in 2012, with only a modest change up to 2016.

Low-income nations, many of which are undergoing important economic development, are under-spending in national allocations to the health sector and remain highly reliant on international aid. A goal of five to six percent of GDP spent on health is widely regarded as a minimum to provide the health care needed in any country. A 2016 study published in Lancet by the

Institute for Health Metrics and Evaluation, indicates that only one of 37 low-income countries, and 36 out of 98 of middle-income countries, are expected to meet the target of five percent. Low rates of national health expenditures in countries will be a serious limiting factor in improved health and universal access, especially if preventive care is unable to compete for resources as compared to clinical and hospital services.

CONCLUSION

All countries face problems of financing, cost constraint, overcoming structural inefficiencies, and funding incentives for high quality and efficiency in health services. National health systems are necessarily complex, but go well beyond medical and hospital care. The quality of the community infrastructure—sewage, water, roads, communication, urban planning—social support such as pensions and welfare for the disabled, widows, orphans and others in need are essential for population health. Attention to the quantity and quality of food (i.e., food and nutritional security), levels of education, and professional organization are all parts of this continuum.

National health systems are not only a matter of adequacy and methods of financing and assuring access to services; they must also address health promotion, national health targets, and adapt to the changing needs of the population, the environment, and with a broad intersectoral approach to health of the population and the individual. The structure, content, and quality of a health system plays a vital role in the social and economic development of a society and its quality of life.

Universal access is increasingly widely accepted as essential to reduce the social inequalities in health. even when income gaps are high. However, vulnerable populations with higher levels of risk than those of the general population are still relatively deprived even under classical universal insurance systems. The key common factors of elevated vulnerability are poverty, isolation by geographic location, physical access by reasons of residency location, ethnicity, education and institutional barriers which reduce access. These inequality factors are the Achilles heel of classical universal health insurance and service systems most of which have sought health promotion measures. There can be little doubt that universal access to health insurance or service systems reduces inequalities, but they require imaginative and outreach-oriented approaches to reach those urban and rural poor, people of aboriginal descent, those with an income lower than the poverty threshold, the unemployed, the homeless, and those who have not completed secondary education.

Societal programs to increase family disposable income for the poor are effective in reducing the health inequities. The two are complementary and equally important in social policy. In the United States more than ten percentages of the population are without any, or have inadequate, health insurance. Loss of health coverage with change of place of employment and the rapidly increasing cost of private health insurance generated widespread pressure for a national health program. The business community, too, loses confidence in voluntary health insurance as costs of health insurance mounted rapidly and as a cost of employment in an increasingly harms the competitive international business climate.

Narrow planning for health systems ignores this message at the risk of missing their targets of improved health indicators, such as those adopted by the United Nations—i.e., the Millennium Development Goals and Sustainable Development Goals. The MDGs and SDGs represent a growing movement of globalization of health with economic and political dimensions and greater stress on human rights to health policy. They are particularly relevant to LMICs (low- and middle-income countries), but high-income countries have health inequalities that require new approaches based on outreach poverty abatement, and health promotion concepts. MDGs and SDGs presented a challenge to establish common data systems for performance measures to monitor effectiveness of policies and programs. This helps to build capacity for target-oriented health planning in low- and middle-income countries (LMICS). A holistic view of Health for All must take into account the many reasons for health disparities and disadvantage to the poor in health status. Insurance to pay for doctors, hospitals, laboratories and imaging centers is necessary, but not sufficient, to raise population health standards for all. The "nontariff barriers"—i.e., issues beyond payment for services which may be addressed with incentives in payment systems, not only to reduce hospital length-of-stay, but to reduce health-care acquired infections, reaching out to chronically ill people with health promotion measures such as nutritional support, pneumonia and influenza immunization, hypertension control, cancer screening, and many other features of public health promotion.

Since the 1880s, when Bismarck introduced national health insurance in Germany as part of Social Security with funding though Sick Funds, many countries have grappled in unique ways with developing health care systems. National health insurance systems developed through social security and social welfare systems, by national health insurance, or options to provide access to health services. In Canada national health insurance provides universal coverage through national support for provincial health plans, paid for by general taxation, with national criteria. In the United States, President Lyndon Johnson established Social Security-based health insurance for the elderly and the poor through amendments to the Social Security Act of 1935, and President Barack Obama extended health insurance through the Affordable Care Act of 2010. The UK National Health Service—with the Northern Ireland, Scottish and Welsh NHS run semi-independently—was established in 1948, providing a state-run system of medical, hospital, preventive, and community health care. Though not discussed here, Nordic and other European health systems provide universal coverage with involvement from all three levels of government, but over 80 percent of expenditures are funded through public sources. In Denmark, Norway and Sweden county councils are central to funding and management; in Finland, the municipalities provide most of the health care.

The former socialist countries have gone through painful periods of transition. Many of these countries have developed free-market systems with dynamic growth in national economies along with health system reform. Health systems in transition have adapted with great gains in longevity and reduced mortality from preventable diseases in many former socialist countries in Central and Eastern Europe. Others have had difficulties addressing the "missed epidemiologic transition" from infectious disease to control of non-communicable disease but have begun to make progress in the 21st century.

Globally, public and private donor partnerships have emerged to help the poorest countries cope with overwhelming health problems of raising immunization coverage levels, reducing child and maternal mortality, managing HIV, tuberculosis, malaria, diarrheal and respiratory diseases and vaccine-preventable diseases in keeping with the MDGs based on a consensus of all member nations of the UN. The objectives and specific targets included: reducing poverty, improving equal access of boys and girls to primary education, reducing child and maternal mortality, managing significant diseases such as HIV, tuberculosis, and malaria, along with improving the environment. Reaching the targets for achieving these goals depends on developing infrastructures of health systems that provide access for all and distribution to meet geographic and social inequities in health. Each country needs to develop its own system, but can learn from the experience of others. The purpose of this case study is to highlight the unique and common features, including positive and negative lessons learned from national health systems. Observing and learning can help in defining needs for countries lacking but aspiring to achieve universal health systems, including positive and negative challenges.

Universal access is an important means of assuring that the economic barrier is removed for the total population, leading to increased access to medical and hospital services for those previously lacking the means to reach these services. Universal access systems have been achieved in most industrialized countries. However, the US has not achieved this goal even with, by far, the highest health expenditures of OECD countries. This is due mainly to political gridlock despite success with its single payer system for Medicare for the elderly. For low-income countries, the rates of health expenditures at present and forecast for the coming decades will be insufficient to achieve universal access systems. There must be a fundamental political change in national policies with health as a higher priority for funding and leadership. Universal healthcare access is still a work in progress.

The goal of universal access is a worthy one: to make health care accessible to all. The advent of universal access, however, is not assured given low levels of funding in many countries most in need of improved access but relying heavily on donors and out-of-pocket payments. The devil is in the details.

RECOMMENDATIONS

1. Universal health insurance (UHI) or national health service systems are essential for advancing population health and should be give high priority in policy and funding by national governments and international aid agencies in middle- and low-income countries in the coming decades.
2. Universal health insurance or service systems cannot be expected to succeed without continuing development of public health and health promotion as equal needs for population health and to achieve SDGs.
3. All countries seeking health development will need to raise public support for financing health systems by raising health expenditures to more than five - six percent of GDP.
4. All countries addressing these issues should endeavor to expand training to include bachelor and master degree training in public health and health systems management in order to raise the professional leadership and management levels to lead in the complexities of health systems in the challenges ahead.
5. Health system development must provide a balance of services from Health Promotion to Hospice care on par with acute and rehabilitation care hospitals as essential, but managed so as to avoid unnecessary economic domination of the health system and potentially damaging health-care infections and trauma.
6. Reaching out to populations-at-risk and in need of preventive care and health promotion by multi-professional and paraprofessional teams—e.g., community health workers, is vital to address chronic care needs and prevent their complications, for remote villages or urban poverty areas, or to groups of people with chronic disease conditions.
7. Health information systems including development and implementation of epidemiology and information technology for monitoring of disease and quality of care require emphasis.
8. Immunization and nutritional support for prevention of infectious diseases, chronic diseases and micronutrient deficiency conditions are crucial for population health and should be given high priority in health system development.
9. Health policy management is vital to achieving universal health coverage to advance population health, but it must be seen as part of Health in All strategies and the SDGs to be effective within financial limitations and cost restraint.
10. Health promotion must be developed in all its aspects to raise population and professional awareness with educational and legal means to reduce risk factors in population health.

STUDENT REVIEW QUESTIONS

1. Describe the major international models of national health systems, including:
   a. Bismarckian—Social Security employment based compulsory health insurance.
   b. Beveridge—National Health Service tax-based—UK, Spain, Italy.
   c. Semashko—Soviet model—state health service plus national health insurance.
   d. National health insurance—Canadian model of tax-based, universal coverage, provincial administration, with federal standards and cost sharing.
   e. Mixed public private insurance systems—US Medicare, Medicaid and Affordable Care Act—with majority holding private insurance through place of work.

2. What is the importance of the following measures in comparing national health systems?
   a. GDP per capita.
   b. Percent GDP spent on health;
   c. Hospital bed to population ratio.
   d. Doctor to population ratio.

3. What statistical monitoring methods may be incorporated into national health systems to promote efficient use of resources and achievement of specified health targets?

4. What methods may be incorporated into national health systems to promote quality of care?

5. How can developing countries achieve universal health care, and at the same time work toward national health targets such as upgrading maternal and child heath, control of infectious diseases and preventing chronic diseases?

6. How can low-income countries address the low public expenditure on health to reduce dependence on global financial aid for Sustainable Development Goals (SDGs)?

RECOMMENDED READINGS

1. Alliance for Health Policy and Systems Research. Strengthening health systems: the role and promise of policy and systems research. Geneva: Global Forum for Health Research, 2004. Available at: http://www.who.int/alliance-hpsr/resources/Strengthening_complet.pdf (accessed 14 June 2017).

2. Alliance for Health Systems Policy and Research. World Health Organization. What is health policy and systems research (HPSR)? 2017. Geneva: World Health Organization. Available at: http://www.who.int/alliance-hpsr/about/hpsr/en/ (accessed 7 July 2017).

3. American College of Physicians. Achieving a high-performance health care system with universal access: What the United States can learn from other countries. Ann Int Med. 2008;148:1–21. Available at: http://www.academia.edu/29544533/Achieving_a_High-Performance_Health_Care_System_with_Universal_Access_What_the_United_States_Can_Learn_from_Other_Countries (accessed 14 June 2017).

4. Anderson GF, Hussey PS, Frogner BK, Waters HR. Health spending in the United States and the rest of the industrialized world. Health Aff. 2005;24(4):903–914. Available at: http://content.healthaffairs.org/content/24/4/903.abstract (accessed 14 June 2017).

5. Anell A. The public–private pendulum—patient choice and equity in Sweden. N Engl J Med. 2015;372(1):2–4. Available at: http://www.nejm.org/doi/pdf/10.1056/NEJMp 1411430 (accessed 2 May 2017).

6. Bambra C. UK health divides–Where you live can kill you 30 December 2016. The socialist health care association. Available at: https://www.sochealth.co.uk/2016/12/30/health-divides-live-can-kill/ (accessed 15 June 2017).

7. Banks J, Marmot M, Oldfield Z, Smith JP. Disease and disadvantage in the United States and in England. JAMA. 2006;295:2037–2045. Available at: http://jamanetwork.com/journals/jama/fullarticle/202788 (accessed 14 June 2017).

8. Blumenthal D, Hsiao W. Lessons from the East—China's rapidly evolving health care system. N Engl J Med. 2015;372:1281–1285. Available at: http://www.nejm.org/doi/full/10.1056/NEJMp1410425 (accessed 2 May 2017).

9. Blumenthal D, Abrams MK, Nuzum R. The affordable care act at five years. N Engl J Med. 2015;371:2451–2458. Available at: http://www.nejm.org/doi/full/10.1056/NEJMhpr1503614#t = article (accessed 14 June 2017).

10. Brekke KR, Nuscheler R, Straume OR. Gatekeeping in health care. J Health Econ. 2007;26:149–170. Available at: https://repositorium.sdum.uminho.pt/bitstream/1822/6828/1/Brekke_Nuscheler_Straume_2007_JHE.pdf (accessed 9 May 2017).

11. Breslow L. The organization of personal health services. Milbank Quart. 2005;83:759–777. Available at: http://onlinelibrary.wiley.com/doi/10.1111/j.1468-0009.2005.00399.x/full (accessed 9 May 2017).

12. Boytsov S. Noncommunicable diseases: stepping up the fight: how the Russian Federation is collaborating with other Commonwealth of Independent States' countries. Bull World Health Org. 2015;93:9–10. Available at: http://www.who.int/bulletin/volumes/93/1/15-030115.pdf (accessed 12 May 2017).

13. Brown LD. Comparing health systems in four countries: lessons for the United States. Am J Public Health. 2003;93:52–56. Available at: https://www.ncbi.nlm.nih.gov/pmc/articles/PMC1447691/pdf/0930052.pdf (accessed 6 May 2017).

14. Busse R, Blümel M. Germany: health system review. Health Syst Tran. 2014;16(2):1–296. Available at: http://www.euro.who.int/__data/assets/pdf_file/0008/255932/HiT-Germany.pdf?ua = 1 (accessed 13 May 2014).

15. Busse R, Blümel M, Knieps F, Bärnighausen T. Germany and health 1: statutory health insurance in Germany: a health system shaped by 135 years of solidarity, self-governance, and competition. Lancet. 2017;390:882–897. Published Online July 3, 2017 https://doi.org/10.1016/S0140-6736(17)31280-1. Available at: http://www.thelancet.com/pdfs/journals/lancet/PIIS0140-6736(17)31280-1.pdf (accessed 13 November 2017).

16. Canadian Broadcasting Corporation. CBC Digital Archives. Available at: http://www.cbc.ca/archives/entry/and-the-greatest-canadian-of-all-time-is (accessed 10 May 2017).

17. Canadian Institute for Health Information. report January 2016. Available at: https://www.cihi.ca/sites/default/files/document/commonwealth_fund_2015_pdf_en.pdf (accessed .How Canada compares: results from the Commonwealth Fund 2015 international health policy survey of primary care physicians. Ottawa, ON: CIHI, 12 May 2017

18. Centers for Disease Control and Prevention. Healthy People 2020: topic areas at a glance. National Center for Health Statistics, last reviewed 6 November 2015. Available at: https://www.cdc.gov/nchs/healthy_people/hp2020/hp2020_topic_areas.htm (accessed 9 May 2017).

19. Centers for Medicare and Medicaid Services (CMS). National health expenditure fact sheet, last modified 21 March 2017. Available at: https://www.cms.gov/research-statistics-data-and-systems/statistics-trends-and-reports/nationalhealthexpenddata/nhe-fact-sheet.html (accessed 9 May 2017).

20. Clarfield M, Bin Nun G, Shvartz S, Azzam Z, Afek A, Basis F, et al. Health and health care in Israel: an introduction. Lancet. 2017. special series May 2017: 7−17. Available at: http://www.thelancet.com/series/health-in-israel (accessed 16 June 2017).

21. Commonwealth Fund. International health care system profiles, 2016. Available at: http://international.commonwealthfund.org/ (accessed 15 June 2017).

22. Commonwealth Fund. 2015 International profiles of health care systems. Available at: http://www.commonwealthfund.org/~/media/files/publications/fund-report/2016/jan/1857_mossialos_intl_profiles_2015_v7.pdf (accessed 15 June 2017).

23. Cylus J, Richardson E, Findley L, Longley M, O'Neill C, Steel D. United Kingdom: Health system review. Health Syst Trans. 2015;17(5):1−125. Available at: http://www.euro.who.int/__data/assets/pdf_file/0006/302001/UK-HiT.pdf?ua = 1 (accessed 13 May 2017).

24. Danishevski K, McKee M. Reforming the Russian health care system. Lancet. 2005;365 (9464):1012−1014. Available at: http://www.thelancet.com/journals/lancet/article/PIIS0140-6736(05)71120-X/fulltext (accessed 13 May 2017).

25. Danishevski K, Balabanova D, McKee M, Atkinson S. The fragmentary federation: experiences with the decentralized health system in Russia. Health Policy Plan. 2006;21 (3):183−194. Available at: https://academic.oup.com/heapol/article/21/3/183/654580/The-fragmentary-federation-experiences-with-the (accessed 13 May 2017).

26. Deber RB. Health care reform: lessons from Canada. Am J Public Health. 2003;93:20−24. Available at: https://www.ncbi.nlm.nih.gov/pmc/articles/PMC1447685/ (accessed 6 May 2017).

27. Declaration of Alma-Ata International Conference on Primary Health Care, Alma-Ata, September 1978, Alma Ata USSR. Available at: http://www.who.int/publications/almaata_declaration_en.pdf (accessed 21 April 2017).

28. DeWitt L. The development of Social Security in America. Social Security Administration. Soc Sec Bull. 2010;70(3). Available at: https://www.ssa.gov/policy/docs/ssb/v70n3/v70n3p1.html (accessed 9 May 2017.

29. Dieleman JL, Templin T, Sadat N, Reidy P, Evans T, Murray CJ, et al. National spending on health by source for 184 countries between 2013 and 2040. Lancet. 2016;387 (10037):2521−2535. Available at: https://www.ncbi.nlm.nih.gov/pubmed/27086174 (accessed 17 May 2017).

30. Ellis A, Fry R. Regional health inequalities in England. UK Office for National Statistics, Department of Health, 2010. Available at: https://link.springer.com/article/10.1057/rt.2010.5 (accessed 16 June 2017.

31. European Parliament. Health care systems in the EU: a comparative study. Directorate General for Research, May 2017. Available at: http://www.europarl.europa.eu/working-papers/saco/pdf/101_en.pdf (accessed 13 June 2017).

32. Evans TG, Kieny MP. Systems science for universal health coverage. Bull World Health Org. 2017;95:484. Available at: http://www.who.int/bulletin/volumes/95/7/17-192542.pdf?ua=1 (accessed 7 July 2017).

33. Feacham R. Health systems special edition. Health systems: more evidence, more debate. Bull World Health Organ. 2000;78(6):715. Available at: http://www.who.int/bulletin/archives/78(6)715.pdf (accessed 9 May 2017).

34. Global Burden of Disease Health Financing Collaborator Network. Evolution and patterns of global health financing 1995−2014: development assistance for health, and government, prepaid private, and out-of-pocket health spending in 184 countries. Lancet. 2017;389:1981−2004. Available at: http://www.thelancet.com/journals/lancet/article/PIIS0140-6736(17)30874-7/fulltext (accessed 15 June 2017).

35. Gotsadze G, Chikovani I, Goguadze K, Balabanova D, McKee M. Reforming sanitary-epidemiological service in Central and Eastern Europe and the former Soviet Union: an exploratory study. BMC Public Health. 2010;10:440. doi:10.1186/1471-2458-10-440. Available at: https://www.ncbi.nlm.nih.gov/pubmed/20663198 (accessed 15 June 2017).

36. Gornick ME, Eggers PW, Reilly TW, Mentnech RM, Fitterman LK, et al. Effects of race and income on mortality and use of services among Medicare beneficiaries. N Engl J Med. 1996;335:791−799. doi:10.1056/NEJM199609123351106. Available at: http://www.nejm.org/doi/full/10.1056/nejm199609123351106#t = article (accessed 9 May 2017).

37. Gostin LO, Friedman EA. Global Health: A pivotal moment of opportunity and peril. Health Aff. 2017;36(1):159−165. doi:10.1377/hlthaff.2016.1492. Abstract available at: http://content.healthaffairs.org/content/36/1/159.abstract (accessed 9 May 2017).

38. Guyatt GH, Devereaux PJ, Lexchin J, Stone SB, Yalnizyan A, Himmelstein D, et al. A systematic review of studies comparing health outcomes in Canada and the United States. Open Medicine. 2007;1:e27−e36. Available at: http://www.pnhp.org/PDF_files/ReviewUSCanadaOpenMedicine.pdf (accessed 24 April 2017).

39. Hussey PS, Anderson GF, Osborn R, Feek C, McLaughlin V, Millar J, et al. How does the quality of care compare in five countries? Health Aff. 2004;23(3):89−99. Available at: http://content.healthaffairs.org/content/23/3/89.full.pdf + html (accessed 24 April 2017).

40. Institute for Health Metrics and Evaluation (IHME). Financing global health 2016: development assistance, public and private health spending for the pursuit of universal health coverage. Seattle, WA: IHME, 2017. Available at: http://www.healthdata.org/policy-report/financing-global-health-2016-development-assistance-public-and-private-health-spending (accessed 11 May 2017).

41. Jamison DT, Breman JG, Measham AR, Alleyne G, Claeson M, Evans B, editors. Disease control priorities in developing countries. 2nd edition. Washington, DC: World Bank, 2006. Available at: http://www.dcp-3.org/sites/default/files/dcp2/DCPFM.pdf (accessed 19 April 2017).

42. Kaiser Family Foundation. US global health policy. Available at: http://kff.org/global-health-policy/ (accessed 24 April 2017).

43. Krug E, Cieza A. Strengthening health systems to provide rehabilitation services. Bull World Health Organ. 2017;95(3):167. doi:10.2471/BLT.17.191809. Available at: https://www.ncbi.nlm.nih.gov/pmc/articles/PMC5328120/pdf/BLT.17.191809.pdf (accessed 9 May 2017).

44. LaLonde M. A new perspective on the health of Canadians. Ottawa, ON: Department of National Health and Welfare, 1974A new perspective on the health of Canadians. Ottawa, ON: Department of National Health and Welfare, 1974. Available at: http://www.phac-aspc.gc.ca/ph-sp/pdf/perspect-eng.pdf (accessed 6 May 2017).

45. Lasser KE, Himmelstein DU, Woolhandler S. Access to care, health status, and health disparities in the United States and Canada: results of a cross-national population-based survey. Am J Public Health. 2006;96:1300−1307. Available at: http://www.pnhp.org/PDF_files/USvCan_AJPH06.pdf (accessed 24 April 2017).

46. Light DW, Liebfried S, Tennstedt F. Social medicine vs professional dominance: the German experience. Am J Public Health. 1986;76:78−83. Available at: https://www.ncbi.nlm.nih.gov/pubmed/3510052 (acessed 25 June 2017).
47. Light DW. Universal health care: lessons from the British experience. Am J Public Health. 2003;93(1):25−30. Available at: https://www.ncbi.nlm.nih.gov/pmc/articles/PMC1447686/ (accessed 6 May 2017).
48. Lewis S. A system in name only—access, variation, and reform in Canada's provinces. N Engl J Med. 2015;372:497−500. doi:10.1056/NEJMp1414409. Available at: http://www.nejm.org/doi/pdf/10.1056/NEJMp1414409 (accessed 2 May 2017).
49. Mackenbach JP, Karanikolos M, McKee M. The unequal health of Europeans: successes and failures of policies. Lancet. 2013;381(1972):1125−1134. Available at: http://thelancet.com/journals/lancet/article/PIIS0140-6736(12)62082-0/fulltext (accessed 24 April 2017).
50. Mackenbach JP, McKee. A comparative analysis of health policy performance in 43 European countries. Euro J Public Health. 2013;23(2):195−344. Available at: https://researchonline.lshtm.ac.uk/768566/1/Eur_J_Public_Health-2013-Mackenbach-195-201.pdf (accessed 19 April 2017).
51. Magnussen J, Vrangboek K, Saltman RB. Nordic health systems: recent reforms and health policy challenges. Copenhagen: WHO Regional Office for Europe on behalf of the European Observatory on Health Systems and Policies, 2009http://www.euro.who.int/__data/assets/pdf_file/0011/98417/E93429.pdf?ua = 1 (accessed 13 May 2017).
52. Making Medicare. The history of health care in Canada, 1914−2007. Available at: http://www.historymuseum.ca/cmc/exhibitions/hist/medicare/medic01e.shtml (accessed 7 July 2017).
53. Marmot M. The Marmot review final report: fair society, healthy lives, 2010. Available at: http://www.who.int/pmnch/topics/economics/20100222_marmotreport/en/ (accessed 16 June 2017).
54. Marshall M. A precious jewel—the role of general practice in the English NHS. N Engl J Med. 2015;372(10):893−897. Available at: http://www.nejm.org/doi/pdf/10.1056/NEJMp1411429 (accessed 2 May 2017).
55. Marchildon GP. Canada health system review. Health Syst Trans. 2013;15(1):1−214. Available at: http://www.euro.who.int/__data/assets/pdf_file/0011/181955/e96759.pdf?ua = 1 (accessed 13 May 2017).
56. MacDougall H. Reinventing public health: a new perspective on the health of Canadians and its international impact. J Epidemiol Commun Health. 2007;61(11):955−959. doi:10.1136/jech.2006.046912. Available at: https://www.ncbi.nlm.nih.gov/pmc/articles/PMC2465617/ (accessed 6 May 2017).
57. Morrissey S, Blumenthal D, Osborn R, Curfman GD, Malina D. International health care systems. N Engl J Med. 2015;372(1):75−76. Available at: http://www.nejm.org/doi/pdf/10.1056/NEJMe1415036 (accessed 2 May 2017).
58. Mossialos E, Wenzl M, Osborn R, Sarnak D, editors. International Profiles of Health Care Systems. Australia, Canada, China, Denmark, England, France, Germany, India, Israel, Italy, Japan, The Netherlands, New Zealand, Norway, Singapore, Sweden, Switzerland, and the US: The Commonwealth Fund, 2015January 2016. Available at: http://www.commonwealthfund.org/~/media/files/publications/fund-report/2016/jan/1857_mossialos_intl_profiles_2015_v7.pdf (accessed 15 June 2017).
59. Murray CJ, Frenk J, Evans T. The global campaign for the health MDGs: challenges, opportunities, and the imperative of shared learning. Lancet. 2007;370(9592):1018−1020.

https://doi.org/10.1016/S01406736(07)61458-5. PMID:17889229. Available at: https://www.ncbi.nlm.nih.gov/pubmed/17889229 (accessed 8 July 2017).

60. Newsholme A, Kingsbury JA. Red Medicine: Socialized Health in Soviet Russia. DoubleDay, Doran & Company, Inc; Garden City, New York, 1933. Available at: https://www.marxists.org/archive/newsholme/1933/red-medicine/index.htm (accessed 6 October 2017).

61. Nolte E, McKee CM. Measuring the health of nations: updating an earlier analysis. Health Aff. 2008;27(1):58−71. Available at: http://content.healthaffairs.org/content/27/1/58.full (accessed 19 April 2017).

62. Organization for Economic Cooperation and Development (OECD) 2016. OECD reviews of health care systems. Available at: http://www.oecd.org/els/health-systems/health-data.htm (accessed 19 April 2017).

63. Organization for Economic Cooperation and Development (OECD). Health at a glance 2015. Available at: http://www.oecd.org/health/health-systems/health-at-a-glance-19991312.htm (accessed 19 April 2017).

64. Organization of Economic Cooperation and Development (OECD). Universal health coverage. Available at: http://www.oecd.org/els/health-systems/UHC-Facts-and-Figures-September-2016.pdf (accessed 13 May 2017).

65. Organization of Economic Cooperation and Development (OECD). Life expectancy at birth. Available at: https://data.oecd.org/healthstat/life-expectancy-at-birth.htm (accessed 8 May 2017).

66. Peters DH, El-Saharty S, Siadat B, Janovsky K, Vujicic M, editors. Improving health services delivery in developing countries: from evidence to action. Washington: World Bank, 2009https://doi.org/10.1596/978-0-8213-7888-5. Available at: http://www.tractionproject.org/sites/default/files/Program%20Design-Peters%2C_Improving_Health_Service_Delivery_in_Developing_Countries.pdf (accessed 6 July 2017).

67. Popovich L, Potapchik E, Shishkin S, Richardson E, Vacroux A, Mathivet B. Russian Federation. Health system review. Health Syst Transit. 2011;13(7):1−190, xiii-xiv. Abstract available at: https://www.ncbi.nlm.nih.gov/pubmed/22455875 (accessed 10 July 2017).

68. Rechel B, McKee M. Health reform in Central and Eastern Europe and the former Soviet Union. Lancet. 2009;374(9696):1186−1195. doi:10.1016/S0140-6736(09)61334-9. Abstract available at: https://www.ncbi.nlm.nih.gov/pubmed/19801097 (accessed 12 May 2017).

69. Roemer MI. National health systems of the world. Volumes 1 and 2. New York: Oxford University Press, 1991;1993.

70. Roemer MI. National health systems throughout the world. Annu Rev Public Health. 1993;14:335−353. Available at: http://www.annualreviews.org/doi/pdf/10.1146/annurev.pu.14.050193.002003 (accessed 20 April 2017).

71. Romanow R.J. Commission on the Future of Health Care in Canada. Building on values: the future of health care in Canada 2002. Available at: http://publications.gc.ca/site/eng/237274/publication.html (accessed 6 May 2017).

72. Sanmartin C, Berthelot JM, Ng E, Murphy K, Blackwell DL, Gentleman JF, et al. Comparing health and health care use in Canada and the United States. Health Aff. 2006;25:1133−1142. Available at: http://content.healthaffairs.org/content/25/4/1133.long (accessed 9 May 2017).

73. Schoen C, Osborn R, Doty MM, Squires D, Peugh J, Applebaum S. A survey of primary care physicians in 11 countries, 2009: a perspectives on care, costs, and experiences.

Health Affairs. 2009;28(6):w1171—w1183. Available at: http://content.healthaffairs.org/
content/28/6/w1171.long (accessed 9 May 2017).

74. Sheiman I. Rocky road from the Semashko to a new health model. Bull World Health
Organ. 2013;91:320—321. http://www.who.int/bulletin/volumes/91/5/13-030513.pdf
(accessed 17 February 2017).

75. Steffen M. Universalism, responsiveness, sustainability—regulating the French health care
system. N Engl J Med. 2016;374:401—405. doi:10.1056/NEJMp1504547. Available at:
http://www.nejm.org/doi/full/10.1056/NEJMp1504547#t=article (accessed 2 May 2017).

76. Stock S. Integrated ambulatory specialist care—Germany's new health care sector. N Engl
J Med. 2015;372:1781—1785. doi:10.1056/NEJMp1413625. Available at: http://www.nejm.
org/doi/pdf/10.1056/NEJMp1413625 (accessed 2 May 2017).

77. Teutsh S, Rechel B. Ethics of resource allocation and rationing Medical care in a time of
fiscal Restraint-US and Europe. Public Health Rev. 2012;34:15. doi:10.1007/BF03391667.
Published: 18 April 2017. Available at: http://publichealthreviews.biomedcentral.com/arti-
cles/10.1007/BF03391667 (accessed 13 May 2017).

78. Tulchinsky TH, Varavikova EA. Addressing the epidemiologic transition in the former
Soviet Union: strategies for health system and public health reform in Russia. Am J Public
Health. 1996;86:313—320. Available at: https://www.ncbi.nlm.nih.gov/pmc/articles/
PMC1380508/pdf/amjph00514-0027.pdf (accessed 9 May 2017).

79. Tulchinsky TH, Varavikova EA. The new public health. 3rd edition. San Diego: Academic
Press/Elsevier, 2014643—728. Chapter 13.

80. United Kingdom National Archives. Brave new world: the Welfare State. Available at:
http://www.nationalarchives.gov.uk/pathways/citizenship/brave_new_world/welfare.htm
(accessed 21 April 2017).

81. United Nations Human Development Report 2016. Human development for everyone.
Available at: http://hdr.undp.org/en/2016-report (accessed 19 April 2017).

82. United Nations, General Assembly. Resolution adopted by the General Assembly on 25
September 2015: Transforming our world., agenda items 15 and 116; paragraph 26.
Available at: http:// www.un.org/ga/search/view_doc.asp?symbol = A/RES/70/1&Lang = E
(accessed 20 April 2017).

83. United Nation. Sustainable Development Goals. 17 goals to transform our world. Available at:
http://www.un.org/sustainabledevelopment/sustainable-development-goals/ (accessed 3 July
2017).

84. World Bank. Healthy development. The World Bank strategy for health, nutrition, and population results. Washington: World Bank, 2007.

85. World Bank. Spotlight on nutrition: unlocking human potential and economic growth, 22
April 2017. Available at: http://live.worldbank.org/spotlight-on-nutrition (accessed 23 April
2017).

86. World Bank. Open data. Washington, DC: World Bank, 2017. Available at: http://data.
worldbank.org (accessed 19 April 2017).

87. World Bank. Life expectancy at birth, total (years). Available at http://data.worldbank.org/
indicator/SP.DYN.LE00.IN (accessed 15 June 2017).

88. World Health Organization. Global health observatory. World Health Statistics 2016:
Monitoring health for the SDGs. Available at: http://www.who.int/gho/publications/world_
health_statistics/2016/en/ (accessed 19 April 2017).

89. World Health Organization. Everybody's business: strengthening health systems to improve
outcomes: WHO's framework for action. Geneva: World Health Organization, 2007.

90. World Health Organization. World health report 2006: working together for health. Geneva: World Health Organization, 2006. Available at: http://apps.who.int/iris/bitstream/ 10665/43432/1/9241563176_eng.pdf (accessed 6 July 2017).

91. World Health Report 2000. Health systems: improving performance. Geneva, Switzerland: World Health Organization, 2000. Available at: http://www.who.int/whr/2000/en/ whr00_en.pdf (accessed 17 May 2017).

92. World Health Organization. European region. European health report 2012: charting the way to well-being. Copenhagen: World Health Organization, 2012. Available at: http:// www.euro.who.int/__data/assets/pdf_file/0004/197113/EHR2012-Eng.pdf?ua = 1 (accessed 19 April 2017).

93. World Health Organization. World Health Report 2013: Research for universal health coverage. Available at: http://apps.who.int/iris/bitstream/10665/85761/2/9789240690837_eng. pdf?ua = 1 (accessed 17 May 2017).

94. World Health Organization. European health for all database (HFADB). Available at: http://data.euro.who.int/hfadb/ (accessed 19 April 2017).

95. World Health Organization. Health systems: health system financing. Available at: http:// www.who.int/healthsystems/topics/financing/en/ (accessed 2 May 2017).

96. World Health Organization. Universal health coverage: sustainable development goal 3, health. Available at: http://www.who.int/universal_health_coverage/en/ (accessed 14 May 2017).

Chapter 9

Joseph Goldberger, Pellagra, and Nutritional Epidemiology

ABSTRACT

During the first decades of the 20th century, pellagra was considered the leading public health problem in the southern United States, where poverty was rampant. In 1916, pellagra was ranked second among the leading causes of death in South Carolina. The medical community generally believed pellagra to be infectious in origin. Pellagra was first reported in the United States in 1906 as an epidemic in a mental hospital in Alabama. In 1914, Joseph Goldberger, an infectious disease medical specialist in the US Public Health Service, was sent to investigate the epidemic. He visited psychiatric hospitals and orphanages with endemic pellagra. He conducted surveys including nutritional assessments and medical examinations of symptomatic patients in South Carolina mill towns, orphanages, prisons and mental hospitals. He was struck by the observation that the staff at the institutions he visited was not affected, suggesting that the disease was not infectious but was more likely due to dietary deficiencies and poverty. In one mental hospital, by adding milk and eggs to the diet he eliminated pellagra and concluded that the disease was due to a dietary deficiencies and preventable by a change in diet alone. Goldberger's investigation disproved the infectious disease theory and the dietary theory became accepted as the true explanation that led to interventions, which along with economic development eradicated pellagra in the United States. Goldberger's innovative clinical epidemiologic and laboratory studies, cut short by his premature death, were major steps forward in nutritional epidemiology and epidemiology at large.

Dr Joseph Goldberger (1874–1929) was sent by the US Public Health Service to investigate a massive pellagra epidemic in southern states of US in 1914. His research determined that pellagra was not infectious, but the result of dietary deficiency in essential nutrients, newly called vitamins, making an important contribution to nutritional epidemiology. Pellagra killed an estimated 100,000 poor Southerners in the early part of the 20th century, and was eradicated by improved diets and fortification of flour with vitamin B group. *Courtesy of the US National Library of Medicine, Image ID: B012870 Available at: https://collections.nlm.nih.gov/catalog/nlm:nlmuid-101416622-img (accessed 20 November 2017).*

Case Studies in Public Health. DOI: http://dx.doi.org/10.1016/B978-0-12-804571-8.00002-0
181

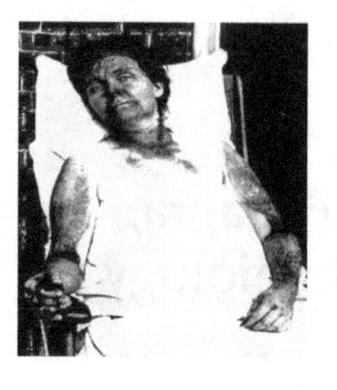

Patient with dermatitis, a symptom of pellagra along with diarrhea, dementia and death (the "Four Ds"). *Courtesy National Institutes of Health, Office of History available at https://history.nih.gov/exhibits/Goldberger/docs/6a.htm (accessed 23 November 2017).*

BACKGROUND

Joseph Goldberger was a child in 1883 when his Hungarian Jewish family emigrated to the United States and settled in the Lower East Side of New York. Goldberger began his studies in engineering, but became interested in medicine and completed his medical degree at the Bellevue Hospital Medical College (now the City College of New York) in 1895 and set up practice in Wilkes–Barre, Pennsylvania. He joined the Public Health Service in 1899 and was involved with efforts to combat yellow fever, typhus, dengue fever, and typhoid fever.

Pellagra is a vitamin deficiency disease due most often to a dietary deficiency of niacin (vitamin B3) and tryptophan. It is often seen in populations whose diet is largely dependent on maize/corn, which is poor in both niacin and tryptophan. Among other symptoms, pellagra presents with the classical "4Ds": diarrhea, dermatitis, dementia, and death (with a fifth, depression added later). First identified among Spanish peasants by Don Gaspar Casal in 1735, pellagra was common in countries in southern Europe where maize/corn, brought over from the New World, became the staple crop. In Europe the term "mal de rosa" was used in Spain, while in Italy it was described as "pelle agra" or farmer's skin, becoming the source of the term pellagra. The disease was also seen in the southern United States in the 19th century and reached epidemic levels there in the early 20th century. Pellagra was first reported as an epidemic in the United States in 1906 in a mental hospital in Alabama. Between 1907–1912, an estimated 25,000 cases were reported in the United States with a 40 percent fatality rate. In the first decades of the 20th century, pellagra was considered the leading public health problem in the southern United States, with hundreds of thousands of cases and nearly 100,000 deaths. In contrast, pellagra is not common in Latin America where corn is a staple diet. In these countries the centuries-old practice of soaking corn in alkaline lime frees the bound niacin and ensures protection from pellagra.

Investigation of the pellagra epidemic by Joseph Goldberger identified nutritional deficiency as the cause of pellagra leading to fortification of cereal grain products with niacin, which all but eradicated the condition from industrialized countries. However, pellagra is still common in India, and in parts of Africa and China, especially where populations are dependent on maize-based diets. Pellagra due to dietary niacin deficiency is a risk for refugee populations living in camps, particularly in Africa.

Originally, pellagra was thought to be due to a toxin in raw corn or produced by digestion in the intestine. In the late 19th century, Cesare Lombroso, in Verona, northern Italy reported many cases of pellagra among mental patients, concluding that it was due to toxic material in corn. One theory was that pellagra was caused by an organism growing in moldy corn affecting people or animals. Despite lack of evidence, laws were passed prohibiting the sale of spoiled or moldy corn, and the association of pellagra with poverty and corn was well established. At the beginning of the 20th century, the corn theory was less accepted and there was a competing hypothesis for the cause of pellagra—an insect-borne infection. This hypothesis was championed by the charismatic Italian investigator Louis W. Sambon. Sambon, discoverer of the role of the tsetse fly in "sleeping sickness" (trypanosomiasis), was consulted in the United States. He strongly advocated the view that pellagra was a insect-borne infectious disease, which was accepted by political and medical authorities in the southern United States. A competing theory was the new "vital amine" hypothesis proposed by Casimir Funk.

A nutritional deficiency was suggested as a potential cause by Casimir Funk, a Polish-Jewish biochemist working in London on beriberi and other nutritional deficiencies. In 1912 Funk published his concept of "vital amines" or essential elements in foods which prevent deficiency conditions such as beriberi, scurvy and rickets, based on previous studies of these conditions, later known as vitamins B1, B2, C, and D. In early 1912 Funk suggested that pellagra could fit with observations that had identified scurvy, rickets and beriberi as nutritional deficiency conditions.

Investigation of the pellagra epidemic became urgent as a result of the dramatic increase in reported cases during the first decade of the 20th century in the southern United States. This was the largest epidemic of a nutritional deficiency disease in US history with almost 100,000 deaths attributed to pellagra in the first four decades of the 20th century, an epidemic which at its peak took over 7,000 lives each year in the 15 southern states. Previous investigation of endemic pellagra in a mental hospital in Illinois led to the conclusion that the disease was due to a microorganism growing in the digestive tract of people living on a diet largely consisting of corn. Another investigating group in South Carolina concluded that pellagra was due to an enteric toxin from contaminated food affecting people suffering from malnutrition.

Two teams of investigators set out to assess pellagra's incidence in cotton-mill villages in South Carolina. The first team, the Thompson–McFadden

Pellagra Commission initiated by New York donors focused on assessing pellagra incidence in cotton mill villages in South Carolina and was led by US Army Medical Corps personnel (1912—14). It concluded that pellagra was likely due to an infectious agent. This was largely due to an emphasis in public health that was focused primarily for decades on microbiologic causes of many diseases. Other diseases then common in the south along with pellagra included the infectious diseases yellow fever, malaria and hookworm which were especially predominant in populations suffering effects of poverty and poor sanitation.

The second team, appointed in 1914 by the US Public Health Service, was led by Dr. Joseph Goldberger, a USPHS epidemiologist who had previously worked on yellow fever, dengue, and typhus. Although the predominant theory of causation of pellagra was that it was infectious in origin, Goldberger was immediately influenced by his observation that the disease struck inmates of affected populations in institutions but not the staff. He was also influenced by finding of surveys as well as by dietary surveys conducted among cotton mill workers in poor southern villages and poverty stricken rural populations. He was cognizant of Funk's theory of vitamin deficiencies and the growing evidence of diseases caused by dietary deficiencies including scurvy, beriberi, rickets, neurological disorders and others. In order to test the dominant infectious disease theory, Joseph Goldberger injected blood from pellagra victims into himself, his wife, and friends in an attempt to transmit pellagra as an infectious disease but without causing pellagra, as evidence against this as an infectious disease.

Goldberger developed a strategic dietary assessment study designed for use in mill towns and in institutions such as prisons, mental hospitals, and orphanages. This was administered in two orphanages in Jackson Mississippi, with a total of 209 pellagra cases among 6—12 year olds. The survey found that their diet was poor in lean meat and other proteins. With no changes made to the sanitary conditions at the facilities, Goldberger ordered milk, eggs, and beans to be added to the children's diet. All cases of pellagra disappeared with only one recurrence during the following year when Goldberger's funding for augmenting institutional diets was used up. Goldberger further tested his dietary hypothesis at the Georgia State Sanitarium, where he enriched the diet of some patients along with a control group of patients who did not receive an improved diet. Patients receiving the enriched diets had no new recurrence of the disease, while the control group saw a 47 percent rate of pellagra recurrence. He visited psychiatric hospitals and orphanages with endemic pellagra and observed that the staff was not affected, suggesting that the disease was not infectious but due to the diet. In one mental hospital, he eliminated pellagra by adding milk and eggs to the diet. From these observations and studies, Goldberger concluded that the disease was due to a lack of vital nutritional elements and therefore preventable.

Goldberger's hypothesis that pellagra was due to poverty and poor nutrition was strongly objected to by the political class in the south, and by the medical community, influenced by Sambon's strongly propagated theory that pellagra was infectious in origin. Rejection of Goldberger's hypothesis was accentuated by local prejudice due to the fact that he was an outsider, a northerner and a Jewish immigrant, implying that the South was poverty stricken and backward. The South was reluctant to recognize epidemiologic evidence that pellagra was due to poor diet and nutritional deficiency. Indications that the disease was thought to be due to poverty and poor diet were considered an insult to the reputation of the South, which was still burdened with economic depression, poverty, and other effects of the defeat in the Civil War (1861−1865) and its enduring aftermath.

By 1917, the evidence produced by Goldberger was convincing. The epidemic peaked after 1925 and then declined rapidly in the late 1920s and 1930s, despite the onset of the Great Depression, along with other diseases then common in the South including malaria, yellow fever, and widespread hookworm infestation. Reduction of these diseases of poverty was due to demographic changes including urbanization as well as public health measures such as extensive educational activities of the US Federal Department of Agriculture (USFDA) extension services, vector control by state and local authorities, as well as projects funded by the Rockefeller Foundation and growing use of fortification of flour. All of these diseases largely disappeared by 1950 in the United States as a result of greater prosperity following the Depression, full employment, and better wages during World War II as well as establishment of federal public health agencies and public health interventions including access to health care. Figure 9.1 shows Pellagra mortality by gender for the period 1920−60 in the

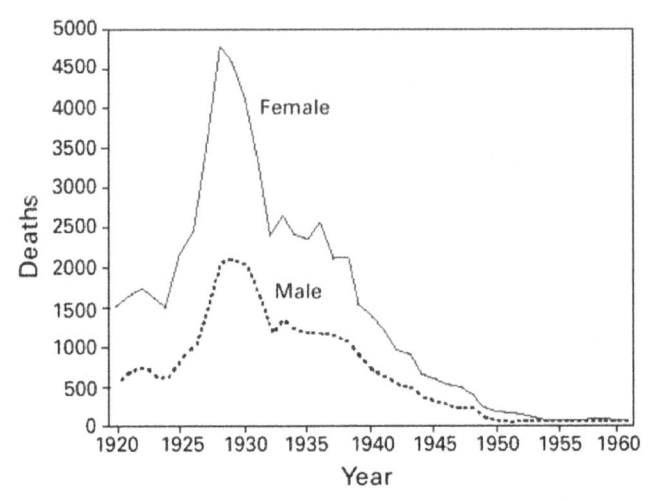

FIGURE 9.1 Pellagra deaths by sex, United States, 1920−60. *Source: Centers for Disease Control and Prevention. Safer and healthier foods. MMWR Morb Mortal Wkly Rep. 1999;48 (40):905−913. Available at: https://www.cdc.gov/mmwr/PDF/wk/mm4840.pdf (accessed 20 August 2016).*

United States with the peak tipping point in 1926–27 followed by a rapid decline. The predominance of African-American deaths was due to severe poverty of sharecroppers and institutionalization rates. Female deaths were commoner than male deaths likely due to food distribution in farm families with males needing more food to carry out the hard conditions of work in agriculture and poor wages for mill workers who were mostly women.

Goldberger, who was trained in infectious disease and epidemiological investigations, identified non-transmission of the disease from patients to staff and went on in a controlled experiment to establish the nutritional, and economic, basis of pellagra. He published his first paper on pellagra less than 3 months after beginning his investigations (followed by a detailed epidemiological paper published in 1915) reporting the findings at the Georgia State Sanitarium. Goldberger continued his studies with laboratory experiments on pellagra in dogs (black tongue) and dietary experiments on volunteer prisoners, as well as in natural disasters such as large scale flooding of the Mississippi River in 1927. Goldberger recommended providing yeast supplements to displaced sharecroppers to prevent the disease. The flood covered most of 12 states; 700,000 people were displaced to Red Cross camps. Pellagra cases soon appeared but yeast distribution resulted in a rapid decline in cases and improvement in symptoms. The pellagra-prevention diet proved effective in a large population in a disaster situation. Shipments of food arranged by Goldberger from Washington provided to children in two Mississippi orphanages and to inmates at the Georgia State Asylum produced dramatic results. Inmates who had fresh meat, milk and vegetables added to the corn-based diet recovered from pellagra. Those without the disease who ate the new diet did not contract pellagra. When the shipments stopped, the disease returned. He identified a deficiency of "water-soluble B vitamin," but he died in 1929 before complete identification of the "pellagra preventive vitamin B" that he had postulated.

Goldberger concluded that pellagra was preventable with an appropriate diet without any alteration in conditions of the hygienic or sanitary environment. He stressed the economic factor of poverty and deprivation as the basis for the disease in mill villages, orphanages, and prisons and among tenant farmers. When prices of cotton fell poverty increased among southern sharecroppers in 1921, Goldberger correctly predicted serious public health consequences with tens of thousands of pellagra cases including thousands of deaths, and even worse for 1922.

By 1938 US bakers widely adopted voluntary enrichment of bread with high-vitamin yeast and later niacin with other vitamins. In 1941, President Franklin D. Roosevelt convened a National Nutrition Conference for Defense. The Conference and the resulting War Order led to increasing voluntary and mandatory enrichment of wheat flour with B vitamins and iron. This led to the first Recommended Dietary Allowances by the Food and Nutrition Board of the National Academy of Sciences as adequate to meet the average daily nutritional needs of most healthy persons according to age group and sex. War Order Number One promoted enrichment of wheat flour with B vitamins and iron (CDC 1999). Following 1942 federal regulations regarding enrichment of flour and farina, Louisiana and South Carolina adopted mandatory fortification of bread and flour. Enactment of fortification of flour in Mississippi was followed by a reduction in the pellagra rate which fell from 101/100,000 in 1946 to less than 1/100,000 in 1947. By the late 1940s, 26 states had enrichment laws, and most wheat flour, cornmeal, and grits were enriched with niacin (Box 9.1).

BOX 9.1 Goldberger's key observations/conclusions

"It is striking therefore that although many inmates develop pellagra after varying periods of institutional residence, some even after 10–20 years of institutional life, and therefore it seems permissible to infer, as the result of the operation within the institution of the exciting cause or causes, yet nurses and attendants living under identical conditions appear uniformly to be immune. If pellagra be a communicable disease, why should there be this exemption of the nurses and attendants? To the writer this peculiar exemption or immunity is inexplicable on the assumption that pellagra is communicable."

"In view of the great uncertainty that exists as to the true cause of pellagra, it may not be amiss to suggest that pending the final solution of this problem it may be well to attempt to prevent the disease by improving the dietary of those among whom it seems most prevalent. In this direction I would urge the reduction in cereals, vegetables, and canned foods that enter to so large an extent into the dietary of many of the people in the South and an increase in the fresh animal food component, such as fresh meats, eggs, and milk."

"In this connection brief reference must be made to two other epidemiological features of pellagra. It is universally agreed (1) that this disease is essentially rural, and (2) associated with poverty. Now there is plenty of poverty and all its concomitants in all cities, and the question naturally arises why its greater predilection for rural poverty?

"It is necessary to keep in mind two considerations of essential importance. The first is that the economic status of this population is bound up in the tenant system, which in turn, is involved in single-crop agricultural production, and the speculative character of agricultural finance as it is practiced in this area, the seasonal fluctuation in income of the tenant ... and other factors of an economic nature" (1), and that "pellagra may be completely prevented by diet" (Goldberger, 1915).

Sources: Goldberger J, Wheeler GA, Sydenstricker E. Pellagra incidence in relation to sex, age, season, occupation, and "disabling sickness" in seven cotton-mill villages of South Carolina during 1916. Public Health Rep. 1920;35(28):1650–1664. Available at: https://www.ncbi. nlm.nih.gov/pmc/articles/PMC1996816/pdf/pubhealthreporig02676-0001.pdf (accessed 19 August 2017).
Goldberger J, Wheeler GA. Experimental pellagra in the human subject brought about by a restricted diet. Public Health Rep. 1915;30(46):3336–3339. Available at: https://www.ncbi. nlm.nih.gov/pmc/articles/PMC1999893/pdf/pubhealthreporig03428-0001.pdf (accessed 19 August 2017).
Goldberger J. The etiology of pellagra: the significance of certain epidemiological observations with respect thereto. Public Health Rep. 1914;29(26):1683–1686. Available at: https://www. ncbi.nlm.nih.gov/pmc/articles/PMC1999934/pdf/pubhealthreporig03461-0001.pdf (accessed 19 August 2016). http://www.ncbi.nlm.nih.gov/pmc/articles/PMC1437745/pdf/ pubhealthrep00159-0087.pdf (accessed 10 August 2017).

He recommended changes in the food supply and dietary habits adding meat and dairy products, with keeping of chickens, cows, and growing diversified vegetable crops among the rural population.

As a result of Goldberger's work and that of others on iodine, vitamins of the B complex, and vitamin D deficiencies common in the early part of the 20th century, there has been increasing public and professional recognition of the role of dietary deficiencies in some diseases. During World War I there was an emphasis on nutritional improvement and availability of nutrients for the general population. Following studies showing high rates of goiter among draftees to the US army and school children in Ohio and other states, food fortification was initiated in 1924, with the addition of iodine to salt to prevent goiter (see Chapter 10).

Despite the knowledge gained from Goldberger's work, as late as 1934, 3,602 cases of death were attributed to pellagra in the United States, with an estimated incidence of 20 clinical cases per death. During the Second World War, food fortification was extended to include enrichment of wheat flour with iron and the vitamins thiamin, niacin, and riboflavin and iodization of salt, milk and margarine with vitamin D, which were well accepted by the food industry and the public.

Goldberger established the cause of pellagra as a nutritional deficiency disease caused by lack of niacin (vitamin B3). This provided important evidence for the then newly defined concept of vitamins in public health. He demonstrated the nutritional basis of this disease, and as James Lind had demonstrated 140 years previously for scurvy (see Chapter 1), establishing nutritional epidemiology as a vital aspect of public health.

In 1936, the Council of Food and Nutrition of the American Medical Association announced it favored a general policy of food fortification and in 1938 bakers began to voluntarily fortify "enriched" bread. Synthetic niacin became available to physicians in the latter half of 1938. Following enactment of US federal enrichment regulation and enactment of mandatory enrichment laws by two southern states, by late 1942 some 75–80 percent of flour used by families and baker's white bread was enriched. By the end of the 1940s, 26 states in the United States had adopted mandatory enrichment of flour or bread, and in five states, fortification included cornmeal and corn grits. Morbidity and mortality from pellagra sharply declined, which was also influenced by general economic improvements and urbanization before, during, and following World War II but also due to widespread fortification of flour in the United States with vitamin B complex and iron.

The CDC recognized food safety and quality as one of the great achievements of public health of the 20th century as follows:

Pellagra is a good example of the translation of scientific understanding to public health action to prevent nutritional deficiency. Pellagra, a classic dietary deficiency disease caused by insufficient niacin, was noted in the South after the Civil War. Then considered infectious, it was known as the disease of the four Ds: diarrhea, dermatitis, dementia, and death. The first outbreak was reported in 1907. In 1909, more than 1,000 cases were estimated based on reports from 13 states. One year later, approximately 3,000 cases were suspected nationwide based on estimates from 30 states and the District of Columbia. By the end of 1911, pellagra had been reported in all but nine states, and prevalence estimates had increased nearly ninefold. During 1906–1940, approximately 3 million cases and approximately 100,000 deaths were attributed to pellagra. From 1914 until his death in 1929, Joseph Goldberger, a Public Health Service physician, conducted groundbreaking studies that demonstrated that pellagra was not infectious but was associated with poverty and poor diet. Despite compelling evidence, his hypothesis remained controversial and unconfirmed until 1937. The near elimination of pellagra by the end of the 1940s has been attributed to improved diet and health associated with economic recovery during the 1940s and to the enrichment of flour with niacin. Today, most physicians in the United States have never seen pellagra although outbreaks continue to occur, particularly among refugees and during emergencies in developing countries.

The growth of publicly funded nutrition programs was accelerated during the early 1940s because of reports that 25 percent of draftees showed evidence of past or present malnutrition; a frequent cause of rejection from military service was tooth decay or loss. In 1941, President Franklin D. Roosevelt convened the National Nutrition Conference for Defense, which led to the first recommended dietary allowances of nutrients, and resulted in issuance of War Order Number One, a program to enrich wheat flour with vitamins and iron. In 1998, the most recent food fortification program was initiated; folic acid, a water-soluble vitamin, was added to cereal and grain products to prevent neural tube defects. (CDC 1999).

An Illinois Pellagra Commission (1909 to 1911) and the Thompson–McFadden Pellagra Commission (1912 to 1917) both concluded that diet did not have a causative role in pellagra. The Thompson–McFadden Commission investigation on the incidence of pellagra failed to produce evidence of pellagra as an infectious disease. The Public Health Services team headed by Goldberger gathered accurate data on diet and socioeconomic factors in the successful second cotton-mill village investigation. The investigation included two key features of effective epidemiology: careful data collection and formulation of analyses that differentiate between alternate hypotheses. In contrast to the Thompson–McFadden Commission, Goldberger integrated administrative and interview data, which was considered unique for its time. Furthermore, Goldberger selected a slightly different set of villages with varying public sanitation services ultimately showing that sanitation was not a factor in pellagra. Mooney suggests this is an early example of multilevel epidemiological analysis. Goldberger's investigation methods included: vital statistics, community surveys, clinical trials, and clinical examination of patients as well as experiments using animals. He studied economic, sanitary, and social conditions. Patients with skin lesions were examined to corroborate the induction of pellagra by diet at a time when laboratory diagnosis was not available. Goldberger's approach to studying pellagra is considered a model to follow in other nutritional epidemiologic studies.

CURRENT RELEVANCE

Pellagra continues to be an issue in some countries such as China, Africa, and India as well as refugee and displaced-person groups. Population groups at risk for pellagra include poor people living in southern and eastern Africa, and people vulnerable to food and nutritional insecurity as a result of displacement as a result of long-term armed conflicts or in some countries (see Table 9.1 pellagra in emergency/displaced populations), with children less

TABLE 9.1 Pellagra Outbreaks in Emergency-Affected Populations

Year	Location	Population	Prevalence (%)
1988[a]	Zimbabwe	–	1.5%
1989[b]	Malawi (11 camps)	285,000	0.5%
1990[c]	Malawi (all camps)	900,000	2.0%
1991[d]	Malawi (Nsanje district)	300,000	0.2%
1994[e] (June)	Nepal (Bhutanese refugees)	85,000	0.5/10,000/day (incidence)
1994[e] (September)	Nepal (Bhutanese refugees)	85,000	0.005/10,000/day (incidence)
1995	Mozambique[f]	200,000	1.4%
1999 (November)	Angola[g]	240,000	2.6/1000/week

[a]Berry-Koch A, Moench R, Kaeewill P, Dualeh M. Alleviation of nutritional deficiency diseases in refugees. Food Nutr Bull. 1990;12(2):106–112.
[b]Moren A, Le Moult D. Pellagra cases in Mozambican refugees [Letter]. Lancet. 1990;335:1403–1404.
[c]Centers for Disease Control. Outbreak of pellagra among Mozambican refugees: Malawi, 1990. MMWR. 1991;40:209–213.
[d]UNHCR, unpublished report.
[e]RNIS Report Nos 5 & 8. ACC/SCN News. June 1994, December 1994.
[f]RNIS February 1996, Report No. 14.
[g]MSF/ICRC Rapid Nutritional Assessment, Kulto province of Bie, Angola, December 1999.
Source: World Health Organization. Pellagra and its prevention and control in major emergencies. Geneva, Switzerland: WHO, 2000. Available at: http://www.who.int/nutrition/publications/en/pellagra_prevention_control.pdf.

vulnerable. Foods provided by international support and aid agencies should be assessed for micronutrient content including niacin. The WHO notes that fortification of foods with niacin is preferable to distribution of vitamin B tablets, although the multivitamin supplements should be included in disaster preparation for short-term measures.

Pellagra can still occur today in high-income countries in patients with alcoholism and anorexia nervosa. Nonspecific symptoms affecting the dermatological, neuropsychiatric, and gastrointestinal systems can manifest before the classical four Ds of diarrhea, dermatitis, dementia, and death (and the fifth, depression). Medical examinations are important, but there is also a role for laboratory tests, which became available by the mid-20th century. Prevention of pellagra as a result of poor nutrition due to chronic diseases is vital for reducing hospitalizations and attendant costs as well as savings in the social costs of illness.

In 1941, "enriched flour" came under federal regulation and by the end of the 1940s, twenty-six states had enrichment laws, and most wheat flour, cornmeal, and grits were enriched with niacin. In Mississippi, the pellagra rate dropped from 101 per 100,000 in 1946 to fewer than 1 per 100,000 in 1947 (Park et al., 2000).

ETHICAL ISSUES

The responses of government and community leaders to Goldberger's conclusions and recommendations were very negative and were also mirrored in the medical community. The findings that the pellagra epidemic was due to dietary insufficiency as a result of poverty was seen as an insult to the reputation of the South, which was still suffering from economic and social distress in the aftermath of the American Civil War (1861–1865). Additionally, the remedy for poor diets was seen as beyond local capacity to resolve. The conclusions and intense lobbying by Sambon and the Thompson–McFadden Commission that pellagra was due to an infection were powerful forces. The fact that Goldberger was a northerner and a Jewish immigrant probably contributed to the intensity of the opposition. However, the stage was set for pellagra and other diseases due to the poverty in the rural south after the US Civil War and the postwar reconstruction period (1863–1877) when many northern "carpet baggers" moved south and profited from the society disrupted by built-in poverty in sharecrop farming and the low-wage cotton industry. In dealing with the pellagra epidemic, it became clear that there is a role to be played by governments and public health to minimize poverty and ameliorate the conditions associated with it.

Globally, two billion people are subject to poor nutrition mainly as micronutrient deficiencies including many essential vitamins and minerals. Food fortification and supplements especially for pregnant women and children are not given the priority they deserve in medium- and low-income countries. Progress has been made especially since the 1990s in mid-level developing countries such as China, India, and Nigeria for salt iodization, and for flour fortification in many other countries, but fortification and supplementation as a whole have not received the global health governmental and public support it needs. Food fortification and supplementation do not receive the full needed support of major donors as priorities for advancing global public health and socioeconomic development.

Pellagra continues to be an issue in certain refugee and displaced-person groups. Refugee populations are growing and nutrition interventions are necessary to prevent long-term damage especially to pregnant women and children but also to all other age groups. Refugees often receive food that is inadequate both in quantity and quality and can suffer from debilitating micronutrient deficiency diseases such as scurvy and beriberi in addition to pellagra. As refugees may be largely dependent on the food provided by governments and donors, food rations should be made more diverse and should be fortified to prevent malnutrition.

ECONOMIC ISSUES

The pellagra epidemic in the United States at the start of the 20th century occurred in most parts of the country, but primarily affected the population in the southern states. In the aftermath of the US Civil War (1861–65), the economy of the South was devastated and sharecropper farming replaced slavery with an emphasis on cotton, tobacco, and corn crops. The effects of this were rural poverty and corn-based diets, which for centuries had also been the basis of pellagra in European countries relying on corn for diets in rural areas. In addition to the pellagra epidemic identified in the early 20th century the American South was also endemic for yellow fever, malaria, and hookworm, affecting mainly children and scarring generations developmentally and also in economic potential. These four diseases disappeared gradually following the Depression and World War II due to public health measures and increased industrial employment bringing prosperity to the south. Food fortification in the United States included iodization of salt starting in the 1920s, fortification of milk with vitamin D in the 1930s, and enrichment of flour and bread in the 1940s.

Studies of long-term fortification programs improving adult productivity are widely accepted in global health promotion, although with lower priority than infectious disease control. The interaction of disease and poverty kept the US South in economic and social poverty until the entry of the United States into World War II, which brought industrialization, full employment, and relative prosperity.

CONCLUSION

From the mid-1910s to the mid-1920s, Dr. Joseph Goldberger of the US Public Health Service was assigned to perform research in a pellagra hospital.

Goldberger hypothesized that the clinical syndrome was the consequence of an inadequate diet and along with his associates conducted surveys and several human experimental studies, demonstrating that pellagra is a dietary deficiency disease associated with poverty and a primarily corn-based diet. He demonstrated that it was a noninfectious disease that can be prevented with dietary modification by adding high-protein foods (milk, eggs, meat, and yeast) to the diet. He then demonstrated that pellagra could be induced and prevented by dietary change in orphanages and prisons. His work was pivotal in the development of nutritional studies with advanced epidemiologic methods.

Goldberger's investigation of the pellagra epidemic in the southern United States is one of the classic examples of public health that defined a strong new direction in prevention of disease and improved public health and epidemiology. The pursuit of an infectious cause of pellagra failed, while a dietary intervention was shown to be effective in treating and preventing pellagra. Nutrition and poverty were clearly shown to be causes of diseases that took tens of thousands of lives in the United States in the first decades of the 20th century. The quality of the investigation eventually proved effective in the face of strong resistance and pressure favoring an infectious theory of pellagra.

The comorbidity of yellow fever, malaria, and hookworm that coexisted with pellagra in the southern states with multidisease epidemics showed the reality that many factors affect the health of people. Public health measures, urbanization, rising stadards of living with economic development were the magic bullets that controlled and eradicated these diseases in that area, and these lessons are applicable today in low- and medium-income countries and for reduction of health inequalities in all countries. The Federal Children's Bureau and the US Sheppard—Towner Act of 1921 provided federal funding for maternity and child care. This fostered development of state and local public health units. The US Department of Agriculture promoted rural nutrition education while the Rockefeller Foundation promoted hookworm control. Public-private initiatives contributed to improve nutrition and public health generally and the decline in pellagra and other diseases in the rural south from the 1920s and beyond.

Goldberger adopted Casimir Funk's vitamin theory taking it to a practical level of addressing a specific disease epidemic. Vulnerable population groups and situations occur in all levels of society in high-, medium-, and low-income countries. Goldberger investigated the situation during the massive Mississippi floods in 1920. He developed survey methods for nutritional epidemiology and his success in investigation and treatment of the epidemic helped to raise professional and public consciousness of the importance of nutrition in human health. With the work of scientists such as Funk, and those working in the same time period with iodine and vitamin D and other micronutrient conditions, Goldberger expanded the field of epidemiology. This expanded public health theory and practice to move forward from the then predominance of the still crucial Germ theory of disease since the late 19th century.

Manmade and natural disasters such as floods, tornadoes, and civil war are part of global health well into the 21st century causing millions to be exposed to substandard nutrition. Refugee populations totaling tens of millions of people living in harsh conditions are found in many parts of the world, and adequate nutritional supplements and interventions are necessary to prevent long-term damage especially to pregnant women and children but also other age groups.

Food fortification, which developed from Goldberger's work and that of others, is as essential for modern public health as pasteurization of milk, chlorination of water, and immunization of children. Micronutrient deficiencies should be seen as occurring together and public health approaches to improving nutrition in both disaster situations and in developing countries with high prevalence of micronutrient deficiency among children and women should be addressed together as an integral part of public health.

Other challenges emerge for nutritional epidemiology even in high-income countries, such as comorbidities with mental health, chronic diseases, and other medical illnesses such as depression, eating disorders, alcoholism, gastrointestinal disorders, immunosuppression by disease or by therapy, cancers, and social isolation. Psychiatric manifestations may be nonspecific such as irritability, poor concentration, anxiety, fatigue, restlessness, apathy, and depression. The occurrence of psychosis in pellagra is an uncommon finding, but advanced stages of encephalopathy are common in chronic alcoholics.

There are controversies about the need for multi-vitamins in the population, and reluctance by authorities to recommend adoption of usage of fortification, and even supplementation except for certain limited population groups. Many nutritional studies indicate low levels of iodine, vitamin D, iron, folate and other essential mineral and vitamins in the general population and in those with special nutrition support in low-, medium-and in high income countries. Suboptimal intake of many vitamins and minerals is a fundamental issue for global health and new policies for supplementation and fortification are needed to achieve the Sustainable Development Goals and to reduce health inequities even in high income countries.

In the 21st century natural disasters, climate change, ethnic cleansing, civil and religious war are creating massive refugee displacement with important public health implications. Not least among the needs for safety, accommodation from the weather, floods, hurricanes, civilian targeting with bombings, starvation and horrific violence is the problem of nutrition and environmental protection such as from mosquitoes carrying malaria, Zika virus and other dreaded diseases. But micronutrient deficiency with multiple essential dietary intake must be addressed in preparation for disasters and dealing with the reality of overt and covert starvation. Niacin, the other B vitamins, iron, Vitamins A and D and others add up to supplements needed especially for children, pregnant women and the elderly. Casimir Funk connected the dots of researchers addressing vitamin B deficiency polyneuro-pathy, scurvy, rickets, and goiter to formulate the concept of vital amines. Joseph Goldberger faced a national crisis and showed the malnutrition origin of pellagra and its cure, against strongly held views that it was an infectious disease. Funk and Goldberger were pioneers, among others addressed in other chapters of this book, in nutritional epidemiology. They prepared the ground for food fortification that has and will continue to save countless people from preventable suffering and premature death. This is public health at it's finest.

The principle of fortification of basic foods to reduce population risk for deficiency diseases, such as pellagra, rickets, osteoporosis and neural tube defects, is also becoming an issue for preventing chronic disease such as car-diovascular diseases, cancer and others. This is not in lieu of promoting healthy diets, but the reality is that many in any population group will con-tinue to eat diets lacking in key micronutrients while producing obesity, or bullemia or anorexia, or who have social or medical realities that make food as their only source of key micronutrients unrealistic. The subject of multivi-tamin supplements is already accepted as needed for large population groups like children, women, the elderly, the poor, refugees, and the homeless. Casimir Funk and Joseph Goldberger pioneered an essential element of pub-lic health nutrition which will continue to evolve. The issues they struggled for are important for all populations in the 21st century for prevention of micronutrient deficiency conditions, cardiovascular diseases, cancer, osteopo-rosis and others.

RECOMMENDATIONS

1. Nutritional epidemiology should be a core component of the training of all public health, medical, paramedical, and social service professions.
2. Public policy should specify nutrition as a major social and economic endeavor to reduce global and national inequalities in health.
3. Global health agencies and donors should recognize and financially sup-port food fortification and supplementation as crucial parts of social, eco-nomic, and health policy.
4. Nutritional deficiencies commonly occur together as groups and should be recognized as comorbidities with infectious and chronic diseases including mental illness.
5. Population health requires both vitamin supplementation to groups at spe-cial risk for deficiency conditions, and food fortification policies with implementation for general population health.
6. Climate change is expected to wreak havoc on agriculture and nutrition in many parts of the world. Wars, civil strife and mass refugee situations in the 21st century will place great demands on the world community to cope with the nutritional insecurity these conditions foster.

7. Political, donors and public health leadership must become more responsive to the micronutrient needs of such situations, not less than addressing communicable diseases and trauma.

STUDENT REVIEW QUESTIONS

1. What were the contributing factors to the pellagra epidemic?
2. Why did the medical community believe that pellagra was an infectious disease until 1914?
3. What was the discovery by Joseph Goldberger that led to a presumptive diagnosis that diet was the key to pellagra?
4. Why was there opposition among medical and state authorities to Goldberger's theory?
5. What convinced the medical community that Goldberger was correct?
6. What were the social and economic impacts of the vitamin deficiency of pellagra on the economy of the southern United States?
7. What was the evidence that led Casimir Funk to define "vital amines" as nutritional element deficiencies as causes of in diseases such as beriberi, scurvy, rickets and possibly pellagra?
8. What is the estimated current prevalence of vitamin and mineral deficiency conditions globally?
9. How should the public health profession respond to this worldwide phenomenon?
10. What priority should be given to reducing the burden of micronutrient deficiency conditions for promoting global health improvement?

RECOMMENDED READINGS

1. Allen L, de Benoist B, Dary O, Hurrell R, editors. Guidelines on food fortification with micronutrients. Geneva, Switzerland: World Health Organization, Food and Agricultural Organization of the United Nations, 2006. Available at: http://www.who.int/nutrition/publications/guide_food_fortification_micronutrients.pdf (accessed 12 August 2017).
2. American Medical Association Committee on Foods. Fortification of foods other than fortification of milk with vitamin D. JAMA. 1935;104(7):563. Available at: http://jama.jamanetwork.com/article.aspx?articleid = 257269 (accessed 19 August 2017).
3. Bishai D, Nalubola R. The history of food fortification in the United States: its relevance for current fortification efforts in developing countries. Econ Dev Cult Change. 2002; 51(1):37–53. Available at: http://web1.sph.emory.edu/users/hpacho2/PartnershipsMaize/Bishai_2002.pdf (accessed 13 August 2017).
4. Bollet AJ. Politics and pellagra: the epidemic of pellagra in the U.S. in the early twentieth century. Yale J Biol Med. 1992;65(3):211–221. Available at: http://www.ncbi.nlm.nih.gov/pmc/articles/PMC2589605/pdf/yjbm00051-0058.pdf (accessed 10 August 2017).
5. Bryan CS, Mull SR. Pellagra Pre-Goldberger: Rupert Blue, Fleming Sandwith, and the "vitamine hypothesis". Trans Am Clin Climatol Assoc. 2015;126:20–45. Available at: https://www.ncbi.nlm.nih.gov/pmc/articles/PMC4530670/pdf/tacca126000020.pdf (accessed 10 August 2017).

6. Carpenter KJ, Lewin WJ. A reexamination of the composition of diets associated with pellagra. J Nutr. 1985;115(5):543−552. Abstract available at: www.ncbi.nlm.nih.gov/pubmed/3998856 (accessed 10 August 2017).

7. Carpenter KJ. The Nobel Prize and the discovery of vitamins, 2004. Available at: http://www.nobelprize.org/nobel_prizes/themes/medicine/carpenter/ (accessed 10 August 2017).

8. Centers for Disease Control and Prevention. Achievements in public health, 1900-1999: safer and healthier foods. MMWR Morb Mortal Wkly Rep. 1999;48(40):905−913. Avialable at: https://www.cdc.gov/mmwr/preview/mmwrhtml/mm4840a1.htm (accessed 10 August 2017).

9. Centers for Disease Control and Prevention. Famine-affected, refugee, and displaced populations: recommendations for public health issues. MMWR Morb Mort Wkly Rep. 1992;41 (No. RR-13):0001. Available at: https://www.cdc.gov/mmwr/preview/mmwrhtml/00019261.htm (accessed 13 September 2017).

10. Delgado-Sanchez L, Godkar D, Niranjan S. Pellagra: rekindling of an old flame. Am J Ther. 2008;15(2):173−175. doi:10.1097/MJT.0b013e31815ae309. Available at: http://www.ncbi.nlm.nih.gov/pubmed/18356638 (accessed 19 August 2017).

11. DesGroseilliers JP, Shiffman NJ. Pellagra. Can Med Assoc J. 1976;115(8):768−770. Available at: https://www.ncbi.nlm.nih.gov/pmc/articles/PMC1878806/ (accessed 9 August 2017).

12. Ellmore JG, Feinstein AR. Joseph Goldberger: an unsung hero of American clinical epidemiology. Ann Intern Med. 1994;121(5):372−375. Abstract available at: https://www.ncbi.nlm.nih.gov/pubmed/8042827 (accessed 10 August 2017).

13. Fairfield KM, Fletcher RH. Vitamins for chronic disease prevention in adults: scientific review. JAMA. 2002;287:3116−3126. Available at: http://jamanetwork.com/journals/jama/fullarticle/195038 (accessed 13 September 2017).

14. Fletcher RH, Fairfield KM. Vitamins for chronic disease prevention in adults: clinical applications. JAMA. 2002;287:3127−3129. Available at: https://www.ncbi.nlm.nih.gov/pubmed/12069676 (accessed 13 September 2017).

15. Gentilcore D. Louis Sambon and the clash of pellagra etiologies in Italy and the United States, 1905−14. J Hist Med Allied Sci. 2016;71(1):19−42. doi:10.1093/jhmas/jrv002. Abstract available at: http://www.ncbi.nlm.nih.gov/pubmed/25740951 (accessed 13 August 2017).

16. Goldberger J, Waring CH, Willets DG. The prevention of pellagra: a test of diet among institutional inmates. Public Health Rep. 1915;30(43):3117−3131. Available at: https://www.ncbi.nlm.nih.gov/pmc/articles/PMC1999890/pdf/pubhealthreporig03425-0005.pdf (accessed 19 August 2017).

17. Goldberger J, Wheeler GA, Sydenstricker E. Pellagra incidence in relation to sex, age, season, occupation, and "disabling sickness" in seven cotton-mill villages of South Carolina during 1916. Public Health Rep. 1920;35(28):1650−1664. Available at: https://www.ncbi.nlm.nih.gov/pmc/articles/PMC1996816/pdf/pubhealthreporig02676-0001.pdf (accessed 19 August 2017).

18. Goldberger J, Wheeler GA. Experimental pellagra in the human subject brought about by a restricted diet. Public Health Rep. 1915;30(46):3336−3339. Available at: https://www.ncbi.nlm.nih.gov/pmc/articles/PMC1999893/pdf/pubhealthreporig03428-0001.pdf (accessed 19 August 2017).

19. Goldberger J. The etiology of pellagra: the significance of certain epidemiological observations with respect thereto. Public Health Rep. 1914;29(26):1683−1686.

Available at: https://www.ncbi.nlm.nih.gov/pmc/articles/PMC1999934/pdf/pubhealthrepor-ig03461-0001.pdf (accessed 19 August 2017).

20. Hegyi J, Schwartz RA, Hegyi V. Pellagra: dermatitis, dementia, and diarrhea. Int J Dermatol. 2004;43(1):1−5. Abstract available at: http://www.ncbi.nlm.nih.gov/pubmed/14693013 (accessed 28 June 2017).

21. Hess AF. Newer aspects of some nutritional disorders. JAMA. 1921;76:693−700. Abstract available at: https://www.cabdirect.org/cabdirect/abstract/19212901640 (accessed 14 September 2017).

22. Humphreys M. How four once common diseases were eliminated from the American South. Health Aff (Millwood). 2009;28(6):1734−1744. doi.10.1377/hlthaff.28.6.1734. Abstract available at: https://www.ncbi.nlm.nih.gov/pubmed/19887414 (accessed 12 August 2017).

23. Jukes TH. The prevention and conquest of scurvy, beri-beri, and pellagra. Prev Med. 1989;18(6):877−883. Abstract available at: http://www.ncbi.nlm.nih.gov/pubmed/2696957 (accessed 13 August 2017).

24. Klevay LM. Medical examination in nutrition surveys. J Nutr. 2005;135(5):1266−1267. Abstract available at: http://jn.nutrition.org/content/135/5/1266.long (accessed 28 July 2017).

25. Langer PL. History of goitre. Endemic goitre. Geneva, Switzerland: World Health Organization, 1960;9−25 (WHO Monograph Series No. 44). Available at: http://apps.who.int/iris/bitstream/10665/38822/1/WHO_MONO_44.pdf (accessed 13 September 2017).

26. Lopez M, Berrios GE. Pellagra encephalopathy in the context of alcoholism: review and case report. Alcohol Alcohol. 2014;49(1):38−41. Available at: http://alcalc.oxfordjournals.org/content/49/1/38.long (accessed 9 August 2017).

27. Martin MG, Humphreys ME. Social consequence of disease in the American South, 1900-World War II. South Med J. 2006;99(8):862−864. Abstract available at: http://www.ncbi.nlm.nih.gov/pubmed/16929881 (accessed 9 August 2017).

28. Method A, Tulchinsky TH. Commentary: Food fortification: African countries can make more progress. Adv Food Technol Nutr Sci Open J. 2015;SE(1):S22−S28. Available at: https://openventio.org/Special-Edition-1/Commentary-Food-Fortification-African-countries-can-make-more-progress-AFTNSOJ-SE-1-104.pdf (accessed 12 September 2017).

29. Mooney SJ, Knox J, Morabia A. Epidemiology in history: the Thompson-McFadden Commission and Joseph Goldberger: contrasting 2 historical investigations in cotton mill villages in South Carolina. Am J Epidemiol. 2014;180(3):235−244. Available at: https://www.ncbi.nlm.nih.gov/pmc/articles/PMC4108042/pdf/kwu134.pdf (accessed 10 August 2017).

30. Morabia A. Joseph Goldberger's research on the prevention of pellagra. JLL Bull. 2006. Commentaries on the history of treatment evaluation. Available at: http://www.jameslindlibrary.org/articles/joseph-goldbergers-research-on-the-prevention-of-pellagra (accessed 13 August 2017).

31. National Academy of Sciences. Overview of food fortification in the United States and Canada. Dietary reference intakes: guiding principles for nutrition labeling and fortification. Washington, DC: National Academies Press, 2003. Available at: http://www.ncbi.nlm.nih.gov/books/NBK208880/ (accessed 13 August 2017).

32. National Institute of Health. Dr Goldberger & the war on pellagra, 2016. Available at: https://history.nih.gov/exhibits/Goldberger/ (accessed 28 July 2017).

33. Otten JJ, Hellwig JP, Meyers LD, editors. Dietary reference intakes: the essential guide to nutrient requirements. Washington, DC: National Academies Press, 2006.

Available at: http://www.nap.edu/catalog/11537/dietary-reference-intakes-the-essential-guide-to-nutrient-requirements (accessed 13 August 2017).

34. Park YK, Sempos CT, Barton CN, Vanderveen JE, Yetley EA. Effectiveness of food fortification in the United States: the case of pellagra. Am J Public Health. 2000;90 (5):727−738. Available at: http://www.ncbi.nlm.nih.gov/pmc/articles/PMC1446222/pdf/10800421.pdf (accessed 10 August 2017).

35. Piro A, Tagarelli G, Lagonia P, Tagarelli A, Quattrone A. Casimir Funk: his discovery of the vitamins and their deficiency disorders. Ann Nutr Metab. 2010;57(2):85−88. doi:10.1159/000319165. Abstract available at: http://www.ncbi.nlm.nih.gov/pubmed/20805686 (accessed 13 August 2017).

36. Prakash R, Gandotra S, Singh LK, Das B, Lakra A. Rapid resolution of delusional parasitosis in pellagra with niacin augmentation therapy. Gen Hosp Psychiatry. 2008;30(6) 581−584. Abstract available at: http://www.ncbi.nlm.nih.gov/pubmed/19061687 (accessed 28 June 2016).

37. Prinzo ZW. Pellagra and its prevention and control in major emergencies. Geneva: World Health Organization, 2000. Available at: http://www.who.int/nutrition/publications/en/pellagra_prevention_control.pdf (accessed 12 September 2017). 5.14 August.

38. Rajakumar K. Pellagra in the United States: a historical perspective. South Med J. 2000;93 (3):272−277. Abstract available at: http://www.ncbi.nlm.nih.gov/pubmed/10728513 (accessed 9 Aug 2017).

39. Rabinowitz SS. Pediatric pellagra. Medscape. 2016. Available at: http://emedicine.medscape.com/article/985427-overview (accessed 12 September 2017).

40. Seal AJ, Creeke PI, Dibari F, Cheung E, Kyroussis E, Semedo P, et al. Low and deficient niacin status and pellagra are endemic in postwar Angola. Am J Clin Nutr. 2007;85:218−224. Available at: http://ajcn.nutrition.org/content/85/1/218.full.pdf + html (accessed 10 August 2017).

41. Semba RD. The discovery of the vitamins. Int J Vitam Nutr Res. 2012;82(5):310−315. doi:10.1024/0300-9831/a000124. Available at: http://econtent.hogrefe.com/doi/pdf/10.1024/0300-9831/a000124 (accessed 14 August 2017).

42. Semba RD. The historical evolution of thought regarding multiple micronutrient nutrition. J. Nutr. 2012;142(1):1435−1565. Available at: http://jn.nutrition.org/content/142/1/143S.full.pdf + html (accessed 14 August 2017).

43. Sydenstricker VP. The history of pellagra, its recognition as a disorder of nutrition and its conquest. Am J Clin Nutr. 1958;6(4):409−414. Available at: http://www.ncbi.nlm.nih.gov/pubmed/13559167 (accessed 20 August 2017).

44. Toole MJ, Waldman RJ. Refugees and displaced persons: war, hunger and public health. JAMA. 1993;5:600−605. Available at: http://cidbimena.desastres.hn/pdf/eng/doc5704/doc5704-contenido.pdf (accessed 13 September 2017).

45. Tulchinsky TH. Micronutrient deficiency conditions: global health issues. Public Health Rev. 2010;32(1):243−255. Available at: https://publichealthreviews.biomedcentral.com/articles/10.1007/BF03391600 (accessed 14 August 2017).

46. Tulchinsky TH, Varavikova EA. The new public health. 3rd edition. San Diego, CA: Academic Press, 2014. Available at: http://store.elsevier.com/The-New-Public-Health/Theodore-Tulchinsky/isbn-9780124157675/ (accessed 12 August 2017).

47. Tulchinsky TH. The key role of government in addressing the pandemic of micronutrient deficiency conditions in Southeast Asia. Nutrients. 2015;7(4):2518–2523. doi:10.3390/nu7042518. Available at: http://www.mdpi.com/2072-6643/7/4/2518/htm (accessed 14 August 2017).

48. Wilcox LS. Worms and germs, drink and dementia: US health, society, and policy in the early 20th century. Prevent Chronic Dis. 2008;5(4):A135. Available at: https://www.ncbi.nlm.nih.gov/pmc/articles/PMC2578784/pdf/PCD54A135.pdf (accessed 23 November 2017).

49. World Health Organization. Pellagra and its prevention and control in major emergencies. 2000. Available at: http://www.who.int/nutrition/publications/emergencies/WHO_NHD_00.10/en/ (accessed 2 September 2017).

Chapter 10

Endemic Goiter and Elimination of Iodine Deficiency Disorders

ABSTRACT

Iodine is an element essential for human growth and development with serious consequences when deficient in human nutrition. Iodine is found in nature universally in soil and water but in highly varying amounts depending on the terrain, with less in many mountainous and plains areas. Iodine deficiency can seriously affect normal fetal development, newborns, and other age groups as a thyroid abnormality. The discovery that iodine supplements prevents thyroid gland enlargement (goiter) in children and adults and prevents serious deficiency in newborns has made a major contribution to public and population health. Successful implementation of a pioneering salt iodization program occurred in France and Switzerland in the 19th century but amid controversy. High rates of goiter were found among US army draftees in 1917. David Marine conducted a large field trial of providing iodine to school children in Akron, Ohio demonstrating effective preventive and curative effects for reducing goiter. Iodized table salt was introduced in Switzerland in 1922 and in the United States in 1924 with widespread use greatly improving the iodine nutritional status of populations. Iodization of salt has been a global health issue promoted by the World Health Organization since the 1970s. In recent decades, iodization of salt on a mandatory basis in China and Nigeria has successfully reduced iodine deficiency dramatically. However, an estimated 38 million newborns in developing countries are vulnerable and unprotected from the lifelong consequences of brain damage associated with iodine deficiency disorders. Even in high-income countries such as in much of Europe iodine insufficiency is far from eliminated. Iodine deficiency control remains a global health challenge.

Case Studies in Public Health. DOI: http://dx.doi.org/10.1016/B978-0-12-804571-8.00001-9

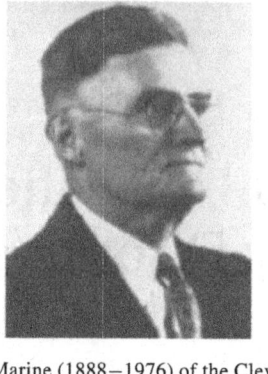

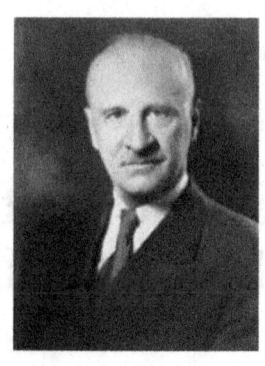

David Marine (1888–1976) of the Cleveland Clinic conducted a large study of school girls in Akron Ohio in 1917–19 of groups who received iodine compared to those who did not. The results were convincing of the effectiveness of preventive and treatment values of iodine supplements for goiter. *Courtesy: US National Library of Medicine; gift of R.H. Follis, Image ID: B027603 at http://resource.nlm.nih.gov/ 101447631 (accessed 23 October 2017).*

David Cowie (1872–1940), first Professor of Pediatrics at the University of Michigan successfully promoted iodization of commercial salt to curb endemic goiter in the United States. *Courtesy: Courtesy of the Image Bank, Bentley Historical Library, University of Michigan. Available at: http://quod.lib.umich. edu/b/bhl/x-hs8464/hs8464 (accessed 16 October 2017).*

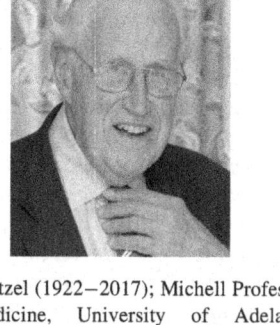

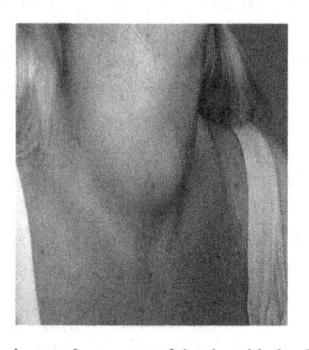

Basil Hetzel (1922–2017); Michell Professor of Medicine, University of Adelaide, Australia; his research into iodine deficiency and brain damage in unborn children had huge global impact; leader and pioneer in international efforts to eradicate iodine deficiency globally. *Photo courtesy of the Basil Hetzel Institute for Translational Health Research, The Queen Elizabeth Hospital, South Australia, September 2017.*

Goiter is an enlargement of the thyroid gland visible at the front and sides of the neck, mostly due to iodine deficiency in the diet; often associated with hypothyroidism. *Source: Wikimedia Commons, the free media repository. Retrieved 09:49, December 8, 2017 from https://commons. wikimedia.org/w/index.php?title=File:Struma _001.jpg&oldid=119199418.*

BACKGROUND

Iodine deficiency in water and soil in many parts of the world creating deficiency conditions in humans with serious health effects. Iodine deficiency is seen in the form of cretinism and goiter in many parts of the world. Iodine was discovered as an element in 1811 by French chemist Barnard Courtois. In 1813 a Swiss doctor, Jean François Coindet, applied a traditional folk medicine using seaweed and treatment with iodine drops to goiter patients and school children with success, stirring medical and public controversy as some suggested this combination was toxic. French chemist Jean Baptiste Boussingault and physician M. Roulin observed in 1835 that some villages in one province of Colombia treated goiter with fluid from sea salt deposits. They demonstrated that salt sent from the goiter-free province reduced the prevalence of goiter in endemic neighboring regions. In 1869 Lancet reported on elimination of goiter in several high-goiter French districts by issuing iodine tablets to school children with reduction in goiter prevalence, but medical opposition continued. Chatin carried out surveys in France and Italy and concluded that low iodine levels in water supplies were the cause of endemic goiter, a view still opposed by the medical establishment of the day with the accepted view that goiter was due to an infectious agent.

In 1917, when the United States was entering World War I, Simon Levin examined draftees for the US army in Houghton County, Michigan and found that some 30 percent showed clinical signs of an enlarged thyroid gland i.e., goiter, 90 percent due to iodine deficiency. More men were disqualified for army service because of goiter than for any other medical reason. Ohio, which is located in the Great Lakes Basin was part of the "Goiter Belt", a high goiter prevalence zone.

David Marine was born in 1880 and grew up on a farm in Maryland. He attended a Liberal Arts College, and at the age of 20 he entered Johns Hopkins University to study zoology, but switched to medicine, graduating high in his class in 1905. He was appointed to a residency in pathology at a hospital linked to Western Reserve University in Cleveland, OH. He reported noticing people and dogs with obvious goiters on his walk to the hospital, and then he indicated his wish to work on the thyroid gland. From 1909, working with fish goiter, he concluded there was no evidence that the disease is infectious, and reduced goiter incidence by adding iodine to the pond. He worked with goiter in farm animals and attributed a decline in goiter as a problem for which local sheep farmers should use iodized salt for their flocks. He gave iodine to goitrous dogs and reported their change from "wizened and listless" to "active and robust." He concluded from his studies that endemic goiter was primarily due to "a compensatory reaction to iodine deficiency." He then convinced the local school authorities to permit his classic study of iodine for prevention and treatment of goiter for school girls in Akron Ohio in 1917. The iodine prophylaxis study in schoolgirls in Akron during 1917–1919 showed a significantly lower frequency of goiter in those treated with iodine five in 2,190 cases (0.2%), compared to a control group with goiter in 495 out of 2,305 girls (21%). In 1924, Marine wrote: "Simple goiter is the easiest and cheapest of all known diseases to prevent and its control may be accomplished by available methods as soon as organized society determines to make the effort.").

David Cowie was born in 1872 in New Brunswick, Canada. His grandfather was a doctor trained in Glasgow, Scotland. He studied at the Battle Creek College, later transferred to study medicine at the University of Michigan and then at the University of Heidelberg, Germany. On return to Michigan he started the Pediatrics Department at the University Hospital. In 1920 he was named the first Professor of Pediatrics at the University of Michigan. He conducted research publishing on many medical topics. His interest in the issue of goiter in the Midwest would lead to his most memorable accomplishment. In 1922, Cowie proposed US iodization of salt to eliminate simple goiter. Advocacy by Marine and Cowie was instrumental in promoting the US iodine supplementation effort. Supported by the American Medical Association (AMA) and the American Public Health Association (APHA), Marine and Cowie persuaded the Morton Salt Company in 1924 to iodize table salt. Public awareness of essential nutrients was growing due to publicity over pellagra, rickets, and cretinism and the productive research findings associated with them in the same time period (see Chapters 9 and 11). Iodized salt became a popular national norm, and with continued support from the medical and public health professions, iodization of table salt became a widely accepted standard in North America. By 1930, 89 percent of total salt sales in Michigan were iodized. Follow-up surveys showed goiter prevalence rates declining rapidly in all parts of the country.

In the lead-up to the US entry into World War II Selective Service reports indicated that 25 percent of army draftees showed evidence of past or present malnutrition leading to rejection from military service for many. In 1941, President Franklin D. Roosevelt convened the first White House National Nutrition Conference for Defense. This led to nationally recommended dietary nutrient allowances, and issuance of War Order Number One to protect civilian health by adopting a program to regulate "enriched" foods, including salt with mandatory levels of iodine; wheat flour with vitamin B complex and iron; and milk with vitamin D. Enriched foods became the popularly accepted norm for most food producers and consumers in the United States due to widespread publicity over medical and public awareness of vitamin deficiencies in the early part of the 20th century. In 1998, folic acid (folate), a water-soluble vitamin, was added to cereal and grain products to prevent neural tube (see Chapters 9, 11 and 20).

Iodization of salt as a preventive measure has become standard public health practice in many countries. It has been compulsory in Canada since 1979 and widespread in Western Europe although not universal and not always at effective levels. Everett Koop, in a 1988 report of the US Surgeon-General on nutrition, noted that the first food fortification of adding iodine to salt in the United States took place in 1924, and that prevention of iodine deficiency is best achieved through the iodization of salt on a national scale as the safest and most cost effective public health measure to prevent iron deficiency disorder (IDD) especially brain damage to newborns.

CURRENT RELEVANCE

Iodine is an essential element in nutrition. Insufficient iodine in natural sources causes clinical or subclinical thyroid disorders with low levels of circulating thyroid hormones and urinary iodine. A deficient or irregular supply of iodine damages fetal development and produces fetal hypothyroidism causing varying degrees of brain damage in infants, including cretinism and in milder forms of mental handicap. Enlargement of the thyroid gland (goiter), indicating suboptimal thyroid function, has been documented in many areas of the world where there are low levels of ground- and surface water iodine.

Basil Hetzel, born and raised in Adelaide, Australia, became a professor of medicine and a medical scientist with an interest in thyroid disorders. In 1964, he was invited by the Papua New Guinea Public Health Department to investigate the goiter and cretinism highly prevalent in the highland villages. He established a plan to give periodic iodine injections and showed reduction in clinical cases. He became an ardent advocate and leading proponent of international efforts to address iodine deficiency globally to prevent goiter, brain damage, and thyroid disorders by tackling iodine deficiency by salt fortification with iodine. He was a key figure in establishing the International Council for the Control of Iodine Deficiency Disorders, working with WHO and UNICEF to help develop national control programs in developing countries. A *Lancet* editorial cited a distinguished American professor of medicine who stated that Hetzel *"helped protect an estimated 80 million newborns from needless brain damage - a major public health triumph comparable to the campaigns to eliminate smallpox and polio."*

During the 1980s the World Health Organization (WHO) expressed growing concern with the widespread nature of iodine deficiency disorders (IDD) affecting an estimated 2.3 billion people especially those in China, the former Soviet Union, Southeast Asia, and in many developing countries. Hetzel, a leading pioneer in promoting global iodine deficiency control and ultimately global elimination in a 1983 editorial in *Lancet*, stated that:

> *"Disorders resulting from severe iodine deficiency affect more than 400 million people in Asia alone. These disorders include stillbirths, abortions, and congenital anomalies; endemic cretinism, characterised most commonly by mental deficiency, deaf mutism, and spastic diplegia and lesser degrees of neurological defect related to fetal iodine deficiency; and impaired mental function in children and adults with goitre associated with subnormal concentrations of circulating thyroxine . . .. Iodised salt and iodised oil (by*

injection or by mouth) are suitable for the correction of iodine deficiency on a mass scale. A single dose of iodised oil can correct severe iodine deficiency for 3–5 years. Iodised oil offers a satisfactory immediate measure for primary care services until an iodised salt programme can be implemented. The complete eradication of iodine deficiency is therefore feasible within 5–10 years."

In 1986, the World Health Assembly called on all nations to introduce iodization of salt or other appropriate technology to reduce this silent pandemic. Dunn in a 1992 editorial in the *New England Journal of Medicine* raised the question of eradication of iodine deficiency. The World Summit for Children meeting at the United Nations in New York in 1990 included the elimination of IDD by the year 2000 in its plan of action. The recommended daily adult iodine intake is about 150 μg/day, about half that for children and infants, but increases to 225 μg/day during pregnancy, because of the ability of the normal thyroid system to compensate for varying levels of supply.

Canada implemented mandatory fortification of salt with iodine in 1979. The Canadian government reported that *"iodine deficiency is among the four major nutritional deficiencies in the world and can lead to several medical disorders, including goiter, stunted physical and intellectual development, stillbirths, and spontaneous abortions. These disorders have been virtually eliminated in Canada through salt iodization."* In the United States, iodine intake was found to have declined between the 1970s and 1990s; about 70 percent of salt sold by grocery stores is iodized but salt consumption has fallen and those on vegan diets may be deficient in iodine especially during pregnancy.

Since 1994 the WHO has recommended iodization of salt as the safest and most cost-effective method to ensure adequate dietary iodine intake. Worldwide household coverage with iodized salt increased from 46 percent in 2000 to 52 percent of homes in 2010 with variation between regions and countries. Coverage increased from 22 percent to 63 percent in Sierra Leone but declined from 75 percent to 65 percent in the Central African Republic. Sub-Saharan Africa, Southeast Asia, Eastern Mediterranean regions, and Eastern Europe have the least access to iodized salt and higher proportions of populations have iodine deficiency. Urinary iodine concentration is a marker for adequate iodine intake with standards recommended by the WHO and the recommended indicator for assessing population-based iodine intake. Dietary iodine is excreted in the urine and spot tests of pregnant women and school children are the recommended indicators of population iodine status. The criteria for assessing the severity of iodine deficiency are shown in Table 10.1.

The WHO and the Food and Agriculture Organization (FAO) of the United Nations recommend addressing IDD of thyroid dysfunction in extreme forms of goiter and cretinism. Other consequences of iodine insufficiency include hypothyroidism, decreased fertility rate, increased perinatal death, and infant mortality. With low iodine intake thyroid hormone production requires

TABLE 10.1 Criteria for Assessing the Public Health Severity of Iodine Deficiency

Severity of Public Health Problem	Indicator	
	Median urinary iodine (μg/L)	Total goiter prevalence (%)
Mild	50−99	5.0−19.9
Moderate	20−49	20−29.9
Severe	<20	>30

Source: Allen L, Dary O, de Benoist B, Hurrel R, editors. WHO guidelines on food fortification with micronutrients. Geneva, Switzerland: WHO, 2006. Available at: http://www.who.int/nutrition/publications/guide_food_fortification_micronutrients.pdf (accessed 18 December 2016).

increased secretion of thyroid stimulating hormone (TSH) resulting in enlargement of the thyroid (goiter). This is the result of thyroid hyperplasia because the thyroid is stressed to produce the needed thyroid hormones.

Deficiency or even mild insufficiency of iodine results in thyroid failure during the critical period of brain development from fetal life up to the third month after birth and will result in irreversible alterations in brain function. In areas of severe endemic iodine deficiency, cretinism may affect up to 5−15 percent of the population. In regions of mild or moderate iodine deficiency the results are milder neurological and intellectual impacts that may cause loss of as much as 15 percent or 8 points of intelligence quotients (IQ) impairment of an iodine deprived person's intellectual potential. Allen et al. in the 2006 *WHO Guidelines on Food Fortification With Micronutrients* reported that: "*A meta-analysis of 19 studies conducted in regions of severe deficiency showed a mean IQ loss of 13.5 points among affected populations. Correction of iodine deficiency at the right time reduces or eliminates all consequences of this readily preventable condition.*"

The global importance of iodine insufficiency disorders including goiter, stillbirths, stunted growth, thyroid deficiency, and mental defects affects 13 percent of the world's population, or 740 million people. From 2003 to 2011, international efforts led to a decrease in the number of iodine-deficient countries from 54 to 32 and the number of countries with adequate iodine intake increased from 67 to 105, with reportedly over 70 percent of the world's population covered by iodized salt since the early 1990s, dramatically reducing the incidence of iodine deficiency.

Nevertheless despite progress in expanding salt iodization, iodine deficiency remains the leading cause of preventable intellectual impairment in the world and may cause as much as 15 percent or 8 points of intelligence quotients (IQ) impairment of an iodine deprived person's intellectual potential. This is especially critical for subclinical hypothyroidism in neonates and goiter in adolescents and adults. Iodized salt programs have been implemented in many countries. UNICEF reports that globally iodine deficiency is the primary cause of preventable brain damage in children, during fetal development and in the first few years of a child's life, with 38 million newborns annually in developing countries at risk of preventable brain damage due to deficiency of iodine.

In 2013, 111 countries and some 70 percent of all households worldwide had access to adequately iodized salt, as defined by surveys of urinary iodine concentration of 100−299 μg/L in school children. Thirty countries remain iodine-deficient, nine are moderately deficient, 21 are mildly deficient, but none are currently considered severely iodine-deficient. However, worldwide iodine deficiency remains a public health problem in 47 countries, and about 1.9 billion people (38 percent of the world's population) live in areas with iodine deficiency. Globally 241 million school children are estimated to have inadequate levels of iodine intake. Surveys of school children show that Southeast Asia has the largest number with low iodine intake (76 million); and progress is slow in Africa, where 39 percent (58 million) have inadequate iodine intake.

Although iodine nutrition has been improving since 2003, global progress may be slowing with nearly one-third of the world's population still living in areas with iodine deficiency. Intervention programs urgently need extension to reach this population still exposed to inadequate iodine, and adequacy of salt fortification alone to achieve iodine adequacy (Table 10.2).

The American Thyroid Association recommends that women take 150 μg of iodine supplements daily during pregnancy and lactation and that all prenatal vitamin/mineral preparations contain 150 μg of iodine. US surveys carried out in 2005−06 and 2007−08 by the National Health and Nutrition Examination (NHANES) studies showed adequate iodine levels in the general population sample with some mild deficiencies in Hispanic populations and higher deficiencies in black population groups.

Some two-thirds of the people living in Western and Central Europe are iodine-deficient. Damage to reproductive function and to the development of the fetus and newborn are the most important consequences of iodine deficiency. The Nordic countries vary widely in regulation and iodine adequacy. Goiter and cretinism were common in pre-iodized salt times especially in some areas in Sweden, but very little occurred in Denmark. Sweden and Finland introduced fortification of table salt 50−75 years ago (1930−46), and Finland as well as Norway adopted iodine fortification of cow fodder. In Denmark iodine has been added to household salt and salt in bread since 2000. Iodine adequacy is excellent in Iceland where fish meal is added to cow fodder. Currently, pregnant and lactating women are reportedly mildly deficient in iodine in some Nordic countries.

TABLE 10.2 The Spectrum of IDD

Fetus	Spontaneous abortions
	Increased risk of stillbirths
	Congenital abnormalities
Neonate	Increased infant mortality
	Cretinism
	Cognitive impairment, neurological disorders, endemic mental retardation
	Hypothyroidism
	Increased susceptibility of the thyroid gland to nuclear radiation
Child, adolescent	Hypothyroidism
	Goiter
	Retarded physical development in child and adolescent
	Impaired mental function
Adult	Spontaneous hyperthyroidism in the elderly
	Goiter with its complications
	Decreased fertility
	Iodine-induced hyperthyroidism in adults
	Increased susceptibility of the thyroid gland to nuclear radiation

Source: Adapted from Allen L, Dary O, de Benoist B, Hurrel R, editors. WHO guidelines on food fortification with micronutrients. Geneva, Switzerland: WHO, 2006. Table 3.8, p. 55. Available at: http://www.who.int/nutrition/publications/guide_food_fortification_micronutrients.pdf (accessed 18 December 2016).

The World Bank assisted China, which until 1993 had the highest levels of iodine deficiency in the world including cretinism with some 400 million people (40% of the global total) estimated to be at risk of IDD; 20 percent of children aged 8−10 in 1995 were estimated to have goiter. In 1993, China launched a national IDD elimination program to address iodine deficiency and increase public consciousness and industry capacity to iodize packaged salt. Monitoring salt quality promoted compliance of the salt industry through enforcement of licensing regulations and legislation banning noniodized salt. Iodized salt in households increased from 80 percent in 1995 to 94 percent in 1999. Salt quality also improved. The World Bank Group reported that the total goiter rates for children aged eight fell from 20.4 percent in 1995 to 8.8 percent in 1999. The progress demonstrated in China shows the high level of political commitment needed for national public health programming. The universal salt iodization (USI) program resulted in improved levels of urinary iodine where the iodized salt was implemented, but as a result of monitoring in 2012, the standard recommended salt iodine concentration was adjusted to 20–30 mg/kg.

In many European countries recent studies of iodine excretion in the urine of adults, adolescents, and newborns and on the iodine content of breast milk indicate a high prevalence of iodine deficiency (moderate in many cases and severe in a few). Although iodized salt is available theoretically in most countries, its quality, availability and consumption are often unsatisfactory. In some countries the iodine content is set too low and salt consumption overestimated. Nearly one-third of the world population still has inadequate iodine intake. Pregnant women in northeast England have 3.5 percent iodine deficiency, and 40 percent borderline. Other UK studies show over 40 percent of pregnant women having inadequate iodine intake with measurable reduction in IQ and school performance in their children. A study in Italy showed mild iodine deficiency in northeast Italy. Adequate iodine status was achieved when iodized salt was combined with daily milk intake in a national iodine program, which led to consumption of iodized salt in 60–70 percent of the Italian households. Studies in Spain and Iran showed benefit in IQ measures for children whose mothers had received an iodine supplement had more favorable psychometric assessment results than children of the other group of mothers. However, iodine fortification in Europe in recent years is showing evidence of undercompensating for deficiency and insufficiency.

Eliminating widespread iodine and other vitamin and mineral deficiencies will not happen without effective governmental public health policies and leadership, not only to fortify salt but also bread, and also to provide supplements for at-risk groups. Nigeria's mandatory salt iodization program provides one example that has been successful. Public health professionals and policy-makers in state and local government, with the support of international agencies, have a moral responsibility to promote aggressive national nutrition policies. Even in many countries in Europe, government leadership is needed to monitor and adjust iodine levels in fortified salt and to mandate fortification of flour with folic acid to prevent neural tube defects. Fortification of salt could also be used in combination with other essential micronutrients such as folic acid, B12, and B6.

India has a 50-year history of salt iodization, but a national policy of USI was not adopted until 1986. Later national and state legislatures enacted subsequent legislation prohibiting sale of noniodized salt for human consumption. Iodized salt coverage varies among the states, but overall 71 percent of households consume iodized salt and surveys show iodine adequacy. However, nearly 250 million Indians including eight million children remain susceptible to IDD (Box 10.1).

From the 1970s onward international efforts to control and ultimately eliminate iodine deficiency conditions were advocated and promoted by international organizations including the WHO, FAO, the World Bank,

BOX 10.1 Historical Milestones From Discovery of Iodine to Elimination of Iodine Deficiency Disorders Globally

1811	Gay–Lussac/Courtois identify and name iodine. Seaweed found effective in treating goiter.
1835	Boussingault and Roulin were the first to recommend iodized salt to prevent goiter.
1916–1919	Marine realized goiter was a serious public health problem in the Great Lakes region of the United States and carried out intervention studies with iodine in schoolchildren in Akron Ohio 1924.
1922	Switzerland's iodized salt program has been operating uninterrupted since 1922.
1924	Cowie promotes manufacture of iodized salt; Morton's iodized salt sweeps America.
1960	WHO's first comprehensive review of goiter on world scale to determine severity of the problem. Successful elimination of IDD in industrialized countries, but progress made in developing countries was very slow.
1970–90	Controlled studies in iodine deficiency in soil and water regions; iodine supplementation eliminated the incidence of cretinism but also improved cognitive function.
1974	The World Food Council is the first of a number of international organizations over the next decade to call for the global elimination of goiter.
1980	First global estimate from WHO on the prevalence of goiter showing 20–60 percent of the world's population suffer from iodine deficiency and/or goiterous, with most of the burden in developing countries.
1983	The concept of IDD is introduced with emphasis on the effects of iodine deficiency on brain function.
1985	UNICEF, WHO, and the Australian government found the International Council for Control of Iodine Deficiency Disorders (ICCIDD) to promote knowledge and its application.
1990–92	The 43rd World Health Assembly in Geneva recognizes IDD elimination as a major priority. The UN World Summit for Children recognized IDD as a public health problem affecting more than two billion people; adopts a plan for virtual elimination of IDD by the year 2000, confirmed by 45th World Health Assembly and WHO-FAO Conference on Nutrition.
1993	The National Advocacy Meeting in China organized with ICCIDD support launches the largest USI and IDD elimination effort in the world with endorsement of the Prime Minister.
2000	Salt 2000 - salt producers endorse USI and IDD elimination. A global network on the sustained elimination of IDD is formed with the ICCIDD, WHO, UNICEF, Salt Institute, EuSalt, Kiwanis International, Micronutrient Initiative, Emory University, and US CDC as member organizations.

(Continued)

BOX 10.1 (Continued)

2001–02	Network for the Sustained Elimination of Iodine Deficiency founded in Paris, France. UN General Assembly Special Session on Children. ICCIDD strongly endorses commitment of Member States on USI as a strategy to eliminate IDD.
2005	The ICCIDD at the World Health Assembly adopts a resolution to require all Member States to report every three years on iodine nutrition status.
2008	Copenhagen Consensus recognizes iodization of salt to eliminate IDD as one of the most economical efforts in international development.
2009	ICCIDD and the ninth International Salt Symposium of private sector salt producers agree to USI and IDD elimination with strategy for progress.
2012–14	Seventy percent of all households worldwide now have access to adequately iodized salt; 111 countries have sufficient iodine intake; 30 countries remain iodine-deficient; 38 million newborns in developing countries every year remain unprotected from the lifelong consequences of brain damage. Iodization of salt to eliminate IDD confirmed as the best investment strategy in international development.
2014 to present	Increasing reports from Europe and elsewhere indicate that inadequate levels of urinary iodine in pregnant women and school children leave newborns and children vulnerable to loss of IQ potential and calls for review of policies to reduce this risk with supplementation as well as modified fortification policies to include industrial as well as table salt.

Sources: Iodine Global Network. Available at: http://www.ign.org/historical-milestones.htm (accessed 18 December 2016); UNICEF. Sustainable elimination of iodine deficiency: progress since the 1990 World Summit for Children. New York: UNICEF; 2008. Available at: http://www.unicef.org/publications/files/Sustainable_Elimination_of_Iodine_Deficiency.pdf (accessed 18 December 2016); Zimmermann MB. Research on iodine deficiency and goiter in the 19th and early 20th centuries. J Nutr. 2008;138:2060–63. Available at: http://jn.nutrition.org/content/138/11/2060.full.pdf + html (accessed 18 December 2016).

UNICEF, the International Council for Control of Iodine Deficiency Disorders, the European Thyroid Association, and Kiwanis International. Some countries (e.g., Canada) and the World Bank have called for national and international action to control this widespread public health problem. The 1990 World Summit for Children called for universal iodization of salt with a target of 95 percent iodization in each country by 1995. By 1994, 94 countries had national plans for iodization of salt, with 58 countries, including almost 60 percent of the world's children, on schedule.

TABLE 10.3 Recommended Dietary Allowances (RDAs) for Iodine

Age	Male	Female	Pregnancy	Lactation
Birth to 6 months	110 mcg[a]	110 mcg[a]		
7–12 months	130 mcg[a]	130 mcg[a]		
1–3 years	90 mcg	90 mcg		
4–8 years	90 mcg	90 mcg		
9–13 years	120 mcg	120 mcg		
14–18 years	150 mcg	150 mcg	220 mcg	290 mcg
19 + years	150 mcg	150 mcg	220 mcg	290 mcg

[a]Adequate Intake (AI). Note: WHO recommends 250 mcg per day for pregnant women.
Source: National Institute of Health. Iodine: fact sheet for health professionals, June 24, 2012.
Available at: https://ods.od.nih.gov/factsheets/Iodine-HealthProfessional/ (accessed 7 August 2016).

Micronutrient Initiatives (MIs), an advocacy and technical nongovernment organization with help from the Canadian government, has promoted iodization initiatives in many developing countries. Although there have been important successes, as of 2015 thirty-five million babies are still born annually without adequate iodine, and half of these will suffer some degree of mental impairment, with the residual problem mainly among the poor. Access to iodized salt is crucial to achieve eradication of IDD. Careful monitoring of access and iodine levels in key population groups is needed to reach the one billion people still subject to this crippling nutritional deficiency. Education to promote public and manufacturer support for regulation and consumption of iodized salt is also vital. Lack of awareness and resistance to government-mandated fortification are very present dangers that will prevent millions from benefitting from this highly effective "magic bullet" of public health (Table 10.3).

The world's highest percentage of desalinated water consumption occurs in Israel with five desalination plants producing 50 percent of the water supply. The process of desalination of seawater results in removal of iodine with the result that populations relying on seawater for potable (drinking) water are at risk for IDD. A case-controlled study of pregnant women and school children in Israel found that 70 percent of participants had iodine intake below the recommended standard. The study concluded that there is an urgent need to investigate the health impact of desalinated water.

Data from the Iodine Global Network and the WHO show that in the decade leading up to 2013 the number of iodine-deficient countries fell from 54 to 30. The number of iodine-sufficient countries increased from 67 to 112, and the number with excessive iodine intake increased from five to 10. In most countries with excess intake overiodization of salt and/or poor monitoring of salt iodization is to blame. Out of 128 countries with household coverage of adequately iodized salt, at least 90 percent of households in 37 countries consume adequately iodized salt, but in 39 countries, coverage rates are below 50 percent.

Addressing iodine deficiency requires advocacy and technical assistance to assist in reaching vulnerable people across the globe. Many international aid agencies, including USAID, UNICEF, the World Bank, and donor governments, such as Canada, are working to assist low income countries to address micronutrient deficiency condition including IDD as essential for health and economic development. This includes advocacy and technical support service to countries wishing to implement food fortification including iodization of salt with financial support from many governments' foreign aid programs. India was helped to protect 2.2 million newborns from mental and physical damage due to iodine deficiency by extending iodized salt use to 108 million people. In Senegal and neighboring countries, 300,000 newborns were protected from IDD by providing 15 million people with adequately iodized salt. African and Asian populations are becoming urbanized with access to manufactured foods. Staple food products are increasingly produced by large-scale industry, enabling successful fortification including monitoring and modification.

Progress is being made, but inertia and complacency are still barriers to achieving the goal of IDD eradication as a public health problem. Iodine deficiency continues to be an important public health problem in Europe as well as in low-income countries. Monitoring of iodine status is crucially important, especially for vulnerable populations, particularly pregnant women, infants, and school children. Monitoring iodization of salt and other dietary iodine sources is important to ensure adequate levels of iodine, thus avoiding iodine excess as well as insufficiency. Finally, it is essential to coordinate interventions designed to reduce population sodium intake with salt iodization programs in order to maintain adequate levels of iodine nutrition as salt intake declines.

ETHICAL ISSUES

The goal of USI is still distant for many countries and requires renewed efforts by governments as well as bilateral and multilateral agencies. Prevention of IDD by setting standards for mandatory fortification of salt and supplements for risk groups may help reduce resistance of some mothers to immunization and public controversy over fluoridation. Some aspects of public health require mandatory regulation (e.g., limiting smoking advertisements or smoking in public places). This can arouse reactions to what some disparagingly called "the Nanny State." A 2014 American Academy of Pediatrics policy statement includes: *"adequate iodine intake is critical in pregnant women and neonates because thyroid hormone is required for brain development in children. Severe, untreated hypothyroidism in infancy results in irreversible cretinism, but milder iodine deficiency can also affect cognitive development of the child."*

While democracy is based on the premise that the rule of law is fundamental to a civil society, which mandates limitations on behavior by a due process of legislation and regulation by elected representatives, monitored by civil service professional staff, under judicial supervision of constitutionality. For example, one cannot drive on the left side of the road except in a designated situation or country, and seat belts and protected child seats are mandatory to protect people from serious injury or death in road crashes. Police and public health officials have the duty to protect public health and safety, with responsibilities to ensure safe and healthful conditions in road and workplace environments, pasteurization of milk, standards and monitoring of food and water quality as well as many other aspects of civil society.

Success in mandatory iodization of salt is not guaranteed. Vietnam experienced serious setbacks, with a decline from 1995 when 90% of households used adequately iodized salt to 45% in 2011 with a decline in urinary iodine concentration among women of reproductive age from the optimal range to levels indicating inadequate iodine intake. This resulted from political backtracking canceling the mandatory regulation of iodized salt (Codling et al., 2015). A similar event in Israel led to cancellation of mandatory fluoridation of water by a new Minister of Health ideologically opposed to fluoridation. Israel also failed to mandate iodization of salt relying on voluntary compliance, but now being revisited. Similarly the UK also relied on voluntary fortification of salt with iodine with the result that iodized salt is not widely available or used and iodine levels in pregnant women are inadequate. Thus the objective of protecting newborns is substandard due to political failure. Unfounded misconceptions occur in the food industry that iodine will interfere with taste and color of food products resulting in lobbying against mandatory iodization and reluctance to comply. Introduction of mandatory fortification requires sustained advocacy by government and academic public health people to stress the need for protecting children from the harm done by iodine inadequacy.

Newborns have a right to be protected by society from the damage done by iodine deficiency. A parent does not have the right to harm the child. A civil society undertakes the responsibility to protect the child from IDD and other vitamin deficiencies just as much as it must protect the child from physical or other abuse. This is an ethical responsibility as well as an economic-driven responsibility, to save the family and society from the cost of caring for sick children.

ECONOMIC ISSUES

The estimated cost of malnutrition to the world economy is 3.5 trillion USD. Studies indicate that every dollar invested in nutritional support, such as in eliminating IDD, yields 16 USD in return value due to improved health and societal effects of work, education, and economic growth. The Copenhagen Conference (2008) evaluated losses due to: reduced physical productivity; indirect losses due to cognitive losses and effects in schooling; and losses due to increased health care costs. The World Bank has long recognized health as a legitimate priority for investment in developing countries and specifically so for nutrition including prevention of iodine deficiency conditions. Elimination of iodine deficiency is deemed one of the most cost-effective programs with a ratio of USD$28 saved per dollar spent. China implemented a program that resulted in reduced goiter rates in children from 20.4 percent in 1995 to 8.8 percent in 1999. The cost of iodine fortification of salt is estimated to be 5−7 ¢/kg, or five percent of the retail price in most countries. In the United States the cost of iodization of salt per person is estimated to be $0.04 annually. Despite the marginal cost of iodized salt, there is a reduction in iodine intake and changes in salt consumption including the use of noniodized salt in manufactured foods in part due to recommendations to reduce salt intake because of the prevalence of hypertension, reduced use of iodized salt in animal supplementation, and a low level of public awareness of iodine deficiency as a public health problem.

Iodine deficiency is highly prevalent in pregnant women in the UK and in other European countries including many that iodize their salt. In the UK, iodization of salt is not mandatory and a low percentage of homes use iodized salt routinely. Iodine supplementation of pregnant women in the UK was shown to be cost-effective and improved the IQ of newborns. A review of IDD in pregnant women in Europe indicates a similar situation even in countries that iodize salt, a reminder that pregnant and lactating women need supplementation of iodine to meet their thyroid hormonal needs to protect the well-being of infants. The cost of iodization and supplementation is minuscule compared to the gain in intelligence and educatability of children in rich and poor countries alike.

CONCLUSION

Iodine deficiency causes serious harm to newborns and infants, resulting in loss of intellectual capacity even when the deficiency is at a subclinical level. Harm to children and adults occurs in terms of enlarged thyroid gland as goiter and disturbed thyroid function. Addressing iodine deficiency is primarily the responsibility of government entities to ensure mandatory fortification of salt or flour with iodine and to monitor urinary iodine levels in pregnant women and school children in order to make adjustments as needed. In addition, professional organizations and medical practitioners should be alerted to the need for routine supplements of iodine for pregnant women either as an independent supplement or in multivitamin preparations to ensure protection of the fetus from inadequate fetal iodine levels and preventable birth defects.

WHO in 2017 states: *"Iodine deficiency is the world's most prevalent, yet easily preventable, cause of brain damage. Today we are on the verge of eliminating it — an achievement that will be hailed as a major public health triumph that ranks with getting rid of smallpox and poliomyelitis"* Despite the remarkable progress cutting the IDD-affected population from two billion people at the beginning of the 21st century to one billion currently, there is growing concern that major difficulties remain in the road to IDD elimination globally. Great progress has been made in implementing the global consensus on fortification of salt with iodine in the reduction of IDD, but much work remains to meet the needs of the nearly one billion people who do not have the protection of fortified foods and suffer the consequences of clinical and subclinical IDD. However, even in advanced countries with long histories of fortified foods, monitoring needs to be strengthened and modifications made to fortification levels to avoid overuse and undersupply of this vitally needed element.

The CDC reports that more than 70 countries, including the United States and Canada, have salt iodization programs. Approximately 70 percent of households worldwide use iodized salt, ranging from almost 90 percent of households in North and South America to less than 50 percent in Europe generally, in the United Kingdom, and the Eastern Mediterranean regions. Recent studies indicate that significant iodine deficiency among pregnant women and school children is found in Europe, the United Kingdom, and many countries, including Israel. Despite the progress, some stagnation has taken hold. A renewed sense of mission and leadership is needed in individual countries and in global initiatives to achieve elimination of IDD as a public health problem globally.

Iodine fortification is indeed a "Magic Bullet" of public health but it must be promoted, used wisely and available to everyone. Education of policy-makers, the general public, manufacturers and professional staff for safe supervision of the monitoring and adjustments needed are vital to success in use of this amazing public health measure. While policies for elimination of IDD have been slow to be adopted or revised in some countries, remarkable progress has been achieved globally since 1990. Successful experience such as seen in China and Nigeria show the potential, so that IDD eradication remains an important public health challenge of high priority in the 21st century.

RECOMMENDATIONS

1. Eradication of iodine deficiency, requires a renewed stress in national and global health policy with strengthening iodine fortification and monitoring of at risk groups.
2. Iodine Supplements: Pregnant and lactating women should receive daily iodine supplements. Prenatal programs should include this in their regular program and manufacturers of supplements should be encouraged (mandated) to include adequate iodine in their products (WHO). Iodine supplements should also be included in routine supplements for infants along with vitamin D and iron. Pregnant women and at-risk groups should be monitored for adequate nutrition status of food micronutrients. Agricultural policies should include providing supplements including iodine as a basic part of animal husbandry for milk and meat production.
3. Universal Iodization of Salt (USI): Strengthen support of and by international organizations and donors for USI with advocacy and guidance for national governments and private sector salt producers in implementing USI. As a member of the Iodine Global Network, UNICEF supports activities in iodization and global policies and standards in iodine nutrition, working to shape the global food fortification agenda and provide guidance on improving monitoring systems. Table salt and industrial salt use in baking food processing should be iodized on a mandatory basis.
4. Monitoring: It is vital to maintain monitoring of urinary iodine levels in pregnant women and school-aged children with regional and socioeconomic variables in order to be able to adjust fortification and supplementation levels. This should include monitoring populations and communities using desalinated water. WHO standards for monitoring should be expanded to include newborns, pregnant women, and school children as well as, milk products, community water supplies, and animal husbandry supplements.
5. Micronutrient Deficiency Conditions: IDD is one of many micronutrient deficiency conditions that can be addressed individually, but must also be seen in the wider context, with fortification and supplementation including multiple essential vitamins and minerals for pregnant and lactating women and for infants and children and other at-risk groups.
6. National governments as well as international health organizations must take initiatives for prevention of iodine deficiency which damages thyroid function and normal development of the fetus, infants and school children and other population groups.

STUDENT REVIEW QUESTIONS

1. Can a nutritional deficiency be eliminated or eradicated as a global public health problem?

2. What are the main methods of control or elimination of IDD as a public health problem?
3. Why has iodization of salt and routine supplements for pregnant women and infants been slow in adoption globally?
4. Should public health focus on iodine or on micronutrient deficits as a group, including iron, vitamins A, B (group), C, D, and essential minerals such as fluoride, sodium, selenium, zinc, and others?
5. What political or societal reactions can occur to slow or impeded progress in implementation of an IDD control program?

RECOMMENDED READINGS

1. Allen L, Dary O, de Benoist B, Hurrel R, editors. WHO guidelines on food fortification with micronutrients. Geneva, Switzerland: WHO, 2006. Available at: http://www.who.int/nutrition/publications/guide_food_fortification_micronutrients.pdf (accessed 18 November 2017).

2. American Academy of Pediatrics. Council on Environmental Health, Policy Statement. Iodine deficiency, pollutant chemicals, and the thyroid: new information on an old problem. Pediatrics. 2014;133(6):1163−1166. Available at: http://pediatrics.aappublications.org/content/pediatrics/133/6/1163.full.pdf (accessed 1 December 2017).

3. Andersson M, de Benoist B, Darnton-Hill I, Delange F. Iodine deficiency in Europe: a continuing public health problem. Geneva, Switzerland: WHO, 2007. Available at: http://www.who.int/nutrition/publications/VMNIS_Iodine_deficiency_in_Europe.pdf (accessed 18 November 2017).

4. Andersson M, Karumbunathan V, Zimmermann MB. Global iodine status in 2011 and trends over the past decade. J Nutr. 2012;142:744−750. Available at: http://jn.nutrition.org/content/142/4/744.full.pdf (accessed 18 November 2017).

5. Bath SC, Button S, Rayman MP. Availability of iodised table salt in the UK − is it likely to influence population iodine intake? Public Health Nutr. 2014;17(2):450−454. Available at: https://doi.org/10.1017/S1368980012005496. Abstract available at: https://www.ncbi.nlm.nih.gov/pubmed/23324480 (accessed 20 October 2017).

6. Bath SC, Rayman MP. A review of the iodine status of UK pregnant women and its implications for the offspring. Environ Geochem Health. 2015;37(4):619−629. Available at: https://www.ncbi.nlm.nih.gov/pmc/articles/PMC4442695/pdf/emss-62337.pdf (accessed 18 November 2017).

7. Bath SC, Sleeth ML, Mc Kenna M, Walter A, Taylor A, Rayman MP. Iodine intake and status of UK women of childbearing age recruited at the University of Surrey in the winter. Br J Nutr. 2014;l112(10):1718−1723. Available at: https://www.ncbi.nlm.nih.gov/pmc/articles/PMC4340577/ (accessed 17 November 2017).

8. Bath SC, Steer CD, Golding J, Emmett P, Rayman MP. Effect of inadequate iodine status in UK pregnant women on cognitive outcomes in their children: results from the Avon Longitudinal Study of Parents and Children (ALSPAC). Lancet. 2013;382:331−337. Available at: http://www.sciencedirect.com/science/article/pii/S0140673613604365 (accessed 17 November 2017).

9. Becker DV, Braverman LE, Delange F, Dunn JT, Franklyn JA, Hollowell JG, et al. Iodine supplementation for pregnancy and lactation—United States and Canada: recommendations of the American Thyroid Association. Thyroid. 2006;16(10):949−951. Available at: http://www.ncbi.nlm.nih.gov/pubmed/17042677 (accessed 17 November 2017).

10. Bishai D, Nalubola R. The history of food fortification in the United States: its relevance for current fortification efforts in developing countries. Econ Develop Cultural Change. 2002;51(1):37−53.   Available   at: http://web1.sph.emory.edu/users/hpacho2/ PartnershipsMaize/Bishai_2002.pdf (accessed 3 November 2017).

11. Caldwell KL, Jones R, Hollowell JG. Urinary iodine concentration: United States National Health and Nutrition Examination Survey 2001−2002. Thyroid. 2005;15:692−699. Abstract available at: http://www.ncbi.nlm.nih.gov/pubmed/16053386 (accessed 18 November 2017).

12. Caldwell KL, Pan Y, Mortensen ME, Makhmudov A, Merrill L, Moye J. Iodine status in pregnant women in the National Children's Study and in U.S. women (15−44 years), National Health and Nutrition Examination Survey 2005−2010. Thyroid. 2013;23(8):927−937. http://dx.doi.org/10.1089/thy.2013.0012. Epub 2013 Jul 20. Available at: http://www.ncbi.nlm.nih.gov/pmc/articles/PMC3752509/ (accessed 18 November 2017).

13. Caldwell KL, Makhmudov A, Ely E, Jones RL, Wang RY. Iodine status of the U.S. population, National Health and Nutrition Examination Survey, 2005−2006 and 2007−2008. Thyroid. 2011;21(4):419−427. doi:10.1089/thy.2010.0077. Abstract available at: http://www.ncbi.nlm.nih.gov/pubmed/21323596 (accessed 5 November 2017).

14. Carpenter KJ. David Marine and the problem of goiter. J Nutr. 2005;135:675−680. Available at: http://jn.nutrition.org/content/135/4/675.long (accessed 24 November 2017).

15. Caulfield LE, Richard SA, Rivera JA, Musgrove P, Black RE. Stunting, wasting, and micronutrient deficiency disorders. In: Jamison DT, Breman JG, Measham AR, et al., editors. Disease control priorities in developing countries. 2nd edition. Washington, DC: The International Bank for Reconstruction and Development/The World Bank, 2006 Co-published by New York: Oxford University Press. Chapter 28. Available at: http://www.ncbi.nlm.nih.gov/books/NBK11761/ (accessed 18 November 2017).

16. Centers for Disease Control. Achievements in public health, 1900-1999: safer and healthier foods. MMWR Morb Mort Wkly Rep. 1999;48(40):905−913. Available at: https://www.cdc.gov/mmwr/preview/mmwrhtml/mm4840a1.htm (accessed 17 November 2017).

17. Centers for Disease Control and Prevention. National report on biochemical indicators of diet and nutrition in the U.S. population 1999−2002. In: Trace elements: iodine; Atlanta GA, 2016, pp. 91−100 Available at: https://www.cdc.gov/nutritionreport/99-02/pdf/ nr_ch4a.pdf (accessed 18 November 2017).

18. Centers for Disease Control and Prevention. Second national report on biochemical indicators of diet and nutrition in the U.S. population. Washington, DC: National Center for Environmental Health, 2012. Available at: http://www.cdc.gov/nutritionreport/pdf/ Nutrition_Book_complete508_final.pdf (accessed 18 November 2017).

19. Center for Global Development. Millions saved: editions 1 and 2, 2016: Case 15: Preventing iodine deficiency disease in China. Available at: http://www.cgdev.org/page/ case-15-preventing-iodine-deficiency-disease-china (accessed 18 November 2017).

20 Codling K, Quang NV, Phong L, Phuong H, Quang ND, Bégin F, et al. The rise and fall of universal salt iodization in Vietnam: lessons learned for designing sustainable food fortification programs with a public health impact. Food Nutr Bull. 2015;36(4):441−454. Available at: https://doi.org/10.1177/0379572115616039. Abstract available at: https://www.ncbi.nlm.nih.gov/pubmed/26578534 (accessed 20 October 2017).

21. Copenhagen Consensus, 2008: malnutrition and hunger, executive summary. Available at: https://www.scribd.com/document/78190561/Copenhagen-Consensus-2008-Summary (accessed 25 November 2017).

22. Costeira MJ, Oliveira P, Santos NC, et al. Psychomotor development of children from an iodine-deficient region. J Pediatr. 2011;159(3):447−453. Available at: http://www.science-direct.com/science/article/pii/S002234761100237X (accessed 18 November 2017).

23. de Benoist B, Andersson M, Egli I, Takkouche B, Allen H, editors. Iodine status worldwide: WHO global database on iodine deficiency. Geneva: Department of Nutrition for Health and Development-World Health Organization, 2004. Available at: http://www.who.int/nutrition/publications/micronutrients/FNBvol29N3sep08.pdf (accessed 20 November 2017).

24. de Benoist B, McLean E, Andersson M, Rogers L. Iodine deficiency in 2007: global progress since 2003. Food Nutr Bull. 2012;29(3):195−202. Available at: http://www.who.int/nutrition/publications/micronutrients/FNBvol29N3sep08.pdf (accessed 18 November 2017).

25. Delange F. Iodine requirements during pregnancy, lactation and the neonatal period and indicators of optimal iodine nutrition. Public Health Nutr. 2007;10(12A):1571−1580. Available at: http://www.ign.org/cm_data/2007_Delange_Iodine_requirement_d_pregnancy_PHN.pdf (accessed 18 November 2017).

26. Delange F, Burgi H. Iodine deficiency in Europe. Bull World Health Organ. 1989;67:317−325. Available at: http://www.ncbi.nlm.nih.gov/pmc/articles/PMC2491245/ (accessed 18 November 2017).

27. Dunn JT. Iodine deficiency—the next target for elimination? New Engl J Med. 1992;326:267−268. Available at: http://www.nejm.org/doi/full/10.1056/NEJM199201233260411 (accessed 18 November 2017).

28. Feyrer J, Politi D, Weil DN. The cognitive effects of micronutrient deficiency: evidence from salt iodization in the United States. National Bureau of Economic Research. NBER Working Paper Series; July 2013. Available at: http://www.nber.org/papers/w19233.pdf (accessed 21 November 2017).

29. Financial Tribune (Iran). Expectant mothers have iodine deficiency: during the last 22 years, iodization of salt has prevented 20,000 goiter cases and increased the average children's IQ by 6. Available at: https://financialtribune.com/articles/people/66362/expectant-mothers-have-iodine-deficiency (accessed 25 October 2017).

30. Food and Agriculture Organization. The state of food and agriculture 2013: food systems for better nutrition. Rome: Food and Agriculture Organization of the United Nations, 2013. Available at: http://www.fao.org/docrep/018/i3300e/i3300e.pdf (accessed 18 November 2017).

31. Goh C. An analysis of combating iodine deficiency: case studies of China, Indonesia, and Madagascar. OED Working Paper Series No. 18. Washington, DC: The World Bank, 2001. Available at: http://ieg.worldbankgroup.org/Data/reports/iodine.pdf (accessed 18 November 2017).

32. Hetzel BS. Iodine deficiency disorders and their eradication. Lancet. 1983;352(8359):1126−1129. Abstract available at: http://www.thelancet.com/journals/lancet/article/PIIS0140-6736(83)90636-0/abstract (accessed 18 November 2017).

33. Hetzel BS. Editorial. The control of iodine deficiency. Am J Public Health. 1993;83:494−495. Available at: http://www.ncbi.nlm.nih.gov/pmc/articles/PMC1694466/pdf/amjph00528-0016.pdf (accessed 17 November 2017).

34. Hetzel BS. Towards the global elimination of brain damage due to iodine deficiency—the role of the International Council for Control of Iodine Deficiency Disorders. Int J Epidemiol. 2005;34(4):762−764. Available at: http://ije.oxfordjournals.org/content/34/4/762.long (accessed 21 November 2017).

35. Hetzel BS. The development of a global program for the elimination of brain damage due to iodine deficiency. Asia Pac J Clin Nutr. 2012;21:164−170. Available at: http://apjcn.nhri.org.tw/server/APJCN/21/2/164.pdf (accessed 30 June 2017).

36. Institute of Medicine, Food and Nutrition Board. Dietary reference intakes: vitamin A, vitamin K, arsenic, boron, chromium, copper, iodine, iron, manganese, molybdenum, nickel, silicon, vanadium, and zinc. Washington, DC: National Academy Press, 2001. Available at: http://www.nap.edu/read/10026/chapter/1 (accessed 18 November 2017).

37. Iodine Global Network. Israel: desalinated seawater linked to iodine deficiency. Available at: http://www.ign.org/p142002523.html (accessed 18 November 2017).

38. Iodine Global Network. Global iodine nutrition scorecard 2015. Available at: http://www. ign.org/cm_data/Scorecard_2015_August_26_new.pdf (accessed 18 November 2017).

39. Iodine Global Network. News, Quick Links. Available at: http://www.ign.org (accessed 18 November 2017).

40. Jaiswal N, Melse-Boonstra A, Sharma SK, Srinivasan K, Zimmermann MB. The iodized salt programme in Bangalore, India provides adequate iodine intakes in pregnant women and more-than-adequate iodine intakes in their children. Public Health Nutr. 2015;18 (3):403−413. doi:10.1017/S136898001400055X. Abstract available at: http://www.ncbi. nlm.nih.gov/pubmed/24762565 (accessed 18 November 2017).

41. Kibirige MS, Hutchison S, Owen CJ, Delves HT. Prevalence of maternal dietary iodine insufficiency in the north east of England: implications for the fetus. Arch Dis Child Fetal Neonatal Ed. 2004;89:436−439. Available at: https://www.ncbi.nlm.nih.gov/pmc/articles/ PMC1721745/pdf/v089p0F436.pdf (accessed 17 November 2017).

42. Koop E. The Surgeon General's report on nutrition and health, summary and recommendations. Washington, DC: US Department Health and Human Services, 1988. Available at: http://www.mcspotlight.org/media/reports/surgen_rep.html (accessed 20 October 2017).

43. Lazarus JH. Iodine status in Europe in 2014. Eur Thyroid J. 2014;3(1):3−6. Published online 2014 Mar 1. doi:10.1159/000358873. Available at: https://www.ncbi.nlm.nih.gov/ pmc/articles/PMC4005253/pdf/etj-0003-0003.pdf (accessed 25 June 2017).

44. Lee L. Iodine deficiency. Medscape. December 16, 2015. Available at: http://emedicine. medscape.com/article/122714-overview#a3 (accessed 18 October 2017).

45. Leung AM, Braverman LE, Pearce EN. History of US iodine fortification and supplementation. Nutrients. 2012;4:1740−1746. doi:10.3390/nu4111740. Available at: http:// www.ncbi.nlm.nih.gov/pmc/articles/PMC3509517/pdf/nutrients-04-01740.pdf (accessed 18 October 2017).

46. Levine R. Preventing iodine deficiency disease in China. Millions saved: proven successes in global health. Washington, DC: Center for Global Development, 2004. Available at: http://www.cgdev.org/page/case-15-preventing-iodine-deficiency-disease-china (accessed 17 December 2016).

47. Markel H. "When it rains, it pours": endemic goiter, iodized salt and David Murray Cowie. Am J Public Heath. 1987;77:219−229. Available at: http://www.ncbi.nlm.nih.gov/pmc/articles/PMC1646845/pdf/amjph00253-0087.pdf (accessed 18 December 2016).

48. Makhmudov AA, Caldwell KL. The challenge of iodine deficiency disorder: a decade of CDC's ensuring the quality of urinary iodine procedures program: EQUIP 10 year anniversary. National Center for Environmental Health (U.S.). Division of Laboratory Sciences. Stephen B. Thacker CDC Library Collection, Centers for Disease Control and Prevention, Atlanta GA, 2011. Available at: https://stacks.cdc.gov/view/cdc/39393 (accessed 30 June 2017).

49. Marine D, Kimball OP. The prevention of simple goiter in man. A survey of the incidence and types of thyroid enlargements in the schoolgirls of Akron (Ohio), from the 5th to the 12th grades, inclusive−the plan of prevention proposed. J Lab Clin Med. 1917;115 (1):128−136. Reprinted and available through: https://www.ncbi.nlm.nih.gov/pubmed/ 1099484 (accessed 30 June 2017).

50. McGuire J, Galloway R. Enriching lives: overcoming vitamin and mineral malnutrition in developing countries. Washington, DC: World Bank, 1994. Available at: http://documents. worldbank.org/curated/en/938771467989505587/pdf/multi0page.pdf (accessed 18 December 2016).

51. Method A, Tulchinsky TH. Commentary: food fortification: African countries can make more progress. Adv Food Technol Nutr Sci Open J. 2015;SE(1):S22−S28. Available at: http://www.openventio.org/AdvancesInFoodTechnologyandNutritionSciencesOpenJournal/ AFTNSOJ-SE1.pdf (accessed 18 December 2016).

52. Monahan M, Boelaert K, Jolly K, Chan S, Bartam P, Roberts TE. Costs and benefits of iodine supplementation for pregnant women in a mildly to moderately iodine-deficient population: a modeling analysis. Lancet Diabetes Endocrinol. 2015;3(9):715−722. Available at: http://www.thelancet.com/journals/landia/article/PIIS2213-8587(15)00212-0/abstract (accessed 17 December 2016).

53. Nystrom HF, Brantsaeter AL, Erlund I, Gunnarsdottir I, Hulthen L, Laurberg P, et al. Iodine status in the Nordic countries past and present. Food Nutr Res. 2016;60:31969. Available at: http://dx.doi.org/10.3402/fnr.v60.31969.

54. Office of Dietary Supplements. Iodine: fact sheet for health professionals. Bethesda, MD: National Institutes of Health, 24 June 2011. Available at: https://ods.od.nih.gov/factsheets/ Iodine-HealthProfessional/ (accessed 18 December 2016).

55. Otten JJ, Hellwing JP, Meyers LD. Dietary reference intakes. Washington, DC: National Academy Press, 2006, 320−327. Available at: https://www.nap.edu/catalog/11537/ dietary-reference-intakes-the-essential-guide-to-nutrient-requirements (accessed 18 December 2016).

56. Ovadia IS, Gefel D, Aharoni D, Turkot S, Fytlovich S, Troen AM. Can desalinated seawater contribute to iodine-deficiency disorders? An observation and hypothesis. Public Health Nutr. 2016;19(15):2808−2817. Available at: https://www.ncbi.nlm.nih.gov/pubmed/ 27149907 (accessed 17 October 2016).

57. Pearce EN, Andersson M, Zimmermann MB. Global iodine nutrition: where do we stand in 2013? Thyroid. 2013;23(5):523−528. doi:10.1089/thy.2013.0128. Available at: http://www. ncbi.nlm.nih.gov/pubmed/23472655 (accessed 18 December 2016).

58. Pearce EN. Iodine deficiency in pregnant women in the UK: the costs of inaction. Lancet Diabetes Endocrinol. 2015;671−672. Available at: http://www.thelancet.com/pdfs/journals/ landia/PIIS2213-8587(15)00228-4.pdf (accessed 18 December 2016).

59. Pincock S. Basil Hetzel: vanquishing iodine deficiency disorders. Lancet. 2013;381 (9868):717. Available at: http://www.thelancet.com/pdfs/journals/lancet/PIIS0140-6736(13) 60569-3.pdf (accessed 9 April 2017).

60. Rah JH, Garg A, Naidu BRG, Dwarka D, Agrawal DD, et al. Reaching the poor with adequately iodized salt through the supplementary nutrition programme and midday meal scheme in Madhya Pradesh, India. Bull World Health Organ. 2013;91:540−544. doi:10.2471/BLT.12.110833. Available at: http://www.who.int/bulletin/volumes/91/7/12-110833/en/ (accessed 18 December 2016).

61. Statistics Canada. Iodine status of Canadians, 2009 to 2011; 2013. Available at: http://www. statcan.gc.ca/pub/82-625-x/2012001/article/11733-eng.htm#n3 (accessed 18 December 2016).

62. Shen H, Su X, et al. Eliminating iodine deficiency in China: achievements, challenges and global Implications. Nutrients. 2017;9(4):361. Available at: https://doi.org/10.3390/ nu9040361. Available at: https://www.ncbi.nlm.nih.gov/pmc/articles/PMC5409700/pdf/ nutrients-09-00361.pdf (accessed 20 November 2017).

63. Tomasson RE. Dr. David Marine, 96, Found goiter's cure. New York Times, November 1976. Available at: http://www.nytimes.com/1976/11/28/archives/dr-david-marine-96-found-goiters-cure-almost-70-years-ago.html (accessed 28 October 2017).

64. Tran TD, Hetzel B, Fisher J. Access to iodized salt in 11 low- and lower- middle-income countries: 2000 and 2010. Bull World Health Organ. 2016;94(2):122−129. Available at: https://www.ncbi.nlm.nih.gov/pmc/articles/PMC4750437/ (accessed 17 November 2016).

65. Trumpff C, De Schepper J, Tafforeau J, Van Oyen H, Vanderfaeillie J, Vandevijvere S. Mild iodine deficiency in pregnancy in Europe and its consequences for cognitive and psychomotor development of children: a review. Med Biol. 2013;27(3):174−183. Available at: http://www.sciencedirect.com/science/article/pii/S0946672X13000047 (accessed 1 December 2017).

66. Tulchinsky TH. Micronutrient deficiency conditions: global health issues. Public Health Rev. 2010;32:243−255. Available at: https://publichealthreviews.biomedcentral.com/articles/10.1007/BF03391600 (accessed 20 November 2017).

67. Tulchinsky TH, Varavikova EA. The new public health. 3rd edition. San Diego, CA: Academic Press/Elsevier, 2014, 442−443.

68. UNICEF. Micronutrients; December 23, 2015. Available at: http://www.unicef.org/nutrition/index_iodine.html (accessed 18 November 2017).

69. UNICEF. Universal salt iodization in Nigeria: processes, successes, and lessons. Available at: http://www.unicef.org/nigeria/ng_publications_USI_in_Nigeria_Report.pdf (accessed 18 November 2017).

70. UNICEF. Sustainable elimination of iodine deficiency. New York: UNICEF, 2008. Available at: https://www.unicef.org/publications/files/Sustainable_Elimination_of_Iodine_Deficiency.pdf (accessed 14 November 2017).

71. UNICEF Nigeria. Nutrition information sheet; June 2006. Available at: http://www.unicef.org/wcaro/WCARO_Nigeria_Factsheets_Nutrition.pdf (accessed 17 November 2017).

72. Velasco I, Carreira M, Santiago P, Muela JA, García-Fuentes E, Sánchez-Muñoz B, et al. Effect of iodine prophylaxis during pregnancy on neurocognitive development of children during the first two years of life. J Clin Endocrinol Metab. 2009;94(9):3234−3241. Abstract available at: https://academic.oup.com/jcem/article/94/9/3234/2596586 (accessed 15 November 2015).

73. Watutantrige FS, Nacamulli D, Pozza D, Giachetti M, Frigato F, Redaelli M, et al. Iodine status in schoolchildren living in northeast Italy: the importance of iodized-salt use and milk consumption. Eur J Clin Nutr. 2013;67(4):366−370. Abstract available at: http://www.ncbi.nlm.nih.gov/pubmed/23462940 (accessed 18 November 2017).

74. Wong EM, Sullivan KM, Perrine CG, Rogers LM, Pena-Rosas JP. Comparison of median urinary iodine concentration as an indicator of iodine status among pregnant women, school-age children, and nonpregnant women. Food Nutr Bull. 2011;32(3):206−212. Available at: https://www.ncbi.nlm.nih.gov/pubmed/22073794 (accessed 17 December 2016).

75. World Health Organization/UNICEF/International Council for the Control of Iodine Deficiency Disorders. Global prevalence of iodine deficiency disorders. Micronutrient Deficiency Information System Working Paper No. 1. Geneva, Switzerland: WHO, 1993. Available at: http://apps.who.int/iris/handle/10665/37149 (accessed 17 December 2016).

76. World Health Organization. Resolution WHA60.21. Sustaining the elimination of iodine deficiency disorders. Sixtieth World Health Assembly, Geneva, 23 May 2007. Geneva, Switzerland: WHO, 2007. Available at: http://who.int/nutrition/topics/WHA60.21_idd_en.pdf (accessed 17 December 2016).

77. World Health Organization. Salt reduction and iodine fortification strategies in public health: report of a joint technical meeting convened by the World Health Organization and the George Institute for Global Health in collaboration with the International Council for the Control of Iodine Deficiency Disorders (ICCIDD) Global Network, Sydney, Australia; March 2013. Available at: http://apps.who.int/iris/bitstream/10665/101509/1/9789241506694_eng.pdf (accessed 17 December 2016).

78. World Health Organization; UNICEF; ICCIDD. Assessment of the iodine deficiency disorders and monitoring their elimination. Geneva, Switzerland: WHO, 2007. Available at: http://apps.who.int/iris/bitstream/10665/43781/1/9789241595827_eng.pdf (accessed 18 December 2016).

79. Zimmermann M. Research on iodine deficiency and goiter in the 19th and early 20th centuries. J Nutr. 2008;138:2060−2063. Available at: http://jn.nutrition.org/content/138/11/2060.full.pdf + html (accessed 18 December 2016).

80. Zimmerman M, Delange F. Iodine supplementation of pregnant women in Europe: a review and recommendations. Eur J Clin Nutr. 2004;58(7):979−984. Available at: http://www.nature.com/ejcn/journal/v58/n7/full/1601933a.html (accessed 18 December 2016).

81. Zimmermann MB. Iodine deficiency in pregnancy and the effects of maternal iodine supplementation on the offspring: a review. Am J Clin Nutr. 2009;89(2):668S−672SS. Available at: http://ajcn.nutrition.org/content/89/2/668S.full.pdf + html (accessed 18 December 2016).

82. Zimmermann MB. The effects of iodine deficiency on pregnancy and infancy. Paediatr Perinat Epidemiol. 2012;26(Suppl 1):108−117. Available at: https://www.ncbi.nlm.nih.gov/pubmed/22742605 (accessed 17 December 2016).

83. Zimmermann MB. Iodine deficiency and excess in children: worldwide status in 2013. Endocr Pract. 2013;19(5):839−846. doi:10.4158/EP13180.RA. Abstract available at: http://www.ncbi.nlm.nih.gov/pubmed/23757630 (accessed 18 December 2016).

84. Zimmermann MB, Boelaert K. Iodine deficiency and thyroid disorders. Lancet Diabet Endocrinol. 2015;3(4):286−295. Available at: https://www.ncbi.nlm.nih.gov/pubmed/25591468 (accessed 17 December 2016).

85. Zimmerman MB, Gizat M, Abbot K, Andersson M, Lazarus JH. Commentary: iodine deficiency in pregnant women in Europe. Lancet. 2015. Available at: http://www.ign.org/cm_data/2015_Zimmermann_Iodine_deficiency_in_pregnant_women_in_Europe.pdf (accessed 18 December 2016).

Chapter 11

Elmer McCollum and Edward Mellanby: Vitamin D and Cod Liver Oil for Prevention of Rickets and Osteoporosis

ABSTRACT

Rickets was pandemic in the early 20th century in industrialized countries among the urban working class and poor. The rapid development of nutritional sciences and Elmer V. McCollum's work on vitamin D during the 1920s revealed the cause to be lack of sunlight exposure and poor nutrition. Edward Mellanby discovered that cod-liver oil treated and prevented rickets, which became an international standard of prevention with rapid decline in rickets prevalence. During World War II, mandatory fortification of "enriched milk" in the United States and Canada virtually eliminated rickets. When it was assumed that rickets was a problem of the past and mandatory fortification cancelled, the disease made a comeback in Canada leading to reintroduction in 1979 of mandatory fortification of milk.

Rickets and osteomalacia are also returning in other high-income countries especially among low birth weight, breastfed infants of dark skinned religiously, covered women, but also in indigenous or poor populations living in remote areas, or socially deprived urban settings. Vitamin D has found recognition as a universally essential vital amine (vitamin) normally produced by sunlight acting on the exposed skin and essential for bone health and other body functions including fighting carcinogenesis, cardiovascular and other diseases associated with aging. Multiple studies carried out around the world show that vitamin D deficiency is common everywhere in many age and gender groups including in sunny countries and is now considered a global pandemic requiring a high priority in public health in high-, medium- and low- income countries around the world. Vitamin D food fortification and supplementation for vulnerable populations such as pregnant and lactating women, infants and toddlers to prevent rickets, as well as adult women to prevent osteoporosis, are increasingly vital for public health policy globally.

Case Studies in Public Health. DOI: http://dx.doi.org/10.1016/B978-0-12-804571-8.00011-1

227

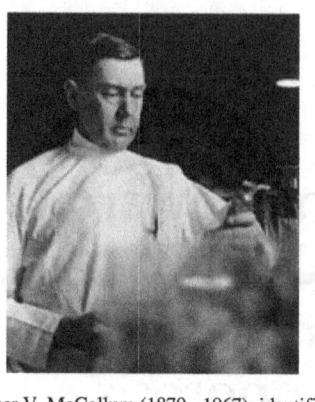

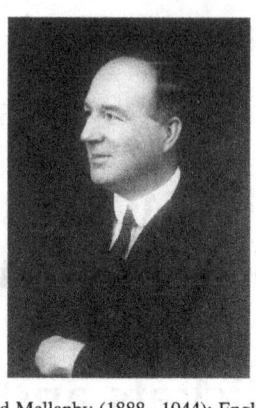

Elmer V. McCollum (1879–1967); identified "anti rachitic" nutritional factor later called Vitamin D and promoted healthy diets in America. *Photo courtesy of US National Library of Medicine ID: 101422517 NLM Image ID: B017820 Available at: http:// resource.nlm.nih.gov/101422517.*

Sir Edward Mellanby (1888–1944); English doctor who in 1919 identified and promoted cod liver oil as effective treatment and prevention of rickets then called "the English disease". *Courtesy: Wellcome Library*

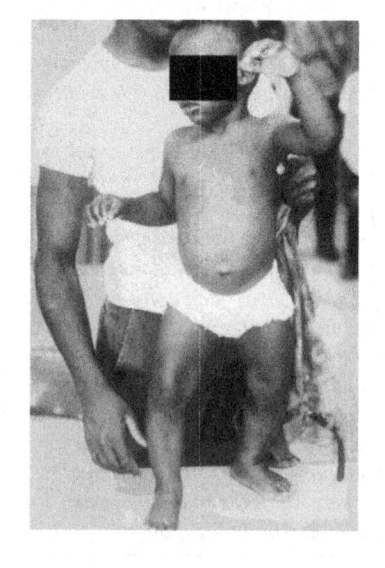

This child is suffering from malnutrition and has manifested symptoms of the disease known as nutritional rickets. Note the bowed legs and enlarged right wrist. Nutritional Rickets is a condition in which children's bones are too soft, and do not develop properly due to a deficiency of vitamin D. *Source: cdc phil at https:// phil.cdc.gov/Details.aspx?pid = 2435.*

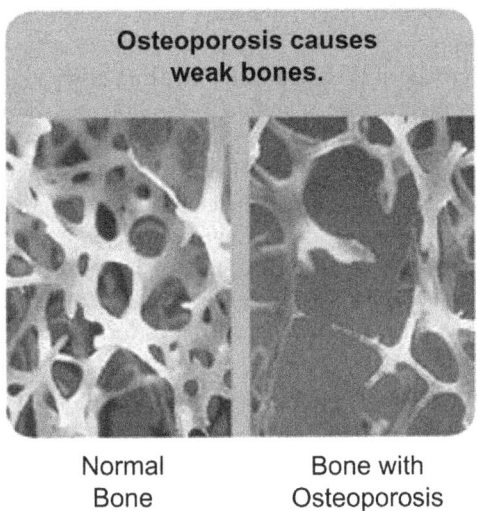

Normal   Bone with
Bone   Osteoporosis

Figure from U.S. Department of Health and Human Services. The 2004 Surgeon General's Report on Bone Health and Osteoporosis: What It Means To You. U.S. Department of Health and Human Services, Office of the Surgeon General, 2004. *National Institutes of Health. Osteoporosis, updated November 2010. Available at: https://report.nih.gov/NIHfactsheets/Pdfs/Osteoporosis (NIAMS).pdf (accessed 3 December 2017).*

BACKGROUND

Vitamin D is an essential micronutrient. It plays a major role in the fixation of calcium in the body and therefore important in the growth and maintenance of bone health. Increasing evidence of other important roles for vitamin D have been discovered in recent decades and are still explored today, such as immunomodulatory (affecting the immune system) and antiproliferative (affecting cell growth) functions.

Lack of vitamin D is divided into two levels of severity: deficiency and insufficiency. These are defined according to the concentration of 25-hydroxy-vitamin-D (25(OH)D) in the serum, the circulating, more stable form of the vitamin. Deficiency status is defined as $0-40\,nmol/L$ while insufficiency includes the range of $40-80\,nmol/L$.

Deficiency, which defines an extreme lack of the micronutrient, is directly related to rickets, a severe childhood disease that causes bone deformities, and to osteomalacia, a painful adulthood disease where the deficient calcium fixation leads to softening of the bones, affecting mainly women following menopause.

Vitamin D insufficiency was found to be related to different long-latency chronic conditions, including those related to calcium such as osteoporosis, muscle pain, and fatigue as well as hypertension/cardiovascular diseases. Due to its antiproliferative and immunomodulatory functions, vitamin D deficiency is also considered to be related to cancer (breast, colon, prostate), diabetes, multiple sclerosis, and lupus.

Vitamin D is produced in the human body from previtamin D3, depending on exposure to sunlight, more specifically to ultraviolet-B (UVB) radiation. Seasonal variations of sun exposure, use of sunscreen, dark skin pigmentation, air pollution, and aging, but mainly lack of regular sun exposure due to lifestyle and cultural issues, all affect the cutaneous production of the vitamin. Vitamin D is also obtained by dietary intake of eggs, liver, and fatty fish as well as supplementation and fortified foods. The dietary requirement for vitamin D is much higher in the absence of adequate exposure to sunlight resulting in the need for recommended standards for dietary intake, nutritional supplements in high-risk groups, and fortification of basic foods. Geographical variation including latitude and seasonality are factors in UVB light exposure affecting vitamin D levels and the need for dietary intake but multiple reports of low vitamin D levels in sunny countries have emphasized the global nature of the problem.

Rickets is one of important diseases of infancy because of its serious complications, including disorders of long bone growth, bowing of legs, pelvic deformity and, in extreme forms tetany and in infants and toddlers with convulsions, heart failure and death in extreme cases.

The early history of rickets begins with ancient medical writings from the first and second centuries CE, describing bone deformities among infants, by Soranus, a Roman physician and Galen, of the same era. In 1650 Francis Glisson, a Cambridge University physician, published a treatise on rickets, describing the clinical features and suggesting treatments. The first report of rickets in infants was published in 1651.

Rickets, along with scurvy and beri-beri, were known for centuries, but their causes were elusive until the twentieth century. The nineteenth century dogma of nutrition was based on influential German chemists led by von Liebig that an adequate diet consisted of 12 percent protein, five percent mineral, 10−30 percent fat, and the remainder as carbohydrate. This belief survived until the early part of the twentieth century when other researchers sought evidence that "accessory food factors" were essential for health and survival. The concept was sharpened by Casimir Funk in 1912 who described these other factors as "vital amines," which as essential nutritional elements that in deficiency conditions result in diseases such as beriberi, scurvy and rickets. Funk adapted it as a new term, "vitamins" (DeLuca, 2014).

Rickets, a childhood nutritional deficiency disease, was widespread in industrialized countries. In 1870, for example, it was believed that as many as one third of the poor children of such cities as London and Manchester suffered from obvious rickets. As late as 1921, rickets affected 75 percent of children in New York City schools, and in the same year, McCollum claimed that probably half of the children in cities in the United States had clinical rickets.

At the turn of the 20th century, rickets was rampant among infants and children living in crowded highly air polluted industrial cities of North America and Europe. The disease had a very common occurrence, and yet its exact etiology and effective treatment were elusive. Antirachitic properties of cod-liver oil were known and used. Dietary animal experiments and epidemiologic understanding of the correlation between sunlight exposure and rickets led to solving the riddle of the disease. In 1919, investigators in Germany showed that exposure to sunlight cured rickets, and that it acted by altering fats to produce vitamin D.

Elmer McCollum (1879–1967) was born in a poor farming family near Redfield, Kansas, and attended a rural single-room school. He was bright, energetic, self-educated and determined to advance his education. Working at numerous jobs he studied in a local high school, then the University of Kansas, graduating in 1903, and finally at Yale University, earning a PhD in organic chemistry in 1906. He joined the University of Wisconsin as an instructor in agricultural chemistry in 1907. He worked at the Agricultural Experiment Station in a study in progress, led by Stephen Babcock, to examine the effects of feeding three commonly used grains on the health and reproductive capacity of dairy cattle. The groups received chemically similar wheat, oats, and corn diets, respectively. The surprise finding was that the corn-fed cattle stayed healthy and strong, while the others languished. This study was pivotal in the development of nutritional science, then in its infancy. McCollum developed methods of chemical analysis of nutritive elements of fats important in healthy nutrition of rats, identifying the fat-soluble "anti rachitic" nutritional factor, then the fourth known vitamin, later to be called vitamin D.

Edward Mellanby (1984–1955) was born in West Hartlepool, the son of a shipyard owner, and educated at Barnard Castle School. He studied physiology at Emmanuel College, Cambridge and then medicine at St. Thomas's Hospital in London, graduating in 1913. As a lecturer at King's College for Women, London (1913–1920), he was asked to investigate the cause of rickets, then so common in the UK it was known as "the English disease." Impressed by the work of McCollum, Mellanby found that feeding caged dogs a diet of porridge induced rickets, which could then be reversed with cod liver oil. He showed in 1919 that the missing dietary "anti rachitic factor" was present in cod liver oil, leading to the promotion of cod liver oil to cure and prevent rickets. McCollum, in 1922, showed that the cod liver oil factor that cures rickets was the new vitamin he called vitamin D. Mellanby, then Sir Edward, guided the development of the British Medical Council, and as Secretary of the British War Cabinet provided control of the food policy during World War II including the policy of fortification of margarine with vitamins A and D along with adding calcium to bread during wartime. Mellanby later served as Chairman on the League of Nations technical nutrition committee, promoting standardization of vitamins.

Rickets declined with growing use of cod liver oil but remained widespread until fortification of milk was introduced in the 1940s, during World War II, in Britain and North America. The prevalence of rickets in the United Kingdom (UK), especially in the industrial cities in northern England and Scotland, declined dramatically with wide use of cod-liver oil and vitamin D fortification of margarine and in 1942, vitamin D had to be added as 400 IU to some foods including breakfast cereals. An isolated incident of overdosing with vitamin D in a nursery in the United Kingdom in the 1950s led to continuing bias against vitamin D fortification of milk in most of Europe despite increasing evidence of recurrence of rickets. In Canada, although antirachitic procedures (cod-liver oil for children and adding vitamin D to milk and margarine) were routine during the 1940s, the practice waned in the 1950s and due to concern of potential excesses of Vitamin D, with a switch from compulsory to voluntary fortification of milk with vitamin D. This led to hospitalizations for rickets, as reported from locations across the country. A 1971 Canadian national nutrition survey found significant vitamin D deficiencies in certain age, sex, ethnic, and geographic population groups. The addition of vitamin D was made mandatory for milk and margarine in Canada in 1975 and in 2011 regulations permitted fortification of other manufactured foods including bread and yeast-leavened baking products on a voluntary basis.

CURRENT RELEVANCE

Since the 1970s, a decline in milk consumption among children and adolescents has been reported in many developed countries, including France, Germany, the UK, Canada and the United States. Much of this is attributed to "milk displacement" with carbonated beverages (sodas) being preferred to milk, a trend increasing worldwide.

Reemergence or greater recognition of rickets has been noted in the United States in recent years and affects mostly black infants and children between four and 54 months of age who were exclusively breastfed over 6 months. Rickets cases reported in the United States between 1996 and 2003 numbered 166, among mostly black breastfed children. The Centers for Disease Control and Prevention (CDC) estimate that five of every million children between six months and five years of age have clinical rickets, with peak prevalence of vitamin D-deficient rickets between six and 18 months of age. The majority of affected children are black or breastfed.

In adults, malabsorption or poor dietary intake of vitamin D can result in osteomalacia with fragile bones and frequent fractures. Among the elderly, who are shut-in especially during winter months or among homebound or institutionalized patients, vitamin D deficiency is common. Air pollution and prolonged rainy seasons as well as greater indoor activity of children and concern that sun exposure leads to cancer of the skin including highly lethal melanomas may also contribute to poor levels of sun exposure.

In 1995, a Canadian report noted that despite the knowledge of benefits of sunlight and enrichment of milk with vitamin D, rickets had not completely disappeared, and that 17 cases of nutritional rickets were diagnosed at the Toronto Sick Children's Hospital from 1990 to 1995. Through the Canadian Pediatric Surveillance Program, pediatricians reported 104 cases of vitamin D deficiency rickets between 2002 and 2004. Severe vitamin D deficiency in the Canadian population has been reduced to less than 10 percent with a mean vitamin D intake of 200−300 IU (international units) compared to the recommended 600−800 IU for different age groups. However, in indigenous populations Vitamin D deficiency in children remains common. Arctic traditional foods can provide 1,000 IU vitamin D in the diet largely consisting of fish and other fatty foods. Hypovitaminosis D remains a public health concern among indigenous children in Canada and the United States. The primary objective in this study was to investigate the Vitamin D supplements for pregnant women which were controversial in the 1950–60s with allegations that they were teratogenic and caused a rare cardiac condition later shown to be of genetic origin (Wagner, 2008).

In the UK, during World War II children were given supplements such as cod-liver oil, but this practice stopped in the 1950s. Rickets in the UK was considered to have disappeared but in recent years there has been an upswing in reported cases. A study in the UK reported that the rate of rickets hospitalization rose tenfold from 0.34 cases per 100,000 children between 1991 and 1996 to 3.16 cases per 100,000 children between 2007 and 2011. Clinical cases of severe rickets including deaths are currently being reported in the UK, primarily in breast-fed infants of dark-skinned immigrant mothers unaware of the need for vitamin D supplements for infants. UK immigrant children with dark skin, e.g., of African, Caribbean, Asian, and Middle Eastern origin, are at risk because of prolonged breast feeding, low vitamin D among the mothers and less sunlight exposure for both mother and child, while they need more sunlight to make vitamin D. Those who are growing rapidly (premature babies, infants, toddlers, adolescents) and overweight children are also more at risk, and need vitamin D supplements. During 20 months of surveillance of rickets between March 2015−March 2017 from 3,500 pediatricians in the UK, 89 cases met the case definition; males 52 percent, females 48 percent. At the time of diagnosis 22 percent were aged under 1 year, 42 percent 1−2 years, 27 percent 2−5 years, and 9 percent 5−15 years. African (30%) and Pakistani (18%) children were a high proportion of the notified cases. (Julies et al., 2017).

In medium- and low-income countries, attaining the Millennium Development Goals (MDGs) is in part dependent on adequate micronutrient intake in the daily diet. A key goal is an increase in breastfeeding. However, as vitamin D content of human milk is extremely low, exclusively breastfed infants not adequately exposed to sunlight are at high risk to develop clinical rickets. In tropical and subtropical countries, urban overcrowding with

TABLE 11.1 Recommended Vitamin D Daily and Upper Limit by Age Group

Life Stage	Recommended Amount	Upper Limit
Birth to 12 months	400 IU	1000–1500 IU
Children 1–13 years	600 IU	2500–3000 IU[a]
Teens 14–18 years	600 IU	4000 IU[b]
Adults 19–70 years	600 IU	4000 IU
Adults 71 years and older	800 IU	4000 IU
4000 Pregnant and breastfeeding women	600 IU	4000 IU

[a]Children 1–8 years
[b]Children 9 years and older.
Source: US National Institutes of Health. Office of Dietary Supplements. Vitamin D, Updated 15 April 2016. Available at: https://ods.od.nih.gov/factsheets/VitaminD-Consumer/ (accessed 7 June 2017).

atmospheric pollution, a lack of vitamin D-fortified foods, long rainy seasons and social customs that limit skin exposure to sunlight are major factors in the development of vitamin D deficiency. Low dietary calcium intake is typically observed as a parallel risk factor. Vitamin D deficiency is common among northern indigenous people, and is attributed to living in high latitudes with long winters and limited sun exposure, but also to darker skin that blocks solar UVB and poor access to dietary sources of vitamin D such as fortified milk.

The importance of vitamin D in pregnancy has largely been ignored despite data that deficiency during pregnancy causes higher risk of maternal preeclampsia, periodontal disease in the mother, and impaired fetal growth increasing the risk of rickets in early infancy. A Global Working Group of the European Society of Pediatric Endocrinology in 2015 established definitions for rickets, vitamin D, and calcium deficiency recommending supplementary routine intake of vitamin D and calcium for infants and pregnant women for prevention and treatment of rickets and osteomalacia including women of childbearing age, and during lactation. They also recommend identification of risk groups who would benefit from screening and supplementation, such as dark skinned immigrant women with total body clothing who are likely to have little sun exposure, and their children. The Consensus Group advocates for eradication of rickets and osteomalacia through implementation of international vitamin D supplementation for infants and pregnant women along with food fortification programs.

The National Institutes of Health (NIH) Office of Dietary Supplements recommends vitamin D supplementation by age group. Table 11.1 presents the current recommended daily intake of vitamin D for different ages, genders, and pregnancy groups. The recommendation is US-based, where most milk and breakfast cereals are already fortified with vitamin D, but not milk products. However, the US national survey (NHANES 2005–06) findings indicate average intake levels for males from foods alone ranged from 204 to 288 IU/day depending on life stage group; for females the range was 144 to 276 IU/day, below the recommended intake levels, and almost no one has levels that are too high. In general, young people have higher blood levels of 25-hydroxyvitamin D than older people and males have higher levels than females. Deficiency levels of vitamin D are higher among African Americans, and people with enteric and endocrine disorders and obesity. Levels of fortification and supplementation will need review and adjustment, especially in view of substantial and mounting evidence of the importance of vitamin D in prevention of cardiovascular disease, asthma, colorectal, breast and other cancers, neurological and immunologic disorders, as well as osteoporosis.

Low levels of vitamin D lead to osteoporosis among postmenopausal women and result in the loss of bone mass, often leading to fractures, including those of the hip and spine. Those fractures are related to significantly higher morbidity and mortality. A 1998 study reported that the prevalence of vitamin D deficiency was common among US hospitalized patients. An editorial in the same issue noted that residents of latitudes 40 degrees north of the equator, due to low levels of sun exposure, make little vitamin D in winter. The editorial goes on to state that *"administration of vitamin D to older subjects with or without low serum 25-hydroxyvitamin D concentrations slow bone turnover and increases bone density. Most important of all, vitamin D and calcium supplementation in older subjects can reduce the rates of hip and other fractures"*. A UK study of seasonality of vitamin D levels in adults indicates that the majority of the population show low levels of vitamin D during and following winter months.

Vitamin D is attracting much attention from researchers due to its role in immune system maintenance and in cancer prevention, and while this is still in the hypothesis-generation stage, the evidence for such roles is mounting. The spread of these diseases across the world makes the issue of adequate vitamin D supply a global concern, affecting people of all ages and socioeconomic classes and stressing the need for supplementation and fortification. With growing stress on breastfeeding alone for infants up to 6 months and continuing following introduction of other foods the potential for low levels of vitamin D in newborns of low birth weight in particular is high, and thus routine vitamin D supplements for pregnant women and for infants is vital in all countries.

Global high prevalence of vitamin D insufficiency, reemergence of rickets and the growing scientific evidence linking low circulating 25(OH)D to increased risk of osteoporosis, diabetes, cancer, and autoimmune disorders have stimulated recommendations to increase sunlight (UVB) exposure as a source of vitamin D. Use of sunscreens blocks exposures to the sun and greatly reduces the amount of vitamin D absorbed. However, concern over increased risk of melanoma with unprotected UVB exposure has led to the alternative recommendation that sufficient vitamin D should be supplied through dietary sources including supplements along with sun exposure for 20−30 minutes between 11 AM to 2 PM five days per week.

Some 70 percent of the US milk supply is fortified voluntarily with vitamin D. However, the American Academy of Pediatrics recommends that all infants and children, including adolescents, have an additional minimum daily intake of 400 IU of vitamin D beginning soon after birth (Wagner and Greer, 2008). As noted above, Canada has mandatory regulation of both milk and margarine; in 2011 regulations were extended to include bread and yeast-leavened food products on a voluntary basis. A survey in Canada reports that 68 percent of Canadians had blood concentrations of vitamin D over 50 nmol/L—the level sufficient for healthy bones while 32 percent were below the cut-off. Children aged 3−5 had the highest rates above the cut-off (89%), while the 20 to 39 year olds had the lowest satisfactory rates (59%) (Statistics Canada, 2013). Healthy children and adolescents should be encouraged to follow a healthy lifestyle associated with a normal body mass index (BMI), including a varied diet with vitamin D-containing foods (fish, eggs, dairy products) and adequate outdoor activities with associated sun exposure.

Vitamin D intake is often too low to sustain healthy circulating levels of 25(OH)D in countries without mandatory staple food fortification, such as with milk and margarine. Even in countries that do fortify, vitamin D intakes are low in some groups due to their unique dietary patterns, such as low milk consumption, vegetarian diet, limited use of dietary supplements, or loss of traditional high fish intake. Finland introduced mandatory fortification of milk and margarine products in 2003. A study reports 50 percent increase in mean vitamin D blood levels in men aged 18−28 after fortification while 4 year olds reached a mean intake of vitamin D near the recommended level. However, adequacy was achieved by less than one-third of the children. Fortification had very little effect of raising the low levels of vitamin D in teen-aged girls in Finland.

The solution to widespread vitamin D deficiency lies in a multi-facetted approach, with both supplementation targeted to higher risk groups and food fortification in order to reach the general population. Despite milk fortification and current supplementation practices, widespread vitamin D deficiency according to current standards recommended by the US Institute of Medicine is still a nutritional problem even in high-income countries. In medium- and low-income countries, where fortification and supplementation are not practiced, vitamin D deficiency (among other micronutrient deficiency conditions such as iodine, iron, folic acid deficiencies) should be considered a serious underlying cause of high mortality rates of mothers, neonates, and others.

The importance of vitamin D in pregnancy has largely been ignored in global public health policy despite data that deficiency during pregnancy is associated with higher risk of maternal preeclampsia, periodontal disease in the mother, and impaired fetal growth increasing the risk of rickets in early infancy. Food fortification has proven to be the most effective means of increasing vitamin D levels across all population age/gender groups, along with screening for rickets and vitamin D levels as key public health programs for high- and especially medium- and low-income countries.

The return of clinical rickets among immigrant children in high income countries, and wide evidence of vitamin D deficiency in countries at all levels of socioeconomic development has made vitamin D a global public health issue of high priority. These issues are particularly challenging in rapidly growing elderly populations with dramatic increases in the number of bone disorders and other diseases beyond rickets, such as osteomalacia, and osteoporosis with multiple life-threatening fractures. The relationships between vitamin D deficiency and a wide range of illnesses including asthma, multiple sclerosis, cancer of the colon, cardiovascular diseases, and others require more investigation, but there is a growing evidence base indicating these relationships exist. The issue requires national and international efforts to screen for vitamin D status, along with implementation of policies or guidelines for vitamin D fortification and/or supplementation. It is also important to reassess recommended dietary intake guidelines, to monitor vitamin D levels in various age groups, and to promote public awareness of the complications of vitamin D deficiency.

ETHICAL ISSUES

Rickets has been shown to be highly prevalent in rich and poor countries including those with high levels of year-long sunlight with both vitamin D and calcium deficiency due to practices limiting sun exposure and lack of vitamin D-containing foods or supplements. Major international organizations including the World Health Organization (WHO), UNICEF, and the Food and Agriculture Organization (FAO) have not included vitamin D deficiency as a major public health issue, possibly due to the fact that internationally there are more acute micronutrient deficiency problems such as iodine, vitamin A, and iron deficiency; however, this does not justify ignoring the problem, especially in northern climate countries where sun exposure is limited seasonally and where no other source of vitamin D is available such as in fortified milk.

Hospitalization rates for rickets in England were low in the 1960s and 1970s, declined further in the 1980s and 1990s, but increased dramatically in the 2000s. Exaggerated concerns for toxicity have restrained policy in most European countries preventing adoption of fortification of milk and strongly promoting vitamin D supplements.

In the United States, 25% of women who are 65 years of age and over have osteoporosis of the femur neck or lumbar spine; for men 5% (NCHS, 2016). Preventing fractures in elderly people is a priority, especially with the increase in the elderly population to possibly a quarter of the population in the industrialized countries over the next two decades, but there is recognition that developing countries are also experiencing significant growth during this time.

The population approach in nutrition has a well-established track record in preventing important micronutrient deficiency conditions and related chronic diseases. Food fortification is essential to reach people who either do not or cannot respond to the individual health education and a healthy diet, due to lack of knowledge or access, or to its higher cost. Thus supplementation is essential for specific high-risk groups including women, infants, children, the elderly and in fact the population in general.

The ramifications of all this are many: fortification of milk products with vitamin D; routine supplements to infants, children, and adolescents; routine supplements for adults especially the elderly; measures to prevent falls among the elderly; education about the need for regular sun exposure for adults and the elderly (avoiding excess for fear of skin cancers); regulation and education among food manufacturers of good fortification and manufacturing practices; and education for good nutrition and increased awareness of nutrition among primary caregivers and the public generally as well as national governments.

The American Academy of Pediatrics (AAP) revised previous 2003 recommendations to increase the daily supplements recommended from 200 to 400 IU/day for all infants and children beginning in the first few days of life, noting increasing reports of rickets in infants due to inadequate vitamin D intake and decreased exposure to sunlight. Supplements should be used throughout childhood and adolescence, because adequate sunlight exposure is reduced by decreased outdoor in activity of children.

In 2015 the Consensus Group of the European Society for Pediatric Endocrinology (ESPE) conducted a thorough literature review of prevalence of rickets worldwide, established definitions for rickets, vitamin D and calcium deficiency, intakes of vitamin D and calcium required for prevention and treatment of rickets as well as for osteomalacia in women of childbearing age, pregnancy and lactation, and identification of risk groups who benefit from screening and supplementation. The ESPE group advocates eradication of rickets and osteomalacia through implementation of international vitamin D supplementation and food fortification programs and recommends specifically that:

- all infants should receive vitamin D (400 IU/day) supplements for the first year of life regardless of method of feeding;
- all pregnant women should take daily supplements of vitamin D (600 IU/day);

- all women in the age of fertility should take vitamin supplements; and
- sun exposure daily for 20−30 minutes.

Aging and lifestyle trends can lead to poor diet and changes in lifestyle habits contributing to important nutrient deficiencies in people of all ages, but particularly in children. Milk and dairy products comprise the main source of calcium intake for most children, but milk consumption has declined in recent decades. Vitamin D insufficiency is widespread among different age groups including children and adolescents in many countries.

Low levels of vitamin D have been found in all age groups in populations around the world. Studies of adults and seniors indicate calcium intake levels well below those recommended by national guidelines. Similarly, alarmingly, lifestyle factors such as excessive lack of sunlight exposure, alcohol consumption, smoking, and high or low body mass index (BMI) also elevate risk of osteoporosis and fractures. Children living in areas of high atmospheric pollution are at risk of developing vitamin D deficiency rickets.

Aging, poverty and lifestyle trends can lead to poor diet, which along with little or no direct sunlight exposure adversely affect bone and muscle health. Among the rapidly increasing elderly population, the impact of inadequate nutrition on falls and fracture prevention is a serious health risk due to osteoporosis. Inadequate protein and micronutrient intake with little or no direct sunlight exposure common in older people can adversely affect bone and muscle health.

Nutrient needs for vitamin D are vital throughout the lifespan even though dietary energy requirements and sun exposure vary with life stages. Lack of food sources of vitamin D without fortification of milk is a crucial factor in population adequacy of vitamin D for bone health. Factors such as reduced acid secretion may reduce absorption of iron and vitamin B12. Detection and management of nutrition−dietary related health conditions require biochemistry analysis for micronutrient deficiencies especially calcium and vitamins A, C, and D. Micronutrient deficiencies can be monitored, detected and managed with biochemical analysis on a selective basis during annual physical examination and in population surveys.

Profound physiological, psychosocial, and environmental changes, such as decreased sense of taste or smell, isolation, loneliness, depression, and inadequate finances, may also impact dietary adequacy and malnutrition in older ages. Counseling and other interventions such as increasing micronutrients in food products can prevent or reverse malnutrition thus improving functional health status and mobility. Lack of daily exposure to the sun is a major factor in low vitamin D levels in the elderly. Counseling can help delay care dependency, improve intrinsic capacity, and reverse frailty status.

Dietary and supportive counseling along with micronutrient supplements and access to fortified foods, for institutionalized people and independent-living elderly, as well as residents of orphanages, prisons, long-term mental facilities is essential. Many health and social conditions can result from lack of sunlight exposure and vitamin D deficiency.

Supplementation and food fortification are critical for prevention of clinical rickets, osteomalacia, and oestoporiosis as well as for improved health status and public health goals. However, the problem is global in scope. Food fortification by government mandate and regulation is essential in high-, medium-, and low-income countries, with cooperation from the private sector, food manufacturers, and in the context of broader policies for poverty reduction, education, and agricultural reform.

ECONOMIC ISSUES

Hypovitaminosis D and related abnormalities in bone chemistry are most common in the elderly residents of Europe but are reported in all elderly populations globally. Adequate exposure to sunlight is essential for vitamin D adequacy for all age groups, but oral intake augmented by both fortification and supplementation is necessary to maintain baseline stores. Although hypovitaminosis D has been detected frequently in virtually all age groups but with special impact on the elderly and housebound people, widespread preventive action has been slow to develop with wide variation in the epidemiology of hip fractures globally and in the European Union.

A 1995 report of hip fractures in 15 European Union (EU) countries estimated 382,000 cases and total care cost of about ECUs (European Currency Unit) 9 billion, indicating "*the need for routine supplementation for people at risk for osteoporosis.*" In 2000 there were nearly 900,000 hip fractures (females, 711,000; males, 179,000) in 27 EU countries. The 2008 EU report notes that among the EU countries, only ten had national guidelines for calcium and vitamin D supplements. A 2010 survey described the epidemiology, burden, and treatment of osteoporosis in the 27 countries of the EU and the high social and economic cost of the disease, with a projected increase of the economic burden due to aging populations. The report noted that: "*use of pharmacological interventions to prevent fractures has decreased in recent years, suggesting that a change in health care policy is warranted.*" In the United Kingdom, hip fractures were found to place great demand on resources and have the gravest impact on patients because of increased mortality, long-term disability, and loss of independence.

In Canada annually between 70 and 90 percent of hip fractures are caused by osteoporosis and primarily in those aged 50 or more years. Osteoporosis Canada reported that the health system costs of treating osteoporosis and fractures (acute and ambulatory care, prescription drugs, and indirect costs) had reached more than $2.3 billion (Canadian) annually as of 2010, rising to $3.9 billion when including the costs of long-term care facilities.

In the United States there are at least 250,000 hospitalizations for fractures in people over the age of 65 years annually, with over 95 percent caused by falls. NIH reports that there are over 40 million people who already have osteoporosis or are at high risk for fractures due to low bone mass. Over 2 million osteoporotic fractures for all sites occurred in the United States at a cost of $19 billion in 2005 with projected increase by 50% by 2025. As longevity increases in high- medium- and low-income countries the projections are that hip fractures will increase. Given the public health implications of osteoporotic fractures, the primary goal of osteoporosis therapy is to prevent fractures by slowing or preventing bone loss, maintaining bone strength, and minimizing or eliminating factors that may contribute to falls.

The consensus from these studies goes on to recommend that steps be taken to increase vitamin D intake, by nutritional advice to patients, planning institutional meals, and alerting physicians to the nearly universal need for more vitamin D. A widespread increase in vitamin D intake is likely to have a greater effect on osteoporosis than many other interventions. Concern about vitamin D deficiency among elderly women with a high risk of fracture particularly in winter months has raised the issue of routine vitamin D supplementation, which is inexpensive and effective and should be considered in people over 70 years of age who have a high risk of fracture including those who live in temperate, northern, and tropical or desert climes as well.

Low vitamin D levels have been demonstrated widely in Europe in a survey that reported that in the 27 original countries of the European Union an estimated 22 million women and 5.5 million men have osteoporosis. Of the 3.5 million new fragility fractures, 610,000 were hip fractures, 520,000 vertebral fractures, 560,000 forearm fractures, and 1,800,000 other fractures. The economic burden of incident and prior fragility fractures was estimated at 37 billion euros ($41.2 billion USD). International Osteoporosis reports that hip fracture costs have doubled or tripled in some EU countries over 10 years due to lack of priority and screening facilities such as bone-mineral density scanners. This screening modality is reimbursed by national insurance plans in only nine of 27 member states. Osteoporosis is part of national public health programs in only 10 of 27 countries. In Sweden, hip fractures account for nearly as many hospital days as acute myocardial infarction and for more than prostate and breast cancers combined.

CONCLUSION

To conclude, vitamin D deficiency not only causes rickets among children but also precipitates and exacerbates osteoporosis among adults and causes the painful bone disease osteomalacia. Vitamin D deficiency has been associated with increased risk of cancers, specifically colorectal cancer, as well as neurological (specifically multiple sclerosis), cardiovascular disease, rheumatoid arthritis, and type 1 diabetes mellitus. A 2017 report of a

Consensus Group of the Food and Nutrition Board, Health and Medicine Division, National Academies of Sciences report that in the US studies of NHANES between 2003-2006, deficient intake of vitamins D, A, E, B6, and C continues at deficiency levels similar to those of the 1970s to the 1990s for most age and racial/ethnic groups, even though deficiencies are less than those in Europe due to long term fortification of basic foods. This report addresses the role of deficiencies for many chronic diseases including cardiovascular diseases and cancer (Kumanyika S et al., 2017).

Although chronic excessive exposure to sunlight increases the risk of melanoma and other skin cancers, the avoidance of all direct sun exposure increases the risk of vitamin D deficiency, which can have serious consequences. Sensible sun exposure (usually 20−30 minutes of exposure of the arms and legs or the hands, arms, and face, two or three times per week) and increased dietary and supplemental vitamin D intake are reasonable approaches to guarantee vitamin D sufficiency.

Prevention of vitamin D deficiency conditions should include routine supplementation of vitamin A and D for infants from 1 to 12 months at least, and according to the American Academy of Pediatrics up to the end of adolescence. Standard pediatric and public health textbooks should promote supplements and fortification of basics foods with vitamin D. It is a problem in the population everywhere whether sunny or not that cannot be addressed by only providing vitamins to high-risk groups, and milk fortification is justified.

The use of milk as the vehicle for supplementation is logical, since vitamin D is a fat-soluble, acid labile substance that requires buffering against the acid milieu of the stomach, and the high calcium content of milk is a bonus. Fortification of baby formulas, infant cereals, and milk products is one of the most important cost-effective public health nutrition measures used. Failure to promote its application internationally has been an important lapse of the international health community. In addition, the recommended adequate intake should be adjusted according to the results of nutrition surveys to meet population needs. To increase intake, the amount of vitamin D in milk, milk substitutes, and milk products or cereal could be increased, but because that is not likely to be effective for adults, fortification of other foods should be considered. The amount of vitamin D in supplemental multivitamins or calcium supplements should be increased substantially, and all adults should be advised to take them.

Osteoporosis and resultant fractures of hip, vertebrae, and other bones are an enormous burden on health and economics of care for increasing elderly populations and must be considered a public health issue of high priority. Screening, education, and vitamin D supplements with calcium and medications are important to preserve health among the elderly and especially those institutionalized. For older persons, supplemental oral intakes of approximately 1,300 IU/day are needed to reach the low end of the optimal range of vitamin D levels. This cannot be monitored clinically because of difficulty in routine clinical measurement of serum 25(OH)D3 concentrations among patients, so a population risk group approach is needed, along with standardization and improved reproducibility and sensitivity of measurements of serum 25(OH)D3 levels.

All countries should adopt and sustain supplementation and fortification policies for vitamin D for the benefit of all age groups including the extremes of life but also the child, adolescent and middle aged. Canada recommends routine vitamin D supplementation for all adults year round. US guidelines for menopausal women include recommendations of calcium intake of 1,200 mg/day for adults age 50 and older and vitamin D_3 of 800−1,000 IU/day.

As discussed, there is mounting evidence that low levels of vitamin D are risk factors in many cancers and neurological, cardiovascular, and endocrine diseases, which require further consideration of recommended vitamin D levels in national policy.

Micronutrient malnutrition is a major public health issue in the developed world, but it is even more important in low-income, developing countries. There has been declining milk consumption in high-income countries with replacement of carbonated flavored beverages in many population groups and in many medium- and low-income countries, milk consumption is not part of the food culture. Vitamin D deficiency, rickets, osteomalacia, and thyroid deficiency are highly prevalent conditions in low-income developing countries. In low-income countries, regardless of the degree of sunlight, vitamin D and calcium levels are very low due to sun avoidance practices, low availability and consumption of vitamin D-rich foods, absence of fortification, and low use of supplements. Food fortification and routine supplements for pregnancy and infancy are crucial for personal and public health including reducing neonatal mortality. Vitamin D deficiency has been described as a global pandemic including in tropical zones. Its ramifications warrant concerted efforts to combat this deficiency with proven and cost-effective fortification and supplementation public health methods, to meet the challenges of rapidly increasing elderly populations and generally less outdoor activity for all age groups.

RECOMMENDATIONS

1. Recognize nutritional rickets, osteoporosis, and vitamin D and calcium deficiencies as preventable global public health problems particularly for infants, children, adolescents, pregnant and lactating women, and all adults including the elderly in high-, medium-, and low-income countries.

2. Public health strategies for rickets prevention include implementation of prevention programs with outreach to populations with a high prevalence of vitamin D deficiency, limited vitamin D, and calcium intakes.

3. Vitamin D supplements should be incorporated into childhood primary health care programs along with other essential micronutrients and immunizations and into pregnancy and post pregnancy care programs along with other recommended micronutrients.

4. In medium- and low-income countries, regardless of degree of latitude or climate, vitamin D and calcium fortification and use of supplements are vital public health measures to promote maternal health and to reduce low birth weight and neonatal mortality in support of the MDG goals.

5. Universally supplement all infants with vitamin D (400 IU/day) from birth to a minimum 24 months of age, independent of mode of feeding, and preferably through to adolescence.

6. Provide vitamin D supplements to pregnant and lactating women, infants, and children up to adolescent years, through public health programs.

7. Monitor and follow up on rickets cases and fractures among the elderly as well as adherence to recommended vitamin D and calcium intakes and implement surveillance for nutritional rickets.

8. Fortify staple foods with vitamin D and calcium, as appropriate, such as cow and other milks, flour, or other foods based on cultural dietary patterns. Food fortification can prevent rickets and improve the vitamin D status of infants, children, and adolescents if appropriate foods are used and sufficient fortification is provided, if fortification is supported by relevant legislation, and if the process is adequately monitored. Indigenous food sources of calcium should be promoted or subsidized in children.

9. Age groups and especially adults age 45 plus should take vitamin D supplements daily and strive for sun exposure of at least 20 minutes per day five days per week. All elderly persons over age 65 should take multivitamins including 1,000 IU of vitamin D per day.

10. All long-term institutionalized persons including patients, students, and prisoners should be given vitamin D supplements daily.

STUDENT REVIEW QUESTIONS

1. Why is vitamin D deficiency described as a global pandemic?
2. Why is clinical rickets returning and why is it an indicator of wider vitamin D deficiency?
3. Why has cod-liver oil been adopted as a widely used preventive measure for children since the 1920s?
4. Why was milk fortification with vitamin D adopted as a mandatory public health measure in the United States and Canada in the 1940s?
5. What role did the American Academy of Pediatrics play in promoting vitamin D supplements for all infants and older children?

6. What risk factors account for an increase in rickets and osteoporosis awareness in the past decade in Europe?
7. Explain why fortification of milk with vitamin D is not widely implemented in Europe and in low-income countries globally.
8. How can rickets and low vitamin D levels occur in countries with high levels of sunlight?
9. What are the risk factors in low vitamin D levels in the middle aged and elderly in a population?
10. What preventive measures should be taken to prevent hypovitaminosis D (i.e., low vitamin D) in the population at large?

RECOMMENDED READINGS

1. Agarwal K, Mughal M, Upadhyay P, Berry J, Mawer E, Puliyel J. The impact of atmospheric pollution on vitamin D status of infants and toddlers in Delhi, India. Arch Dis Child. 2002;87(2):111–113. Available at: http://www.ncbi.nlm.nih.gov/pmc/articles/PMC1719192/ (accessed 9 October 2017).
2. Al-Mustafa Z, Al-Madan M, Al-Majid H, Al-Muslem S, Al-Ateeq S, Al-Ali A. Vitamin D deficiency and rickets in the Eastern Province of Saudi Arabia. Ann Trop Paediatr. 2007;27(1):63–67. Abstract available at: http://www.ncbi.nlm.nih.gov/pubmed/17469734 (accessed 9 October 2017).
3. Atapattu N, Shaw N, Hogler W. Relationship between serum 25-hydroxyvitamin D and parathyroid hormone in the search for a biochemical definition of vitamin D deficiency in children. Pediatr Res. 2013;74(5):552–555. Abstract available at: http://www.ncbi.nlm.nih.gov/pubmed/23999068 (accessed 9 October 2017).
4. Babu U, Calvo M. Modern India and the vitamin D dilemma: evidence for the need of a national food fortification program. Mol Nutri Food Res. 2010;54(8):1134–1147. Abstract available at: http://www.ncbi.nlm.nih.gov/pubmed/20440690 (accessed 9 October 2017).
5. Black L, Seamans K, Cashman K, Kiely M. An updated systematic review and metaanalysis of the efficacy of vitamin D food fortification. J Nutr. 2012;142(6):1102–1108. Available at: http://jn.nutrition.org/content/142/6/1102.long (accessed 9 October 2017).
6. Braegger C, Campoy C, Colomb V, Decsi T, Domellof M, Fewtrell M, et al. Vitamin D in the healthy European paediatric population. J Pediatr Gastroenterol Nutr. 2013;56(6):692–701. Abstract available at: http://www.ncbi.nlm.nih.gov/pubmed/23708639 (accessed 9 October 2017).
7. Baggerly CA, Cuomo RE, French, Garland CF, Gorham ED, Grant WB, et al. Sunlight and vitamin D necessary for public health. J Am Coll Nutr. 2015;34(4):359–365. Available at: https://www.ncbi.nlm.nih.gov/pmc/articles/PMC4536937/ (accessed 9 October 2017).
8. Black R. Micronutrient deficiency-an underlying cause of morbidity and mortality. Bull World Health Organ. 2003;81(1):79. Available at: https://www.ncbi.nlm.nih.gov/pmc/articles/PMC2572405/pdf/12751414.pdf (accessed 10 October 2017).
9. Burge R, Dawson-Hughes B, Solomon DH, Wong JB, King A, Tosteson A. Incidence and economic burden of osteoporosis-related fractures in the United States, 2005–2025. J Bone Miner Res. 2007;22(3):465–475.
10. Calvo MS, Whiting SJ, Barton CN. Vitamin D fortification in the United States and Canada: current status and data needs. Am J Clin Nutr. 2004;80(suppl):1710S–1716S. Available at: http://ajcn.nutrition.org/content/80/6/1710S.full (accessed 7 June 2017).

11. Calvo MS, Whiting SJ, Barton CN. Vitamin D intake: a global perspective of current status. J Nutr. 2005;135(2):310−316. Available at: http://ajcn.nutrition.org/content/80/6/1710S.full (accessed 10 October 2017).

12. Cantorna MT, Zhu Y, Froicu M, Wittke A. Vitamin D status, 1,25-dihydroxyvitamin D3, and the immune system. Am J Clin Nutr. 2004;80(6 Suppl):1717S−1720S. Available at: http://ajcn.nutrition.org/content/80/6/1717S.long (accessed 10 October 2017).

13. Cashman KD, Dowling KG, Skrabáková Z, Gonzalez-Gross M, Valtueña J, De Henauw S, et al. Vitamin D deficiency in Europe: pandemic? Am J Clin Nutr. 2016;103 (4):1033−1044. First published February 10, 2016, https://doi.org/10.3945/ajcn.115.120873. Available at: http://ajcn.nutrition.org/content/103/4/1033.full.pdf + html (accessed 3 October 2017).

14. Cauley JA. Public health impact of osteoporosis. J Gerontol A Biol Sci Med Sci. 2013;68 (10):1243−1251. Available at: https://www.ncbi.nlm.nih.gov/pmc/articles/PMC3779634/ (accessed 9 November 2017).

15. Centers for Disease Control and Prevention. Achievements in public health, 1900−1999. Safer and healthier foods. Morb Mort Wkly Rep. 1999;48(40):905−913. Available at: https://www.cdc.gov/mmwr/preview/mmwrhtml/mm4840a1.htm (accessed 10 November 2017).

16. Centers for Disease Control and Prevention. Home and recreational fact sheet—older adult falls. Available at: http://www.cdc.gov/HomeandRecreationalSafety (accessed 9 November 2017).

17. Centers for Disease Control and Prevention. Division of nutrition, physical activity, and obesity. Breastfeeding: vitamin D supplementation. Updated 17 June 2015. Available at: http://www.cdc.gov/breastfeeding/recommendations/vitamin_D.htm (accessed 15 November 2017).

18. Cesur Y, Doğan M, Ariyuca S, Basaranoglu M, Bektas MS, Peker E, et al. Evaluation of children with nutritional rickets. J Pediatr Endocrin Metab. 2011;24:35−43. Abstract available at: http://www.ncbi.nlm.nih.gov/pubmed/21528813 (accessed 9 October 2017).

19. Chapman T, Sugar N, Done S, Marasigan J, Wambold N, Feldman K. Fractures in infants and toddlers with rickets. Pediatr Radiol. 2010;40(7):1184−1189. Abstract available at: http://www.ncbi.nlm.nih.gov/pubmed/20012034 (accessed 9 October 2017).

20. Cheney M. Canadian experience with food fortification. In: Tulchinsky TH, editor. Proceedings of the Israeli-Palestinian conference on micronutrient deficiency conditions and their prevention. Public Health Rev. Tel Aviv, Israel: Tel Aviv International Scientific Publ, 2000, pp. 171−177.

21. Darnton-Hill I, Darnton I, Nalubola R. Fortification strategies to meet micronutrient needs: successes and failures. Proc Nutr Soc. 2002;61(2):231−241. Abstract available at:http://www.ncbi.nlm.nih.gov/pubmed/12133205 (accessed 10 October 2017).

22. Davies JH, Shaw NJ. Preventable but no strategy: vitamin D deficiency in the UK. Arch Dis Child. 2011;96(7):614−615. Abstract available at: http://adc.bmj.com/content/early/2010/07/22/adc.2010.191627 (accessed 8 November 2017).

23. Dawson-Hughes B, Harris SS, Krall EA, Dallal GE. Effect of calcium and vitamin D supplementation in men and women 65 years of age or older. N Engl J Med. 1997;337 (10):670−676. Abstract available at: http://www.nejm.org/doi/full/10.1056/NEJM199709043371003 (accessed 10 October 2017).

24. Dawodu A, Saadi H, Bekdache G, Javed Y, Altaye M, Hollis B. Randomized controlled trial (RCT) of vitamin D supplementation in pregnancy in a population with endemic vitamin D deficiency. J Clin Endocrinol Metab. 2013;8:2337−2346. Abstract available at: http://www.ncbi.nlm.nih.gov/pubmed/23559082 (accessed 9 October 2017).

25. DeLuca HF. History of the discovery of vitamin D and its active metabolites. BoneKEy Rep. 2014;3:1−8. doi:10.1038/bonekey.2013.213. Available at: https://www.nature. com/bonekeyreports/2014/140108/bonekey2013213/full/bonekey2013213.html (accessed 4 June 2017).

26. Dhanwal DK, Dennison EM, Harvey NC, Cooper C. Epidemiology of hip fracture: world-wide geographic variation. Indian J Orthop. 2011;45(1):15−22. Available at: http://www. ncbi.nlm.nih.gov/pmc/articles/PMC3004072/ (accessed 8 November 2017).

27. El Hayek J, Egeland E, Weiler H. Vitamin D status of Inuit preschoolers reflects season and vitamin D intake. J. Nutr. 2010;140(10):1839−1845. Available at: http://jn.nutrition. org/content/140/10/1839.full.pdf+html (accessed 10 October 2017).

28. Ekbote V, Khadilkar A, Chiplonkar S, Hanumante N, Khadilkar V, Mughal M. A pilot randomized controlled trial of oral calcium and vitamin D supplementation using fortified laddoos in underprivileged Indian toddlers. Eur J Clin Nutr. 2011;65 (4):440−446. Available at: http://www.ncbi.nlm.nih.gov/pubmed/21245882 (accessed 9 October 2017).

29. European Union. Report on osteoporosis in the European community-action for prevention. Luxembourg, 1998. Available at: https://ec.europa.eu/health/sites/health/files/state/docs/eu-report-1998.pdf (accessed 9 October 2017).

30. Farrar MD, Webb AR, Kift R, Durkin MT, Allan D, Herbert A, et al. Efficacy of a dose range of simulated sunlight exposures in raising vitamin D status in South Asian adults: implications for targeted guidance on sun exposure. Am J Clin Nutr. 2013;97(6):1210−1216. Available at: http://ajcn.nutrition.org/content/97/6/1210.long (accessed 9 October 2017).

31. Flynn A, Moreiras O, Stehle P, Fletcher RJ, Muller DJ, Rolland V. Vitamins and minerals: a model for safe addition to foods. Eur J Nutr. 2003;42(2):118−130. Abstract available at: http://www.ncbi.nlm.nih.gov/pubmed/12638033 (accessed 10 October 2017).

32. Ford ND, Stein AD. Risk factors affecting child cognitive development: a summary of nutrition, environment, and maternal−child interaction indicators for sub-Saharan Africa. Dev Orig Health Dis. 2016;7(2):197−217. Available at: https:// www.ncbi.nlm.nih.gov/pmc/articles/PMC4800975/pdf/nihms764641.pdf (accessed 23 November 2017).

33. Fox A, DuToit G, Lang A, Lack G. Food allergy as a risk factor for nutritional rickets. Pediatr Allergy Immunol. 2004;15(6):566−569. Abstract available at: http://www.ncbi.nlm. nih.gov/pubmed/15610373 (accessed 9 October 2017).

34. Frost P. Vitamin D deficiency among northern native peoples: a real or apparent problem? Int J Circumpolar Health. 2012;71:18001. doi:10.3402/IJCH.v71i0.18001. Available at: http://www.ncbi.nlm.nih.gov/pmc/articles/PMC3417586/ (accessed 10 October 2017).

35. Funk C. The chemical nature of the substance that cures polyneuritis in birds produced by a diet of polished rice. J Physiol (London). 1911;43:395−402. Available at: https://www. ncbi.nlm.nih.gov/pmc/articles/PMC1512869/pdf/jphysiol02546-0049.pdf (accessed 20 November 2017).

36. Gennari C. Calcium and vitamin D nutrition and bone disease of the elderly. Public Health Nutr. 2001;4(2B):547−559. Abstract available at: http://www.ncbi.nlm.nih.gov/pubmed/ 11683549 (accessed 10 October 2017).

37. Godel JC. Position statement, Canadian Pediatric Society, First Nations, Inuit and Métis Health Committee. Vitamin D supplementation for Canadian mothers and infants. (reaf-firmed January 30, 2015). Paediatr Child Health. 2007;12(7):583−589. Available at: http:// www.cps.ca/documents/position/vitamin-d (accessed 10 October 2017).

38. Goldacre M, Hall N, Yeates DG. Hospitalisation for children with rickets in England: a historical perspective. Lancet. 2014;383(9917):597−598. Available at: http://www.thelancet. com/pdfs/journals/lancet/PIIS0140-6736(14)60211-7.pdf (accessed 3 December 2017).

39. Greer F. Defining vitamin D deficiency in children: beyond 25-OH vitamin D serum concentrations. Pediatrics. 2009;124:1471−1473. Available at: http://pediatrics.aappublications. org/content/124/5/1471.extract (accessed 9 October 2015).

40. Haider N, Nagi A, Khan K. Frequency of nutritional rickets in children admitted with severe pneumonia. J Pak Med Assoc. 2010;60(6):729−732. Available at: http://jpma.org. pk/full_article_text.php?article_id=2289 (accessed 9 October 2017).

41. Harvard School Public Health. The nutrition source. Vitamin D and health. Available at: http://www.hsph.harvard.edu/nutritionsource/vitamin-d/ (accessed 7 November 2017).

42. Hawgood BJ. Sir Edward Mellanby (1884−1955) GBE KCB FRCP FRS: nutrition scientist and medical research mandarin. J Med Biogr. 2010;18(3):150−157. Available at: http:// www.ncbi.nlm.nih.gov/pubmed/20798415 (accessed 7 November 2017).

43. Heaney RP. Functional indices of vitamin D status and ramifications of vitamin D deficiency. Am J Clin Nutr. 2004;80(6 Suppl):1706S−1709S. Available at: http://ajcn.nutrition. org/content/80/6/1706S.long (accessed 10 October 2017).

44. Health Canada. Vitamin D and calcium: updated dietary reference intakes. Ottawa, 2012. Available at: http://www.hc-sc.gc.ca/fn-an/nutrition/vitamin/vita-d-eng.php (accessed 14 November 2017).

45. Hemlund E, Svedbom A, Ivergård, Compston J, Cooper C, Stenmark J, et al. Osteoporosis in the European Union: medical management, epidemiology and economic burden. Arch Osteoporos. 2013;8:136. Available at: http://www.ncbi.nlm.nih.gov/pmc/articles/PMC3880487/ (accessed 10 November 2017).

46. Holick MF, Binkley NC, Bischoff-Ferrari HA, Gordon CM, Hanley DA, Heaney RP, et al. Evaluation, treatment and prevention of vitamin D deficiency: an Endocrine Society clinical practice guideline. J Clin Endocrinol Metab. 2011;96(7):1911−1930. Abstract available: http:// www.ncbi.nlm.nih.gov/pubmed/21646368 (accessed 9 October 2017).

47. Holick MF. Environmental factors that influence the cutaneous production of vitamin D. Am J Clin Nutr. 1995;61(3 Suppl):638S−645S. Available at: http://www.ncbi.nlm.nih.gov/ pubmed/7879731 (accessed 9 October 2017).

48. Holick MF. Sunlight and vitamin D for bone health and prevention of autoimmune diseases, cancers, and cardiovascular disease. Am J Clin Nutr. 2004;80(6 Suppl):1678S−1688S. Available at: http://ajcn.nutrition.org/content/80/6/1678S.full.pdf+html (accessed 10 October 2017).

49. Holick MF. The vitamin D deficiency pandemic: a forgotten hormone important for health. Public Health Rev. 2010;32. BF03391602. doi:10.1007/BF03391602. Available at: https://publichealthreviews.biomedcentral.com/track/pdf/10.1007/BF03391602? site=publichealthreviews.biomedcentral.com (accessed 2 June 2017).

50. Hollis B, Johnson D, Hulsey T, Ebeling M, Wagner C. Vitamin D supplementation during pregnancy: double-blind, randomized clinical trial of safety and effectiveness. J Bone Miner Res. 2011;26:2341−2357. Available at: https://www.ncbi.nlm.nih.gov/pmc/articles/ PMC3183324/pdf/nihms306620.pdf (accessed 9 October 2017).

51. Ioannou C, Javaid M, Mahon P, Yaqub M, Harvey N, Godfrey K. The effect of maternal vitamin D concentration on fetal bone. J Clin Endocrinol Metab. 2012;97:E2070−E2077. Available at: https://www.ncbi.nlm.nih.gov/pmc/articles/PMC3485609/ (accessed 9 October 2017).

52. International Osteoporosis Foundation. Osteoporosis in the European Union in 2008: ten years of progress and ongoing challenges, 2008. Available at: https://www.iofbonehealth. org/sites/default/files/PDFs/EU%20Reports/eu_report_2008.pdf (accessed 9 October 2017).

53. International Osteoporosis Foundation. Osteoporosis facts and statistics, 2015. Available at: http://www.iofbonehealth.org/facts-and-statistics/index.html (accessed 15 November 2017).

54. Institute of Medicine. Dietary reference intakes: guiding principles for nutrition labeling and fortification. Washington, DC: National Academies of Science Press, 2003. Available at: https://www.nap.edu/download/10872 (accessed 23 November 2017).

55. Institute of Medicine. Dietary reference intakes for calcium and vitamin D. Washington, DC: National Academies Press, 2011. Available at: http://iom.nationalacademies.org/Reports/ 2010/Dietary-Reference-Intakes-for-Calcium-and-Vitamin-D.aspx (accessed October 28, 2017).

56. Jorde R, Grimnes G. Vitamin D and health: the need for more randomized controlled trials. J Steroid Biochem Mol Biol. 2015;148:269−274. Abstract available: http://www.ncbi.nlm. nih.gov/pubmed/25636723 (accessed 10 October 2017).

57. Julies P, Blair M, Pall K, Lynn R. G145 Nutritional rickets presenting to secondary care in children (<16 years): a UK surveillance study. Arch Dis Child. 2017;102:A59−A60. Abstract available: http://adc.bmj.com/content/102/Suppl_1/A59.3 (accessed 9 June 2017).

58. Kalra P, Das V, Agarwal A, Kumar M, Ramesh V, Bhatia E. Effect of vitamin D supplementation during pregnancy on neonatal mineral homeostasis and anthropometry of the newborn and infant. Br J Nutr. 2012;108:1052−1058. Abstract available: http://www.ncbi. nlm.nih.gov/pubmed/22212646 (accessed 9 October 2017).

59. Kaluski DN, Tulchinsky TH, Haviv A, Averbuch Y, Rachmiel S, Berry EM, et al. Addition of essential micronutrients to foods: implication for public health policy in Israel. Isr Med Assoc J. 2003;5(4):277−280. Available at: https://www.ima.org.il/FilesUpload/ IMAJ/0/53/26858.pdf (accessed 10 and 11 October 2017).

60. Kanis JA, Odén A, McCloskey EV, Johansson H, Wahl DA, Cooper C. IOF working group on epidemiology and quality of life. A systematic review of hip fracture incidence and probability of fracture worldwide. Osteoporos Int. 2012;23(9):2239−2256. Available at: https://www.ncbi.nlm.nih.gov/pmc/articles/PMC3421108/ (accessed 9 October 2017).

61. Khadgawat R, Marwaha R, Garg M, Ramot R, Oberoi AK, Sreenivas V, et al. Impact of vitamin D fortified milk supplementation on vitamin D status of healthy school children aged 10−14 years. Osteoporos Int. 2013;24(8):2335−2343. Abstract available at: http:// www.ncbi.nlm.nih.gov/pubmed/23460234 (accessed 9 October 2017).

62. Kiely M, Black L. Dietary strategies to maintain adequacy of circulating 25-hydroxyvitamin D concentrations. Scand J Clin Lab Invest Suppl. 2012;243:14−23. Abstract available at: http://www.ncbi.nlm.nih.gov/pubmed/22536758 (accessed 9 October 2017).

63. Kift R, Berry J, Vail A, Durkin M, Rhodes L, Webb A. Lifestyle factors including less cutaneous sun exposure contribute to starkly lower vitamin D levels in U.K. South Asians compared with the white population. Br J Dermatol. 2013;169(6):1272−1278. Abstract available at: http://www.ncbi.nlm.nih.gov/pubmed/23855783 (accessed 9 October 2017).

64. Kozlov A, Khabarova Y, Vershubsky G, AteevaY, Ryzhaenkov V. Vitamin D status of northern indigenous people of Russia leading traditional and "modernized" way of life. Circumpolar Health. 2014;73 (December). Available at: http://www.tandfonline.com/doi/full/ 10.3402/ijch.v73.26038 (accessed 9 October 2017).

65. Kramer MS, Kakuma R. The optimal duration of exclusive breast feeding: a systematic review. Geneva, Switzerland: WHO, 2002. Available at: http://www.who.int/nutrition/publications/optimal_duration_of_exc_bfeeding_review_eng.pdf (accessed 11 November 2017).

66. Kumanyika S, Oria MP (editors). Food and Nutrition Board, Health and Medicine Division. Guiding principles for developing dietary reference intakes based on chronic disease: a consensus study report of the committee on the development of guiding principles for the inclusion of chronic disease endpoints in future dietary reference intakes. The National Academies Press. Washington DC, 2017. Available at: https://www.nap.edu/download/24828 (accessed 28 November 2017).

67. Lamberg-Allardt C, Brustad M, Meyer H, Steingrimsdottir L. Vitamin D: a systematic literature review for the 5th edition of the Nordic Nutrition Recommendations. Food Nutr Res. 2013;3:57. Available at: https://www.ncbi.nlm.nih.gov/pmc/articles/PMC3790913/ (accessed 9 October 2017).

68. Laaksi IT, Ruohola JP, Ylikomi TJ, Auvinen A, Haataja RI, Pihlajamäki HK, et al. Vitamin D fortification as public health policy: significant improvement in vitamin D status in young Finnish men. Eur J Clin Nutr. 2006;60(8):1035−1038. Available at: https://www.ncbi.nlm.nih.gov/pubmed/16482069 (accessed 24 November 2017).

69. Lazol J, Cakan N, Kamat D. 10-year case review of nutritional rickets in Children's Hospital of Michigan. Clin Pediatr (Phila). 2008;47(4):379−384. Available at: http://www.ncbi.nlm.nih.gov/pubmed/18192641 (accessed 9 October 2017).

70. Leal J, Gray AM, Bristo-Alhambra D, Arden NK, Cooper C, et al. Impact of hip fracrure on hospital care costs: a population based study. Osteoporos Int. 2015;27(2):549−558. Available at: https://link.springer.com/content/pdf/10.1007%2Fs00198-015-3277-9.pdf (accessed 9 November 2017).

71. Leffelaar E, Vrijkotte T, van Eijsden M. Maternal early pregnancy vitamin D status in relation to fetal and neonatal growth: results of the multi-ethnic Amsterdam born children and their development cohort. Br J Nutr. 2010;104:108−117. Available at: http://www.ncbi.nlm.nih.gov/pubmed/20193097 (accessed 9 October 2017).

72. Mahon P, Harvey N, Crozier S, Inskip H, Robinson S, Arden N, et al. Low maternal vitamin D status and fetal bone development: cohort study. J Bone Miner Res. 2010;25:14−19. Available at: https://www.ncbi.nlm.nih.gov/pmc/articles/PMC4768344/pdf/emss-64964_amend.pdf (accessed 9 October 2017).

73. Maiya S, Sullivan I, Allgrove J, Yates R, Malon M, Brain C, et al. Hypocalcaemia and vitamin D deficiency: an important, but preventable, cause of life-threatening infant heart failure. Heart. 2008;94(5):581−584. Available at: http://heart.bmj.com/content/heartjnl/94/5/581.full.pdf (accessed 9 October 2017).

74. Mayor S. NICE issues guideline to prevent falls in elderly people. BMJ. 2004;329(7477):1258. Available at: https://www.ncbi.nlm.nih.gov/pmc/articles/PMC534478/ (accessed 10 October 2017).

75. McAuley KA, Jones S, Lewis-Barned NJ, Manning P, Goulding A. Low vitamin D status is common among elderly Dunedin women. NZ Med J. 1997;110(1048):275−277. Available at: http://www.ncbi.nlm.nih.gov/pubmed/9269291 (accessed 10 October 2017).

76. McCollum EV, Davis M. The necessity of certain lipins in the diet during growth. J Biol Chem. 1913;25:167−175.

77. McCollum EV, Simmonds N, Becker JE, Shipley PG. An experimental demonstration of the existence of a vitamin which promotes calcium deposition. J Biol Chem. 1922; 53:293−298.

78. McCollum EV, Simmonds N, Kinney M, Shipley PG, Park EA. Studies on experimental rickets. The effects of diets deficient in calcium and in fat-soluble A in modifying the histological structure of the bones. 1921 [classic article reprinted]. Am J Epidemiol. 1995;141:280−296. Available at: http://www.ncbi.nlm.nih.gov/pubmed/ 7840105.

79. Meikeljohn AP. Sir Edward Mallenby (1885−1955). Am J Clin Nutr. 1955;3(3):246−247. Available at: http://ajcn.nutrition.org/content/3/3/246.full.pdf+html (accessed 7 November 2015.

80. Melanby E. An experimental investigation on rickets. 1919 [classic article]. Nutrition. 1989;5(2):81−87. Available at: http://www.ncbi.nlm.nih.gov/pubmed/2520279 (accessed 10 October 2015).

81. Meller Y, Kestenbaum RS, Galinsky D, Shany S. Seasonal variations in serum levels of vitamin D metabolites and parathormone in geriatric patients with fractures in southern Israel. Isr J Med Sci. 1986;22(1):8−11. Abstract available at: http://www.ncbi.nlm.nih.gov/ pubmed/3485617 (accessed 10 October 2017).

82. Method A, Tulchinsky TH. Commentary: food fortification: African countries can make more progress. Adv Food Technol Nutr Sci Open J. 2015;(SE(1)), 22−28. Available at: http:// www.openventio.org/Special-Edition-1/Commentary-Food-Fortification-African-countries-can-make-more-progress-AFTNSOJ-SE-1-104.pdf (accessed 3 June 2017).

83. Mishal AA. Effects of different dress styles on vitamin D levels in healthy young Jordanian women. Osteoporos Int. 2001;12(11):931−935. Available at: http://www.ncbi. nlm.nih.gov/pubmed/11804019 (accessed 10 October 2017).

84. Mitchell JP, Cooper C, Dawson-Hughes B, Gordon CM, Rizzoli R. Life course approach to nutrition. Osteoporos Int. 2015;26(12):2723−2742. Available at: http://link.springer. com/article/10.1007/s00198-015-3288-6/fulltext.html (accessed 10 October 2017).

85. Miyako K, Kinjo S, Kohno H. Vitamin D deficiency rickets caused by improper lifestyle in Japanese children. Pediatr Int. 2005;37(2):142−146. Available at: http://www.ncbi.nlm. nih.gov/pubmed/15771690 (accessed 9 October 2017).

86. Munns CF, Shaw N, Kiely M, Specker BL, Thacher TD. Global consensus recommendations on prevention and management of nutritional rickets. J Clin Endocrinol Metab. 2016;101(2):394−415. Available at: https://www.ncbi.nlm.nih.gov/pmc/articles/ PMC4880117/ (accessed 1 June 2017).

87. Munns CF, Simm PJ, Rodda CP, Garnett SP, Zacharin MR, Ward LM, et al. Incidence of vitamin D deficiency rickets among Australian children: an Australian Paediatric Surveillance Unit study. Med J Aust. 2012;196(7):466−468. Available at: https://www. ncbi.nlm.nih.gov/pmc/articles/PMC4880117/ (accessed 9 October 2017).

88. Nahoo T, Holmes CP, Ostry A. An analysis of the development of Canadian food fortification policies: the case of vitamin B. Health Promot. Int. 2005;20(4):375−382. Available at: http://heapro.oxfordjournals.org/content/20/4/375.full (accessed 17 November 2017).

89. National Center for Health Statistics. Osteoporosis, 2016. Available at: https://www.cdc. gov/nchs/fastats/osteoporosis.htm (accessed 23 October 2017).

90. National Health Service NHS. Rickets, last reviewed 21 December 2015. Available at: http:// www.nhs.uk/Conditions/Rickets/Pages/Introduction.aspx (accessed 7 November 2017).

91. National Institutes of Health. Osteoporosis, updated November 2010. Available at: https:// report.nih.gov/NIHfactsheets/Pdfs/Osteoporosis(NIAMS).pdf (accessed 3 December 2017).

92. North American Menopause Society. Management of osteoporosis in post-menopausal women: 2010 position statement of the North American Menopause Society. Menopause. 2010;17(1):25−54; quiz 55−56. Available at: http://www.ncbi.nlm.nih.gov/ pubmed/20061894 (accessed 9 October 2017).

93. Nowson CA, Margerison C. Vitamin D intake and vitamin D status of Australians. Med J Aust. 2002;177(3):149–152. Available at: https://www.mja.com.au/journal/2002/177/3/vitamin-d-intake-and-vitamin-d-status-australians (accessed 10 October 2017).

94. Oberhelman S, Meekins M, Fischer P, Lee BR, Singh RJ, Cha SS, et al. Maternal vitamin D supplementation to improve the vitamin D status of breast-fed infants: a randomized controlled trial. Mayo Clin Proc. 2013;88(12):1378–1387. Available at: https://www.ncbi.nlm.nih.gov/pmc/articles/PMC3923377/pdf/nihms-531463.pdf (accessed 9 October 2017).

95. Osteoporosis Canada. Bone health and osteoporosis. Available at: https://osteoporosis.ca/bone-health-osteoporosis/ (accessed 7 November 2017).

96. Ozkan B. Nutritional rickets. J Clin Res Pediatr Endocrinol. 2010;2(4):137–142. Available at: http://www.ncbi.nlm.nih.gov/pmc/articles/PMC3005686/ (accessed 9 October 2017).

97. Park YK, Sempos CT, Barton CN, Vanderveen JE, Yetley EA. Effectiveness of food fortification in the United States: the case of pellagra. Am J Public Health. 2000;90 (5):727–738. Available at: https://www.ncbi.nlm.nih.gov/pmc/articles/PMC1446222/pdf/10800421.pdf (accessed 10 October 2017).

98. Paterson CR. Vitamin D deficiency rickets and allegations of non-accidental injury. Acta Pediatr. 2009;98(12):2008–2012. Available at: http://www.ncbi.nlm.nih.gov/pubmed/19572990 (accessed 9 October 2017).

99. Pettifor J. Calcium and vitamin D metabolism in children in developing countries. Ann Nutr Metabl. 2014;64(Suppl 2):15–22. Available at: https://www.karger.com/Article/FullText/365124 (accessed 30 October 2017).

100. Pettifor JM. How should we manage vitamin D deficiency rickets? Indian J Pediatr. 2014;51:259–260. Available at: http://medind.nic.in/ibv/t14/i4/ibvt14i4p259.pdf (accessed 10 October 2017).

101. Piirainen T, Laitinen K, Isolauri E. Impact of national fortification of fluid milks and margarines with vitamin D on dietary intake and serum 25-hydroxyvitamin D concentration in 4-year-old children. Eur J Clin Nutr. 2007;61(1):123–128. Available at: http://www.nature.com/articles/1602506 (accessed 9 October 2017).

102. Raiten DJ, Picciano MF. Vitamin D and health in the 21st century: bone and beyond. Executive summary. Am J Clin Nutr. 2004;80(6 Suppl):1673S–1677S. Available at: http://ajcn.nutrition.org/content/80/6/1673S.long (accessed 10 October 2017).

103. Rajakumar K. Vitamin D, cod-liver oil, sunlight and rickets: a historical perspective. Pediatrics. 2003;112(2):132–135. Available at: http://pediatrics.aappublications.org/content/112/2/e132.full (accessed 10 October 2017).

104. Ramason R, Selvaganapathi N, Ismail NHB, Wong WC, Rajamoney GN, Chong MS. Prevalence of vitamin D deficiency in patients with hip fracture seen in an orthogeriatric service in sunny Singapore. Geriatr Orthop Surg Rehab. 2014;5(2):82–86. Available at: http://www.ncbi.nlm.nih.gov/pmc/articles/PMC4212370/ (accessed 7 November 2015).

105. Rosenfeld L. Vitamins: the early years of discovery. Clin Chem. 1997;43(4):680–685. Available at: http://www.ncbi.nlm.nih.gov/pubmed/9105273 (accessed 10 October 2015).

106. Ross AC, Manson JE, Abrams SA, Aloia JF, Brannon PM, Clinton SK, et al. The 2011 report on dietary reference intakes for calcium and vitamin D from the Institute of Medicine: what clinicians need to know. J Clin Endocrinol Metab. 2011;96(1):53–58. Available at: http://www.ncbi.nlm.nih.gov/pmc/articles/PMC3046611/ (accessed 9 October 2015).

107. Royal Society of Chemistry. Chemistry in its element: vitamin D. Available at: https://www.thenakedscientists.com/podcasts/chemistry-its-element/vitamin-d-chemistry-its-element (accessed 3 June 2017).

108. Saadi H, Dawodu A, Afandi B, Zayed R, Benedict S, Nagelkerke N, et al. Effect of combined maternal and infant vitamin D supplementation on vitamin D status of exclusively breastfed infants. Matern Child Nutr. 2009;5(1):25−32. Available at: http://www.ncbi.nlm.nih.gov/pubmed/19161542 (accessed 9 October 2015).

109. Scharla SH. Prevalence of subclinical vitamin D deficiency in different European countries. Osteoporos Int. 1998;8(Suppl. 2):S7−S12. Available at: http://www.direct-ms.org/sites/default/files/Scharla.pdf (accessed 7 November 2015).

110. Sempos CT, Vesper HW, Phinney KW, Thienpont LM, Coates PM, Vitamin D, Standardization Program (VDSP). Vitamin D status as an international issue: national surveys and the problem of standardization. Scan J Clin Lab Invest. 2012;243:32−40. Available at: http://www.ncbi.nlm.nih.gov/pubmed/22536760 (accessed 9 October 2015).

111. Senniappan S, Elazabi A, Doughty I, Mughal Z. Case 2: fractures in under-6-month-old exclusively breast-fed infants born to immigrant parents: nonaccidental injury? (case presentation). Diagnosis: pathological fractures secondary to vitamin D deficiency rickets in under-6-months-old, exclusively breast-fed infants, born to immigrant parents. Acta Pediatr. 2008;97(7):836−837. Available at: https://www.ncbi.nlm.nih.gov/pubmed/24886848 (accessed 3 June 2017).

112. Shakur YA, Lou W, L'Abbe MR. Examining the effects of increased vitamin D fortification on dietary inadequacy in Canada. Can J Public Health. 2014;105(2):e127−e132. Available at: https://www.ncbi.nlm.nih.gov/pubmed/24886848 (accessed 3 June 2017).

113. Spiro A, Buttriss JL. Vitamin D: an overview of vitamin D status and intake in Europe British Nutrition Foundation, London, UK. Nutr Bull. 2014;39:322−350. Available at: http://www.ncbi.nlm.nih.gov/pmc/articles/PMC4288313/pdf/nbu0039-0322.pdf (accessed 24 October 2015).

114. Statistics Canada. Vitamin D levels of Canadians 2012−2013, 27 November 2015. Available at: http://www.statcan.gc.ca/pub/82-625-x/2014001/article/14125-eng.htm (accessed 14 November 2015).

115. Svedbom A, Hemlund B, Ivergård M, Compston J, Cooper C, Stenmark J, et al. Osteoporosis in the European Union: a compendium of country-specific reports. Arch Osteoporos. 2013;8(1−2):137. Available at: http://www.ncbi.nlm.nih.gov/pmc/articles/PMC3880492/ (accessed 7 November 2015).

116. Taylor J, Geyer L, Feldman K. Use of supplemental vitamin D among infants breastfed for prolonged periods. Pediatrics. 2010;125:105−111. Available at: http://www.ncbi.nlm.nih.gov/pubmed/19948571.

117. Terushkin V, Bender A, Psaty E, Engelsen O, Wang S, Halpern A. Estimated equivalency of vitamin D production from natural sun exposure versus oral vitamin D supplementation across seasons at two US latitudes. J Am Acad Dermatol. 2010;62(6):e921−e929. Available at: http://www.ncbi.nlm.nih.gov/pubmed/20363523 (accessed 9 October 2015).

118. Thacher TD, Fischer PR, Strand MA, Pettifor JM. Nutritional rickets around the world: causes and future directions. Ann Trop Paediatr. 2006;26:1−16. Available at: http://www.ncbi.nlm.nih.gov/pubmed/16494699 (accessed 9 October 2015).

119. Thacher TD, Fischer PR, Pettifor JM. Vitamin D treatment in calcium-deficiency rickets: a randomized controlled trial. Arch Dis Child. 2014;99(9):807−811. Available at: http://www.ncbi.nlm.nih.gov/pubmed/24748637 (accessed 9 October 2015).

120. Thacher TD, Pludowski P, Shaw NJ, Mughal MZ, Munns CF, Hogler W. Nutritional rickets in immigrant and refugee children. Public Health Rev. 2016;37:3. doi:10.1186/s40985-016-0018-3. Available at: http://publichealthreviews.biomedcentral.com/articles/10.1186/s40985-016-0018-3 (accessed 2 June 2017).

121. Thomas MK, Lloyd-Jones DM, Thadham RI, Shaw AC, Deraska DJ, Kitch BT, et al. Hypovitaminosis D in medical inpatients. N Engl J Med. 1998;338(12):777−783. Available at: http://www.ncbi.nlm.nih.gov/pubmed/9504937 (accessed 10 October 2015).

122. Tulchinsky TH, editor. Proceedings of the Israeli-Palestinian conference on micronutrient deficiency conditions and their prevention. Public Health Reviews. Tel Aviv, Israel: Tel Aviv International Scientific Publ, 2000.

123. Tulchinsky TH, Nitzan Kaluski D, Berry EM. Food fortification and risk group supplementation are vital parts of a comprehensive nutrition policy for prevention of chronic diseases. Eur J Public Health. 2004;14(3):226−228. Available at: http://www.ncbi.nlm.nih.gov/pubmed/15369023 (accessed 10 October 2015).

124. Uday S, Kongjonaj A, Aguiar M, Tulchinsky T, Högler W. Variations in infant and childhood vitamin D supplementation programmes across Europe and factors influencing adherence. Endocr Connect. 2017;6(8):667−675. Available at: https://www.ncbi.nlm.nih.gov/pmc/articles/PMC5655685/ (accessed20 November 2017).

125. Utiger RD. The need for more vitamin D. N Engl J Med. 1998;338(12):828−829. Available at: http://www.ncbi.nlm.nih.gov/pubmed/9504945 (accessed 10 October 2015).

126. United States. Public Health Service. Office of the Surgeon General. Surgeon General's report on nutrition and health. Publication No 88-50210. Washington, DC: Department of Health and Human Services (DHH) Public Health Service (PHS), 1988. Available at: http://profiles.nlm.nih.gov/ps/access/NNBCQH.pdf (accessed 9 October 2015).

127. US Department of Health and Human Services. The 2004 surgeon general's report on bone health and osteoporosis: what it means to you. Office of the Surgeon General, 2004. Available at: https://www.bones.nih.gov/health-info/bone/SGR/surgeon-generals-report (accessed 3 December 2017).

128. US Department of Health and Human Services National Institutes of Health, Office of Dietary Supplements. Vitamin D fact sheet for health professionals (vitamin D deficiency), reviewed 10 November 2014. Available at: https://ods.od.nih.gov/factsheets/VitaminD-HealthProfessional/#h5 (accessed 9 October 2015).

129. US Preventive Services Task Force. Final recommendation statement: vitamin D deficiency: screening, 2014. Available at: http://www.uspreventiveservicestaskforce.org/Page/Document/RecommendationStatementFinal/vitamin-d-deficiency-screening (accessed 28 October 2015).

130. Vidailhet M, Mallet E, Bocquet A, Bresson JL, Briend A, Chouraqui JP, et al. Vitamin D: still a topical matter in children and adolescents. A position paper by the Committee on Nutrition of the French Society of Paediatrics. Arch Pediatr. 2012;19(3):316−328. Available at: http://www.ncbi.nlm.nih.gov/pubmed/22284232 (accessed 9 October 2015).

131. Viljakainen H, Saarnio E, Hytinantti T, Miettinen M, Surcel H, Mäkitie O, et al. Maternal vitamin D status determines bone variables in the newborn. J Clin Endocrinol Metab. 2010;95(4):1749−1757. Available at: http://www.ncbi.nlm.nih.gov/pubmed/20139235 (accessed 9 October 2015).

132. Wagner CL, Greer FR. American Academy Pediatrics, Section on Breastfeeding; American Academy of Pediatrics Committee on Nutrition. Prevention of rickets and vitamin D deficiency in infants, children, and adolescents. Pediatrics. 2008;122(6):1142–1152. Available at: http://pediatrics.aappublications.org/content/pediatrics/122/5/1142.full.pdf (accessed 29 October 2017).

133. Wagner CL, McNeil R, Hamilton SA, Winkler J, Rodriguez-Cook CR, Warner G, et al. A randomized trial of vitamin D supplementation in 2 community health center networks in South Carolina. Am J Obstet Gynecol. 2013;208(2):e131–e137. Available at: http://www.ncbi.nlm.nih.gov/pubmed/23131462 (accessed 9 October 2015).

134. Ward LM, Gaboury I, Ladhani M, Zlotkin S. Vitamin D-deficiency rickets among children in Canada. CMAJ. 2007;177(2):161–166. Available at: http://www.ncbi.nlm.nih.gov/pubmed/17600035 (accessed 9 October 2015).

135. Webb AR, Kift R, Durkin MT, O'Brien SJ, Vail A, Berry JL, et al. The role of sunlight exposure in determining the vitamin D status of the U.K. white adult population. Br J Dermatol. 2010;163(5):1050–1055. Available at: http://www.ncbi.nlm.nih.gov/pubmed/20716215 (accessed 9 October 2015).

136. WebMD. Slideshow: A visual guide to osteoporosis. Available at: http://www.webmd.com/osteoporosis/ss/slideshow-osteoporosis-overview. (accessed 3 June 2017).

137. Weiler H for Canadian Council of Food and Nutrition. Vitamin D: the current state in Canada. CCFN report, August 2008. Available at: https://www.cfdr.ca/Downloads/CCFN-docs/Vitamin-D-Report---final---Aug3-08-revAug9-_2_.aspx (accessed 10 October 2015).

138. Weisberg P, Scanlon KS, Li R, Cogswell ME. Nutritional rickets among children in the United States: review of cases reported between 1986 and 2003. Am J Clin Nutr. 2004;80 (6 Suppl):1697S–1705S. Available at: http://www.ncbi.nlm.nih.gov/pubmed/15585790 (accessed 10 October 2015).

139. Wharton B, Bishop N. Rickets. Lancet. 2003;362:1389–1400. Available at: http://www.ncbi.nlm.nih.gov/pubmed/14585642?dopt = Abstract.

140. Whiting SJ, Langlois KA, Vatanparast H, Greene-Finestone LS. The vitamin D status of Canadians relative to the 2011 dietary reference intakes: an examination in children and adults with and without supplement use. Am J Clin Nutr. 2011;94:128–135. Available at: http://ajcn.nutrition.org/content/94/1/128.full.pdf (accessed 7 November 2015).

141. Wilton P. Cod liver oil, vitamin D and the fight against rickets. CMAJ. 1995;152 (9):1516–1517. Available at: http://www.ncbi.nlm.nih.gov/pubmed/7728707 (accessed 10 October 2015).

142. World Health Organization. Diet, nutrition and the prevention of chronic diseases. World Health Organ Tech Rep Ser. 2003;916(i–viii):1–149. Available at: http://www.who.int/dietphysicalactivity/publications/trs916/download/en/; http://www.who.int/dietphysicalactivity/publications/trs916/en/gsfao_introduction.pdf (accessed 10 October 2015).

143. World Health Organization. The optimal duration of exclusive breastfeeding: report of an expert consultation. Geneva, Switzerland: WHO, 2002. Available at: http://www.who.int/nutrition/publications/optimal_duration_of_exc_bfeeding_review_eng.pdf (accessed 9 November 2015).

144. Zhang M, Shen F, Petryk A, Tang J, Chen X, Sergi C. "English Disease": historical notes on rickets, the bone–lung link and child neglect issues. Nutrients. 2016;8(11):722. https://doi.org/10.3390/nu8110722. Available at: https://www.ncbi.nlm.nih.gov/pmc/articles/PMC5133108/ (accessed 23 November 2017).

Chapter 12

Norman Gregg and Congenital Rubella Syndrome

ABSTRACT

Dr. Norman McAlister Gregg, an ophthalmologist practicing in Sydney Australia in 1941 observed an unusually large number of cases of congenital cataract in newborns. His inquiries revealed that the cases were mostly associated with a history of rubella in the mother during the first trimester of pregnancy. Subsequent investigation demonstrated that intrauterine death, spontaneous abortion, and birth defects including congenital heart disease, deafness, and other birth defects are frequently associated with rubella occurring early in pregnancy.

Gregg reported on his findings, which were received with skepticism by the medical community. However, his hypothesis was confirmed and for this discovery, Gregg was knighted by Queen Elisabeth in 1953, and received many other honors. With the 1979 development of improved rubella vaccine and its inclusion in MMR vaccine with measles and mumps and its increasingly widespread use around the world, this cause of birth defects is being gradually reduced. In 2012, the WHO made rubella part of its disease eradication program along with measles to prevent congenital rubella syndrome (CRS) globally. CRS remains an important cause of serious birth defects and mortality especially in low-income countries struggling to strengthen their immunization programs. CRS is one cause of birth defects for which public health interventions can make a huge impact in reducing the burden of morbidity, disability and mortality of children.

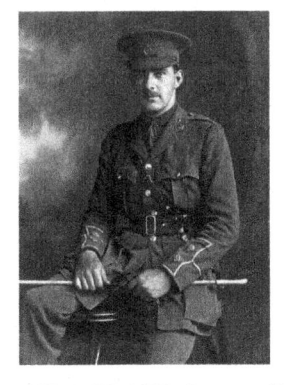

Norman McAlister Gregg (1892–1966), in World War I army uniform; Ophthalmologist in Sydney, Australia. In 1941 he recorded many cases of cataracts in newborns born from mothers who had rubella during pregnancies, thus discovering Congenital Rubella Syndrome. *Photo courtesy of the University of Sydney Archive.*

Case Studies in Public Health. DOI: http://dx.doi.org/10.1016/B978-0-12-804571-8.00012-3

BACKGROUND

Norman Gregg was born in Sydney, Australia, youngest of six children, whose father was an auctioneer. Norman grew up excelling in academics and many sports including tennis, cricket, baseball, and others. He graduated from medical school at the University of Sydney and joined the British army fighting on the Western Front where he was awarded the Military Cross. He trained in opthalmology in England after the war, returning to Sydney opening his opthalmology practice in 1923.

Gregg was a senior ophthalmic surgeon practicing in Sydney, and a lecturer in ophthalmology at the University of Sydney. Following a major epidemic of rubella in 1940, Gregg, then aged 48, noted an unusual increase in his practice of congenital cataract cases of unusual appearance often associated with congenital heart defects, including 78 infants born following maternal rubella infection in early pregnancy. In October 1941, Gregg delivered a paper titled, "Congenital Cataract Following German Measles in the Mother," to the Ophthalmological Society of Australia in Melbourne, published in its journal *Transactions* (see Figure 12.1).

Gregg's paper focused on rubella during pregnancy associated with cataracts and congenital heart diseases. However, following media reports, some mothers also reported deafness as an isolated defect in infants following rubella in their pregnancies. A 50-year follow-up indicated long-term sequelae including cardiovascular disease, deafness, and diabetes. In the United States, the Helen Keller Center described follow-up among patients aged between 16 and 36 years with higher than expected rates of glaucoma and diabetes, hypo- and hyperthyroidism, hormone imbalances, premature aging, and esophageal and gastrointestinal problems.

Rubella (German measles) is generally a mild viral contagious disease with lymphadenopathy and a diffuse, raised red rash. low-grade fever, malaise, common cold-like symptoms; and swollen glands characterize the early clinical (prodromal) period. The incubation period typically lasts two-three weeks after exposure. Differentiation from scarlet fever, measles, or other

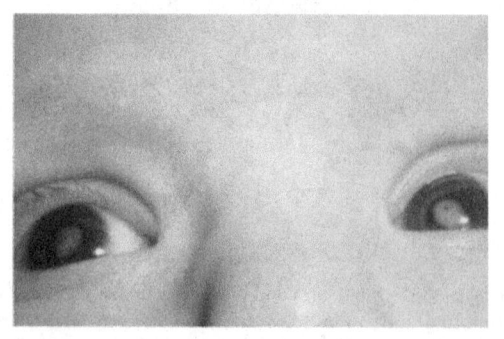

FIGURE 12.1 Child with cataracts due to congenital rubella syndrome. *PHIL Photo ID #4284. Available at: https://www.cdc.gov/rubella/about/photos.html*

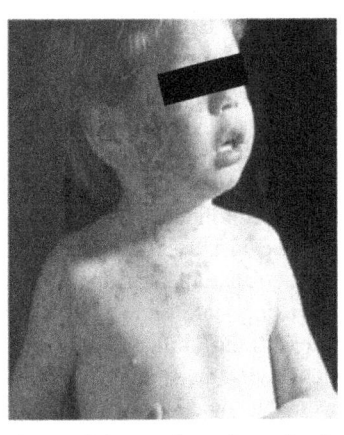

FIGURE 12.2   Child with characteristic maculopapular rash of rubella. *Source: Centers for Disease Control and Prevention. Available at: http://www.vaccineinformation.org/photos/ rubecdc007.jpg (accessed 6 October 2017).*

febrile diseases with rash may require laboratory testing and recovery of the virus from nasopharyngeal, blood, stool, and urine specimens. The rash is lighter than that of measles and may last three-four days. Arthralgia is common in primarily adult female patients and may last up to one month. Deafness is most common, resulting from direct cochlear damage and cell death. Hearing loss is mild to severe with incidence ranging from 12 to 19 percent of cases (Figure 12.2).

Traditionally considered a variant of measles, rubella was first described in 1814 in Germany as a separate condition and called rubella or German measles. The rubella virus first isolated in 1962 is officially classified as a togavirus of genus rubivirus (human virus). It is an enveloped RNA virus, with a single antigenic type that does not cross-react with other members of the same togavirus group. Rubella is usually a mild illness, with a low-grade fever, sore throat, and a rash that starts on the face and spreads to the rest of the body. Some people may also have a headache, conjunctivitis, and general discomfort before the rash appears, thyroid dysfunction, inflammation of the lungs, and other hormone problems. The viremia lasts five-seven days and readily passes the placental barrier to transfer from an infected mother to the fetus. Humans are the only known reservoir of rubella virus. If a woman is infected with rubella virus early in pregnancy there is a 90 percent chance of passing the virus on to her fetus. This can cause miscarriage, stillbirth, or severe birth defects known as congenital rubella syndrome (CRS).

Rubella virus is relatively unstable and readily inactivated by a variety of methods. Rubella virus was grown by Paul Parkman and Harry Meyer at the NIH (Biological Standards) and developed as a live, attenuated vaccine by Maurice Hilleman at Merck and licensed in 1969. It was integrated with measles mumps rubella vaccine in 1971, but in 1979, an improved live rubella vaccine was developed by Stanley Plotkin with high efficacy and safety. This strain was added by Hilleman to the Measles Mumps Rubella (MMR) vaccine approved by FDA with a second dose recommended since 1989. MMR has become a widely used global standard (see Chapter 19). Rubella vaccine was initially used in Europe primarily to protect non-pregnant adult women but this was found to be complex and ineffective. Rubella vaccination policy then focused on elimination of viral circulation by immunizing both boys and girls in childhood. Before 1962, no formal nationwide immunization program existed in the United States. Vaccines were administered in private medical practices and local health departments and paid for out-of-pocket or provided using state or local government funds with some support from federal maternal and child health block grant funds. In 1962, the Vaccination Assistance Act of the Public Health Service Act was adopted to promote vaccine-preventable disease control nationally. In the 1964–65 rubella epidemic, the Centers for Disease Control and Prevention (CDC) (WER 2011) reported 12.5 million rubella cases and 20,000 CRS newborns including 3,580 cases of blindness and deafness, 11,250 fetal and 2,100 neonatal deaths, with total economic cost estimated at US $1.5 billion.

CRS is associated with single or multiple congenital anomalies including cataracts, deafness, microophthalmia, congenital heart defects, mental/intellectual disability, congenital glaucoma, microcephaly, meningo-encephalitis, and others such as autism, diabetes mellitus, thyroid dysfunction inflammation of the lungs, and other hormone problems. Long-term functional status factors indicate social and occupational handicaps as common in CRS survivors. Insulin-dependent diabetes is also suspected as a late consequence of congenital rubella.

The European Region is working on the elimination of rubella circulation and CRS eradication. Progress in the elimination of rubella has been successful since the 1990s in western European countries and in most Eastern European countries since 2005, with some countries having cases up to 2014. Countries of the former Soviet Union (CIS) have been making progress since 2005. Each European country has an immunization program, monitoring systems and laboratory support, which creates problems of standardization of reporting. The European Center for Disease Control (ECDC) monitors European rubella outbreaks on a monthly basis.

Moderate and severe CRS cases are recognizable at birth, but mild cases may not be detected for months or years after birth. In 2008, the WHO estimated more than 110,000 CRS births occurred with the highest burden in the Southeast Asia (46%) and African regions (39%). By 2012 few countries in either region had introduced rubella vaccine. Between 2000 and 2014 adoption of rubella vaccine increased from 12 to 24 of the 27 countries but rubella cases were reported by only 16 countries. Before vaccination became available and widely used rubella was an endemic disease with epidemics every six-nine years with a cumulative buildup of susceptible people in the population facilitating spread of the virus. In areas where children are well-vaccinated, adolescent and young adult infection is more apparent, with

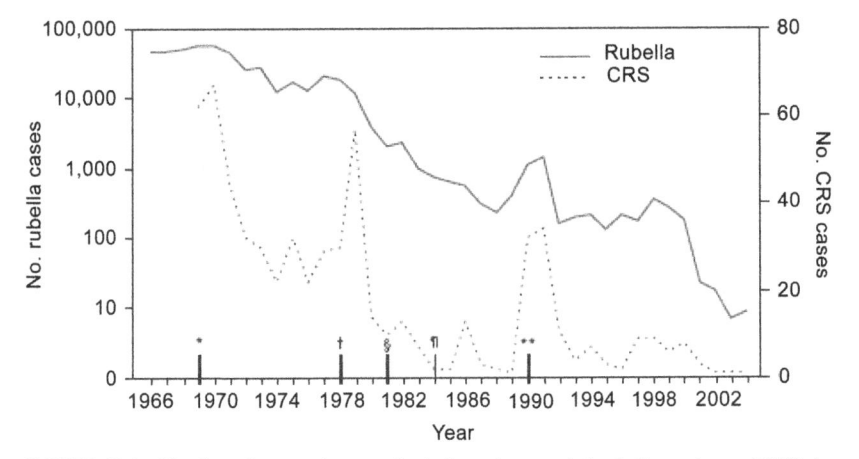

FIGURE 12.3   Number of reported cases of rubella and congenital rubella syndrome (CRS), by year, and chronology of rubella vaccination recommendations by the Advisory Committee on Immunization Practices, United States, 1966–2004. *1969—First official recommendations are published for the use of rubella vaccine. Vaccination is recommended for children aged 1 year to puberty. †1978—Recommendations for vaccination are expanded to include adolescents and certain adults, particularly females. Vaccination is recommended for adolescent or adult females and males in populations in colleges, certain places of employment (e.g., hospitals), and military bases. §1981—Recommendations place increased emphasis on vaccination of susceptible persons in training and educational settings (e.g., universities or colleges) and military settings, and vaccination or workers in health-care settings. ¶1984—Recommendations are published for vaccination of workers in day care centers, schools, colleges, companies, government offices, and industrial sites. Providers are encouraged to conduct prenatal testing and postpartum vaccination of susceptible women. Recommendations for vaccination are expanded to include susceptible persons who travel abroad. **1990—Recommendations include implementation of a new 2-dose schedule for measles-mumps-rubella vaccine. *Source: Centers for Disease Control and Prevention. Achievements in public health: elimination of rubella and congenital rubella syndrome — United States, 1969–2004. MMWR Morb Mort Wkly Rep. 2005;54(11);279–282. Available: https://www.cdc.gov/mmwr/preview/mmwrhtml/mm5411a5.htm (accessed 17 July 2017).*

declining epidemics in institutions, colleges, and among military personnel (see Figure 12.3).

CURRENT RELEVANCE

Rubella infection of pregnant women during their first trimester of pregnancy is the primary public health implication of this disease. The emotional and financial burden of CRS, including the cost of treatment of its congenital defects, makes this vaccination program cost-effective and critical. Its inclusion in a modern immunization program is fully justified. Elimination of CRS syndrome should be one of the primary goals of a program for prevention of vaccine-preventable diseases (VPDs) in developed and developing countries. Adoption of MMR and the two-dose policy will gradually lead to eradication of rubella and rubella syndrome but immunization of young adults will be needed to reduce the population of unprotected who were not immunized as children or whose immunity has waned.

A sharp reduction of rubella cases was seen in the United States following introduction of the vaccine in 1970, but rates increased in 1978, following rubella epidemics in 1976–78. A further reduction in cases was followed by a sharp upswing of rubella and CRS in 1988–90. An outbreak of rubella among the Amish in the United States, who refuse immunization on religious grounds, resulted in seven cases of CRS in 1991. Since 1994, vaccination recommendations in the United States have been coordinated with the CDC, the US Public Health Service, and professional organizations such as the American Academy of Pediatrics (AAP) to achieve high coverage and herd immunity to prevent measles and rubella outbreaks, which can affect children before the age of immunization and young adults. It is now thought that vaccination of sufficient numbers in the United States reduced circulation of the virus and protected the most vulnerable groups in the population. Improved access to vaccines will be helped by increased health insurance coverage and preventive care measures under the Patient Protection and Affordable Care Act (Obamacare) of 2010.

Most industrialized countries adopted MMR in the 1990s and subsequently, a two-dose policy. Rubella and CRS incidence dropped dramatically. Controversy occurred in the United Kingdom resulting from published allegations that MMR vaccine causes autism. Despite proof that this was disproven, immunization rates fell due to parental refusals to below 90 percent but later gradually improved. In the early 2000s reduced MMR usage resulted in an increase in outbreaks, cases, and circulation of rubella, mumps, and measles. This was subsequently improved by providing incentive payments for general practitioners with 100 percent age-specific immunization coverage.

Some parts of Europe failed to adopt MMR vaccine use and have suffered recurrent outbreaks of these diseases. A number of outbreaks were reported in 2005–07. Poland reported 7,946 cases of rubella in 2005 (20.8/100,000 population), an increase of 64 percent compared to 2004. MMR was added to the routine immunization schedule at the end of 2003. In 2003, Italy approved a national plan for the elimination of measles and congenital rubella, with the aim of reducing and maintaining the incidence of CRS to less than one case per 100,000 live births by 2007, then extended to 2015, but a review study still showing low levels of rubella protective antibodies among young adults including women in the age of fertility.

Despite the common program recommended by the European Region of WHO, childhood immunization programs vary widely across the European Union and the European Region of the WHO. In some countries where regional autonomy for immunization is permitted programs vary. Coverage with a first dose of a measles-containing vaccine (usually MMR) was 82 percent in the UK, 84 percent in Ireland, 87 percent in France, and 88 percent in Belgium in 2005, all well below the herd immunity levels required for measles control. Former socialist countries vary in their programs, coverage is generally high but in some countries adoption of relatively more recent vaccines is slow. Until 2009, some countries in the 53-member region covered by WHO Europe targeted rubella immunization to adolescent girls and women of child-bearing age. This has left many adolescents and young adults vulnerable to rubella with outbreaks in Poland and Romania. Since 2009, all 53 countries in WHO European Region adopted two doses of rubella containing for all children as part of routine immunization programs. The WHO considers eradication of measles and rubella a higher priority than mumps and strongly recommends that the combination MMR vaccine be used.

The WHO's global measles and rubella strategic plan 2012−2020 recommends universal use of rubella-containing vaccine (RCV) in childhood. Immunization coverage has increased from 83 countries in 1996 to 130 of the 193 WHO Member States in 2009. Grant et al. (2015), and (CDC) report substantial progress toward global rubella and CRS control and elimination during 2000−2014. Rubella cases declined by 95 percent, from 670,894 cases in 102 countries in 2000 to 33,068 cases in 162 countries in 2014, although case recording is problematic. RCVs were used in national immunization schedules in only two of 46 countries in the African Region, 35 out of 35 in the Region of the Americas, 4 of 11 countries in the Southeast Asia Region, 53 of 53 in the European Region, 15 of 21 in the Eastern Mediterranean Region, and 21 of 27 countries in the Western Pacific Region (WPR). In 2016, coverage with first dose of rubella-containing vaccine varied widely by region: globally 46 percent; African region 13 percent; Americas 92 percent; Eastern Mediterranean 46 percent; European 93 percent; South East Asia 15 percent; Western Pacific 96 percent (Feldstein et al, MMWR 2017). Coverage with one dose of measles containing vaccine (MCV1) in 2016 was the same as RCV1 in the Americas and European Regions, but markedly lower than MCV1 globally and in African and South East Asian Regions (see Table 12.1).

In Latin America and the Caribbean before wide-scale rubella vaccination an estimated 16,000−20,000 CRS cases were reported each year. Since adoption of widespread immunization in routine child immunization with RCV and special initiatives for older ages it is estimated that more than 112, 500 CRS cases have been prevented over a 15-year period in Latin America and the Caribbean, resulting in a cost savings of around $3 billion USD. Before the introduction of the vaccine, up to four babies in every 1,000 live births were born with CRS. The addition of MMR in many countries on a large scale has practically eliminated rubella and CRS in many developed and in some developing countries. The WHO Region of the Americas has since 2009 had no endemic (locally transmitted) cases of rubella infection.

In 2003, the Pan American Health Organization (PAHO) adopted a resolution calling for rubella and CRS elimination in the Americas by the year 2010. The PAHO advanced rubella and CRS elimination strategy including introduction of RCVs into routine vaccination programs was adopted with the goal of high immunization coverage of children and adults to eliminate

TABLE 12.1 Vaccination Coverage of RCV1 (Rubella First Dose) by World Health Organization Region—Worldwide, 2016

WHO Regions	RCV1 Percent Coverage 2016	MCV1 Percent Coverage 2016
Global	47	85
Africa	13	72
America	92	92
Eastern Mediterranean	46	77
Europe	93	93
South East Asia	15	87
Western Asia	96	96

Note: RCV1, rubella containing vaccine 1 dose; MCV1, measles containing vaccine 1 dose
Source: Feldstein LR, Mariat S, Gacic-Dobo M, Diallo MS, Conklin LM, Wallace AS. Global Routine Vaccination Coverage, 2016. MMWR Morb Mort Wkly Rep. 2017;66(45):1252-1255. Available at: https://www.cdc.gov/mmwr/volumes/66/wr/mm6645a3.htm (accessed 9 December 2017).

occurrence and transmission along with heightened surveillance. By 2009, all countries in the Americas routinely vaccinated children against rubella, and local and regional rubella transmission was interrupted. However, many low-income countries did not adopt rubella vaccines until 2016 nor could they reach the target of immunization programs to achieve herd immunity of over 90 percent.

During 2012—14, a rubella-elimination goal was established in the Western Pacific Region. In the Southeast Asia Region rubella and CRS control was targeted as an initial step toward establishing an elimination goal. However, in the Eastern Mediterranean Region lack of priority, and widespread civilian displacement are delaying rubella-elimination goals. In the African and Southeast Asian regions low rates of immunization coverage make it difficult to reach rubella and CRS control by 2020. As of December 2014, countries of four WHO regions had met rubella control and elimination goals.

In the early days of rubella immunization, many countries adopted a strategy focused on prevention of rubella in women before and during the age of fertility. Immunization strategy for rubella control in this model was to vaccinate schoolgirls aged 12 and up and women after pregnancy to provide protection throughout the period of fertility. This was a problematic strategy in that immunization during early pregnancy was thought to endanger the fetus, and thus testing of women was required. In addition, this strategy failed to reduce circulation of the virus as boys, and adult men were unprotected. Strategies thus were gradually revised to the goal of eradication of the virus in the total population creating the herd immunity which was needed to protect women in the age of fertility.

In 2015, the WHO Region of the Americas became the first in the world to be declared free of endemic transmission of rubella. In the same year, CDC reported an increase in countries using a rubella-containing vaccine from 99 (51 percent) countries in 2000 to 152 (78 percent) by the end of 2016 of the 194 WHO countries. WHO's 2016 Midterm Review of the Global Vaccine Action Plan in March 2017 reports that global coverage was estimated at 47 percent. Further *"rubella control is lagging as 45 Member States still have not introduced the vaccine and two regions (African and Eastern Mediterranean) have not yet set rubella elimination or control targets."* But WHO hopes for eradication of CRS along with measles by the year 2020 in at least five regions of WHO. This requires political and professional motivation, organization, funding, and dedicated follow-up, but should be achievable by this target date or a few years later, making the world a much safer place for babies.

ETHICAL ISSUES

In order to reach maximum herd immunity and prevent circulation of rubella virus, eradication strategies in high-income countries include routine immunization of boys and girls, primarily using two doses of MMR vaccine. Additional emphasis is placed on immunization of adults such as health care personnel, people in group settings such as colleges, armed forces, and prisons as well as personnel in other professions working with children, such as doctors, nurses, teachers, kindergarten, and other caregivers. The current approach is to give a routine dose of MMR in early childhood, followed by a second dose at early school age to reduce the pool of susceptible persons. Young adults should be considered for MMR immunization as they may not have been adequately immunized in childhood. Women of reproductive age should be tested to confirm immunity prior to pregnancy and receive the immunization if not already immune. Should a woman become infected during pregnancy, termination of pregnancy as previously recommended is now managed with hyperimmune globulin.

In 1999, both the WHO and CDC recommended eradication of diseases that cause serious harm as feasible technically by the use of currently licensed vaccines for general use. There are many short term feasible targets for regional elimination or total eradication, including polio, measles and rubella, along with some "neglected tropical diseases" which are also nearing eradication. Eradication where feasible is seen as cost-effective, sustainable, and essential to promote social justice. Vaccine development has and can be expected to create improvements with further possibilities of future eradication of vaccine preventable diseases (VPDs) and even non-communicable diseases (see Chapters 10 and 19). Other viral diseases are associated with birth defects such as mumps with deafness. In 2015-16 a viral origin of birth defects was seen most dramatically in the Zika virus epidemic spreading from Brazil to the Caribbean and southern US.

The possibilities are there but depend on many factors that can hasten or slow the process. Public health and political advocacy for immunization is a fundamental responsibility to achieve the Millenium and Sustainable Development Goals (MDGs and SDGs) for children. Congenital anomalies are important causes of childhood death, chronic illness, and disability in many countries. In 2010, the World Health Assembly adopted a resolution on birth defects calling all member states to promote primary prevention and improve the health of children with congenital anomalies by:

- Developing and strengthening registration and surveillance systems;
- Developing expertise and building workforce capacity;
- Promoting national responsibility for funding universal immunization, universal access to health care, and adequate public funding for health;
- Developing new vaccines and strategies for disease control;
- Strengthening research and studies on etiology, diagnosis, and prevention; and
- Promoting sustained international cooperation.

At the same time the larger picture of child disabilities appears to be growing in the United States, with nonphysical disabilities predominating and appearing more often in poorer sections of society but also in upper levels of education and income. Public health needs more research for public health and societal interventions to prevent such disabilities. Success with CRS is one element but many more issues including nutrition and socioeconomic, genetic, and environmental factors also need to be addressed. Progress with decreased incidence of CRS is remarkable, but it is only one step in the continuing challenges of child health.

ECONOMIC ISSUES

A review of economic analyses published by Hinman et al. in 2002 examined five cost benefit studies of rubella eradication in high-income and five in low-income countries. They concluded that inclusion of rubella vaccine in the routine immunization programs of both developing and developed countries produced positive economic benefits comparable to those associated with hepatitis B, rotavirus and hemophilus influenza type b (Hib) vaccine which are increasingly adopted by low-income countries. A 2013 systematic literature review of the economics of eradication of rubella and CRS also reported that treatment of CRS is costly and rubella vaccination programs are highly cost-effective (Babigumira et al., 2013).

Data for the 2009 birth cohort in the United States by Zhou et al. (2014) was used to develop costs of all diseases covered by routine immunizations used in the United States. They estimated that rubella immunization prevented nearly 2 million cases of rubella and 632 cases of CRS. Deaths prevented were estimated at 15 for rubella and 70 for CRS. The total costs (direct and indirect) were calculated at US $908 million for rubella and US $390 million for CRS, far exceeding costs of immunization. The rubella epidemic of 1964–65 had resulted in some 20,000 infants with CRS. Complacency and parental refusal have led to reduced concern and funding for measles with a resurgence of the virus due to importation and local spread among the unprotected. Furthermore, local health departments have not always been able to ensure full immunization, including two doses of MMR vaccine, in preschool children. This epidemic also resulted in more than 2,000 cases of encephalitis, deafness in 8,000 persons, 3,580 deaf and blind children, and mental retardation in a further 1,800 children. Patients were categorized in three groups of CRS severity with one-third needing institutional care.

Annually there are about four million births in the United States at risk for vaccine preventable diseases. A review of immunization programs shows that parental refusal is an increasing problem, while some providers miss giving measles vaccine to some children during office visits and fail to refer disadvantaged children to clinics offering immunization at no cost. However, overall the US has done well with increasing vaccination coverage. During the years 1994–2013, routine child immunization resulted in net cost savings of more than $1.36 trillion. Rubella cases declined in the United States from 47,745 cases annually in the prevaccination era to six cases annually currently i.e., by more than 99 percent. Congenital rubella syndrome cases declined from 152 average annual cases to one case in recent years, or by 99 percent.

A systematic literature review of studies on costs of rubella and CRS treatment and the costs, cost-effectiveness or cost-benefit of rubella vaccination was published by Babigumira et al. (2013). This included 20 studies in high-income countries as well as seven in middle-income countries, but found none in low-income countries. CRS cases were found to cost (in 2012) up to US$140,000 over a lifetime in high-income countries. Other effects noted were spontaneous and surgical abortions, fetal death and CRS with multiple defects of the brain, heart, eyes, physical growth and hearing of an estimated 110,000 infants annually. Vaccination programs reduce this physical, financial, and emotional burden, as well as being highly cost-effective. CRS is an important cause of hearing and visual impairment and mental handicap, often causing lifelong physical and mental disability requiring costly institutional care and special schools with costly health care and societal resources. Economic studies of the impact of rubella in low-income countries which bear the greatest burden of CRS are needed.

A study in Korea examined different immunization program models and concluded that measles-rubella vaccine catch-up campaigns in addition to the routine two-dose MMR vaccination program are the preferred economic and public health program policy in Korea. The CDC reported that rubella and CRS was endemic with epidemics about every five years in Japan until the early 2000s with seasonal increases during the spring and summer. Reported rubella cases remained at record low levels until 2010, and a few outbreaks in 2011 were reported in the workplace among adult males. In 2012, there was a sharp increase to 2,392 cases, a rate of 18.7/1,000,000 population, approximately double the reduction target of the Western Pacific region (WPR). In the first quarter of 2013 there were 5,442 rubella cases with 72 percent laboratory confirmed, with 77 percent of cases in adult males.

An outstanding US-based nongovernment organization (NGO), the March of Dimes (MOD), long active in the field of preventing birth defects now concentrates on preventing low birth weight. According to the MOD, 15 million babies are born prematurely each year around the world, one million will die, and the average medical cost of care for a healthy baby in the United States is $4,389 and for a premature baby $54,194.

Many countries, especially in the Africa and Southeast regions of the WHO, are currently struggling to maintain immunization, averaging less than 75 percent coverage of infants even with financial assistance from the Global Alliance for Vaccine Initiative (GAVI) and the Bill and Melinda Gates Foundation. The GAVI has support from many organizations including the WHO, CDC, Gates Foundation, Lions Club International, UNICEF and many others. In 2011 the GAVI announced a plan to vaccinate 300 million children in 30 countries by 2015 and strive for eradication of rubella virus during the 21st century.

The public health model for CRS eradication is based on experience with routine immunization of children and special immunization activities (SIAs) to reach other vulnerable groups such as young adults along with outbreak control measures, similar to measles eradication efforts. The experience of measles re-emerging in Europe since 2010 with secondary transmission to the Americas and other parts of the world revealed weaknesses in immunization coverage and lack of sufficient herd immunity as a result of growth of vaccine rejectionist attitudes, but also due to past weaknesses in vaccine policy.

CONCLUSION

Sir Norman Gregg's astute 1941 clinical observation and documentation of bilateral cataracts in 78 newborns whose mothers in 68 cases reported having rubella during their pregnancies led to identification of CRS. Rubella infection was a nearly universal disease of children until the introduction of an effective vaccine in 1969. The growing use of rubella-containing vaccine (RCV) in MMR, MR or rubella alone in two doses in recent decades is reducing the global incidence of rubella and CRS. The potential for control and over time elimination of these diseases and their serious effects on affected newborns can be achieved. The African and Southeast Asian regions of the WHO have the longest way to go to reach this target.

The WHO reports that rubella control of endemic rubella in the Americas has been achieved with the last rubella and CRS cases documented in 2009. The number of WHO member states using RCV has grown from 99 in 2000 to 152 in 2016, but there is still nonuse in 42 countries. In the European Region of the WHO all countries use RCV and reported cases have declined from 621,039 in 2000 to 609 cases in 2014. The WHO 2012−20 global plan recommendations for eradication of rubella and CRS to be achieved by the end of 2015 included: reduce global measles deaths by at least 95 percent compared with 2000 levels; achieve regional measles and rubella/CRS elimination goals; and achieve measles and rubella elimination in at least five WHO regions.

However, the return of measles to Europe and America in 2010−17 suggests that it may be too early to claim total victory while the disease is still endemic in many countries even if at lower levels. Global travel is thought to have brought measles from Europe to Disneyland, California, US in 2014. Subsequent rapid spread of measles to many parts of California, especially affected infants under the age of routine vaccination with MMR. However, there is a an increase in cases as well among young adults who may not have had full immunization or whose immunity had waned. Most worrying is the slow rate of adoption of rubella-containing vaccine in the most affected low-income countries in Africa and Asia. In addition there is a growing trend of parental refusal of vaccination in the United States and Europe based on false and disproved allegations that MMR vaccine causes autism (see Chapter 19). Another concern is the levelling off of donor funding, and although some recipient countries assume full financial responsibility for funding their own immunization programs, there may be setbacks in funding ahead. Nevertheless, the target of elimination of this preventable cause of birth defects is achievable with extension of rubella vaccine to countries not yet using it at all or sufficiently, increased surveillance, and recognition of the vital health responsibility and issues involved by national governments.

CRS is only one of the causes of birth defects or anomalies that cause structural or functional anomalies (e.g., neural tube defects, preterm birth, and genetic metabolic or hematologic disorders) that occur during intrauterine life and can be identified prenatally, at birth or later in life. Rubella is one of the infectious disease causes of birth defects but nutritional, genetic, environmental, and socioeconomic result in approximately four million babies dying from birth defect complications, which are a significant part of total neonatal and child deaths. Public trust in the importance of immunization to provide individual and herd immunity is a governmental and an individual responsibility and a continuing challenge for public health (see Chapter 19).

Prevention of birth defects has advanced dramatically with control and elimination of CRS along with prevention of neural tube defects by fortification of basic foods with folic acid. Other infectious causes of birth transmission of infections from mother to newborn include hepatitis C, and HIV. In early 2015, reports from Brazil indicated that the Zika mosquito-borne virus causing mild illness in pregnant women was associated with a sudden increase in microcephaly and other birth defects in the newborn of infected mothers. This was declared a public health emergency by WHO as Zika virus is a major issue for protection of newborns as this virus, transmitted by a specific vector, Aedes aegypti mosquitoes, is spreading rapidly from previous local habitats. Prevention of infectious diseases and nutritional deficiency during pregnancy, which may harm newborns with serious birth defects, are major challenges for public health even beyond the current challenge of CRS. But success in eradicating CRS will open the way for further successes in promoting infant health and safety.

The discovery of CRS by Norman Gregg followed by the development of inexpensive, safe and effective vaccines created the potential for eradication of CRS, which is a preventable disease caused by a virus solely affecting humans. The vision of eradication of CRS is still a challenge for the global health community. Setbacks include the re-emergence of measles in 2010–17, increasing parental resistance to immunization, and resurgence of vaccine preventable diseases (VPDs) such as diphtheria and pertussis which require adjustments of immunization practices to include pregnant women in order to protect young infants before their immunization can take effect. Eradication of rubella and congenital rubella syndrome is achievable in most regions of the world by 2020 and globally within a short number of years following depending on the rate of expansion of coverage in countries lagging in rubella vaccination uptake. Final eradication of CRS will be a great achievement for public health and for humanity.

RECOMMENDATIONS

Rubella and CRS eradication should be seen as key to a broader approach for improving child health that includes the following:

1. Recognition that prevention of birth defects is a vital global public health objective.
2. Recognition that birth defects include low birth weight and nutritional, infectious, environmental as well as genetic causes.
3. Recognition that prevention of CRS is a prime target for global public health achievement of eradication.

4. Measles, mumps, and rubella (MMR) vaccine should be adopted and given routinely as two doses for all infants and children as integral parts of immunization programs in all countries with priority to achieve this in low- and medium-income countries in Africa and Asia.

5. Immunization should be similarly assured for young adults including college and other postsecondary students, members of the armed forces, woman of childbearing age, caregivers in hospital or other medical and non medical group settings, people who travel internationally, and passengers on cruise ships, holiday resorts, or other group settings.

6. Monitoring of rubella and CRS using effective surveillance to evaluate programmatic efforts and adaptation with strategies to ensure outbreak control and progress in eradication of rubella virus.

7. Achieve and maintain high vaccination coverage with two doses of measles and RCVs for a total population and individual immunity including young adults who may not have been immunized as children.

8. Develop and maintain outbreak preparedness to respond rapidly to control outbreaks and prevent further spread of rubella by selected local and regional immunization campaigns to reduce population susceptibility.

9. Communicate and engage to build public confidence and demand for immunization; mandatory vaccination with 2 doses of MMR should be considered.

10. Perform the research and development needed to support cost-effective operations and improve vaccination and diagnostic tools.

STUDENT REVIEW QUESTIONS

1. How did Norman Gregg identify CRS?
2. What are the main birth defects associated with CRS?
3. What are the forms of rubella vaccine used for vaccinating children?
4. What is the burden of disease and disability for birth defects and particularly for CRS?
5. Who should be immunized with RCVs?
6. How can rubella recur in areas deemed clear of the disease?
7. What other strategies along with CRS eradication should be used to reduce birth defects?

RECOMMENDED READINGS

1. Babigumira JB, Morgan I, Levin A. Health economics of rubella: a systematic review to assess the value of rubella vaccination. BMC Public Health. 2013;13:406. http://dx.doi.org/10.1186/1471-2458-13-406. Available at: http://www.ncbi.nlm.nih.gov/pmc/articles/PMC3643883/ (accessed 14 July 2017).

2. Bae GR, Choe YJ, Go UY, Kim YI, Lee JK. Economic analysis of measles elimination program in the Republic of Korea, 2001: a cost benefit analysis study. Vaccine. 2013;31(24):2661–2666. http://dx.doi.org/10.1016/j.vaccine.2013.04.014. Abstract available at: http://www.ncbi.nlm.nih.gov/pubmed/23602654 (accessed at 12 July 2017).

3. Black RE, Laxminarayan R, Temmerman M, Walker N, editors. Reproductive, maternal, newborn, and child health: disease control priorities, 3rd edition, volume 2. Washington, DC: World Bank, 2016. Available at: https://www.ncbi.nlm.nih.gov/books/NBK361907/pdf/Bookshelf_NBK361907.pdf (accessed 26 July 2017).

4. Burki T. GAVI alliance to roll out rubella vaccine. Lancet. 2012;12:15−16. Available at: http://www.thelancet.com/pdfs/journals/laninf/PIIS1473-3099(11)70362-0.pdf (accessed 17 July 2017).

5. Castillo-Solóranzo C, Marsigli C, Bravo-Alacántara P, Flannery B, Matus CR, Tambini G, et al. Elimination of rubella and congenital rubella syndrome in the Americas. J Infect Dis. 2011;204(Suppl 2):S571−S578. Available at: http://jid.oxfordjournals.org/content/204/suppl_2/S571.full.pdf + html (accessed 17 July 2017).

6. Centers for Disease Control and Prevention. Nationwide rubella epidemic—Japan, 2013. Morb Mortal Wkly Rep. 2013;62(23):457−462. Available at: http://www.cdc.gov/mmwr/preview/mmwrhtml/mm6223a1.htm (accessed 17 July 2017).

7. Centers for Disease Control and Prevention. Global progress toward rubella and congenital rubella syndrome control and elimination—2000−2014. MMWR Morb Mort Wkly Rev. 2015;64(37);1052−1055. Available at: https://www.cdc.gov/mmwr/preview/mmwrhtml/mm6437a5.htm (accessed 20 July 2017).

8. Centers for Disease Control and Prevention. Vaccines and immunizations: rubella epidemiology and prevention of vaccine-preventable diseases. The Pink Book: Course Textbook-13th Edition, 30 July 2015. Available at: http://www.cdc.gov/vaccines/pubs/pinkbook/rubella.html# (accessed 17 July 2017).

9. Chrstianson A, Howson CP, Modell B. Global report on birth defects: the hidden toll of dying and disabled children. White Plains, NY: March of Dimes Birth Defects Foundation, 2006. Available at: http://www.marchofdimes.org/materials/global-report-on-birth-defects-the-hidden-toll-of-dying-and-disabled-children-executive-summary.pdf (accessed 17 July 2017).

10. Cohen BE, Durstenfeld A, Roehm C. Viral causes of hearing loss: a review for health professionals. Trends Hear. 2014;18:1−17. Available at: http://www.ncbi.nlm.nih.gov/pmc/articles/PMC4222184/ (accessed 17 July 2017).

11. Colzani E, McDonald SA, Carrillo-Santistevea P, Busana MC, Lopalco P, Cassini A. Impact of measles national vaccination coverage on burden of measles across 29 Member States of the European Union and European Economic Area, 2006−2011. Vaccine. 2014;32(16):1814−1819. Abstract available at: http://www.ncbi.nlm.nih.gov/pubmed/24530930 (accessed 17 July 2017).

12. Cooper LZ, Larson HJ, Katz SL. Protecting public trust in immunization. Pediatrics. 2008;122:149−153. Available at: http://fearlessparent.org/wp-content/uploads/2014/11/Protecting-Public-Trust-Vaccines-Cooper-Pediatrics-2008.pdf (accessed 17 July 2017).

13. Dunn PM. Perinatal lessons from the past: Sir Norman Gregg, Ch M, MC, of Sydney (1892−1966) and rubella embryopathy. Arch Dis Child Fetal Neonatal Ed. 2007;92(6):F513−F514. Available at: http://www.ncbi.nlm.nih.gov/pmc/articles/PMC2675410/ (accessed 17 July 2017).

14. Dyer O. Zika virus spreads across Americas as concerns mount over birth defects. BMJ. 2015;351:h6983s. Available at: http://www.bmj.com/content/bmj/351/bmj.h6983.full.pdf (accessed 17 July).

15. European Centre for Disease Prevention and Control. Survey on rubella, rubella in pregnancy and congenital rubella surveillance systems in EU/EEA countries. Stockholm: ECDC, 2013. Available at: http://ecdc.europa.eu/en/publications/Publications/survey-rubella-pregnancy-congenital-surveillance-systems-may-2013.pdf (accessed 17 July 2017).

16. European Center for Disease Control. Surveillance report: measles and rubella monitoring, August 2012. Available at: https://ecdc.europa.eu/sites/portal/files/media/en/publications/Publications/SUR-Monthly-measles-and-rubella-Aug-2012.pdf (accessed 4 July 2017).

17. Feldstein LR, Mariat S, Gacic-Dobo M, Diallo MS, Conklin LM, Wallace AS. Global routine vaccination coverage, 2016. MMWR Morb Mort Wkly Rep. 2017;66 (45):1252−1255. Available at: https://www.cdc.gov/mmwr/volumes/66/wr/mm6645a3.htm (accessed 9 December 2017).

18. Forrest JM, Turnbull FM, Sholler GF, Hawker RE, Martin FJ, Doran TT, et al. Gregg's congenital rubella patients 60 years later. Med J Austr. 2002;177(11−12):664−667. Abstract available at: https://www.mja.com.au/journal/2002/177/11/greggs-congenital-rubella-patients-60-years-later (accessed 17 July 2017).

19. Gallone MS, Gallone MF, Larocca AMV, Cinzia G, Tafuri S. Lack of immunity against rubella among Italian young adults. BMC Inf Dis. 2017;17:199. Available at: https://bmcinfectdis.biomedcentral.com/articles/10.1186/s12879-017-2295-y (accessed 23 July 2017).

20. Grant GB, Reef SE, Dabbagh A, Gacic-Dobo M, Peter M, Strebel PM. Global progress toward rubella and congenital rubella syndrome control and elimination 2000−2014. Morb Mortal Wkly Rep. 2015;64(37):1052−1055. Available at: http://www.cdc.gov/mmwr/preview/mmwrhtml/mm6437a5.htm (accessed at 17 July 2017).

21. Grant GB, Reef SE, Dabbagh A, Gacic-Dobo M, Strebel PM. Rubella and congenital rubella syndrome control progress, 2000−2014. Wkly Epidemiol Rec WER. 2015;90 (39):510−516. Available at: http://www.who.int/wer/2015/wer9039.pdf?ua51 (accessed 17 July 2017).

22. Gregg NM. Congenital cataract following German measles in the mother. 1941. Trans Opthalm Soc Aust. 1942;3:35−46. Available at: http://www.ncbi.nlm.nih.gov/pmc/articles/PMC2272051/pdf/epidinfect00028-0013.pdf (accessed 17 July 2017).

23. Helen Keller National Center. Congenital rubella syndrome, 2015. Available at: https://www.helenkeller.org/hknc/common-causes-0 (accessed 17 July 2017).

24. Hinman A. Eradication of vaccine-preventable diseases. Ann Rev Public Health. 1999;20:211−229. Abstract available at: http://www.ncbi.nlm.nih.gov/pubmed/10352857 (accessed 17 July 2017).

25. Hinman AR, Irons B, Lewis M, Kandola K. Economic analyses of rubella and rubella vaccines: a global review. Bull World Health Organ. 2002;80(4):264−270. Available at: http://www.who.int/bulletin/archives/80(4)264.pdf (accessed 17 July 2017).

26. Hinman AR, Orenstein WA, Schuchat A. Vaccine-preventable diseases, immunizations and MMWR-1961 2011. Morb Mortal Wkly Rep Suppl. 2011;60(04):49−57. Available at: http://www.cdc.gov/mmwr/preview/mmwrhtml/su6004a9.htm?s_cid = su6004a9_w (accessed 20 July 2017).

27. Houtrow AJ, Larson K, Olson LM, Newacheck PW, Halfon N. Changing trends of childhood disability, 2001−2011. Pediatrics. 2014;134(3):530−538. Available at: http://pediatrics.aappublications.org/content/134/3/530.long (accessed 17 July 2017).

28. Kurbanov B, Musabaev E, Latipov R. The economic burden of congenital rubella syndrome and rubella vaccination in Tashkent City, Uzbekistan. EpiNorth. 2012;13:18−24. Available at: http://www.epinorth.org/eway/default.aspx?pid = 230&trg = Area_5268 &MainArea_5260 = 5263:0:15,2946:1:0:0:::0:0&Area_5263 = 5268:44984::1:5264:1:::0:0 &Area_5268 = 5273:47949::1:5266:3:::0:0 (accessed 17 July 2017).

29. Lambert N, Strebel P, Orenstein W, Icenogle J, Poland GA. Rubella. Lancet. 2015;385 (9984):2297−2307. doi:10.1016/S0140-6736(14)60539-0. Abstract available at: http://www.thelancet.com/journals/lancet/article/PIIS0140-6736(14)60539-0/abstract (accessed 17 July 2017).

30. Lancaster PAL Gregg, Sir Norman McAlister (1892–1966), Australian Dictionary of Biography, National Centre of Biography, Australian National University, 1966. Available at: http://adb.anu.edu.au/biography/gregg-sir-norman-mcalister-10362/text18351, (accessed 9 August 2017).

31. Lanzieri TM, Pinto D, Prevots DR. Impact of rubella vaccination strategy on congenital rubella syndrome. J Pediatr (Rio J). 2007;83(5):415–421. Available at: http://www.scielo.br/pdf/jped/v83n5/en_v83n5a04.pdf (accessed 17 July 2017).

32. Mackey DA. 2005 Gregg Lecture: congenital cataract—from rubella to genetics. Clin Experiment Ophthalmol. 2006;34(3):199–207. Abstract available at: http://www.ncbi.nlm.nih.gov/pubmed/16671898 (accessed 17 July 2017).

33. March of Dimes. Annual report, 2014. Available at: http://www.marchofdimes.org/mission/annual-report.aspx (accessed 17 July 2017).

34. Martinez-Quintana E, Castillo Solerzano C, Torner N, Rodriguez-Gonzalez F. Congenital rubella syndrome: a matter of concern. Rev Panam Salud Publica. 2015;37(3):179–186. Available at: http://www.scielosp.org/pdf/rpsp/v37n3/v37n3a08.pdf (accessed 17 July 2017).

35. McLean H, Redd S, Abernathy E, Icenogle J, Wallace G. Chapter 14: Rubella. In: Manual for the surveillance of vaccine-preventable diseases. Available at: http://www.cdc.gov/vaccines/pubs/surv-manual/chpt14-rubella.html (accessed 17 July 2017).

36. Muscat M, Shefer A, Den Mamou M, Spataru R, Jankovic S, Deshevoy S, et al. The state of measles and rubella in the WHO European Region, 2013. Clin Microbiol Infect. 2014;20(5):12–18. Available at: http://www.clinicalmicrobiologyandinfection.com/article/S1198-743X(14)60170-1/pdf (accessed 17 July 2017).

37. Orenstein W.A., Hinman A., Nkowane B., Olive J.M., Reingold A. Measles and rubella global strategic plan 2012–2020: mid term review. Available at: http://www.who.int/immunization/sage/meetings/2016/october/ (accessed 23 November 2017).

38. Plotkin SA. The history of rubella and rubella vaccination leading to elimination. Clin Inf Dis. 2006;43(Suppl. 3):S164–S168. doi:10.1086/505950. Available at: https://academic.oup.com/cid/article-lookup/doi/10.1086/505950 (accessed 8 August 2017).

39. Plotkin SA, Farquhar JD, Katz M, Buser F. Attenuation of RA 27/3 rubella virus in WI-38 human diploid cells. Am J Dis Child. 1969;118(2):178–185. doi:10.1001/archpedi.1969.02100040180004 Abstract available at: http://jamanetwork.com/journals/jamapediatrics/article-abstract/503157 (accessed 8 August 2017).

40. Plotkin SA, Orenstein WA, Offit PA, editors. Vaccines. 6th edition. Philadelphia, PA: Saunders, 2013.

41. Strebel PM, Gacic-Dobo M, Reef S, Cochi SL. Global use of rubella vaccines, 1980–2009. J Infect Dis. 2011;204:S579–S584. Available at: https://academic.oup.com/jid/article/204/suppl_2/S579/871488 (accessed 17 July 2017).

42. Whitney C, Zhou F, Singleton J, Schuchat A. Benefits from immunization during the vaccines for children program era, United States, 1994–2013. Morb Mortal Wkly Rep. 2014;63(16):352–355. Available at: http://www.cdc.gov/mmwr/preview/mmwrhtml/mm6316a4.htm (accessed 17 July 2017).

43. Williams J, Mai CT, Mulinare J, Isenberg J, Flood TJ, Ethen M, et al. Updated estimates of neural tube defects prevented by mandatory folic acid fortification—United States 1995–2011. Morb Mort Wkly Rep. 2015;64(1):1–5. Available at: https://www.cdc.gov/mmwr/preview/mmwrhtml/mm6401a2.htm (accessed 17 July 2017).

44. World Health Organization. Integrated management of pregnancy and child birth (IMPAC). Standards for maternal and neonatal care: prevention of congenital rubella

syndrome (CRS), 2006. Available at: http://www.who.int/reproductivehealth/publications/maternal_perinatal_health/prevention_crs.pdf (accessed 17 July 2017).

45. World Health Organization Regional Office for Europe. Eliminating measles and rubella: framework for the verification process in the WHO European Region, 2014. Available at: http://www.euro.who.int/__data/assets/pdf_file/0009/247356/Eliminating-measles-and-rubella-Framework-for-the-verification-process-in-the-WHO-European-Region.pdf (accessed 17 July 2017).

46. World Health Organization. Rubella vaccines: WHO position paper. Wkly Epidemiol Record WER. 2011;86(29):301−306. Available at: http://www.who.int/wer/2011/wer8629.pdf (accessed 17 July 2017).

47. World Health Organization. Rubella and congenital rubella syndrome control progress 2000−2014. Wkly Epidemiol Rec WER. 2015;90(39):510−516. Available at: http://www.who.int/wer/2015/wer9039.pdf?ua = 1 (accessed 17 July 2017).

48. World Health Organization. Congenital anomalies fact sheet No. 370, updated September 2016. Available at: http://www.who.int/mediacentre/factsheets/fs370/en/ (accessed 17 July 2017).

49. World Health Organization. Rubella fact sheet, updated November 2017. Available at: http://www.who.int/mediacentre/factsheets/fs367/en/ (accessed 17 November 2017).

50. World Health Organization European Region. Health for all data base. Available at: http://data.euro.who.int/hfadb/ (accessed 17 July 2017).

51. World Health Organization. Immunization, vaccines and biologicals. Rubella, 3 November 2016. Available at: https://www.cdc.gov/vaccines/pubs/pinkbook/rubella.html (accessed 4 July 2017).

52. World Health Organization. Measles and rubella global strategic plan 2012−2020: mid term review. Available at: http://www.who.int/immunization/sage/meetings/2016/october/1_MTR_Report_Final_Color_Sept_20_v2.pdf?ua = 1&ua = 1 (accessed 4 July 2017).

53. World Health Organization Regional Office for South East Asia. Strategic plan for measles elimination and rubella and congenital rubella syndrome control in the South-East Asia Region 2014−2020, 2015. Available at: http://www.searo.who.int/entity/immunization/documents/sear_mr_strategic_plan_2014_2020.pdf (accessed 26 July 2017).

54. Zhou F, Shefer A, Wenger J, Messonier M, Wang Y, et al. Economic evaluation of the routine childhood immunization program in the United States, 2009. Pediatrics. 2014;133 (9):577−585. Available at: http://pediatrics.aappublications.org/content/pediatrics/133/4/577.full.pdf (accessed 17 July 2017).

Chapter 13

Ethical Issues in Public Health*

ABSTRACT

The field of public health includes a wide scope of activities and professional disciplines, ranging from sanitation, health protection, epidemiology, environmental health, financing, health promotion, including supervision, or the provision of clinical care. Each of these disciplines works in systems that face ethical dilemmas, making it important that public health workers have motivation to understand and practice within the ethical guidelines of their profession, thus making ethics an important component of training and practice. The dangers of ethical lapses are overwhelmingly apparent in the case of the Eugenics movement of the early 20th century which metamorphosed from forced sterilizations in many liberal democratic countries into mass murder of physically and mentally handicapped children and adults in Nazi Germany. Between 1939 and 1941, 180 thousand psychiatric patients along with an equivalent number of handicapped children and adults were killed in an organized extermination program in Germany by lethal gassing. This method was then applied to the industrialized murder or Holocaust of six million Jews and millions of other "untermenschen" (sub human) in the greatest genocide in human history. Shortly after World War II ended the Nuremberg Trials of Nazi war criminals were conducted including medical doctors, and some were executed for crimes against humanity. This was followed by the 1948 United Nations Declaration on Human Rights and by the World Medical Association's Helsinki Declaration. Both are widely accepted as cornerstone documents—the latter specifically governing ethical standards related to human experimentation—and are revised regularly since being issued in 1964. But genocide has not disappeared, nor has unscrupulous experimentation such as the Tuskegee experiment on black Americans infected with syphilis and left untreated even after the availability of a cure, penicillin. Ethical standards are now required by "Helsinki Committees"—ethical review boards—in most medical facilities worldwide. Ethical frameworks have evolved in part due to bitter experience of ethical failures later recognized and affecting public health standards of practice. Future generations of public health leaders and staff will face many ethical issues such as mandatory immunization of health workers and school children, and assisted death of terminally ill patients.

---

* This case report is largely derived and modified from Tulchinsky T.H., Varavikova E.A., The new public health, 3rd edition. Academic Press/Elsevier: San Diego, 2014, chapter 15 pages 804–816.

Case Studies in Public Health. DOI: http://dx.doi.org/10.1016/B978-0-12-804571-8.00027-5

277

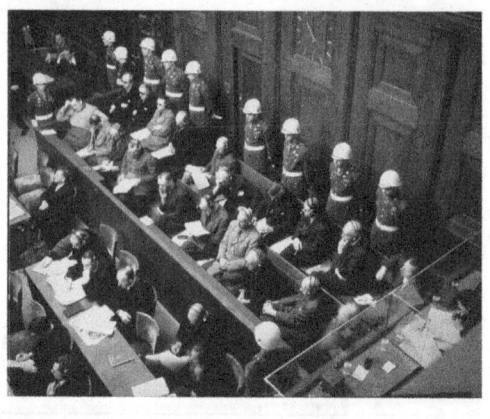

Nuremberg Trial of Nazi war criminals, 1945−46. Available at: https://fcit.usf.edu/holocaust/resource/gallery/N1945.htm.

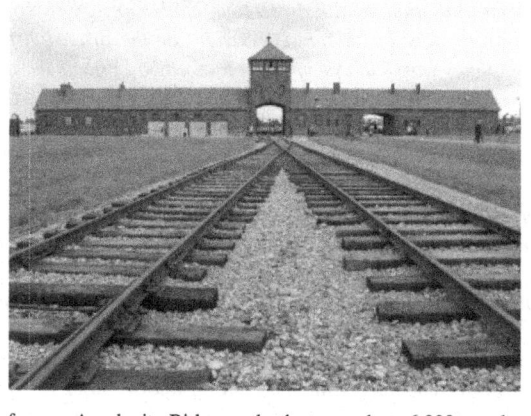

Entrance to the infamous Auschwitz-Birkenau death camp where 6,000 people were put to death in gas chambers daily by the Nazi regime in World War II. *Source: The Holocaust, public domain available at: http://www.history.com/topics/world-war-ii/the-holocaust/pictures/holocaust-concentration-camps/poland-auschwitz-birkenau-death-camp*

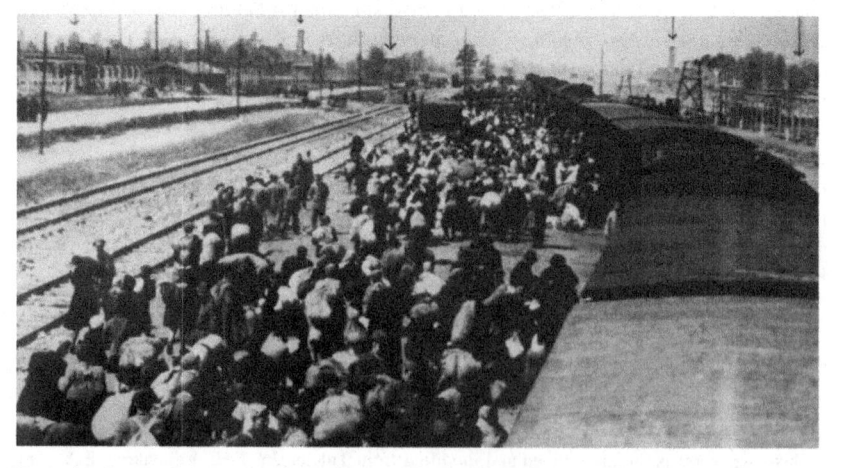

Hungarian Jews arriving at Auschwitz near end of WWII for immediate gassing/extermination. *Source: The Holocaust, public domain available at: http://www.history.com/topics/world-war-ii/the-holocaust/pictures/holocaust-concentration-camps/arriving-at-auschwitz*

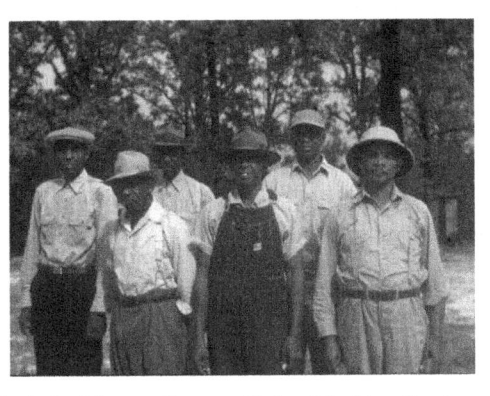

Tuskegee Syphilis Study Participants. *Courtesy: National Archives Catalogue, Tuskegee Syphilis Study Administrative Records, 1929−72.*

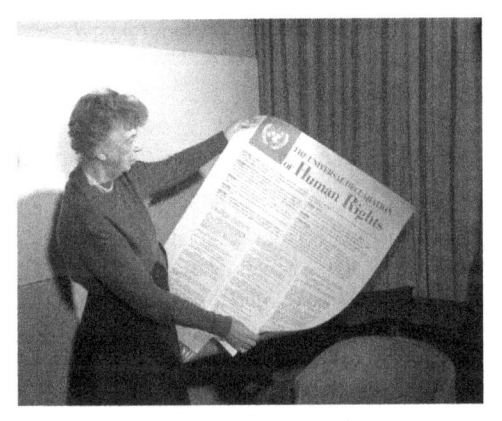

Eleanor Roosevelt (1884−1962) former First Lady of the US, leading human rights diplomat reading the Universal Declaration of Human Rights, United Nations November 1949, United Nations, Lake Success, New York. Photo # 117539, United Nations Photo Library at http://www.unmultimedia.org/photo/.

BACKGROUND

The Universal Declaration of Human Rights (UDHR) is a milestone document in the history of human rights. Proclaimed by the United Nations General Assembly in 1948 it provides a "Magna Carta" as a common standard for all peoples and all nations. Arising from the horrors of genocide and mass civilian casualties of World War II, the Declaration of Human Rights sets out, for the first time, fundamental human rights to be universally protected. It also provides a context for the complex topic of ethics in public health.

Ethics is a branch of philosophy that deals with the distinction between right and wrong—with the moral consequences of human actions. The ethical principles that arise in epidemiologic practice and research include:

- Informed consent
- Confidentiality

- Respect for human rights
- Scientific integrity

The Centers for Disease Control (CDC) in the US defines public health ethics: "*As a field of study, public health ethics seeks to understand and clarify principles and values which guide public health actions. Principles and values provide a framework for decision making and a means of justifying decisions. Because public health actions are often undertaken by governments and are directed at the population level, the principles and values which guide public health can differ from those which guide actions in biology and clinical medicine (bioethics and medical ethics) which are more patient or individual-centered.*

As a field of practice, public health ethics is the application of relevant principles and values to public health decision-making. Public health ethics inquiry carries out three core functions,

1. *identifying and clarifying the ethical dilemma posed*
2. *analyzing it in terms of alternative courses of action and their consequences*
3. *resolving the dilemma by deciding which course of action best incorporates and balances the guiding principles and values (CDC).*"

Ethics in health is based on the fundamental values and concepts of a society. Medical ethics of the Hippocratic Oath hold the first obligation of a physician is to do no harm. The principle that saving a life is valued above all other religious considerations is of Biblical origins (i.e., Sanctity of Life or *Pikuah Nefesh*), where the saving of a life is equivalent to saving the world. This implies that all measures available are to be used, irrespective of the condition of the patient or the cost. But if sickness and death are seen as acts of God, possibly as punishment for sin, then prevention and treatment may be considered to be interfering with the Divine will, and ethical obligation may be limited to relief of suffering. Humanism balances these two ethical imperatives: saving of life and relief of suffering. Materialism may see health care as primarily a function to preserve health for societal well-being and economic prosperity.

The role of society in protecting the health of the population evolved during the latter 19th century with the sanitation movement and the gradual development of safe water supply, safe management of sewage and waste, and food safety with pasteurization, improving living conditions as well as medical care and the widespread implementation of national health insurance. Countries in Europe and the Americas began to recognize public health as societal obligations at municipal, state and national levels as part of fundamental values and concepts of a society. The astonishing success of public health over the past century increased life expectancy in high-income countries by some 30 years, mostly through improved sanitation, nutrition, living conditions and disease control measures, as well as societal and medical advances making care available to all. In the 1970s, the Lalonde concept emerged that individual behavior was one of the key health determinants, along with human biology, environment and medical care (see Chapter 21). This placed much of the responsibility for illness and its prevention on individual behavior, but at the same time fostered the development of health promotion as an essential component of public health theory and practice. All these points of view are involved in the ethical issues of the New Public Health (see Box 13.1).

BOX 13.1 Values and Ethical Principles of Public Health

1. **Nonmalfeasance**: Hippocratic Oath—do no harm.
2. **Sanctity of human life**: Biblical edict—saving a life comes before all other religious acts.
3. **Universal Declaration of Human Rights**: All humans deserve protection of life, health and well-being.
4. **Individual human rights**: Liberty, privacy, protection from harm.
5. **Solidarity**: Sharing the burden of promoting and maintaining health.
6. **Beneficence**: Reduce harm and burdens of disease and suffering.
7. **Proportionality**: Restriction on civil liberties must be legal, legitimate, necessary, and use the least restrictive means available.
8. **Reciprocity**: All have a right to just treatment but share responsibility to ensure justice especially for those facing heavy social and health burdens.
9. **Transparency**: Honest and truthfulness in the manner and context in which decisions are made must be clear and accountable.
10. **Precautionary**: Duty to take preventive action to avoid harm even before scientific certainty has been established.
11. **Responsibility to Act**: Public health officials and policy-makers have a duty to act and implement preventive health measures demonstrated to be effective, safe, and beneficial to population health. Failure to enforce public health regulations with resulting disease or deaths may constitute negligence on the part of responsible officials with civil or even criminal penalties.
12. **Equity**: Reduce gender, ethnic, social, economic, geographic inequities.
13. **Cost and benefits**: Economic analysis and consideration of priorities.
14. **Stewardship**: Responsibility of governance to act in a trustworthy and ethical manner.
15. **Trust**: Cooperation between the many public and non governmental stakeholders in health.
16. **Evidence based**: Decisions should be evidence-based, and revised, considering new evidence.
17. **Responsive to needs**: Address challenges as they may be anticipated and occur with close monitoring of health status.

Source: Adapted from Tulchinsky TH, Varavikova EA. The new public health, 3rd edition. San Diego. CA: Academic Press/Elsevier, 2014. Chapter 15, page 809.

Resources for health care are limited even in high-income countries, so that priority setting and judicious allocation of resources is always an issue. Money spent on new technology with only marginal medical advantages is often at the expense of well-tried and proven lower-cost techniques to prevent or treat disease. The potential benefits gained by the patient from more interventions are sometimes very limited in terms of length- or quality of life. These are difficult issues when the commitment to do all to preserve the life of the patient conflicts with the patient's concept of quality of life and his or her right to decline, or terminate heroic measures of intervention. Terminally ill patients may endure suffering during radical treatment, which may prolong life by only hours or days, clashing with the physician's ethical obligation to do no harm to the patient. The ethical value of sustaining the life of a suffering, terminally ill patient is a growing medical dilemma. The issue is even more complex when economic values are part of the equation. There is a potential conflict between the economic issues, the role of the physician in preserving life, the physician's obligation to do no harm, the felt needs of the patient and his or her family, and the needs of the community. The right of patients to seek euthanasia or assisted suicide in end-of-life situations is increasingly recognized and practiced in some jurisdictions.

The state represents organized society and has, among its responsibilities, a duty to promote healthful conditions and to provide access to both medical care and public health services. The dissonance between individual rights and community needs is a continuous issue in public health. Application of accepted public health measures for the benefit of people in society may require applying an intervention to everyone in a community or a nation. A democratic society ruled by law and legal protection of human rights may justifiably need to place limits on individual liberties to achieve the goal of reducing disease or injury in the population. Raising taxes and other restrictions on alcohol and tobacco products, laws on mandatory speed limits, driving regulations including seat belt usage, car seats for children and mandatory immunization for school attendance are examples of public health restrictive interventions which place limits on individuals but protect those individuals, their neighbors and the community-at-large from harm.

Some forms of mass medication are accepted methods of public health practice to reduce the risk of disease in the population. Chlorination of community water supplies is a well-established, effective, and safe intervention to protect the public health. Fluoridation of drinking water to prevent tooth decay in children means that other persons are also drinking the same fluoridated water, which is of less direct benefit to them. Mandatory pasteurization of milk is an important standard for public health. Fortification of basic foods with vitamins and minerals is also a cost-effective community health measure and banning of trans fats to reduce heart disease, are all topics with advocates and opponents. The addition of folic acid to food as the most effective way to prevent neural tube defects (NTDs) in newborns is an intervention mandated by the US Food and Drug Administration (USFDA) and in over 80 other countries since 1998 (see Chapter 20). Use of mass immunization is essential for infectious disease control and mass medication is successful for control of "Neglected Tropical Diseases".

Individual and Community Health

Confidentiality to assure the right of the individual to privacy involves ethical issues in the use of health information systems. Records of birth, death, reportable communicable and selected noncommunicable conditions (such as cancers, birth defects, neurological conditions), and hospitalization data—e.g. admissions by cause, length of stay—are essential data bases providing basic tools of epidemiology and health management. The use of detailed individual data, such as in mandatory reporting of infectious diseases and birth defects, e.g., is needed for case-finding and follow-up activities which is vital for population health monitoring and good epidemiologic management of disease outbreaks and routine monitoring functions of public health. However, caution is needed in data use to avoid individual identification to prejudice privacy, or that could be used punitively, such as in denial of access to health insurance or employment for smokers, alcoholics, or AIDS patients on the grounds that these are known causes of health damage that may be attributed to self-inflicted risk factors or preexisting conditions. This may become even more important if preexisting conditions or genetic susceptibility come to be used as determining factors to access health insurance or employment. Reporting is mandatory for physical for sexual abuse and criminally linked injuries as a measure essential for protection of vulnerable groups such as children, women, elderly, ethnic minority groups, or the general public from serious harm from bullying, abuse, violence or incitement to genocide.

Protection of the individual's rights to privacy, and freedom from arbitrary and harmful medical procedures or experiments may clash with the rights of the community to protect itself against harmful health issues. This conflict comes into much of what is done in public health practice, which has both an enforcement basis in law and practice as well as a humanitarian and protective aspect based on education, persuasion, and incentives. Society permits, indeed requires its governments to act for the common good, but sets limits that are protected by the constitution, laws, courts and administrative appeal mechanisms.

Democratic societies have the right and obligation to legislate work, including mine and construction safety regulations, and traffic safety including speed permitted, wearing seat belts, use of car seats for small children and non-use of cellphones during driving. Offenders may be punished by significant fines and be subjected to strict educational efforts to persuade them to comply. Similarly, the community must ensure sanitary conditions to prevent hazards or nuisances for neighbors. Society must act to protect the environment against the unlawful poisoning of the atmosphere, water supply, or earth. Enforcement is a legitimate and necessary activity of the public health network to protect the community from harm. Table 13.1 shows topics where individual rights and responsibilities

TABLE 13.1 Individual and Community Rights and Responsibility in Health: Ethical/Legal Issues

Ethical/Legal Issues	Individual Rights and Responsibilities	Community Rights and Responsibilities
Sanctity of human life	Individuals responsible to avoid behavior damaging their own health and that of others	Responsible for providing a feasible basket of service; equitable access for all
Individual vs. community rights	Immunization for individual protection	Immunization for herd immunity and community protection; education; community may mandate immunization
Right to health care	All are entitled to needed emergency, preventive, and curative care	Community right to care regardless of location, age, gender, ethnicity, medical condition, and economic status
Personal responsibility	Individual responsible for health behavior, diet, exercise, and nonsmoking	Community education for health-promoting lifestyles; avoid "blame the victim"
Corporate responsibility	Management accountability to criminal and civil action	Producer, purveyor of health hazard accountablity for individual and community damage
Provider responsibility	Professional, ethical care, and communication with patient	Ensure access to well-organized health care, accredited to accepted standards
Personal safety	Protection from individual, family, and community violence	Public safety, law enforcement, protection of women, children, vulnerable groups and elderly, safety from terrorism
Freedom of choice	Choice of health provider, limitations of gatekeeper functions, control costs function, right to second opinion, and right of appeal	Confidentiality, informed consent, birth control ensuring individual rights, limitations of self-referrals to specialist
Euthanasia	Individual's right to assisted death within limitations by societal, ethical, and legal standards	Assure individual and community interests; prevention of abuse by family or others with conflict of interest

(Continued)

TABLE 13.1 (Continued)

Ethical/Legal Issues	Individual Rights and Responsibilities	Community Rights and Responsibilities
Confidentiality	Individual's right to privacy, limitation of information	Mandatory reporting of specified diseases; data for epidemiological analysis
Informed consent	Right to know, risks vs. benefits; agree or disagree to treatment or participation in experiments	Helsinki Committee approval of research; regulate fair practice in right to know; Patient's Bill of Rights
Birth control	Right to information and access to birth control and fertility treatment; woman's rights over her body	Political, religious limited promotion of fertility; alternatives to abortion; legal protection of women's right to choose
Access to health care	Universal access, prepayment; individual contribution through workplace or taxes	Solidarity principle and adequate funding; right to cost containment, limitations on service benefits
Regulation and incentives to promote preventive care	Social security for hospital delivery, attendance for prenatal care; primary care, ambulatory care; home care	Incentive grants to assist communities for programs of national interest; limit institutional facilities
Global health	Human rights and aspirations; economic development, health, education, and jobs	Reduction of health risks; occupational hazards and environmental damage
Rights of migrants and minorities	Equality in universal access	Pro-active outreach for high-needs groups
Prisoners' health	Human rights	Security and human rights; reduce inequalities in sentencing convicts, harsh dangerous conditions in prisons; prohibition of torture and execution
Allocation of resource	Lobbying, advocacy for equity and innovation	Adequate resources for health; equitable distribution, targeting high-risk groups; cost containment

Source: Adapted from Tulchinsky TH, Varavikova EA. The new public health, 3rd edition, San Diego, CA; Academic Press/Elsevier, 2014. Chapter 15, page 807.

predominate, and a second set of rights that are the prerogative of the community to protect its citizens against public health hazards. Sometimes the issues overlap with political, advocacy, or legal action so that court decisions or new laws are needed to adjudicate precedents for the future.

Genocide

The 20th century was replete with mass murders, executions, and genocide with nationalistic, ideological, and racist motives perpetrated by fascist, Stalinist, and radical xenophobic political movements when gaining governmental power by election or by revolution, in some cases using then-common public health terminology and concepts. In the 21st century, radical jihadist terrorist groups and governments such as in Syria not only conduct mass killing of civilians, but also target ethnic minorities and religious groups with active genocide including deliberate use of chemical weapons, mass starvation, rape, murder and enslavement against civilians with bombings of civilians, medical workers, and hospital facilities.

Public health policy is guided by two distinct but interactive paradigms; the biotechnological disease and the social-ecological health paradigms. In the 19th century these were the Germ Theory and the Miasma Theories, long at loggerheads, yet both produced enormous gains in public health. The biomedical paradigm addresses alleviation of disease risk or manifest diseases, with immunizations, screening and risk-factor reduction. The social health paradigm addresses the improvement of the physical and socioeconomic environment and healthy living, with the objectives of reducing disease and inequities in health between socioeconomic and regional population health disparities.

During the early part of the twentieth century, a segment of the social hygiene movement adopted ideas of racial improvement by compulsory termination of pregnancies and sterilization of the mentally ill, retarded, and other "undesirable persons." By 1935, when the Nazi sterilization laws were passed, about 20 states in America already had sterilization laws in effect with concurrence of the US Supreme Court. American eugenics policies were praised by Hitler, and these ideas were adopted in Nazi Germany leading to execution of half a million "undesirables" under the eugenics concept, and were adapted for mass extermination of Jews, Gypsies, homosexuals, and others during the Holocaust.

The policies of eugenics were widely promoted by medical professionals in Sweden, the United States and Canada. This led to adoption of policies and programs to force legally sanctioned sterilization of mentally handicapped or mentally ill patients. This practice was attractive to Nazi policy before and after its rise to power in 1933, with wide support among the medical and psychiatric professions. Between 1939 and 1941, 180,000 psychiatric and physically handicapped patients were killed in Germany with the active participation by medical doctors, psychiatrists, nurses, and ancillary personnel under direct guidance of the so called T4 program, named after the address of Hitler's headquarters from where it was directed.

This corruption of public health distorted a socially oriented concept of public health to a racially oriented policy with horrendous actions of mass murder in the name of racial purity as a public health policy. This policy was supported and implemented by leading psychiatrists in a number of western liberal democratic countries providing a precedent adopted and expanded in monstrous manners in Nazi Germany with nearly total support and participation of a highly Nazified medical profession. The T4 program utilized starvation and gassing to kill helpless people and these methods became the direct antecedent to the mass murder of Jews, Gypsies, homosexuals, Soviet prisoners, and other "undesirables."

A noted Cambridge professor of modern history, Sir Richard Evans wrote:

> "At the heart of German history in the war years lies the mass murder of millions of Jews in what the Nazis called "the final solution to the Jewish question in Europe". This book provides a full narrative of the development and implementation of this policy of genocide, while also setting it in the broader context of Nazi racial policies toward the Slavs, and toward Gypsies, homosexuals, petty criminals and 'asocials'." (preface xiv).

> Evans continues: "For many years, and not merely since 1933, the medical profession, particularly in the field of psychiatry, had been convinced that it was legitimate to identify a minority of handicapped as 'a life unworthy of life', and that it was necessary to remove them from the chain of heredity if all the many measures to improve the health of the German race under the Third Reich were not to be frustrated. Virtually the entire medical profession has been actively involved in the sterilization programme, and from here it was but a short step in the minds of many to involuntary euthanasia" (page 82). "By the time the main killing programme had ended, in August 1941, a large part of the medical and caring professions had been brought in to operate the machinery of murder.... the circle of those involved had grown inexorably wider, until general practitioners, psychiatrists, social workers, asylum staff, orderlies, nurses and managers, drivers and many others had become involved, through a mixture of bureaucratic routine, peer pressure, propaganda and inducements and rewards.... Having proved itself in this context, it was ready to be applied in others, on a far larger scale." (p. 101).

> The T4 euthanasia program was administered directly from Hitler's main office "The euthenasia program was preceded by mass sterilization of nearly 400,000 'unfit' Germans before the war broke out" (p. 105).

> (Evans RJ. The Third Reich at War. New York: Penguin Press, 2006).

The human and national cost of genocide lasts for generations. The hatred and fear may wane, but the trauma goes deep. It lasts with the victims and their descendants, but also with the perpetrating country and its culture. The Nazi Holocaust has downstream effects in public health in German-speaking countries over 65 years since the events took place. The eugenic theory assumption was that a healthy population must be "free" of "racially contaminated" individuals and inferior groups which led to a public policy to eliminate racially "unclean" members through forced sterilization and murder opening the door to a euthanasia program of mass execution of mentally and physically handicapped Germans and others in psychiatric facilities, which provided a working model for the industrialized murder of the Holocaust. This was in direct conflict to a 200-year tradition of Germany's socially-oriented public health grounded in the political philosophy of human rights and social justice, many of whose advocates were mostly exiled or murdered. Many of the Nazi oriented academic medical leaders during World War II remained in key positions in the German public sector for many following decades.

The Nuremberg Doctors Trial in 1946−47 convicted many leading Nazi physicians of crimes against humanity with severe punishments including hanging or long prison terms. However, many in the medical profession aligned with these horrors remained in leading positions in the medical community—one even being elected to head the World Medical Association then discussing the Helsinki Declaration of Ethics in Biomedical Research before being forced to resign. The Nuremberg Trials and the subsequent Helsinki Declaration laid the fundamentals of biomedical ethics with regulations and requirements of ethical procedures and the Institutional Research Board, often referred to as Helsinki Committees. These were established by individual research centers, universities, hospitals, and other health care facilities to supervise and approve (or refuse) applications seeking funding, conducting, and publishing research involving human subjects.

The reappearance of genocide in the late twentieth century in the Balkans and Rwanda and in the twenty-first century in Darfur with over 300,000 deaths and 2.5 million displaced persons highlight this as a public health concern and its prevention as a public health and international political responsibility. Incitement to genocide is now considered a crime against humanity and was the basis for trials and convictions of leaders of the Rwandan Tutsi tribe, as well as inciters to ethnic violence and the political leaders and perpetrators of mass murders in the former Yugoslav republic. The threat and practice of genocide is still present, whether it is the murderous raids of Sudanese Janjaweed militias in Darfur and South Sudan, or the threats of genocide by Iran and associated terrorist organizations against Israel and Jews in general, the killing of Christians in northern Nigeria, Muslims in Myanmar and the genocidal civil war in Syria. Incitement to genocide is now accepted as part of international discourse, including the United Nations, which acted to accommodate the Rwanda massacres in 2003.

The risk of "silent" genocide is present in the 21st century with forced migration, limiting access rights of refugees to host countries, use of chemical weapons against civilian targets, use of starvation, mass rape and abuse of civilian displaced persons, and persecution including mass murder, expulsion, and slavery of minority ethnic, religious and refugee populations.

The UNICEF report of 2017 states: *"2016 was one of the most dangerous years to be a child in recent memory. Millions of children were threatened and displaced by crises around the world. Millions more faced poverty, deprivation, violence, exploitation and discrimination."* There are 66 million displaced persons in the world in 2017 who are refugees from war, endemic violence, terror, sexual violence and slavery, ethnic violence, chemical warfare, bombing civilians and medical facilities, hazardous journeys to "safety," and starvation as a tool of warfare, all forms of genocide. All of this in the 21st century when "Never Again: was the slogan following the Holocaust and other horrors of the 20th century.

Genocide represents the most extreme assault on human rights and protection for life. In the 20th century, an estimated 200 million have perished from genocide. An outline of genocides of the past 100 years is seen in Box 13.2. The Turkish genocide of Armenians in 1917 was followed by horrific genocides carried out under the flag of communism in Soviet USSR in the 1920s, in the Peoples' Republic of China under Chairman Mao in the 1950s and the Khmer Rouge in Cambodia in the 1980s, nationalism in the former Yugoslav republics in the 1990s and ethnic hatred in Darfur in the early years of the 21st century, and in civil war in Syria in the second decade of the 21st century. Totalitarian dictatorships, past war and defeat, ideologies of exclusiveness, ethnic purity and religious fundamentalism increase risks for genocide. Perpetrators use dehumanizing, demonizing and delegitimizing hate speech to desensitize or intimidate bystanders and to incite, mobilize, order and instruct followers to carry out mass murder.

The UN Convention on Prevention and Punishment of the Crime of Genocide (UNPPCG) of 1948 defines acts committed with intent to destroy, in whole or in part, members of a national, ethnical, racial or religious group as crimes against humanity. The UNPPCG specifies that incitement to genocide is itself a crime against humanity. Legal action should focus on state-sanctioned incitement as a recognized early warning sign. The UNPPCG convention defines genocidal acts including the following as punishable under international law:

- Genocide.
- Conspiracy to commit genocide.
- Direct and public incitement to commit genocide.
- Attempt to commit genocide.
- Complicity in genocide.

Genocide prevention requires international surveillance networks for monitoring and reporting incitement and hate speech in media, textbooks, places of worship, and the internet. Surveillance should monitor and identify the sources, and map their distribution and spread. Dehumanization,

BOX 13.2 Eugenics and Genocide: "the Slippery Slope"

Eugenics was a movement within the "Social Hygiene" concept of the early part of the 20th century. It was widely promoted to improve the population by reducing births among mentally ill and handicapped people. Legislation in some states in the US was upheld in decisions of the Supreme Court.

In 1942, the *American Journal of Psychiatry* published three articles, one arguing that "feebleminded" people should be killed (i.e., euthanasia). A rebuttal argued against euthanasia. An unsigned editorial position was that "euthanasia" would be appropriate in some cases, and that parents' opposition to this procedure should be the subject of psychiatric concern. The arguments referred to the context of eugenics and the murder of mental patients in Germany. The editorial pointed out that those genetic theories in psychiatry could be a precursor for future similar proposals. Forced sterilization was also practiced in Canada and Sweden.

This idea was promoted by Hitler in *Mein Kampf* and adopted by the Nazi party, which was legally elected to office in 1933. Organized massacres of mentally-ill and handicapped children and adults led to practices of various modes of killing, including starvation and gas chambers. These methods were then applied in concentration camps and the Holocaust murder of six million Jews and millions of others.

Genocide represents the most extreme assault on the respect for life. During the 20th century, an estimated 200 million have died during genocide. Totalitarian dictatorships, past wars and defeat, ideologies of exclusiveness, ethnic purity, and religious fundamentalism increase risks for genocide. Perpetrators use dehumanizing, demonizing, delegitimizing incitement by hate speech and propaganda to desensitize or intimidate bystanders and to promote, organize, order, and instruct followers ready to carry out mass murder. Consider the following list:

- 1915–17: Armenian genocide by Ottoman Turkish Empire—1.2 million killed.
- 1920–40s: Eugenics movement—United States, Sweden, Canada.
- 1920s: Mass executions, deportations, starvation as policy in Soviet Union Stalinist regimes killed millions.
- 1930–40s: Mass sterilization of "defectives" in the US and Sweden.
- 1930–40s: Mass murder of "defectives" in Nazi Germany (750,000).
- 1940s: Quarantining as pretext for ghettos by Nazis.
- 1940s: Concentration camps, human experimentation.
- 1940s: Holocaust; six million Jews and genocide in Nazi occupied Poland and the Soviet Union.
- 1947: Nuremberg Trials; convictions and capital punishment for crimes against humanity, genocide and criminal experimentation on humans by Nazi leaders and medical doctors.
- 1950s: Mass starvation in Maoist China—estimated deaths of 21 million people.
- 1948: Convention on the Prevention and Punishment of the Crime of Genocide.
- 1975–79: Cambodian political genocide of 1.7 million; genocide of Hmong in Laos.
- 1988: Iraqi genocide of Kurds in town of Halabja by poison gas.

(Continued)

BOX 13.2 (Continued)

- 1988: Brazil genocide of Tikuna people.
- 1992−95: Serbian rape, starvation and massacres in Srebrenica in Bosnia, Croatia and Herzegovina.
- 1994: Rwandan genocide of Tutsi tribe with 800,000 killed over a 100-day period from April to July.
- 2003−12: Sudanese genocide in Darfur (400,000 plus).
- 2011−17: Sudanese genocide of Nuba people.
- 2012−17 Iran incitement to genocide of Israel.
- 2012−17: Syria: Civil war; mass civilian deaths by bombardment and gas, displacement of millions; genocide of Yazidis and Christians.
- 2012−17: Democratic Republic of Congo massacres of Kivu minority; mass violence and refugee flow from South Sudan.
- 2017 Expulsion and mass violence against over 600,000 Rohingya Muslim population of Myanmar.

Source: Adapted from Tulchinsky TH, Varavikova EA. The new public health, 3rd edition. San Diego, CA: Academic Press/Elsevier, 2014, chapter 15 page 810. United Nations. Convention on the Prevention and Punishment of the Crime of Genocide. Available at: http://www.hrweb.org/ legal/genocide.html (accessed 4 May 2017). Richter ED. Commentary. Genocide: can we predict, prevent, and protect? J Public Health Policy. 2008;29(3):265−274. Available at: http://www. genocidewatch.org/images/Articles_Can_we_prevent_genocide_by_preventing_incitement.pdf. United to Prevent Genocide. The Bosnian war and Srebrenica. Available at: http://endgenocide.org/ learn/past-genocides/the-bosnian-war-and-srebrenica-genocide/ (accessed 15 April 2017). Joseph J. The 1942 'euthanasia' debate in the American J Psychiatry. Hist Psych. 2005;16(62 Pt 2): 171−179. Abstract available at: https://www.ncbi.nlm.nih.gov/pubmed/16013119 (accessed 16 April 2017).

demonization, delegitimization, disinformation, and denial are danger signs of potential genocidal actions. Genocide results from human choice and bystander indifference. One lesson of the Holocaust and subsequent genocides is that silence by nations and international organizations constitutes complicity. The public health community has a responsibility to speak out publicly on genocidal threats and its early warning signs (See Box 13.1).

Human Experimentation

Human experimentation has been a subject of great concern since the Nazi and Imperial Japanese armed forces' horrific experiments on prisoners and concentration camp victims during World War II. The Nuremberg trials set forth ten principles of professional responsibility to comply with internationally acceptable medical behavior in regard to research on humans (see Table 13.2).

The Helsinki Declaration was first adopted by the World Medical Assembly in 1964, and amended in 1975, 1983, 1989, 1996, and 2013. It delineates standards of medical experimentation and requires informed consent from subjects subjecting themselves to medical research. These

TABLE 13.2 Ethical Issues of Medical Research Derived from the Nuremberg Trials, the Universal Declaration of Human Rights and Declaration of Helsinki

Nuremberg Doctors Trial, 1946–47	The voluntary consent of a human subject is absolutely essential, with the exercise of free power of choice without force, fraud, deceit, duress, or coercion
	Experiments should be such as to bear fruitful results, based on prior experimentation and the natural history of the problem under study. They should avoid unnecessary physical and mental suffering
	The degree of risk should not exceed the humanitarian importance of the experiment
	Persons conducting experiments are responsible for adequate preparations and resources for even the remote possibility of death or injury resulting from the experiment
	The human subject should be able to end his participation at any time
	The scientist in charge is responsible to terminate the experiment if continuation is likely to result in injury, disability, or death
Universal Declaration of Human Rights, 1948	Everyone has the right to a standard of living adequate for the health and well-being of himself and of his family, including food, clothing, housing, and medical care and necessary social services
Declaration of Helsinki, 1964	Research must be in keeping with accepted scientific principles, and should be approved by specially appointed independent committees
	Biomedical research should be carried out by scientifically qualified persons, only on topics where potential benefits outweigh the risks, with careful assessment of risks, where the privacy and integrity of the individual is protected, and where the hazards are predictable. Publication must preserve the accuracy of research findings
	Each human subject in an experiment should be adequately informed of the aims, methods, anticipated benefits, and hazards of the study. Informed consent should be obtained, and a statement of compliance with this code
	Clinical research should allow the doctor to use new diagnostic or therapeutic measures if they offer benefit as compared to current methods

(Continued)

TABLE 13.2 (Continued)	
	In any study, the patient and the control group should be assured of the best available methods. Refusal to participate should never interfere with the doctor–patient relationship. The well-being of the subject takes precedence over the interests of science or society

Note: Summarized from the Nuremberg Trials (1948) and World Medical Association, Declaration of Helsinki.
Source: Adapted from Tulchinsky TH, Varavikova EA. The new public health, 3rd edition. San Diego, CA: Academic Press/Elsevier, 2014, chapter 15 page 812. United Nations. Universal Declaration of Human Rights. Available at: http://www.un.org/events/humanrights/2007/hrphotos/declaration%20_eng.pdf. World Medical Association. Available at: http://www.wma.net/ (accessed 3 May 2017).

standards have become the international norm for experiments, with national-, state-, and hospital-Helsinki committees regulating research proposals within their jurisdiction. Funding agencies require standard approval by the appropriate Helsinki committee, sometimes called Institutional Review Boards (IRBs) or Ethical Review Boards (ERBs), before considering any proposal, with informed consent on any research project. The process recognizes that medical progress is based on research that must include studies involving human subjects, but medical research is subject to ethical standards that promote and ensure respect for human subjects and protect their health and rights. The key issues examined include:

- Research objectives should outweigh the risks and burdens to the research subjects.
- Research should conform to generally accepted scientific principles and literature.
- Participants are volunteers.
- Informed consent must be obtained including warning of potential risks.
- Risks are minimized and monitored.
- Respect for privacy and confidentiality.
- Respect for human rights.
- Scientific integrity.
- Social solidarity and paternalism.
- Fairness and equity.
- If the results are definitively positive, the research should be stopped.

The Tuskegee experiment (see Box 13.3) conducted in Alabama from 1932 to 1972 by the US Public Health Service (USPHS) was a grave and tragic violation of medical ethics. It was initiated in the context of the 1930s and consistent with widespread and institutionalized racism, detached from

---

BOX 13.3 The Tuskegee Experiment

The Tuskegee experiment was carried out by the US Public Health Service between 1932 and 1972. It was meant to follow the natural course of syphilis in 399 infected African-American men in Alabama and 201 uninfected men. The men were not told that they were being used as research subjects. The experiment had been intended to show the need for additional services for those infected with syphilis. However, when penicillin became available in 1942, the researchers did not inform or offer the men treatment, even those who were eligible when drafted into the army in 1942. The experiment was stopped in 1972 as "ethically unjustified" when the media exposed it to public scrutiny.

The case is considered unethical research practice because, in the time it was conducted, it did not provide the patients with information on the research nor on the availability of curative care when it became available. The patients' well-being was put aside in the interest of a descriptive study.

A similar experiment was conducted by the US Public Health Service in full cooperation with the Guatemala Ministry of Health during 1946–1948 in which soldiers, prisoners, and others were deliberately exposed to prostitutes known to be infected with syphilis. This experiment was terminated when it was revealed in the US media by a historian.

In 1997, President Bill Clinton apologized to the survivors and families of the men involved in the experiment on behalf of the US government. The Tuskegee experiment is the source of widespread lingering suspicion of public health in the African-American community to the present time.

Source: Adapted from Tulchinsky TH, Varavikova EA. The new public health, 3rd edition. San Diego, CA: Academic Press/Elsevier, 2014, chapter 15 page 813. (accessed 5 May 2017). Reverby SM. Ethical failures and history lessons: the U.S. Public Health Service research studies in Tuskegee and Guatemala. Public Health Rev. 2012;34(1):189206. Available at: https:// publichealthreviews.biomedcentral.com/articles/10.1007/BF03391665 (accessed 3 December 2017).

---

humanist values and historical medical ethics of "first, do no harm." The Tuskegee experiment, and a following similar study conducted by the USPHS in conjunction with the Ministry of Health in Guatemala, are remembered as important ethical transgressions which have had repercussions until the present time resulting in suspicion of public health endeavors, particularly among the African-American community in the US, even after a public apology in 1997 by then president Bill Clinton.

Ethics in Public Health Research

The line between practice and research is not always easy to define in public health, which has surveillance of population health as one of its major tasks. This surveillance is mostly anonymous, but relies on individually identifiable data needed for reportable and infectious disease control as well as for causes of death, birth defects, mass screening programs, and other special disease registries. It may also be necessary to monitor the effects of chronic disease, for example, to ascertain repeat hospitalizations of patients with congestive heart failure to assess the long-term effects of treatment, and the effects strengthening ambulatory and outreach services to sustain chronic patients at a safe and functional level in their own homes.

Preventive care practices—e.g., sanitation, healthy and safe food and diets, health promotion, immunizations, prenatal care, newborn screening, Pap smears, mammography, and colonoscopies—as well as access to medical care and hospital utilization, are all part of public health. Monitoring and impact assessment of preventive programs may require special surveys, such as those conducted by the US National Health and Nutrition Studies (NHANES) and are important to assess health and nutritional status as well as other measures of health status and risk factors such as smoking and exercise. Every effort in public health research must be made to preserve anonymity and privacy for the individual, but in some cases such as reporting of contagious diseases or birth defects, case contact is crucial. This can entail identifying people who attended an event or were on an airplane where an infected person may have been — such as with measles or antibiotic resistant tuberculosis — so as to take appropriate preventive measures.

The general distinction between research and practice has to do with the intent of the activity. Clinical research uses experimental methods to establish the efficacy and safety of new or unproven interventions; many drugs and procedures in common use have never been subjected to randomized controlled trials. In practice, many methods are devised that are held to be effective and safe by expert opinion and documented as such. Researchers comparing HIV or hepatitis B transmission rates among intravenous drug users not using needle exchange programs would be doing unethical research, according to accepted current standards, by giving safe needles to the experimental group and withholding them from the control group. The scientific justification of an experiment must be made explicit but would not likely be approved by an Ethical Review Board (Helsinki Committee). In some cases of new therapy for life threatening conditions, the FDA will "fast track" what are called "orphan drugs" urgently needed as happened with the NIH recommendation for antiretroviral (ART) drugs for HIV/AIDS. This turned out to be a major success for treatment and prevention of HIV (Faucci, 2014). Clinical equivalence is a necessary condition of all clinical and public health research and provision of standard of care treatment to control groups is a minimal requirement for most research ethics boards. Determination of the standard, and whether it should be place, time, and community specific, is an area of ongoing controversy.

A 1996 US Public Health Service study supported by the US National Institutes of Health (NIH) and WHO compared a short course of zidovudine

(AZT) to a placebo given late in pregnancy to HIV-positive women in Thailand, measuring the rate of HIV infection among the newborns. The experiment was terminated when a protest editorial appeared in a prominent medical journal. This study confirmed previous findings that AZT given during late pregnancy and labor reduced maternal-fetal HIV transmission by half. The findings indicate that AZT should be used in developing countries, and the manufacturers agreed to make it available at reduced costs. The result has been a major success with more recent medications to reduce maternal–fetal transmission of IIIV in many places in Africa with important financial and professional support from the Global Alliance for Vaccine Initiatives (GAVI), international donors, and a slowing of the spread of HIV- and AIDS-related deaths.

An outstanding case of breach of ethics in public health research occurred with the "Wakefield Effect" as described in Box 13.4. The importance of responsible medical journalism to keep a watchful eye on the possibilities of misleading scientific publications is of great importance for the ethical and legal aspects of public health.

CURRENT RELEVANCE

A preeminent ethical issue in public health is that of assuring universal access to services, and/or the provision of services according to need. While all industrialized countries except the United States have universal health care insurance or national health service evolving since the 19th century (see Chapter 8); the United States is still struggling with the issue in the 21st century. The solidarity principle of societal shared responsibility for funding universal access to health care is based on equitable prepayment for health care for all by nationally regulated mechanisms through place of work or general revenues of government. A society may see universal access to health care as a positive value, and at the same time utilize incentives to promote or place limits on use of services or benefits to the individual such as hospital care, immunization, screening programs, prescription drugs and others. Some services may be arbitrarily excluded from health insurance, such as dental care, although this is to the detriment of children and a financial hardship for many. Strategies for program inclusion are often based on historical precedent rather than cost-effectiveness or evidence. While efforts are being made to include more children in the program, the Medicaid system in the US defines eligibility at income levels up to 133 percent of the poverty line, thus excluding a high percentage of the working poor. This is a topic of current and continuing political importance in electoral platforms in the US to address the challenge of the uninsured and poorly insured working poor population (i.e., Obamacare versus Trumpcare). Health is also a political issue in countries with universal health systems where funding may be inadequate or patient dissatisfaction common.

BOX 13.4 The Wakefield Effect

In 1998, one of the top medical journals in the world, *Lancet*, published an article by a number of well-known researchers headed by Dr. Andrew Wakefield. The article reported on 12 cases of autistic children and allegedly showed a connection to immunization with MMR vaccine (measles-mumps-rubella).

The immediate effect of this "revelation" was widespread alarm in the United Kingdom and abroad concerning MMR vaccine and a drop in immunization coverage with measles-containing vaccines in the United Kingdom and elsewhere. This was mainly triggered by mothers refusing to have their child vaccinated with the "risk of autism". As a result, measles epidemics occurred in the United Kingdom and in many other countries with the disease again becoming endemic in many parts of Europe and spreading to North and South America by travelers and tourists.

After a long series of investigative journalism in the British press, the article came under scientific scrutiny and the withdrawal of many of the coauthors, but consistent insistence by the lead author of its authenticity. Coauthors admitted to having been credulous and insufficiently vigilant in agreeing to be associated with the paper. British medical authorities later found Dr. Wakefield guilty of medical fraud and the UK General Medical Council withdrew his license to practice medicine. In 2000, 12 years after the original publication, *Lancet* formally withdrew the article. This fraudulent scientific publication caused a serious loss of the credibility of immunization in general, and especially regarding MMR vaccine, one of the greatest life savers of public health.

The return of measles in Europe to endemicity with frequent international transmission, fostered loss of confidence by mothers in immunization. Measles-containing vaccines were particularly affected due to the publicity given to the Wakefield case and issues of scientific integrity. Fraud and conflict of interests were proven in this case. The journal editors failed to ensure the scientific integrity of the lead author and coauthors, and were negligent in failure of the journal to retract fraudulent and disproven publications in real time, instead of waiting 12 years after publication.

In other public health issues, single publications of findings of small sample and poorly assessed studies published in haste without adequate critical review occur frequently. In electronic media, the problem of disinformation provokes great anxiety and rejection of well-established successful public health interventions such as fluoridation, and folic acid fortification of flour, with unsubstantiated and disproven claims that they may cause cancer, asthma, and other ill effects.

The interface between ethics, law, and science in public health requires continuous sensitivity to the downstream effects of reducing public trust and reduced parental compliance with immunization of their children and putting other children at risk.

Source: Adapted from Tulchinsky TH, Varavikova EA. The new public heath, 3rd edition. San Diego, CA: Academic Press/Elsevier, 2014, chapter 15, Box 15.18, page 814. Wakefield AJ, Murch SH, Anthony A, Linnell J, Casson DM, Malik M, et al. Ileal lymphoid nodular hyperplasia, non-specific colitis, and pervasive developmental disorder in children [retracted]. Lancet. 1998;351:637–641. (accessed 17 April 2017). Office of Research Integrity. Definition of research misconduct. Available at: http://ori.hhs.gov/misconduct/definition_misconduct.shtml. Murch SH, Anthony A, Casson DH, Malik M, Berelowitz M, Dhillon AP, et al. Retraction of an interpretation. Lancet. 2004;363:750. Available at: https://www.ncbi.nlm.nih.gov/pubmed/15016483 (accessed 21 April 2017). Godlee F, Smith J, Marcovitch H. Editorial. Wakefield's article linking MMR vaccine and autism was fraudulent. BMJ 2011;342:c7452. Available at: http://www.bmj.com/content/342/bmj.c7452 (accessed 17 April 2017). Tulchinsky TH, Varavikova EA. The new public health, 3rd edition. San Diego, CA: Academic Press/Elsevier, 2014. Page 814.

The HIV/AIDS epidemic which appeared suddenly in the early 1980s and became a global pandemic in 1990s raised a host of medical and public health ethical issues. Management of the epidemic was in some respects in conflict with the long-established role of public health of contacting and quarantining persons suffering from selected communicable diseases. It was not acceptable or feasible in modern society to require follow-up of case contacts or to isolate HIV carriers, at a time when there was no clinical cure with medications. However, this led to failure or delay of public health authorities, even in the late 1980s, to close public bathhouses in New York and other US cities where exposure to multiple same-sex partners promoted spread of a lethal disease, which could have been interpreted as negligence. During the 1980s, the politics of HIV/AIDS in the US centered on concerns in the community of men who have sex with men (MSM) that HIV testing could be used in a discriminatory manner. AIDS was initially addressed as a civil liberties issue and not as a public health problem. Screening, reporting, and case contact follow-up were seen as an invasion of privacy and counterproductive by increasing resistance to and avoidance of testing.

In these political circumstances, the educational approach was adopted as most feasible and acceptable. The AIDS epidemic and public anxiety about contracting AIDS through casual sexual contact reinforced the need for public education on safe sex. This has been raised as an ethical issue because such education may be construed as condoning teenage and extramarital relations. The issue of HIV screening of pregnant women in general or in high-risk groups took on a new significance with the findings that treatment of the pregnant woman reduces the risk of HIV infection of the newborn, and that breastfeeding may be contraindicated.

A similar issue arose anew in the past decade in the context of using the new human papillomavirus (HPV) vaccine for prevention of cancer of the cervix. Initially the vaccine was recommended for preteen girls to create protective antibodies to the virus before they became sexually active to prevent the possibility of sexually transmitted infection of the virus. Controversy arose over concern that this immunization of young girls might promote early onset of sexual activity. Gradually acceptance increased and other age groups of women were urged to take the vaccine. Boys were added to the recommended immunization target groups so as to reduce transmission of the virus, and to address male-to-male transmission via oral and anal sex. Inclusion of HPV vaccination requirement for school entry is under debate in the US, but parental refusals are increasing. CDC reports that HPV infects a large proportion of people in the US. Among adults aged 18−59 it was 45 percent in men and 40 percent in women. Nearly 10,000 women in the US are diagnosed with cervical cancer each year and 3,700 women die. Cancer of the cervix has been massively reduced by routine Pap smears for early case-finding and treatment. The advent of an effective HPV vaccine promises to lower cancer of cervix rates even further. The disease is much more common in low-income countries where screening and HPV immunization are still very low on the health priorities list, so that cervical cancer is the second leading cancer killer of women worldwide. A recent survey conducted by the American Academy of Pediatrics result indicated that nearly 90 percent of pediatricians reported that they experienced parental vaccine refusals in 2013 compared to 75 percent in 2006. The vaccines most likely to be refused, mainly due to misinformation, are HPV, influenza, measles, mumps, and rubella vaccines, all strongly recommended by public health and clinicians.

Choices in health policy are often between one "good" and another. Limitations in resources may make this issue even more difficult in the future, with aging populations, increasing population prevalence of physical disabilities, and rapid increases in technology and its associated costs. For example, the UK's National Health Service at one point refused to provide dialysis to persons over age 65. When computed tomography (CT) was first introduced, Medicare in the US refused to insure this service as an untested medical technique. Due to a lack of facility resources such as incubators and poor prospects for the survivors, the Soviet health system considered newborns as living only if they weighed over 1,000 grams and survived more than seven days. Those under 1,000 grams who would be considered living by other international definitions, would be placed in a freezer to die. At the opposite extreme, many western medical centers use extreme and costly measures to prolong life in terminally ill patients, preserving life temporarily, but often with much suffering for the person and at great expense to the public system of financing health care.

In many countries, such as those in the former Soviet system, spending for hospital services, in some cases was grossly overemphasized and in excess of need, accompanied by lack of funds for community care such as adding new vaccines for the immunization program for children, although coverage rates were high. In the US, there was a lack of funds for immunization of poor children, but this has gradually improved over the past decade with changes in health insurance for the poor as well as by using food supplement programs to promote immunization.

Research Misconduct

The Office of Research Integrity of the US Department of Health and Human Services defines research misconduct as: "fabrication, falsification, or plagiarism in proposing, performing, or reviewing research, or in reporting research results:

- *Fabrication* is making up data or results and recording or reporting them.
- *Falsification* is manipulating research materials, equipment, or processes, or changing or omitting data or results such that the research is not accurately represented in the research record.

- *Plagiarism* is the appropriation of another person's ideas, processes, results, or words without giving appropriate credit.
- *Research misconduct* does not include honest error or differences of opinion."

The prevalence and publication of erroneous information and compromised research findings is an ongoing issue in the 21st century, which can spread false information in the media such as the internet. This can have serious negative consequences for population health. Pseudoscience can feed populist movements with tragic consequences in public health.

Helsinki Research Ethics Committees (or Institutional Review Committees) are responsible to ensure that ethical principles are maintained in research proposals and publication of results of such research. These principles include informed consent, confidentiality, and scientific integrity. Publication in peer-reviewed journals is essential for establishing and advancing the evidence base for public health practice. Poor, or fraudulent science, can have a substantial adverse impact on public opinion both on health issues and on the priorities in the allocation of resources. It is essential that journal editors and reviewers adhere to high ethical and professional standards. They must be vigilant to avoid allowing poor professional standards of articles to be published or allowing non-professional factors or conflicts of interest to distort decision-making processes. Professional integrity and high scientific standards are vital to advance public health practice.

Ethics in Patient Care

Ethical issues between the individual patients and health care providers are important in health systems. A doctor is expected to use diligence, care, knowledge, skill, discretion, and caution in keeping with practice standards accepted at the time by responsible medical opinion, and to maintain the basic medical imperative to "do no harm" to the patient. Patients should have the right to free choice of provider and treatment, to observance of quality standards, access to high quality health services, to be informed of his or her condition, give informed consent, to confidentiality of personal and health information, and to physical privacy during care and diagnosis, to available alternatives for treatment, to be informed of the risks and benefits involved, and to complain and seek compensation for negligence. Ideally, patients have the right of access to high quality health services, to safety and freedom from harm caused by lack of resources, geographic inequality, poor functioning of health services, and from medical malpractice and errors. Patients' rights include the right of access to innovative procedures, including diagnostic procedures, according to international standards and independent of economic or financial considerations. Patients may seek alternative medical opinions, but this right is not unlimited, as any insurance plan or health service may place restrictions on payment for further opinions and consultation without the agreement of a primary care provider, which is called "the gatekeeper" role.

Health insurance providers have responsibility beyond that of payment for health service and individual care by a physician, in institutions, or through services in the community or the home. The contract for service is becoming less between an individual physician and the patient, but increasingly among a health system provider group staff and a client. This places a new onus on the physician to ensure that patients receive the care they require. Conversely, the US provider often faces the dilemma of knowing that a patient may not access needed services because of a lack of adequate health insurance, and the terrible practice of exclusions due to "prior health conditions".

Sanctity of Life Versus Euthanasia

The imperative to "save a life" is an important ethical and practical issue in health care. Principles of physician-assisted euthanasia were based on a legal process including psychiatric assessment. Physician-aided suicide of a patient is facilitated by providing the means or information—e.g., indication of a lethal medication dosage—provided by a physician who is aware of the patient's intent. Both are based on the right of the patient to decide to die with dignity when their illness is terminal and the individual is suffering excessively. This is not a medical decision alone. It is also an agonizing issue for society to address.

The Nazi euthanasia program in Germany in the 1930s and its subsequent application as mass extermination in the Holocaust with grossly unethical human experimentation provided the direst of warnings to societies of what may follow when the principle of the sanctity of individual human life is breached. The issue, however, returned to the public agenda in the 1980s and 1990s as advances in medical science have allowed the prolongation of human life beyond hope of recovery.

Legislation in the Netherlands, Belgium, the US ("assisted suicide" in six US states, Washington DC, Oregon, Vermont, California, Colorado, and Montana as of April 2017), northern Australia and Canada legally sanctioned passive euthanasia (i.e., withdrawing medical assistance) with various safeguards in a variety of circumstances, such as long-term comas or late stages of terminal illnesses. The legislation in Canada, known as "dying with dignity", is the federal regulatory framework with strict criteria for eligibility and procedures, provides for medical assistance in dying for those persons with a "grievous and irremediable medical condition; they have made a voluntary request for medical assistance in dying that, in particular, was not made as a result of external pressure; and they give informed consent to receive medical assistance in dying after having been informed of the means that are available to relieve their suffering." The person must be eligible for government-funded health services and be over 18 years. Doctors, patients, relatives, and health care organizations need clear guidelines, orientation, procedures, legal protection, and limitations where failure to take the utmost steps to "save" the patient by intubation, resuscitation, or transplantation may cause legal jeopardy. Protection of the elderly or chronically ill from malicious application of this form of merciful death must ensure that it is truly the patients' wish. This requires well defined procedures with legal, social, psychiatric and medical participation.

Even though a distinction can be drawn theoretically between permitting and facilitating death, in practice, doctors in intensive care units face such decisions regularly where the line is often blurred. Hospital doctors routinely take extreme measures to prolong the life of hopeless cases. Such decisions should not be considered for economic reasons alone, but in practice the costs of care of the terminally ill will be a driving force in debate of the issue. Living wills allow a patient to refuse heroic measures such as resuscitation, with "do not resuscitate" standing orders and assignment of power of attorney to family members to make such decisions. Family attitudes are important, but the social issue of redefining the right of a patient to opt for legal termination of life by medical means will be an increasingly important issue in the 21st century.

The Imperative to Act in Public Health

As in other spheres of medicine and health, in public health the decision whether to intervene in an issue is based on identification and interpretation of the problem. A case must be made of importance even if a rare condition, establishing evidence of the potential of the intervention to improve the situation, to do no harm, and to convince the public and political leaders of the need for such intervention along with the resources to carry it out. This process requires patience and a longer time frame than many other fields in health.

Some interpretations of ethics in health consider that the only purpose for which power can be rightfully exercised over any member of a democratic community, without asking individual permission and possibly against their will, is to prevent harm to others. However, this is a dictum that is not always applied to public health, which is obliged to act to protect health in so many spheres such as water, sanitation, food and drug safety, and environmental health on a spectrum that extends to banning smoking in public places, mandating food fortification, and many other areas for improved population health in a civil society.

Failure to act is an action, and when there is convincing evidence of a problem that can be alleviated or prevented entirely by an accepted and demonstrably successful intervention, then the onus is on the public health leader/authority to advocate such action and to implement it as best as possible under the existing conditions. Failure to do so is a breach of "good standards of practice" and could be unethical. Inertia of the public health system in the face of evidence of a demonstrably effective modality such as adoption of state-of-the-art vaccines or fortification of flour with folic acid to prevent birth defects would come under this categorization and may even constitute neglect and unethical practice. This is not an easy categorization because there is often disagreement and even opposition to public health interventions, as was the case in opposition to vaccination long after Jenner's crucial discovery of this procedure in the late eighteenth century. This idea is also a significant problem true today with opposition to many proven measures such as immunization, fluoridation or fortification of basic foods. Box 13.5 shows the ethical standards of the American Public Health Association of 2002.

The problem of refusals of vaccination has become an issue in the US mainly among upper middle class families. In Western Europe delay in updating immunization programs such as the two doses of measles policy in the past has created a situation of measles outbreaks across Europe since 2010 with many cases among unimmunized children or among young adults or those with only one dose and waning immunity. In many low- and medium-income countries funding levels for health are minimal leading to the delay in professional or governmental acceptance of "new" vaccines. This has been a serious issue but international donors have helped countries in sub-Saharan Africa to expand the range of vaccines in their routine programs with important life saving vaccines such as rotavirus and hemophilus influenza B. Underfunding for health is an ethical dilemma in many low- and medium-income countries. In former Soviet countries including the Russian Federation much of the overall low level of funding for health is due to their declining, but still relatively high, acute-care hospital bed supply with much longer average length of hospital stay leaving primary care and upgrading of immunization lagging.

Closure of hospitals involves difficult political and ethical decisions and is a source of dispute between central health authorities, the medical professions, and local communities. Health reforms in many industrialized countries, such as reducing hospital bed supplies, managed care systems, promoting cost containment, and reallocation of resources raise ethical and political issues often based on vested interests such as private insurance systems, hospitals, and private medical practitioners (see Chapters 8 and 15).

Where there is a high level of cumulative evidence from professional literature and from public health practice in "leading countries" with a strong scientific base and case for action on a public health issue, when does it become bad practice or even unethical public health practice to ignore and fail to implement such an intervention? Such ethical failures occur frequently and widely. For example, is it unethical to not fortify grain products with folic acid and salt with iodine when there is overwhelming evidence of safety and cost effectiveness? Should there be a recommended European

BOX 13.5 Principles of Ethical Public Health Practice: American Public Health Association, 2002

1. Public health should address the fundamental causes of disease and requirements for health, aiming to prevent adverse health outcomes.
2. Public health should achieve community health in a way that respects the rights of individuals in the community.
3. Public health policies, programs, and priorities should be developed and evaluated through processes that ensure an opportunity for input from community members.
4. Public health should advocate and work for the empowerment of disenfranchised community members, aiming to ensure that the basic resources and conditions necessary for health are accessible to all.
5. Public health should seek the information needed to implement effective policies and programs that protect and promote health.
6. Public health institutions should provide communities with the information they have that is needed for decisions on policies or programs and should obtain the community's consent for their implementation.
7. Public health institutions should act in a timely manner on the information they have within the resources and the mandate given to them by the public.
8. Public health programs and policies should incorporate a variety of approaches that anticipate and respect diverse values, beliefs, and cultures in the community.
9. Public health programs and policies should be implemented in a manner that most enhances the physical and social environment.
10. Public health institutions should protect the confidentiality of information that can bring harm to an individual or community if made public. Exceptions must be justified on the basis of the likelihood of significant harm to the individual or others.
11. Public health institutions should ensure the professional competence of their employees.
12. Public health institutions and their employees should engage in collaborations and affiliations in ways that build the public's trust and the institution's effectiveness.

Source: American Public Health Association. Principles of the ethical practice of public health Version 2.2, 2002. Available at: https://www.apha.org/~/media/files/pdf/membergroups/ ethics_brochure.ashx (accessed 15 April 2017).

immunization program; should milk be fortified with vitamin D; should vitamin and mineral supplements be given to pregnant and lactating women, and children; should all newborns be given vitamin K intramuscularly routinely? Other examples include the issues of fluoridation of water supplies and opposition to genetically modified crops or generic drugs in African countries. These issues are continuously debated and the responsibility of the trained public health professional is to review the international literature on a topic and formulate a position based on the cumulative weight of evidence. It is not possible to wait for indisputable evidence because in epidemiology and public health, this rarely occurs. This is another reason that guidelines established by respected agencies and professional bodies free from financial obligations to vested interest groups are essential to review evidence which accumulates on a continuing basis on many issues thought to have been resolved or which appear de novo.

A recent public health issue has been the banning of trans fats in baking and cooking, with legislation in New York City and some upstate New York State counties. The US Food and Drug Administration (USFDA) has declared trans fats, found in many popular processed foods, like baked goods and frozen foods, to be unsafe for consumption as they contribute to heart disease. The USFDA promotes manufacturer compliance and will regulate banning of use of trans fats by 2018, which is expected to reduce coronary heart disease and prevent thousands of fatal heart attacks every year. The USFDA reports that between 2003 and 2012, consumer trans fat consumption decreased about 78 percent and that the labeling rule and industry reformulation of foods were key factors in informing healthier consumer choices and reducing trans fat in foods. While trans fat intake has significantly decreased, the current intake remains a public health concern. The Institute of Medicine (IOM) recommends that consumption of trans fat be as low as possible while consuming a nutritionally adequate diet.

The WHO European Region reports that five European countries are in the process of banning trans fats through regulation, while others have decided to use self-regulatory mechanisms. On the other hand, virtually no countries in the European Region fortify flour with folic acid to prevent birth defects (neural tube defects), a lapse in current international public health standards. Along with rising incidence of rickets in infancy due to lack of sun exposure and lack of vitamin D supplements in pregnancy care, birth defects and severe rickets are increasing especially among dark skinned mothers in full body clothing for religious reasons. Most consumers do not know that some processed food categories contain large amounts of trans fats. Consumption in some population groups, particularly poorer people, can be very high. Removing trans fats from the food supply is one of the most straightforward public health interventions for reducing the risk of cardiovascular diseases and some cancers, and improving diets. A study comparing myocardial infarctions in New York counties that banned trans fat usage to counties that did not showed a greater reduction in acute myocardial infarctions in the counties that had banned trans fats. The ethical issue will be to see the rate of acceptance of this finding in other jurisdictions versus traditional opposition to too much interference by the state. The same issue regarding folic acid fortification of flour to reduce birth defects is similarly both a professional and ethical question. Virtually all European countries have ignored the evidence and fail to adopt mandatory fortification thus harming poorer population groups with less money to buy healthier foods. The delay in implementation of proven safe and effective public health measures is one of the key ethical issues in public health practice.

ETHICAL ISSUES

Coleman et al. discuss global issues in public health ethics with emphasis on disparities in health status; access to health care and the benefits of medical research; responding to the threat of infectious diseases; efforts to contain the spread of infectious diseases; international cooperation in health monitoring and surveillance (e.g., International Health Regulations); exploitation of individuals in low-income countries; health promotion, participation, transparency, and accountability. The global Millennium Development Goals (MDGs) and the follow-up Sustainable Development Goals (SDGs) reflect a consensus on objectives and a respectable degree of international support by donor countries. Strong networks such as the Global Vaccine Alliance involve international organization (e.g., WHO, UNICEF, World Bank), donor countries and private donors (e.g., Bill and Melinda Gates Foundation, Carter Foundation, Rotary Club and many others), with a strong track record of mobilizing funds and cooperation with private industry to raise immunization coverage and inclusion of new vaccines in many low income countries and in NTD elimination programs.

Recent public health emergencies involving anthrax, severe acute respiratory syndrome (SARS), Ebola, and Zika viruses have been declared "public health emergencies" and dramatized the need for restrictive public health measures. These include quarantine, isolation, and rationing of vaccines in short supply. Policy-makers and front-line care providers face difficult ethical questions in such cases which can be expected to occur with new challenges in the future. Support during the Ebola outbreak in West Africa in 2014–16 and Zika spreading out from Brazil in 2016–17 has been criticized as bumbling and inadequate, but did indicate strong levels of international cooperation and shared global concern. This most recent Ebola epidemic was the longest and most deadly in history, resulting in nearly 29,000 cases and over 11,000 deaths in Guinea, Liberia, and Sierra Leone. Several potentially useful therapeutic agents were available in 2014 that had been tested on animals, and limited early studies of the safety of vaccine candidates for humans. However, the affected countries struggled to deal with the rapidly escalating epidemic and the growing number of patients. Médecins sans Frontiére (MSF) provided the front-line treatment and infection control, and warned that the epidemic was "out of control" and would require a massive international response. First responders in many settings show the way in ethical behavior in calamitous situations such as the Syrian civil war where civilians as well as medical facilities are bombed and gassed deliberately by government and foreign forces.

National, international, and local representatives play a critical role in preparing the global community for unexpected epidemics. Research, with sound clinical trials based on best practices for improving clinical care and vaccines for prevention to protect at risk populations, are needed during and between public health emergencies. Research efforts to develop vaccines for these emerging infectious diseases and others such as malaria and dengue are impressive and will hopefully bring forth lifesaving vaccines on large scales in the coming decade. In the case of Ebola, none of the clinical trials have reached definitive conclusions about efficacy in the search for therapeutics, but vaccine trials have identified vaccines that are safe and effective. The availability of financial, organizational, and professional resources to tackle such issues is an underlying problem of priority decision-making with professional, ethical, and moral standards.

Public health may face the challenge of pandemic influenza—such as the avian flu—with decisions regarding allocation of vaccines, treatment of massive numbers of patients arriving at hospitals in acute respiratory distress with very limited resources to cope, coping with sick or absent staff, and many other issues such as not only individual life-and-death situations, but large scale mortality. The ethical questions will be replaced by struggles to cope. Preparation for such potential catastrophic events will be a challenge to public health organizations and the health system generally.

Public health is tasked with monitoring population health and implementing measures to reduce morbidity or mortality of the population within ethical norms of societal acceptability. Advancing public health goals, with minimal restriction of individual liberties, will reduce the burden of disease and mortality, while reducing inequities and advancing social justice. This requires trained professionals to monitor population-based data and research with translation of new science into practice. Programs to achieve these objectives must be evidence-based to substantiate that they will achieve these goals with minimal restrictions, but with public support for those vital to ethical and successful public health.

Teaching Public Health Ethics

The aim of ethics education in public health should be to enhance the ability of public health professionals, policy makers and citizens to reason rationally about the moral dilemmas and value conflicts inherent to human rights, social justice, and the application of knowledge and technology in the health sciences and in public health measures.

Ethics analysis typically involves the capability to identify the public health issue and its contribution to health of the population. This requires a review of the professional literature to know the state-of-the-art techniques and to be able to articulate the factual information to the decision-makers and the public. This requires identification of the ethical issues of the case and to identify the "stake-holders"—those whose rights and interests will be most directly affected by the decisions made and the values, concerns, and information at stake in the case. The ability to identify options available to decision-makers in the case is vital to making the "case for action" and the decision-making process, before, during and after a public health event or process as in pandemic preparedness. The cost of action versus inaction is a vital factor.

Training current faculty on public health ethics issues should be mandatory in schools of public health in order to incorporate ethics into existing courses of formal educational programs. This requires specific and mandatory courses on public health ethics along with incorporation of discussion of ethical issues in core courses in the program.

CONCLUSION

Defining and applying ethical and high standards of practice of medical care as well as public health requires an ideological commitment to individual and community sanctity of life. Ethics in health also requires commitment to advancement of health care and use of best practices of international standards to the maximum extent possible under the local conditions in which the professional is working. This is not an easy commitment as there is often dispute and outright hostility to public health activities in part because of past ethical distortions of great magnitude. But this is an optimistic field of activity by virtue of the great achievements it has brought to humankind. Preparation for disasters and unanticipated health emergencies can raise issues of security, quarantine, isolation, rationing of vaccines due to insufficient supplies—e.g., in influenza epidemics—or restrictions on community events or family burials as in the case of Ebola in West Africa in 2014–16.

Public health also faces slow responses to advances in the science of vaccines or in health promotion measures with proven efficacy. Addressing current issues is a vital part of the "New Public Health" and our ethical and professional commitments. The role of public health in climate change is both a professional and ethical issue, as are many other topics such as food fortification, fluoridation of community water supplies, access to birth control and other longstanding and new topics. Advancement in global health requires consensus of national governments and international bodies working together to alleviate poor health conditions with available professional standards and resource mobilization to achieve this goal. Most issues in public health have ethical aspects so that education on future public health requires adequate attention to the topic, perhaps best presented in case studies.

Ethical issues in public health include both definition of, and decisions to act on a problem, but also delay, avoidance, or inaction when best evidence available indicates action prevents harm to the population. Failure to act in a timely fashion or to allocate resources to meet clear health needs of a population can be unethical just as much as acting in a harmful way. While resource allocation is a political decision, failure to act can be as injurious and unethical as being directly responsible for harmful acts. Public health as a profession and a movement or ideology must be willing to point out the effects of nonaction as well as of ethical or nonethical acts. Compliance with evil is unethical and the preparation of public health workers requires understanding of how to differentiate, and to how to advocate for the better choices in policy and its implementation.

RECOMMENDATIONS

1. Ethics should be incorporated in all courses in public health as well as health policy and management programs.
2. Dedicated courses in ethics should be included in public health education curricula to provide interested students with an opportunity for more in-depth study.
3. Public health ethics along with public health law should be included in criteria for curricula as "cross cutting" courses required by accreditation agencies.
4. Public health ethics orientation workshops should be provided to help teachers in all topic areas of the curriculum, core and elective, incorporate ethics in their teaching material.
5. The topic of public health ethics should be incorporated in ongoing educational programs for practitioners in the broad multi-disciplinary fields of public health.
6. Public awareness and engagement efforts that accompany public health programs and interventions should incorporate some measure of ethics education.
7. Critical thinking about the values involved in a public health controversy is vital to combat the public health problem in question.
8. Recognition that the concepts of social solidarity and obligations as well as individual rights are fundamental in public health practice.
9. Recognition that emergency preparedness and response includes mandatory immunizations such as measles and other public health measures as in influenza or cholera control immunization.
10. Training in ethical studies should be part of public health training at all levels including continuing education.
11. Curriculum development should include awareness of ethical issues of artificial and natural catastrophes of the past century as well as current topics.
12. Case studies are valuable teaching tools and incorporated and examined in class discussion.

13. Teachers of other aspects of public health including epidemiology and health promotion should include ethics in their syllabi and course content.
14. Consideration should be given to development of Helsinki Committee procedures and review criteria for public health-related research based on data sets without individual identification in public health research proposals.
15. Teachers of ethics in public health should have dual training in public health and ethics.

STUDENT REVIEW QUESTIONS

1. Why was eugenics a popular topic in western countries among intellectuals during the early part of the 20th century?
2. How was eugenics practiced in liberal democratic countries?
3. How did the eugenics idea become translated into mass murder of the handicapped in Germany, and then adapted to genocide of Jews and others in the Holocaust?
4. Why is incitement to genocide seen as a precursor and crime against humanity?
5. Why is approval of a "Helsinki Committee" needed before applying for a research grant?
6. Why is assisted death permitted in some jurisdictions, and what steps are needed to ensure this is solely based on the patient's wishes?
7. Discuss the ethics of requiring children to be fully immunized before they can attend school.
8. What is the "Wakefield Effect", and how is it affecting attitudes to immunization?
9. How should practicing doctors and public health explain mandatory chlorination, and fluoridation of community water supplies?
10. Is banning cigarette smoking in public places an infringement of individual rights?
11. Is parental refusal of immunization without a valid medical reason ethical?
12. Discuss what you think are ethical issues in public health.
13. Discuss what you think are ethical issues in medical practice.
14. Discuss public health ethics issues in global health.
15. Discuss ethical issues in medical and public health research.
16. Describe the historical and current meaning of the Nuremberg Trials, the Universal Declaration of Human Rights, the Helsinki Declaration and the Tuskegee experiments on public health and medical research ethics.

17. Discuss the role of the news and social media in investigation of public health issues and in spread of "pseudoscience" disinformation on public health topics such as vaccination, fluoridation, and food fortification.

18. Describe the lasting implication of the Tuskegee experiment for attitudes towards the public health profession in the US.

RECOMMENDED READINGS

1. Aceijas C, Brall C, Schröder-Bäck P, Otok R, Maeckelberghe E, Stjernberg L, et al. Teaching ethics in schools of public health in the European Region: findings from a screening survey. Public Health Rev. 2012;34(1). Available at: https://link.springer.com/journal/40985/34/1/page/1 (accessed 22 June 2017).

2. Anikeeva O, Braunack-Mayer A, Rogers W. Requiring influenza vaccination for health care workers. Am J Public Health. 2009;99(1):24−29. http://dx.doi.org/10.2105/AJPH.2008.136440. Available at: https://www.ncbi.nlm.nih.gov/pmc/articles/PMC2636609/ (accessed 15 April 2017).

3. American Public Health Association. Principles of the ethical practice of public health, version 2.2, 2002. Available at: https://www.apha.org/~/media/files/pdf/membergroups/ethics_brochure.ashx (accessed 22 June 2017).

4. Bachrach S. In the name of public health—Nazi racial hygiene. New Engl J Med. 2004;351(5):417−420. Available at: http://content.nejm.org/cgi/content/full/351/5/417?ijkey=8bee5b41cf11cadc3a826ad16fc2deef59aa8f32&keytype2 = tf_ipsecsha (accessed 4 May 2017).

5. Birn AE, Molina N. In the name of public health. Am J Public Health. 2005;95 (7):1095−1097. Available at: https://www.ncbi.nlm.nih.gov/pmc/articles/PMC1449322/ (accessed 14 April 2017).

6. Brandt EJ, Myerson R, Perraillon MC, Polonsky TS. Hospital admissions for myocardial infarction and stroke before and after the trans-fatty acid restrictions in New York. JAMA Cardiol. 2017;2(6):617−625. Abstract available at: http://jamanetwork.com/journals/jama-cardiology/currentissue (accessed 22 June 2017).

7. Callahan D, Jennings B. Ethics and public health: forging a strong relationship. Am J Public Health. 2002;92(2):169−176. Available at: https://www.ncbi.nlm.nih.gov/pmc/articles/PMC1447035/pdf/0920169.pdf (accessed 16 April 2017).

8. Centers for Disease Control and Prevention. Technology and innovation, 31 January 2017. Available at: https://www.cdc.gov/od/science/technology/ (accessed 17 April 2017).

9. Centers for Disease Control and Prevention. CDC and public health ethics. Available at: https://www.cdc.gov/od/science/integrity/phethics/ (accessed 4 May 2017).

10. Centers for Disease Control and Prevention. Good decision making in real time: practical public health ethics for local health official, students manual. 1 August 2012. Available at: https://www.cdc.gov/od/science/integrity/phethics/trainingmaterials.htm (accessed 15 April 2017).

11. Centers for Disease Control and Prevention. US Public Health Service syphilis study at Tuskegee. The timeline, last updated 8 Dec 2016. Available at: http://www.cdc.gov/tuskegee/timeline.htm (accessed 14 April 2017).

12. Centers for Disease Control and Prevention. Ebola Virus Disease: Ebola outbreak in West Africa 2014−2016. Last reviewed 21 October 2016. Available at: https://www.cdc.gov/vhf/ebola/outbreaks/2014-west-africa/ (accessed 14 April 2017).

13. Centers for Disease Control and Prevention. National Health and Nutrition Examination Survey (NHANES). Last update 25 January 2017. Available at: https://www.cdc.gov/nchs/nhanes/ (accessed 17 April 2017).

14. Coleman CH, Bouësseau MC, Reis A. The contribution of ethics to public health. Bull World Health Organ. 2008;86(8):578. Available at: http://www.who.int/bulletin/volumes/86/8/08-055954/en/ (accessed 14 April 2017).

15. Convention on the Prevention and Punishment of the Crime of Genocide. United Nations, 1948. Available at: http://www.hrweb.org/legal/genocide.html (accessed 14 April 2017).

16. Coughlin SS, Katz WH, Mattison DR. Ethics instruction at schools of public health in the United States for the Association of Schools of Public Health Education Committee. Am J Public Health. 1999;89(5):768–770. Available at: http://www.ncbi.nlm.nih.gov/pmc/articles/PMC1508720/ (Accessed 15 May 2015).

17. Coughlin SS. Ethical issues in epidemiologic research and public health practice. Emerg Themes Epidemiol. 2006;3:16. Available at: https://ete-online.biomedcentral.com/articles/10.1186/1742-7622-3-16 (accessed 14 April 2017).

18. Dawson A, Paul Y. Mass public health programmess and the obligations of sponsoring and participating organisations. J Med Ethics. 2006;32(10):580–583. Available at: https://www.ncbi.nlm.nih.gov/pmc/articles/PMC2563318/ (accessed 16 April 2017).

19. European Patient's Forum. EPF strategic plan 2014–2020. Available at: http://www.eu-patient.eu/globalassets/library/strategic-planning/epf-strategic-plan-2014-2020-final.pdf (accessed 17 April 2017).

20. Evans J. The third reich at war. New York: Penguin Press, 2009.

21 Faucci AS. Preface: evolving ethical issues over the course of the AIDS pandemic. Public Health Rev. 2012;34(1):19–24. Available at: https://publichealthreviews.biomedcentral.com/track/pdf/10.1007/BF03391654?site = publichealthreviews.biomedcentral.com (accessed 3 December 2017).

22. Frumkin H, Hess J, Luber G, Malilay J, McGeehin M. Climate change: the public health response. Am J Public Health. 2008;98(3):435–445. Available at: http://gis.geog.queensu.ca/CODIGEOSIM/SecureInternalPage/Literatures/pdfFiles/WNV/Climate%20Change%20Public%20Health%20Response.pdf (accessed 14 April 2017).

23. Gamble VN. Under the shadow of Tuskegee: African Americans and health care. Am J Public Health. 1997;87:1773–1778. Available at: https://www.ncbi.nlm.nih.gov/pmc/articles/PMC1381160/pdf/amjph00510-0023.pdf (accessed 14 April 2017).

24. Genocide Watch. Available at: http://genocidewatch.net/ (accessed 5 May 2017).

25. Godlee F, Smith J, Marcovitch H. (editorial). Wakefield's article linking MMR vaccine and autism was fraudulent. BMJ. 2011;342:c7452 Available at: http://www.bmj.com/content/342/bmj.c7452.full.print (accessed 16 April 2017).

26. Gray S. The ethics of publication in public health. Public Health Rev. 2012;34(1). Available at: https://link.springer.com/content/pdf/10.1007%2FBF03391664.pdf (accessed 22 June 2017).

27. Grodin M, Annas GJ. (editorial). Legacies of Nuremberg: medical ethics and human rights. JAMA. 1996;276:1682–1683. Abstract available at: http://jamanetwork.com/journals/jama/article-abstract/411077 (accessed 16 April 2017).

28. Gruskin S, Dickens B. (editorial). Human rights and ethics in public health. Am J Public Health. 2006; 96(11):1903–1905. Available at: https://www.ncbi.nlm.nih.gov/pmc/articles/PMC1751819/pdf/0961903.pdf (accessed 16 April 2017).

29. Guttman N, Salmon CT. Guilt, fear, stigma, and knowledge gaps: ethical issues in public health communication interventions. Bioethics. 2004;18(6):531−552. Abstract available at: https://www.ncbi.nlm.nih.gov/pubmed/15580723 (accessed 4 May 2017).

30. Health Law Institute, Dalhousie University. End-of-Life law and policy in Canada. Available at: http://eol.law.dal.ca/ (accessed 3 May 2017).

31. Hyder AA, Merritt M, Ali J, Tran NT, Subramaniam K, Akhtar T. Integrating ethics, health policy and health systems in low- and middle-income countries: case studies from Malaysia and Pakistan. Bull World Health Organ. 2008;86(8):606−611. Available at: https://www. ncbi.nlm.nih.gov/pmc/articles/PMC2649452/pdf/08-051110.pdf (accessed 5 May 2017).

32. Jennings B, Kahn J, Mastroianni A, Parker LS, editors. Ethics and public health: model curriculum. Washington DC: Association of Schools of Public Health, 2003. Available at: https://s3.amazonaws.com/aspph-wp-production/app/uploads/2014/02/EthicsCurriculum.pdf (accessed 4 May 2017).

33. Joseph J. The 1942 'euthanasia' debate in the American Journal of Psychiatry. Hist Psych. 2005;16(62 Pt 2):171−179. Available at: https://hal.archives-ouvertes.fr/hal-00570816/document (accessed 16 April 2017).

34. Kass NE. An ethics framework for public health. Am J Public Health. 2001;91 (11):1776−1782. Abstract available at: http://ajph.aphapublications.org/doi/abs/10.2105/ AJPH.91.11.1776 (accessed 15 April 2017).

35. Ethical issues in public health research. In: Last JM A dictionary of epidemiology. New York: Oxford University Press, 2000.

36. Lo B, Katz MH. Clinical decision making in public health emergencies: ethical considerations. Ann Intern Med. 2005;143:493−498. Abstract available at: https://www.ncbi.nlm. nih.gov/pubmed/16204162 (accessed 16 April 2017).

37. Lee LM. Public health ethics theory: review and path to convergence. J Law Med Ethics. 2012;40(1):85−98. Abstract available at: https://www.ncbi.nlm.nih.gov/pubmed/22458465 (accessed 22 June 2017).

38. Lemon SM, Hamburg MA, Sparling PF, Choffnes ER, Mack A, editors. Ethical and legal considerations in mitigating pandemic disease: forum on microbial threats. Washington, DC: National Academies Press, 2007. Available at: https://www.ncbi.nlm.nih.gov/books/ NBK54167/ (accessed 14 April 2017).

39. Lombardo PA, Dorr GM. Eugenics, medical education and public health: another perspective on the Tuskegee syphilis experiment. Bull Hist Med. 2006;80(2):291−316. Available at: https://www.researchgate.net/publication/6974743_Eugenics_Medical_Education_and_the _Public_Health_Service_Another_Perspective_on_the_Tuskegee_Syphilis_Experiment (accessed 16 April 2017).

40. Mariner WK. Public confidence in public health research ethics: counterpoint on human subjects research. Public Health Rep. 1997;112(1):33−36. Available at: https://www.ncbi. nlm.nih.gov/pmc/articles/PMC1381835/pdf/pubhealthrep00042-0035.pdf (accessed 16 April 2017).

41 McKee M. A preface: How ethics failed: lessons for public health for all time. Public Health Rev. 2012;34(1):93−95. Available at: https://publichealthreviews.biomedcentral. com/articles/10.1007/BF03391659 (accessed 3 December 2017).

42. Murch SH, Anthony A, Casson DH, Malik M, Berelowitz M, Dhillon AP, et al. Retraction of an interpretation. Lancet. 2004;363(9411):750. Available at: http://www.thelancet.com/ pdfs/journals/lancet/PIIS0140-6736(04)15715-2.pdf (accessed 4 May 2017).

43. National Conference of State Legislatures. HPV vaccine: state legislation and statutes, 10 May 2017. Available at: http://www.ncsl.org/research/health/hpv-vaccine-state-legislation-and-statutes.aspx (accessed 22 June 2017).

44. Nuremberg Code. Trials of war criminals before the Nuremberg military tribunals under control council law no. 10. Permissible medical experiments. Washington, DC: U.S. Government Printing Office, 1949. Available at: https://www.loc.gov/rr/frd/Military_Law/pdf/NT_war-criminals_Vol-II.pdf (accessed 16 April 2017).

45. Palermoa T, Peterman A. Undercounting, overcounting and the longevity of flawed estimates: statistics on sexual violence in conflict. Bull World Health Organ. 2011;89:924–925. Available at: http://www.who.int/bulletin/volumes/89/12/11-089888.pdf (accessed 4 March 2017).

46 Pūras D. Human rights and the practice of medicine. Public Health Rev. 2017;38(9). Available at: https://publichealthreviews.biomedcentral.com/articles/10.1186/s40985-017-0054-7 (accessed 3 December 2017).

47. Reverby SM. Ethical failures and history lessons: the U.S. Public Health Service research studies in Tuskegee and Guatemala. Public Health Rev. 2012;34(1):189–206. Available at: https://publichealthreviews.biomedcentral.com/articles/10.1007/BF03391665 (accessed 3 December 2017).

48. Richter ED, Stein Y, Barnea A, Sherman M. Genocide: can we predict, prevent, and protect? J Public Health Policy. 2008;29(3):265–274. Available at: https://www.researchgate.net/publication/242486019_Can_we_prevent_Genocide_by_preventing_Incitement (accessed 4 May 2017).

49. Rothstein M. (editorial). The future of public health ethics. Am J Public Health. 2012;102 (1): 9. Available at: https://www.ncbi.nlm.nih.gov/pmc/articles/PMC3490560/ (accessed 16 April 2017).

50. Shuster E. Fifty Years Later: the significance of the Nuremberg Code. N Engl J Med. 1997;337:1436–1440. Available at: http://www.nejm.org/doi/full/10.1056/NEJM199711133372006#t = article (accessed 22 June 2017).

51. Sidel V. The social responsibilities of health professionals: lessons from their role in Nazi Germany. JAMA. 1996;276(20):1679–1681. Abstract available at: http://jamanetwork.com/journals/jama/article-abstract/411071 (accessed 16 April 2017).

52. Sofair AN, Kaldjian LC. Eugenic sterilization and a qualified Nazi analogy: the United States and Germany, 1930–1945. Ann Intern Med. 2000;132(4):312–319. Abstract available at: https://www.ncbi.nlm.nih.gov/pubmed/10681287 (accessed 10 June 2017).

53. Stanton G. The international alliance to end genocide. Available at: http://genocidewatch.net/ (accessed 22 June 2017).

54. Stern AM. Sterilized in the name of public health. Am J Public Health. 2005;95:1128–1138. Available at: https://www.ncbi.nlm.nih.gov/pmc/articles/PMC1449330/pdf/0951128.pdf (accessed 16 April 2017).

55. Strous RD. Psychiatry during the Nazi era: ethical lessons for the modern professional. Ann Gen Psych. 2007;6(8). http://dx.doi.org/10.1186/1744-859X-6-8 Available at: https://www.ncbi.nlm.nih.gov/pmc/articles/PMC1828151/pdf/1744-859X-6-8.pdf (accessed 16 April 2017).

56. Teutsch S, Rechel B. Ethics of resource allocation and rationing medical care in a time of fiscal restraint-US and Europe. Public Health Rev. 2012;34(1). Available at: https://link.springer.com/content/pdf/10.1007/BF03391667.pdf (accessed 22 June 2017).

57. Thieren M, Mauron A. Nuremberg code turns 60. Bull World Health Organ. 2007;85 (8):573. Available at: https://www.ncbi.nlm.nih.gov/pmc/articles/PMC2636392/ (accessed 3 March 2017).

58. Thomas JC, Sage M, Dillenberg J, Guillory VJ. A code of ethics for public health. Am J Public Health. 2002;92:1057–1060. Available at: https://www.ncbi.nlm.nih.gov/pmc/articles/PMC1447186/ (accessed 22 June 2017).

59. Tulchinsky TH, Flahault A. Editorial: why a theme issue on public health ethics? Public Health Rev. 2012;34(1):7–17. Available at: https://link.springer.com/article/10.1007/BF03391653 (accessed 22 June 2017).

60. Tulchinsky T, Jennings B, Viehbeck S. Integrating ethics in public health education: the process of developing case studies. Public Health Rev. 2015;36:4. vvv. Available at: http://publichealthreviews.biomedcentral.com/articles/10.1186/s40985-015-0002-3 (accessed 3 March 2017).

61. United Nations. Universal Declaration of Human Rights. Available at: http://www.un.org/en/universal-declaration-human-rights/ (accessed 28 March 2017).

62. US Department of Health and Human Services, Office of Research Integrity. Definition of research integrity. Available at: https://ori.hhs.gov/definition-misconduct (accessed 22 June 2017).

63. US Food and Drug Administration. The FDA takes step to remove artificial trans fats in processed foods. Available at: https://www.fda.gov/newsevents/newsroom/pressannouncements/ucm451237.htm (accessed 28 April 2017).

64. US National Academies of Sciences, Engineering, and Medicine. Fostering integrity in research. Washington, DC: The National Academies Press, 2017 https://doi.org/10.17226/21896. Available at: https://www.nap.edu/catalog/21896/fostering-integrity-in-research (accessed 17 April 2017).

65. US National Academies of Sciences, Engineering, and Medicine. Integrating clinical research into epidemic response: the Ebola experience. Washington, DC: The National Academies Press, 2017. Available at: https://www.nap.edu/catalog/24739/integrating-clinical-research-into-epidemic-response-the-ebola-experience (accessed 18 April 2017).

66. Varmus H, Satcher D. Ethical complexities of conducting research in developing countries. New Engl J Med. 1997;337(14):1003–1005. Abstract available at: http://www.nejm.org/doi/full/10.1056/NEJM199710023371411 (accessed 4 May 2017).

67. von Cranach M. The killing of psychiatric patients in Nazi Germany between 1939–1945. Isr J Psychiatry Rel Sci. 2003;40(1):8–18. Abstract available at: https://www.ncbi.nlm.nih.gov/pubmed/12817666?dopt=Abstract (accessed 3 March 2017).

68. Wakefield AJ, Murch SH, Anthony A, Linnell J, Casson DM, Malik M, et al. Ileal lymphoid nodular hyperplasia, non-specific colitis, and pervasive developmental disorder in children [retracted]. Lancet. 1998;351(9103):637–641. Available at: http://www.thelancet.com/journals/lancet/article/PIIS0140-6736(97)11096-0/fulltext (accessed 4 May 2015).

69. Wharam B, Lazarou L. Ethical considerations in an era of mass drug administration. Parasit. Vec. 2013;6:234. Available at: https://doi.org/10.1186/1756-3305-6-234. Available at: https://www.ncbi.nlm.nih.gov/pmc/articles/PMC3750652/ (accessed 3 December 2017).

70. World Health Organization. Genomics Resource Centre. Patients' rights. Posted 2012. Available at: http://www.who.int/genomics/public/patientrights/en/ (accessed 25 April 2017). (accessed 4 May 2017).

71. World Health Organization. Ethical considerations in developing a public health response to pandemic influenza. Geneva: WHO, 2007. Available at: http://www.who.int/csr/resources/publications/WHO_CDS_EPR_GIP_2007_2c.pdf [accessed on 7 July 2008].

72. World Health Organization. Global Network of WHO Collaborating Centres for Bioethics. Global health ethics: key issues. Luxembourg: WHO, 2015. Available at: http://www.who. int/ethics/publications/global-health-ethics/en/ (accessed 4 May 2017).

73. World Health Organization, European Region. Europe leads the world in eliminating trans fats. Copenhagen, 18 September 2014. Available at: http://www.euro.who.int/en/media-centre/sections/press-releases/2014/europe-leads-the-world-in-eliminating-trans-fats (accessed 28 April 2017).

74. World Medical Association. Declaration of Helsinki; Ethical principles for medical research involving human subjects. Bull World Health Organ. 2001;79(4):373–374. Available at: http://www.who.int/bulletin/archives/79(4)373.pdf (accessed 4 May 2017).

75. World Medical Association. Declaration of Helsinki: ethical principles for medical research involving human subjects; amended by 64th WMA General Assembly, 2013. JAMA. 2013;310(20):2191–2194. http://jamanetwork.com/journals/jama/fullarticle/1760318, (accessed 4 May 2017).

76. Yoshida EM. Selecting candidates for liver transplantation: a medical ethics perspective on the microallocation of a scarce and rationed resource. Can J Gastroenterol. 1998;12(3):209–215. Abstract available at: https://www.ncbi.nlm.nih.gov/pubmed/9582546 (accessed 4 May 2017).

77 Yox S.B., Offit P.A. Stories of science gone wrong: Paul Offit discusses his new book. Offit PA. Pandora's Lab: Seven Stories of Science Gone Wrong. National Geographic, 2017, Medscape, June 12, 2017. Available at: http://www.medscape.com/viewarticle/ 881347 (accessed 21 June 2017).

78. Zambon MC. Ethics versus evidence in influenza vaccination. Lancet. 2004;364:2161–2163. Available at: http://www.thelancet.com/journals/lancet/article/PIIS0140-6736(04)17608-3/ fulltext.

79. Zusman SP. Water fluoridation in Israel: ethical and legal aspects. Public Health Rev. 2012;34. epub ahead of print. Available at: https://publichealthreviews.biomedcentral.com/ articles/10.1007/BF03391658 (accessed 25 June 2017).

80. Sofair AN, Kaldjian LC. Eugenic sterilization and a qualified Nazi analogy: the United States and Germany, 1930–1945. Ann Intern Med. 2000;132(4):312–319. Available at: https://www.ncbi.nlm.nih.gov/pubmed/10681287 (accessed 10 June 2017).

81. Yox S, Offit PA. Stories of science gone wrong: Paul Offit discusses his new book-Medscape-Jun 12, 2017. Available at: http://www.medscape.com/viewarticle/881347? nlid = 115740_804&src = WNL_mdplsfeat_170620_mscpedit_infd&uac = 107534HX&spon-=3&impID = 1371926&faf = 1 (accessed 21 June 2017).

82. UNICEF Annual Report 2016. Available at: https://www.unicef.org/publications/index_96412. html?utm_source = newsletter&utm_medium = email&utm_campaign = annual_report (accessed 22 June 2017).

83. Offit PA. Pandora's lab: seven stories of science gone wrong. National Geographic Press, 2017.

Chapter 14

Framingham and North Karelia: Studies that Changed the Cardiovascular Disease Pandemic

ABSTRACT

Cardiovascular disease (CVD) mortality increased dramatically until the mid-1960s in the industrialized countries, but has declined in the past half century. CVDs remain in the top leading causes of mortality in high-, medium-, and low-income countries, accounting for nearly one-third (32.3%) of all deaths globally in 2013. Stroke mortality began a steady slow decline in the early part of the 20th century and coronary heart disease mortality since the mid-1960s. These changes resulted from many factors including improved public health, treatment and access to medical care, improved education, standards of living and evidence-based prevention and management, reduction of smoking, cholesterol and improved control of hypertension. Major population based studies in Framingham, Massachussets USA and North Karelia, Finland along with other studies advanced the evidence base for identifying risk factors amenable to prevention care and health promotion. Future reduction will require increased application of health promotion for helping people and populations-at-risk to alter their diets, lifestyle, smoking habits, and to reduce the growing prevalence of obesity, diabetes type II, lack of exercise, and alcohol excess. An underemphasized issue is discovery and management of still undertreated hypertension. Global efforts to reduce the burden of CVD mortality and morbidity still have a long way to go to reduce avoidable mortality, to prolong healthful years of life, and to reduce global and national disparities adversely affecting the socially and economically disadvantaged.

Case Studies in Public Health. DOI: http://dx.doi.org/10.1016/B978-0-12-804571-8.00013-5

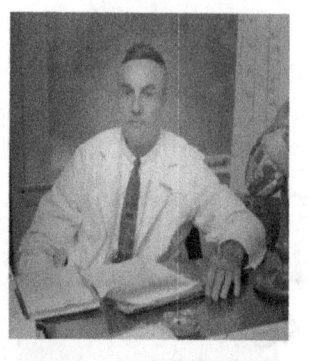

Dr. Thomas Royal (Roy) Dawber, (1913–2005), Founding Director Framingham Heart Study 1949–1966 : *Courtesy of the Framingham Heart Study Archives, Boston University School of Medicine, and the US National Heart, Lung and Blood Institute.*

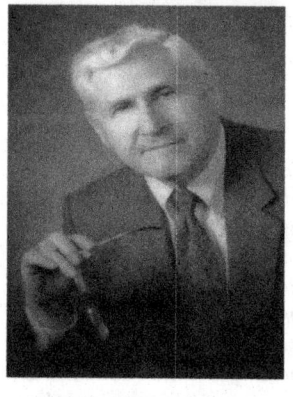

Dr. William B. Kannel (1923–2011), Study Director Framingham Heart Study 1966–1994: *Courtesy of the Framingham Heart Study Archives, Boston University School of Medicine, and the US National Heart, Lung and Blood Institute.*

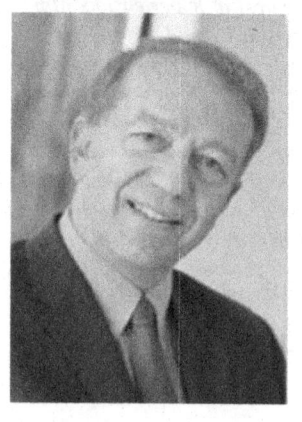

Dr. Pekka Puska (1945-), Founder of North Karelia Project, 1972–1978, Finland: *Courtesy of Dr Pekka Puska.*

BACKGROUND

The epidemiologic transition from infectious to non-infectious diseases seen in the developed countries in the 20th century is being followed by a similar transition in lower-income countries even as all countries still wrestle with infectious diseases new and old. The change from the predominance of infectious diseases to non-infectious diseases as leading causes of premature mortality during the 20th century have accelerated since the end of World War II. Antibiotics and vaccines, along with improved living standards, sanitation, nutrition, and safe water and food, brought about reduction in morbidity and mortality rates from infectious diseases and an increase in life expectancy. Infectious diseases, while still important, are no longer the primary issues in population health in the developed countries, and similar trends are appearing in the developing countries.

Pioneering Epidemiologic Studies

Coronary heart disease (CHD) reached epidemic proportions in the 1950s, peaking in the early 1960s in the United States, but later in other developed countries. Studies in the late 1940s in the UK such as those of Jeremy Morris of London transport workers comparing rates between bus conductors and bus drivers showed that physical activity was a key factor in differences in coronary heart disease mortality rates. This was followed by the UK Whitehall Studies (from 1947 to 1972), led by Michael Marmot, of civil servants showing marked differences in cardiovascular disease (CVD) mortality rates between higher-level and lower-level civil servants, which were attributed to social class differences in risk factors and degree of independence in the work settings and living conditions of these groups.

A growing body of studies and evidence from the 1930s and onward showed the harmful effects of smoking which had reached large proportions of US, UK and other populations before, during and following World War II. The pioneering studies of Richard Doll and Bradford Hill (British epidemiologists) reported in 1954, convincingly demonstrated the strong relationship between smoking and lung cancer. Controversy followed with doubts cast on the these conclusions, while epidemiology was absorbing the complexities of causation of non-communicable diseases being less conclusive than those of infectious disease models. However, the Doll and Hill classic study encouraged other cohort studies during the 1950s to the 1970s leading to the same conclusion, i.e., smoking causes lung and other cancers, along with causal links to cardiovascular diseases.

Many studies conducted since the mid-1950s such as those by Ancel Keys (1904—2004) at the University of Minnesota focused on blood lipids in the early case-control and cohort studies or integrating with blood pressure from population studies. Keys initiated comparative international studies of dietary pattern and the prevalence of coronary heart disease. The Seven Countries Study, which included Finland, United States, Netherlands, Italy, Yugoslavia, Greece, and Japan, finding elevated blood lipids (Finland and United States were high, while Greece and Japan low), identifying high levels of cholesterol along with high rates of cigarette smoking as key public health issues. High levels of cholesterol were observed in clinical studies, including evidence of high rates of atherosclerosis lesions found in autopsied young soldiers killed in the Korean War (1950–1953). These studies placed primary emphasis on diet and cholesterol control as the key modalities in coronary heart disease care.

The Framingham Heart Project was launched in 1948 by Boston University and the National Institutes of Health. The study focused on identifying multiple associated predisposing factors for cardiovascular diseases in a community population cohort. The North Karelia Project in the 1970s focused on interventions at the community and regional interventions to reduce the complex known multiple risk factors.

Decreasing smoking, reducing hypertension, healthful dietary changes, daily low dose aspirin and treatment to reduce cholesterol levels together made the greatest contribution to the observed decline in mortality rates from the peak and "tipping point" in the late 1960s and early 1970s. The evidence that high blood pressure, high cholesterol, and lack of physical exercise were key factors in cardiovascular disease was increasingly accepted as crucial to primary prevention and control of the epidemic. More recent trends in child and adult obesity and growing prevalence of diabetes indicate the vital importance of early intervention in childhood and among adults for prevention of cardiovascular disease.

The Framingham Heart Study in the United States identified key risk factors, and the North Karelia project developed community and national health promotion interventions to reduce the high risk factors for CVD in the region's population. Finland's North Karelia project, along with many other epidemiologic and clinical studies were also enormously important to the development of epidemiology of chronic disease and prevention of cardiovascular diseases. The Stanford Community Study starting in 1974 followed the community health-promotion approach in two intervention groups and one control group town with information campaigns and individual counseling. The project showed reduced fat content of diets in the intervention communities with reduced cholesterol levels as compared to the control town population.

In 1978, a conference organized by the US National Institutes of Health (NIH) in Bethesda reviewed the reasons behind the substantial decline in cardiovascular and total mortality seen since the mid-1960s. This led the World Health Organization (WHO) to organize an international epidemiologic investigation system, called MONICA (Multinational **MONI**toring of trends and determinants in **CA**rdiovascular disease). MONICA was conducted from the mid-1980s to the mid-1990s with 38 projects in 12 countries worldwide. During the 10-year period 13 million people were monitored with 166,000 myocardial infarction patients registered.

Noncommunicable diseases (NCDs) account for a growing proportion of total causes of death globally increasing from 60 percent (31 million) in 2000 to 68 percent of all deaths (38 million) in 2015 (see Figure 14.1). Ischemic heart disease, cerebrovascular and lung disease, and cancer are leading causes of death worldwide in high-, medium-, and low-income countries.

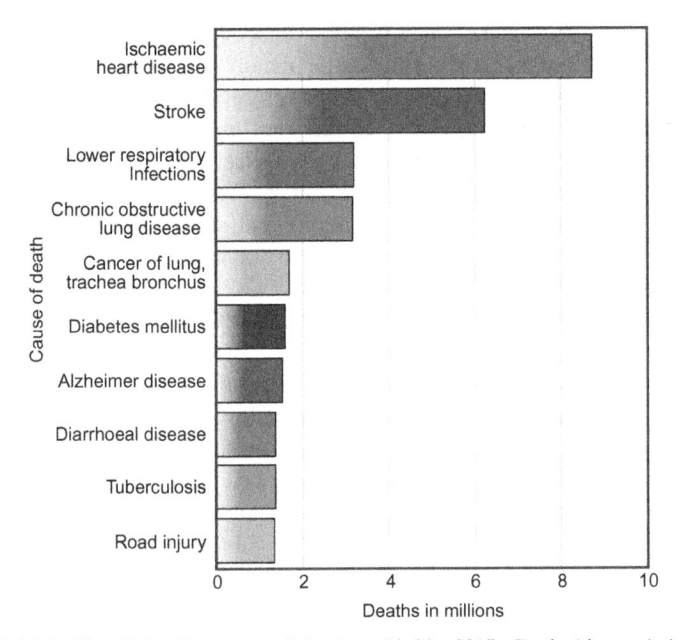

FIGURE 14.1   Top 10 leading causes of death worldwide, 2015. *Cited with permission of the World Health Organization. Source: World Health Organization: The top ten causes of death, Updated 17 January 2017. Available at: http://www.who.int/mediacentre/factsheets/fs310/en/* (accessed 20 July 2017).

In the WHO European Region, heart attacks and stroke cause 90 percent of CVD deaths and one quarter of all deaths. Former Soviet countries have high mortality from cardiovascular diseases which in aging populations threaten economic and social development. Medical and epidemiological research was needed and succeeded in identifying many of the causes and mechanisms of NCDs and demonstrated that many of these causes of death can be prevented.

Epidemiological, biochemical, genetic and animal studies, clinical and intervention trials, and especially large-scale, community-based preventive studies have led to evidence that lifestyle factors are crucial in the pandemic of CVD. Unhealthy nutrition, smoking, physical inactivity, excess use of alcohol, poverty, and psychosocial stress are the major lifestyle issues, while control of elevated blood pressure, blood lipids, and clinical management over time are the main medical care issues i.e., secondary prevention of an existing condition to prevent further progression to a clinical disease. Adverse physical and social environmental conditions are also key contributors to the burden of NCDs, particularly CVDs, as well as lung, liver, mental, and other chronic diseases. These are risk factors for cardiovascular diseases which could be reduced by changes in personal lifestyle habits and good medical care.

During the 1960s there was a growing understanding that smoking, high cholesterol, and hypertension were major factors in cardiovascular disease. Other contributing factors included: high triglycerides, lower "good" cholesterol (HDL); blood with tendency to clot and block narrowed coronary or arteries supplying the brain or heart. Damaged cells that line the blood vessels along with the buildup of plaque (fat, cholesterol, calcium, and other substances) in blood vessels and thickening and narrowing of blood vessels result in reducing or stopping blood flow to the heart muscle and the brain causing tissue death.

Stimulated by an appeal from the American Cancer Society, American Heart Association, the National Tuberculosis Association, and the American Public Health Association, President John Kennedy appointed a commission of experts to review the evidence. This led to the groundbreaking US Surgeon−General (Luther Terry) 1964 report on smoking and health, specifically linking cigarette smoking with lung cancer, heart disease and emphysema. This landmark document was widely publicized in the news media promoting an enormous response in the United States and internationally. This led many countries to begin adoption of health-promotion activities such as antismoking legislation and changing social norms with smoking reduction, which continue today and have resulted in remarkable reductions in lung cancer deaths along with vital impact in reduction of cardiovascular disease mortality and other diseases in the industrialized countries. During the 1950s and onward many important epidemiologic studies were carried out in the United States, Britain, and other countries that extended the evidence base for the harmful effects of smoking and other risk factors associated with cancer, cardiovascular and lung diseases.

The Framingham Heart Study

The Framingham Heart Study, was established in 1948 as a prospective study of a population cohort in Framingham, Massachusetts, with a sample of 5,209 men and women between the ages of 30 and 62 from this community, a small town near Boston, Massachusetts. Initial extensive physical examinations and lifestyle interviews were conducted for later analysis in the search for common patterns related to CVD development. Since 1948, the subjects have continued to return to the study every two years for a detailed medical history, physical examination, and laboratory tests. In 1971, a second generation - 5,124 of the original participants' adult children and their spouses - was recruited to participate in similar examinations. The project funded by the National Heart, Lung, and Blood Institute (NHLBI) and operated in cooperation with Boston University, and with frequent reports of findings was soon recognized as a leader in cardiovascular health studies. The objective was *"to identify the common factors or characteristics that contribute to CVD by following its development over a long period of time in a large group of participants who had not yet developed overt symptoms of CVD or suffered a heart attack or stroke*". In 1994, a new study group (Omni) reflecting a more diverse community of Framingham was enrolled, and in 2002 a new phase enrolled a third generation of participants, consisting of grandchildren of the original cohort and in 2003, a second group of Omni participants was added.

The early findings became widely cited in the literature as a model fostering epidemiologic approaches for other studies worldwide. The Framingham study added the term *risk factor* and associated concepts to the public health lexicon fundamentally moving away from the focus on 'single causation of disease', which dominated medical thinking in that period of time with findings that profoundly advanced cardiovascular epidemiology and clinical practice. The Framingham study continues to the present time and now includes the third generation of the original study population. Table 14.1 includes key findings of the epidemiology of CVDs as found in the Framingham Heart Study over the nearly 70 years that the study has been continuously conducted.

TABLE 14.1 Research Milestones of the Framingham Heart Study: A Project of the National Heart, Lung, and Blood Institute and Boston University

1960	Cigarette smoking found to increase the risk of heart disease
1961	Cholesterol level, blood pressure, and electrocardiogram abnormalities found to increase the risk of heart disease
1967	Physical activity found to reduce the risk of heart disease and obesity to increase risk of heart disease
1970	High blood pressure found to increase the risk of stroke
	Atrial fibrillation increases stroke risk five-fold
1976	Menopause found to increase the risk of heart disease
1978	Psychosocial factors found to affect heart disease
1988	High levels of HDL cholesterol found to reduce risk of death
1994	Enlarged left ventricle shown to increase the risk of stroke
1996	Progression from hypertension to heart failure described
1998	Atrial fibrillation is associated with an increased risk of all-cause mortality
1998	Simple coronary disease prediction of risk factor categories to allow physicians to predict multivariate coronary heart disease risk in patients without overt CHD
1999	Lifetime risk at age 40 years of developing coronary heart disease one in two for men and one in three for women

(Continued)

TABLE 14.1 (Continued)

2001	High-normal blood pressure associated with an increased risk of cardiovascular disease
2002	Lifetime risk of developing high blood pressure in middle-aged adults 9 in 10
2002	Obesity a risk factor for heart failure
2004	Serum aldosterone levels predict future risk of hypertension in normotensives
2005	LIfetime risk of becoming overweight exceeds 70 percent
2006	A new genome-wide association study launched ("SHARe project")
2007	Biologic and behavioral trait and social ties associated with obesity
2008	Social networks exert key influences on decision to quit smoking
	Four risk factors raise probability of precursor of heart failure and serious cardiac events
2009	Genome-wide Association Study of Blood Pressure and Hypertension identifies eight gene sites associated with blood pressure
	A new genetic variant associated with increased susceptibility to atrial fibrillation, a major risk factor for stroke and heart failure
	Parental dementia may lead to poor memory in middle-aged adults
2009	High leptin levels may protect against Alzheimer's disease and dementia
2010	Sleep apnea tied to increased risk of stroke
	New genes identified that may play a role in Alzheimer's disease
	Having first-degree relative with atrial fibrillation increases risk for this disorder
	Framingham study contributed to discovering hundreds of new genes underlying major heart disease risk factors: body mass index, blood cholesterol, cigarette smoking, blood pressure, and glucose/diabetes
	First definitive evidence of occurrence of stroke by age 65 years in a parent with a three-fold increased risk of stroke in offspring

Cited with permission of the National Heart, Lung, and Blood Institute; National Institutes of Health; U.S. Department of Health and Human Services.
Source: Hajar R. Framingham Contribution to Cardiovascular Disease. Heart Views. 2016; 17(2):78–81. http://dx.doi.org/10.4103/1995-705X.185130 (accessed 20 July 2017).

The findings of the Framingham study of risk factors for heart disease and stroke have stimulated large numbers of epidemiologic studies to confirm and expand the knowledge base in this crucial field of epidemiology and policy for prevention and clinical care. These studies in aggregate have been enormously influential in determining public health policies in health promotion, in screening, and in patient care in the US and globally.

The North Karelia Project

In the early 1960s, Finland's rates of coronary heart diseases and stroke were among the highest in the world (especially for men), with even higher rates in the Finnish province of North Karelia, a rural area of 180,000 persons. In 1972 the North Karelia community intervention project was launched with the objective of reducing morbidity and mortality from CVDs focusing on the then known risk factors, in comparison with a non-intervention similar province. Finnish scientists and decision-makers launched educational and promotional programs aiming to change this situation and extensive scientific research in this field was conducted. Risk factors already identified by US and other researchers, included smoking reduction, hypertension control, and reducing serum cholesterol level, closely linked with diet, especially the high dietary saturated fat intake of Finns. The intervention project hypothesized that this was amenable to change by community health promotion addressing change of smoking and dietary habits that would result in reduction of serum-cholesterol levels followed by a decline in disease and death rates from CHD.

The North Karelia project was an intervention program launched in order to bring this theory into practice. North Karelia, a relatively poor province of Finland, faced many socioeconomic issues, and had high rates of CHD mortality, even in comparison to the very high Finnish national levels. The project was launched in response to growing public concern and to a petition of provincial representatives aware of the exceptionally high morbidity and mortality rates in their region. As described by Openheimer and Puska (Public Health Reviews, 2011), this intervention program was designed and carried out in cooperation with local and national authorities and professionals as well as WHO experts. The project was a comprehensive community-prevention intervention through local organizations with the objective of empowering individuals in the community to make needed dietary, smoking reduction, and other lifestyle changes. Five years after the North Karelia project was launched, its principal focus on community prevention was adopted throughout Finland, and became highly influential in Western Europe, leading to implementation of similar policies for reducing cardiovascular risk factors in the following years.

The project included action promoting healthier nutrition, smoking cessation, and physical activity and over the years expanded to include objectives of other integrated prevention of other major noncommunicable diseases (NCDs) and health promotion. The project was continued for 25 years and in order to ensure continuity and sustainability, the North Karelia Center for Public Health was established in 2000 as a national center for prevention and health promotion.

The North Karelia program developed integrated community approaches for individuals, institutions, and community organizations, which expanded into a national program. During the 1970s and 1980s, many clinical trials demonstrated the efficacy of antihypertensive and lipid-lowering drugs.

Community-based trials, such as the North Karelia project adopted health promotion approaches to reduce risk factors. The combination of individual medical care for high risk patients along with the population-wide approach, produced great success in reducing CVD and provided guidance for addressing many non-communicable diseases, including cancer.

During the 25-year period of the North Karelia project, major changes in risk factors took place as measured by key risk indicators such as smoking, blood pressure, and cholesterol for middle-age men and women, at 5-year intervals between 1971 and 2006. Dietary habits were markedly changed and smoking among males declined from 52 to 31 percent, whereas among females it nearly doubled to 18 percent. Serum cholesterol and blood pressure declined comparably for both genders (see Table 14.2).

Mortality among middle-age males declined by nearly two-thirds in cardiovascular, coronary heart disease (CHD), and lung cancer was reduced by 79, 85, and 80 percent, respectively (Table 14.3). The annual decline in mortality from ischemic heart disease in men averaged 2.9 percent in North Karelia, as compared to two percent in the rest of Finland. For women the respective average annual reduction in mortality were 4.9 percent and three percent.

Prevalence of risk factors and CHD mortality both declined in North Karelia soon after implementation of the intervention program and were adopted nationally. Over the years, parallel changes were observed in CHD mortality trends but were greater in North Karelia than in the rest of

TABLE 14.2 Risk Factor Changes in North Karelia, Men and Women Aged 30–59 Years, 1972–2007

Year	Men			Women		
	Smoking (%)	Serum cholesterol (mmol/L)	Blood pressure (mmHg)	Smoking (%)	Serum cholesterol (mmol/L)	Blood pressure (mmHg)
1972	52	6.9	149/92	10	6.8	153/92
1977	44	6.5	143/89	10	6.4	141/86
1982	36	6.3	145/87	15	6.1	141/85
1987	36	6.3	144/88	16	6.0	139/83
1992	32	5.9	142/85	17	5.6	135/80
1997	31	5.7	140/88	16	5.6	133/80
2002	33	5.7	137/83	22	5.5	132/78
2007	31	5.4	138/83	18	5.2	134/78

Source: Cited with permission of the International Diabetes Federation Puska P. The North Karelia project: 30 years successfully preventing chronic diseases. Diabetes Voice. 2008;53:26–29. Available at: https://pdfs.semanticscholar.org/0ff2/a9381edf12ee04f762e37af08ffd90efddf6.pdf.

Finland. By 2006 CHD mortality among men declined in all of Finland by 80 percent as compared to an 85 percent decline in North Karelia (Figure 14.2). Lung cancer mortality declined in North Karelia by 80 percent to 2006 as compared to 65 percent for total cancer mortality (see Table 14.3). Most of these reductions in CHD and lung cancer mortality were mostly explained by reduction in serum cholesterol level and smoking but dietary change also occurred in the type and amount of fat with increased intake of fresh vegetables and fruit.

The North Karelia project had a major influence on regional, national, and international policy by showing the effectiveness of health promotion in reduced levels of blood lipids, and smoking, and improved dietary habits in the province and in the whole country, but also beneficially influencing health policies in other countries. Pekka Puska, founding director of the North Karelia project, was later director of NCD prevention and health promotion at the WHO and then director general of the National Public Health Institute, Helsinki, Finland.

Lung cancer mortality declined in North Karelia by 80 percent to 2006 as compared to nearly 60 percent in all of Finland (see Table 14.3). Most of these reductions:

TABLE 14.3 Mortality Rates, Selected Causes, North Karelia, 1970 and 2006 (per 100,000), Men, Aged 35−64 Years, Age Adjusted

	Rate in 1970	Rate in 2006	% change 1970−2006
All causes	1509	572	−62%
All cardiovascular	855	182	−79%
Coronary heart disease	672	103	−85%
All cancers	271	96	−65%
Lung cancer	147	30	−80%

Cited with permission of the International Diabetes Federation. Source: Puska P. The North Karelia project: 30 years successfully preventing chronic diseases. Diabetes Voice. 2008;53:26−29. Available at: https://pdfs.semanticscholar.org/0ff2/a9381edf12ee04f762e37af08ffd90efddf6.pdf.

Other Major Research Projects

In 1972 researchers in the Stanford School of Medicine began a field experiment in two communities with a third as a control group in northern California with a total population of 30,000. The purpose was to study modification of cardiovascular risk factors, particularly average fat content in diets through the Community Education Model. The Stanford program used mass media and face-to-face instruction, or in combination, to promote

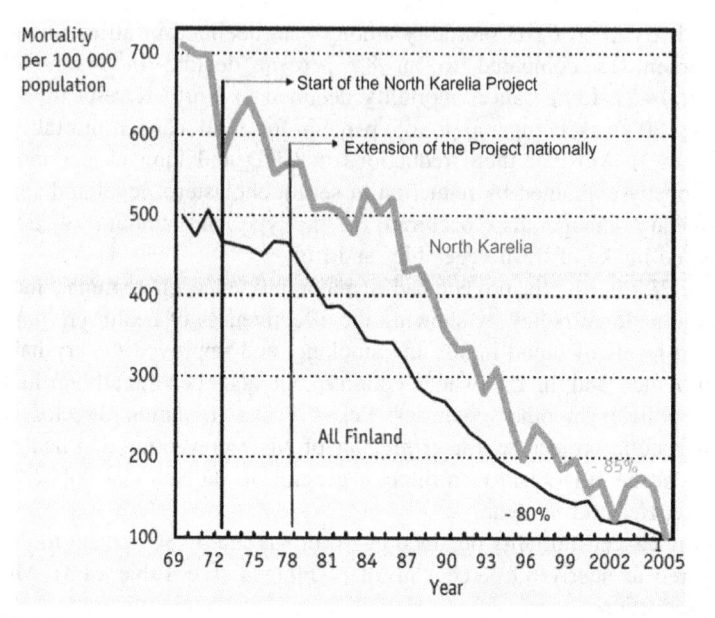

FIGURE 14.2 Coronary Heart Disease age-adjusted mortality rates, North Karelia and Finland, males aged 35−64 years, 1969−2006. *Source: Cited with permission of Prof Pekka Puska. Puska P, Vartiainen E, Laatikainen T, Jousilahti P, Paavola M, editors. The North Karelia Project: From North Karelia to National Action. Helsinki: The National Institute for Health and Welfare (THL), 2009 Chapter 10; and Oppenheimer GM, Blackbuen H, Puska P. From Framingham to North Karelia to US community prevention programs: negotiating research agenda for coronary heart diseases in the second half of the 20th century. Public Health Reviews. 2011;33:450−83. Available at: https://publichealthreviews.biomedcentral.com/articles/ 10.1007/BF03391646 (accessed 23 September 2017).*

wellbeing to improve lifestyle behaviors and health. After two years of the intervention—including both intensive information campaigns and individual counseling—a reduction in the average fat content in diets of 25 grams/day was demonstrated in the two intervention areas, compared to three grams/day in the reference area and a significant drop in the population's cholesterol count in both intervention towns.

Beginning in 1980, the Minnesota Heart Health Program and a parallel project in Pawtucket, (Rhode Island, US) studied health-promotion activities in selected communities as compared to similar communities without special intervention, with results suggesting such studies should be done among high-risk populations, including people with family genetic risk factors, minorities, migrants, low-income groups, remote-area residents, and those with chronic diseases including mental health and occupational groups with high stress settings (e.g., prison guards).

The WHO sponsored a Multinational MONItoring of Trends and Determinants in CArdiovascular Disease (MONICA) from 1982 to 1994, which implemented CVD surveillance in 21 countries, mainly in Europe, but also included centers in the United States, Canada, China, and Australasia. It included mortality, morbidity, coronary care, and population-based risk factor surveillance with well-defined methods and high-quality data. Ten years of standardized data in areas of varying resources and disease patterns showed large differences in policies, resource allocation, and outcomes in the centers in 21 countries. MONICA provided information for disease treatment and prevention and international awareness of the importance of CVD epidemiology and health-promotion interventions.

Public Health Importance

The cumulative effect of these research projects, which were highly publicized in the press and other media, improved the knowledge base for medical self-care. The growing emphasis on Health Promotion as a part of Public Health, brought improvement of health and quality of life to the study populations. The North Karelia project provided a model for further implementation of the intervention program on a national scale, bringing favorable improvements to the public health in Finland as a whole, also raising awareness more widely in Europe. The project also became affiliated with the development of the WHO CINDI (Countrywide Integrated Noncommunicable Disease Intervention), which focused on population health using evidence-based theory and policy approaches with international and health services collaboration in many countries.

The CINDI program showed considerable success in certain countries (e.g., Finland, Lithuania, Russia, and Canada) and even actively contributing to efforts of closing the east-west health gap in Europe. The Framingham, North Karelia, CINDI, and many other community-based epidemiologic studies brought the focus of prevention in medical care and health promotion to changes in lifestyle—smoking cessation, dietary change, physical exercise, hypertension control, and moderation in lifestyle. At the same time major improvements in medical care contributed to greater recognition and management of hypertension as a core issue in cardiovascular health. Improvements with early treatment and successful intervention in acute coronary syndromes, strokes and long-term care brought important advances in this same time period for patients with CVDs.

Fruit and vegetable consumption has been shown to reduce atherosclerosis, improve serum lipid levels, lower blood pressure, and increase antioxidants, especially if consumed regularly early in adult life, and to reduce coronary heart disease risk of mortality. Lack of exercise and poor diets associated with work-related stress contribute to about one-third of CHD cases among middle-age male people. Poverty and chronic illness along with social and mental distress are frequently associated with low socioeconomic status (SES) and self esteem as factors in high rates of CVD morbidity and mortality. Poverty in rural and urban settings has social, economic and physical conditions resulting in lack of availability, knowledge, or financial and physical access to quality food stores and transportation that must be considered as harmful to healthy behavior in diet, smoking, medical care and self-respect. High numbers of low nutritional value fast food and neighborhood convenience stores are social determinants impacting on the health of the poor, especially for CVDs.

National Trends in Cardiovascular Mortality

The rates of decline in CVD and stoke mortality rates in EU member countries (those joining before and after 2004) along with Finland and Israel from 1970 to 2013 is shown in Figures 14.3 and 14.4. The remarkable three-to-six-fold reductions in western countries from the 1970s were followed more recently by declining rates in the countries of Central and Eastern Europe and later by Russia and Ukraine. The Eastern countries of the European region began to show falling CVD mortality rates after 1990 and Russian Federation rates falling after 2003. The east-west mortality and gaps remain high for CVD mortality as important causes of similar gaps in life expectancy between Western and East Europe and also between countries in the eastern part of the Region where smoking, hypertension and alcohol binge drinking remain high risk factors.

The American Heart Association (AHA) reports that cardiovascular disease is the leading global cause of death, accounting for 17.3 million deaths per year, and expected to grow to more than 23.6 million by 2030. Cardiovascular diseases are also the leading cause of mortality with over 800,000 deaths in the United States in 2013 including more than 375,000 deaths from CHD and 130,000 from strokes. Although coronary heart disease and stroke death rates have declined steadily since the mid-1960s, CHD remains the leading cause of death accounting for nearly half of these deaths with stroke in third place. Stroke mortality rates have declined about 34 percent, yet stroke remains a leading cause of disability costing an estimated USD $33 billion annually. Heart failure mortality has also declined due to the effectiveness of secondary prevention by good medical and family care in the community. The decline in cardiovascular disease mortality is one of the most important achievements of both public health and clinical medicine in the past century (CDC 1999) (see Figure 14.5).

However, important social class and ethnic differences are clear throughout the epidemiology of CVD. African Americans have twice the risk

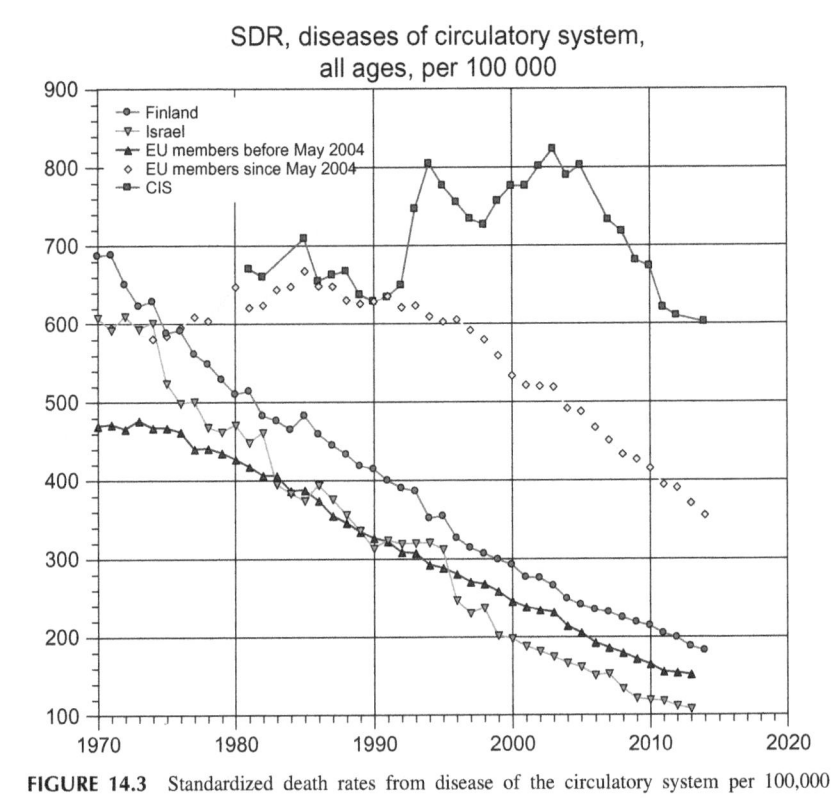

FIGURE 14.3 Standardized death rates from disease of the circulatory system per 100,000 population, selected European Region countries and groups of countries, 1970–2014. Note: CIS is the Commonwealth of Independent States including the Russian Federation, Ukraine and other countries of the former Soviet Union. EU members before 2004 include most of Western Europe and EU countries after 2004 include those countries of central and Eastern Europe which joined the European Union after 2004 (Poland, Hungary, etc.). *Source: WHO European Region. Health for All Database, 2016. Available at: http://www.euro.who.int/en/data-and-evidence/databases/european-health-for-all-database-hfa-db* (accessed 20 July 2017).

compared to white people for mortality from stroke and coronary heart disease; regional differences in CVD mortality are pronounced with the southern states in the United States ("The Stroke Belt") having higher rates of stroke mortality than the rest of the country. The United States identifies stroke as the leading cause of eminently preventable disability, with repeated strokes associated with deaths and disability. The 2020 health goal is to reduce deaths from CVD by 20 percent. Figure 14.5 shows the trend in mortality rates from 1900 to 2010 for total cardiovascular disease, heart disease, coronary heart disease, and stroke. Stroke mortality has declined slowly and steadily in the United States since 1900, probably due to improved societal conditions and medical care. For heart disease the trends are different with rapidly rising rates seen from 1920 to 1960 followed by a "tipping point" with a unexpectedly dramatic and continuing decline since the 1960s up to 2016.

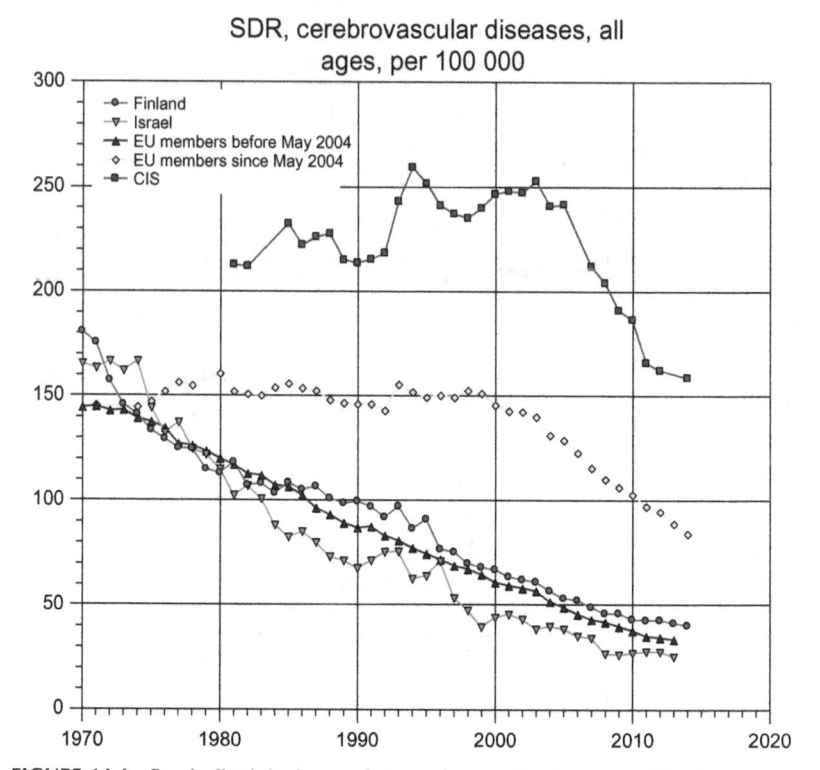

FIGURE 14.4   Standardized death rates from cerebrovascular disease per 100,000 population, selected European Region countries and Groups of Countries, 1970–2014. Note: see footnote of Figure 14.3. *Source: WHO European Region. Health for All Database, 2016. Available at: http://www.euro.who.int/en/data-and-evidence/databases/european-health-for-all-database-hfa-db (accessed 20 July 2017).*

Lackland et al. representing the American Heart Association cited the decline in stroke mortality in the United States as a "major public health and clinical medicine success story". This is attributed to a combination of factors including; smoking reduction, improving discovery and management of hypertension, lipid reduction in the diet, physical exercise, and widespread use of aspirin for prophylaxis. Early and improved medical care and hospital treatment for acute coronary events and strokes have been implemented successfully, with many advances in tertiary prevention ie., preservation of maximum function for chronic disease by effective long term care. Despite the remarkable progress since the 1960s, CDC estimates that in 2010, 200,070 avoidable deaths from heart disease, stroke, and hypertensive disease occurred in the United States. Nearly one-fourth of all cardiovascular disease deaths were avoidable. This includes deaths from arrhythmia, especially atrial fibrillation and congestive heart failure, both treatable conditions with medications under close medical supervision. Medications, electronic pacemakers and other medical devices in process of development can keep patients

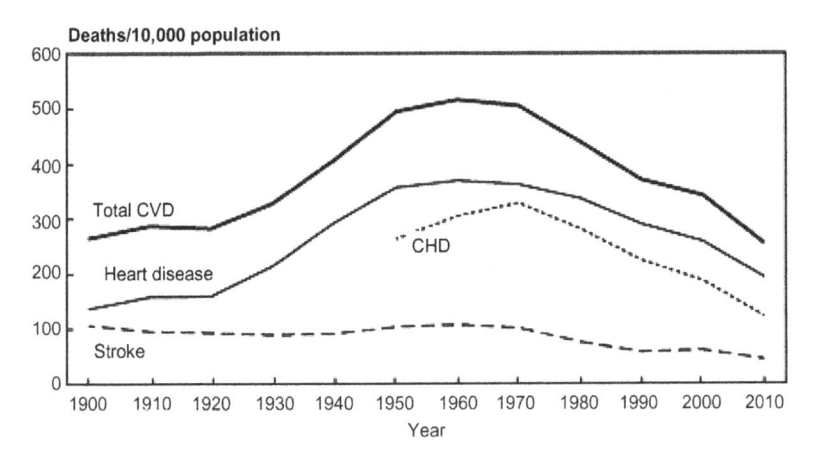

FIGURE 14.5 Death rates for cardiovascular diseases, United States, 1900–2010. *Source: Vital Statistics of the United States, NCHS; cited in: National Institutes of Health, National Heart, Lung and Blood Institute, US Department of Health and Human Services Fact book, 2012. Disease statistics. Available at: https://www.nhlbi.nih.gov/about/documents/factbook/2012/chapter4#gr7 (accessed 20 July 2017).*

alive and functional for long periods. CVD avoidable mortality in the US disproportionately affect non-Hispanic blacks and residents of the South.

CURRENT RELEVANCE

The main factors considered as risk factors for non-communicable disease (NCDs) are still increasing in most of the world, and are at very high levels, especially in European regions. Alcohol consumption levels are rising, physical inactivity is widespread, and obesity and type II diabetes mellitus are a new epidemic of the last few decades, with more than a half of the population in most European countries being overweight and 20–30 percent of adults categorized as obese. Those risk factors are also found to be elevated in children, compared to the past, suggesting future increases in NCDs.

In the European Region most countries have risk-prevention strategies in many ministries of government with formal intersectoral coordination mechanisms. The European Region with the highest burden of NCDs estimates that as much as 80 percent of heart disease and stroke are preventable. Former socialist countries in Eastern Europe have made significant progress in CVD control, but mortality from CHD and stroke remain higher than in the countries of Western Europe. Countries of the former Soviet Union have also made progress since 2005, but the gap between them and western countries is still very large (4 to 1 ratios).

Obesity, smoking and alcohol abuse rates are high in former Soviet republics. Mandatory checkups have improved with cardiovascular risk assessment but effective management of hypertension and diabetes are significantly lower than in Western European standards. Health system reforms are slow to progress along with national development agendas and health plans with low overall expenditure on health as percent of GDP, at seven percent or less as compared to over 10 percent in original EU countries, and with growing social inequality and rural poverty. Worldwide, 17.7 million deaths in 2015 (7.4 million due to coronary heart disease and 6.7 million to stroke), cardiovascular deaths including those resulting from elevated blood pressure are largely caused by high usage of salt from increasing use of processed foods even in low- and middle-income countries. The WHO recommended goals to reduce mortality from CVDs and other NCDs promote reduction in salt intake from 10 grams/day to less than five grams/day. The American Heart Association and the American College of Cardiology lowered the recommended blood-pressure target to less than 120/80 mg Hg. Comprehensive policies of legislation, fiscal measures, information, and cooperation are needed as processed foods including bread account for about 70−75 percent of salt intake. Public health measures can reduce cardiovascular risk by reducing excessive use of sugar and salt, reducing obesity through promotion of exercise, dietary moderation, and by national measures to restrict use of transfats.

WHO estimates that tobacco use (smoking and smokeless) is currently responsible for the death of about six million people across the world each year mostly occurring prematurely, including some 600,000 people from the effects of second-hand smoke. Smoking is mainly associated with ill-health, disability and death from CVDs, cancer, chronic respiratory conditions, and other noncommunicable chronic diseases, as well as increased risk of death from communicable diseases. WHO's MPOWER program refers to: M for monitoring tobacco use and prevention policies; P for protecting people from tobacco smoke; O for offering help to quit tobacco use; W for warning about the dangers of tobacco; E for enforcing bans on tobacco advertising, promotion and sponsorship, and R for raising taxes on tobacco. WHO also attributes 3.7 million deaths or 6.7% of total deaths worldwide in 2012 to ambient air pollution. This includes 29% of deaths due to heart disease and stroke, as well as 16% of lung cancer deaths, and 11% of chronic obstructive pulmonary disease-related deaths.

Success in reducing cardiovascular mortality requires a balance including both individual and population health strategies including reducing air pollution. Changes in risk status occur over time. National-level policymakers have a responsibility to determine the most appropriate emphasis for strategic programming. Tobacco control and smoking reduction programs have been effective at national levels in reducing smoking, a major risk factor in cardiovascular disease. The US *Healthy People 2020* notes that a reduction in the risk of Americans for CVD morbidity and mortality would result if improvements were made across the US population in lifestyle measures and blood pressure control. The report also suggests that depression and other mental health chronic conditions be addressed as a risk factor for cardiovascular disease. Similarly national policies for reducing trans fats by banning their use in some jurisdictions and limiting distribution of high sugar and salt containing prepared foods are vital to further reduction in CVD morbidity and mortality. The UK has been emphasizing reduction in salt content of food products and less use of salt at the dining table. These measures are as important as the regulations for speed limits and seat belts to reduce road traffic deaths or other population-based public health strategies.

The examples of the North Karelia and Framingham projects and other study and intervention programs that followed within the framework of MONICA and CINDI show that primary prevention, focusing on the improvement of lifestyle factors, within integrated and sustainable programs can have a great impact over time and therefore the greatest potential for positive long-term change. But secondary prevention to limit damage from underlying disease such as hypertension, atherosclerosis, diabetes and others require up-to-date medical care which has advanced dramatically in recent decades with effective interventions to prevent and treat cardiovascular events and their long term follow-up.

In 2015 the US Preventive Health Services Task Force reported that community interventions making use of community health workers (*promotores*, community health guides) can play important roles in reducing CVD morbidity in the community. Key activities envisioned include screening and health education; outreach; enrollment, and information; team-based care; patient navigation; and community organization. This kind of public health intervention has proven successful in many settings in low- and medium-income countries but also in the United States as specific public health tasks such as in directly observed therapy for tuberculosis and in many aspects of care for HIV/AIDS patients to enhance and support but not replace medical care. The rising toll of morbidity and mortality of NCDs and especially CVDs as the major causes of death in medium- and low-income countries has led to calls for wider adaptation of community health workers with central roles in primary care as a major strategy to reduce this burden of disease.

Focusing on high-risk groups may bring more immediate gains in disease prevention. Such interventions are also cost-effective, when considering the cost of prevention against the cost of medical care and hospitalization, loss of healthy life years, and subsequent loss of productivity and the burdens these diseases bring.

Although decline in mortality rates for heart disease has been observed in different countries in the last few decades, the case of Finland shows an extremely rapid decline, accompanied by overall improvement in the population's health. The experience of the North Karelia project and the CINDI program as a whole shows the importance of a community-based approach, with multisectoral participation, political commitment implying public policy, and legislation allowing long-term sustainability and producing favorable results. The example of North Karelia showed that a national "demonstration project" can provide a strong basis for national-scale development.

In 2013, OECD reported that CVD is the number one cause of mortality in member countries accounting for around a third of all deaths. Survivors of acute events suffer considerable loss in quality of life due to CVD, particularly after stroke and congestive heart failure. Increasing levels of obesity, high cholesterol and undiscovered or undertreated hypertension, and diabetes, and their increasing combinations (called "metabolic syndrome"), provides the perfect storm of risk factors for serious CVD consequences. Hypertension-related deaths during 2000–13 were due to heart disease, hypertension, stroke, cancer, and diabetes. During this period, hypertension-related deaths with heart disease as the underlying cause of death decreased from 34 percent to 28 percent, and the proportion with stroke as the underlying cause of death decreased from 15 percent to nine percent. The WHO 2014 targets include:

- Reduction in mortality from CVDs, cancer, diabetes and chronic respiratory diseases;
- Reduction in 1.7 million deaths attributed to excess salt intake by reducing salt from 10 grams /day to less than five grams/day;
- Reduction in the prevalence of hypertension by 25 percent as hypertension is associated with over nine million deaths per year and seven percent of the total burden of disease.

In 2017 the American Heart Association and the American College of Cardiology lowered the threshold definition of normal blood pressure from 140/90 to 120/80 raising the bar on this crucial topic. This will substantially increase the population needing follow-up and lifestyle changes; those with higher than borderline hypertension will also need medications. Education of medical care providers and the general public on the importance of blood pressure testing and control has to be high on the agenda of health promotion and medical practice in the coming years.

Despite its number one ranking, mortality rates have shown dramatic improvement over recent decades. On average, OECD member countries have reduced their CVD mortality rate by 42 percent over the 20-year period to 2005. However, the improvements are not uniform across countries, with some countries able to reduce CVD-related mortality by more than 50 percent and others reducing their rates by less than 30 percent. These figures raise important questions on why success has varied so much across countries and to what degree health care systems and policies contribute to this variation. The prevalence of overweight in the US population is far greater than other risk factors as shown in Figure 14.6.

Personal care and lifestyle issues at the center of risk factor reduction are vital to the control of this set of diseases. Millions of lives are at stake

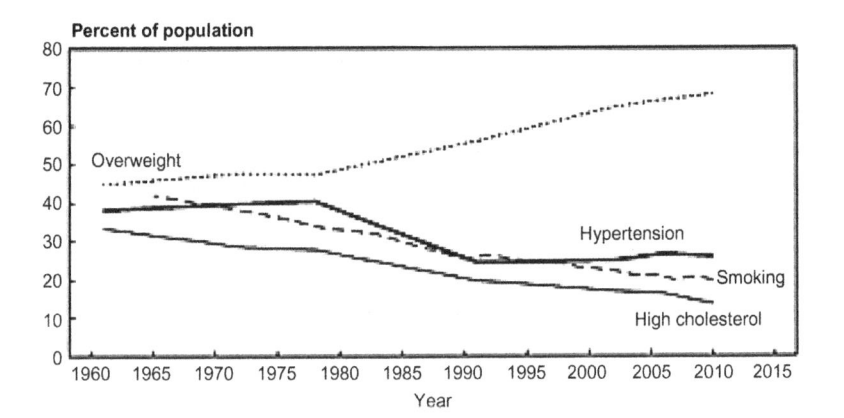

FIGURE 14.6 Age-adjusted prevalence of cardiovascular disease risk factors in adults, U.S., 1961−2011.
Notes: Hypertension is defined as systolic blood pressure 140 mmHg or diastolic blood pressure 90 mmHg, or being on antihypertensive medication. High cholesterol is 240 mg/dL. Overweight is BMI 25 kg/m^2. *Source: NIH NHLIB (NHIS for smoking, ages 18, NCHS; NHANES for the other risk factors, ages 20−74, NCHS). Available at: https://www.nhlbi.nih.gov/about/documents/factbook/2012/chapter4#4_5 (accessed 3 April 2017).*

and the potential for avoiding premature deaths from CVDs has been demonstrated unequivocally since the peak of coronary heart disease in the mid-1960s and the continuing decline of CHD and stroke mortality over many decades. Although there are advances and improvements in high-income countries, much more needs to be done worldwide to apply the positive experience of preventive intervention programs for adaptation and implementation in medium- and low-income countries.

Once thought to be diseases of upper-class men, it is now clear that poverty and social stress are important factors in CVD and that women are at risk as well as men, albeit at later ages but with symptoms less clear-cut than for men. Personal and societal issues increase risks of premature mortality from CVDs including poverty; low educational levels; unemployment; downward social mobility or immobility; lack of support systems and sense of community; life changes such as divorce, death of partners, children, and friends; chronic illness, especially mental illness; social isolation, life dissatisfaction and despair.

This multifactorial mix presents opportunities and challenges for health service providers and social support systems. Prevention and treatment complement each other. Treatment modalities for secondary prevention i.e., reducing the risk of progression of risk factors to serious disease currently available make a major difference in survival from initial risk factors and acute coronary events. Assessment includes recognition of emotional and social factors in causation of CVDs; early diagnosis of risk factors especially of family history, hypertension, diabetes, high blood lipids, and weight loss; aspirin as a routine intake for CVD-risk persons; antihypertensive therapy; beta blockers, ACE inhibitors, and calcium channel blockers and other equivalent medications as routine preventive measures; nitroglycerin and other nitrates; low dose aspirin, and statins and other cholesterol-lowering drugs; and diuretics. Studies reported in the spring of 2016 indicate that a combination of both antihypertensive and statin drugs benefit patients with a statistically significant reduction of cardiovascular events (3.6% vs 5.0%). In an intermediate-risk population, suggestions of benefits for risk groups and age groups have been proposed.

The US National Heart Lung and Blood Institute (NHLBI) and the US Preventive Task Force approach to prevention and treatment of coronary heart disease include heart-healthy lifestyle changes, medicines, medical procedures and surgery and cardiac rehabilitation. Prevention consists of heart-healthy lifestyle changes including: healthy diet; maintaining a healthy weight; managing hypertension and stress; regular physical activity; and cessation of smoking. Treatment goals include: lowering high blood pressure and cholesterol, reducing the risk of blood clots forming which can cause a heart attack or stroke; reducing risk factors to slow, stop, or reverse plaque formation in coronary and other arteries; relief of symptoms; preventing complications of heart muscle damage; and by widening or bypassing clogged arteries.

Clinical management of hypertension, heart disease and stroke have developed and play vital roles in secondary prevention by limiting damage from existing disease. This is important in reducing mortality from CHD. Major advances in clinical care for cardiac or stroke events include advances in emergency care defibrillation, cardio pulmonary resuscitation including rapid transportation for treatment of acute coronary events, and early anti-clotting therapy. Cardiac procedures include valve repair or replacement mainly for rheumatic heart disease, now rare in high-income countries, but still frequent in medium- and low-income countries. Coronary artery bypass procedures are done less frequently than previously largely due to the success of stents and balloon angioplasty. Surgery for congenital heart diseases and transplantation requires high level resources but are effective in saving lives. Valve repair and replacement, heart transplantation, congenital heart operations and life saving medical devices are required to treat some CVDs. Such devices include pacemakers, prosthetic valves, and patches for closing holes in the heart, measures to open blocked coronary arteries with anti-clotting drugs and placement of stents which are wire tubes at the site of the blockage to keep the blood flowing. Longer term management includes cardiac rehabilitation long-term use of aspirin, hypertension and cholesterol control, diet, exercise weight control, and in some cases anti-coagulant therapy and long-term monitoring for all at risk of coronary heart disease and strokes. Cardiac resuscitation and defibrillators available for cardiac arrest cases in the community is another life saving procedure which can be performed by trained first responders including ambulance personnel, police, fire and sport facility personnel.

A proposal for routine use for the general population over age 50 of a "polypill" combining a fixed-dose of blood pressure- and cholesterol-lowering and antiplatelet medications in a single pill, is one suggested strategy for primary prevention in asymptomatic people on the basis of age alone to reduce the global burden of CVD. This concept has not been accepted even as age alone is a key risk factor for CVD. However, routine daily use of aspirin, antihypertensive and statin prophylaxis are widely recommended for persons with clinical and family history of cardiovascular disease and other risk factors. Advances in cardiovascular diagnostics, medical and surgical care are giving better results with short hospital stays and long-term follow-up with effective secondary preventive care, with fewer patients undergoing open-heart surgery, and with improved survival.

The remarkable success seen in recent decades in reducing cardiovascular mortality in many countries resulted from a balance between individual and population health strategies applying knowledge gained from the classic studies. The Framingham epidemiologic study defined the risk factors while the North Karelia community intervention study and many other studies of cardiovascular disease have played enormous roles in defining the issues and promoting new approaches of health promotion to stem the epidemics. Changes in risk factor status were adopted by public health and clinical medicine affecting important changes in population health globally. These changes occur over time and the challenges still ahead are to apply these measures in medium- and low-income countries where CVDs are still extremely high and in all countries facing demographic changes and ageing populations.

National-level policy-makers have a responsibility to determine the most appropriate emphasis for strategic programming. Tobacco control and smoking reduction programs have been effective at national levels in reducing smoking, a major risk factor in CVD. Similarly introduction of national policies for reducing trans fats, sugar, and salt content of prepared foods are vital for further reduction in CVD morbidity and mortality. These are as important as speed limits and seatbelts to reduce road traffic deaths or other population-based public health strategies.

Public health approaches provide attractive strategic opportunities to interrupt and prevent the costly cycle of managing hypertension and its complications. Reducing calories, saturated fat, and salt in processed foods can reduce overall blood pressure and CVD morbidity and mortality by as much or more than, treatment alone. Improving intake of healthy foods such as fruit, vegetables, nuts, and olive oil along with increased regular physical exercise could reduce the burden of chronic disease even more than reducing intake of unhealthy foods.

Complementary strategies for population health and individual patient care include. health promotion to improve cardiovascular health at the population level while targeting those individuals at high CVD risk improves secondary prevention. CVD cuts across all sectors of society but affects poorer sectors of society who are at higher risk largely due to lifestyle issues such as diet and obesity as well as poor ambient air quality and inadequate access to health care. Smoking and exposure to secondhand smoke are still important with almost one-third of coronary heart disease deaths attributable to smoking and exposure to secondhand smoke. Reduction in cigarette consumption may be threatened by increasing promotion and popularity of e-cigarette and nargila (hooka) usage.

The dramatic reduction seen in stroke mortality and improved outcomes are largely the result of reduced cardiovascular risk factors by control of high blood pressure and other health promotion interventions. The World Heart Federation estimates a prevalence of hypertension of over 970 million people worldwide which is expected to increase to over 1.5 billion adults with hypertension in 2025. Hypertension control, smoking reduction and dietary change efforts expanded in the 1970s having a powerful effect on blood pressure level distributions in the population and the decline in stroke mortality. Recent evidence shows health benefits of lowered cardiac events and mortality as well as all cause mortality by reducing target figures for blood pressure control to less than 120 mm systolic and 80 mm Hg diastolic, compared with less than 140 mm and 90 mm Hg (mercury).

In November 2017 Guidelines for the prevention, detection, evaluation, and management of high blood pressure in adults of the American College of Cardiology/American Heart Association Task Force on Clinical Practice Guidelines were published based on a large US population study (SPRINT 2015). The guidelines reported that in the United States, for *"an adult 45 years of age without hypertension, the 40-year risk for developing hypertension is 93% for African Americans, 92% for Hispanics, 86% for whites, and 84% for Chinese adults. Hypertension is the leading cause of death and disability-adjusted life-years worldwide.., High blood pressure is associated with increased risk for CVD, angina, myocardial infarction (MI), heart failure (HF), stroke, peripheral arterial disease, and abdominal aortic aneurysm."* The report categorizes normal BP as $<120/<80$ mm Hg; elevated BP 120–129/<80 mm Hg; hypertension stage 1 as 130–139 or 80–89 mm Hg, and hypertension stage 2 as ≥140 or ≥90 mm Hg. Diagnosis requires an average of two or more readings on separate occasions. Self-monitoring of BP measurement is recommended to confirm the diagnosis and monitor effects of medication, along with clinical and telehealth counseling. The CDC considers that one third of US adults have hypertension with just over half of these well controlled. High blood pressure is undertreated and underdiagnosed among all races and genders, and those with high blood pressure often face serious cardiovascular problems such as stroke, heart attack, or heart failure. Lower blood pressures are strongly associated with a lower incidence of heart disease and stroke. Some controversy remains on blood pressure targets among people over age 60.

Population-based strategies are effective and cost-efficient in improving cardiovascular health of populations in recent decades, but the challenge is still huge in high-, and especially, medium- and low-income countries. These strategies include hypertension identification and control through education of the public and health care providers and easy access to blood pressure measurement in the community. Follow-up is important with management of lifestyle-related issues (e.g., physical activity and smoking cessation, reduced salt and sugar consumption), reduction of salt content in food products as well as in catered and restaurant foods; reduction or elimination of trans fats in processed foods; and labeling of caloric and other nutrient contents of processed and menu-listed foods. Use of low-dose aspirin is widely recommended for routine daily use among adults. Community training of cardiopulmonary resuscitation (CPR) and wide access to defibrillation is recommended. The AHA stresses the importance of reducing salt (and sugar) for all ages but especially those aged two to 19 years, a group in which average daily intake exceeds 3,100 mgm consumed from processed "junk food" and processed food items such as those from grocery stores and fast food restaurants.

Health system approaches should encourage, facilitate, and reward efforts by providers to improve health behaviors and health factors. Population approaches to reducing the burden of CVD requires lifestyle changes of diet, exercise, smoking cessation, and limitations of alcohol consumption. This depends on cultural changes and social change with interventions in schools or workplaces, local communities, and states, as well as nationally. Lifestyle reinforcement by medical care can be enhanced by inclusion of community health workers in health-promotion development.

ETHICAL ISSUES

Education along with restrictions on advertising and smoking in public places have been more effective than expected as the public absorbed the message that "smoking kills." Restrictions on smoking in public places including pubs, bars, and restaurants have been accepted and implemented to a high degree in many countries despite the direct impact on personal "freedom of choice." This has been one of the outstanding achievements of the health promotion component of "the New Public Health".

Legal victories against the tobacco industry related to cigarette promotion, marketing, and compensation for health care costs and compensation payments for personal damage caused by direct and indirect nicotine exposure along with increasing acceptance by smokers to quit the addiction in order to save their own lives are at the heart of the dramatically reduced smoking habits in high-income populations. But the cigarette industry compensated itself by promoting smoking which is still highly prevalent in medium- and low-income countries and in many pockets in high-income countries as well. An outstanding achievement contributing to this progress was the WHO-negotiated Tobacco Framework Convention on Tobacco Control adopted by the World Health Assembly in effect since 2005 *"to protect present and future generations from the devastating health, social, environmental, and economic consequences of tobacco consumption and exposure to tobacco smoke."* The Framework Convention was the first global public health treaty on health to combat the promoters of smoking, but the struggle is far from over with important unresolved issues with increasing efforts and success of tobacco companies to promote smoking in low-income countries and smoking among young people and the surge of smoking e-cigarettes and nargilas.

Hypertension Standards

Hypertension remains a serious risk factor with poor levels of awareness in the general public of the widespread prevalence and the dangers of hypertension when undiscovered or inadequately managed. While population levels of blood pressure have been declining in some high-income countries, the data are highly variable. Recent estimates suggest that one-third of all American adults have hypertension, with one-third not aware, one-third diagnosed but undertreated, and one-third adequately managed. Because of increasing obesity and aging, the prevalence of hypertension in US adults is expected to increase to over 40 percent by 2030. WHO estimates that the prevalence of hypertension is increasing in low- and middle-income countries and is the leading risk factor for global mortality and disability at a cost of USD $94 billion per year.

In 2017, based on a large study published in the New England Journal of Medicine new standards for defining hypertension were adopted by the American Heart Association and the American College of Cardiology. Hypertension is now considered to be present when repeated measures are over 120 systolic and 80 diastolic mm of mercury. This is a lower threshold than the previously accepted 140 and 90. The lower thresholds for hypertension diagnosis will increase the number of people classified as having hypertension and eligible for drug therapy. For those over age 65 the threshold is considered 130 mm systolic.

The importance of this new standard for all age groups is to increase the hypertensive population requiring follow-up, lifestyle change and two kinds of medication.

Access to competent and timely medical care is an important part of public health and requires health insurance or service systems, high-quality training, and tertiary care facilities as well as alert and well-staffed primary and secondary care services. WHO reports that national capacity for prevention and control of CVD suffers from a serious lack of trained personnel with the needed expertise; for example, only two-thirds of health personnel have training for management of high blood pressure. Lessons learned in coping with the CVD epidemic need to be incorporated into basic health policies in low- and medium-income countries as well as for disadvantaged people in high-income countries. This will require education, employment, empowerment and backup of community health workers in outreach programs in deprived or under-served population groups with poor access to medical care and lacking awareness of CVD health threats. This will require development of new, innovative, and possibly controversial, paradigms of health care systems.

ECONOMIC ISSUES

WHO reports that in 2015, cardiovascular deaths accounted for 17.7 million deaths or 31 percent of all global deaths; of these 80 percent occurred in low- and middle-income countries. Stroke was the second-leading global cause of death after heart disease, accounting for 11.8 percent of total deaths worldwide. Because of population growth, rising life expectancy and increasing CVD disease in medium- and low-income countries, cardiovascular mortality is expected to reach 23.6 million deaths globally by 2030.

Heart disease death and disability fell in the United States between 2003 and 2013 by 38 percent, yet the health risks and economic burden remain high. Even with a sharp decline in the mortality rate the 2013 total costs (health and lost productivity) for CVD were more than USD $316 billion. The AHA estimates that by 2030 the costs of high blood pressure as a risk factor will double to USD $416 billion and emphasizes the need for comprehensive population-based strategies incorporating public health and treatment programs reaching out and targeting individuals, workplaces, and communities

Hypertension is the leading cause of one in six deaths among the 75 million Americans with elevated blood pressure. This constitutes an enormous burden of avoidable disease and an important financial and social challenge for the health system. The economic burden is estimated at over USD $73 billion for both direct and indirect costs annually, with CVD and stroke accounting for 14 percent of total health expenditures in 2012 to 2013 and expected to rise from $863 billion in 2010 to $1,044 billion by 2030. The leading contributing factors for stroke include many which can be effectively and inexpensively modified, such as hypertension, excess intake of sodium, calories and trans fats, smoking, lack of physical exercise and weight control to prevent obesity and diabetes.

Hypertension occurs mostly without symptoms but is readily recognized by routine examination and responds to follow-up care in the community which can prevent, diagnose, and treat important complications of heart disease, stroke, kidney, eye, and peripheral vascular complications. National and state policies to reduce the burden of CVD include educational and regulatory measures to eliminate trans fats, and reduce sugar and salt content of manufactured food products, commercial meals, and homecooked foods.

The US Institute of Medicine (IOM) in 2000 reported that hypertension prevalence could be reduced by as much as 22 percent if Americans consumed less salt in their diet and ate more vegetables, fruit, fish and chicken, turkey and meat sources of lean protein. Reducing salt intake from 3,400 mg to the currently advised maximum intake level of 2,300 mg/day could reduce the number of US hypertensive persons by over 11 million and result in approximately $17.8 billion in health care cost savings annually. The Institute also recommends initiatives for weight loss and exercise promotion which are also essential for impact on reducing the burden of CVD and its costs.

The US Food Drug Administration (USFDA) estimates the benefits of elimination of partially hydrogenated oils at $117−242 billion as compared to the $12−14 billion needed to implement the measures. Trans fat reduction is an ongoing process in the United States, although the US FDA reports that average consumption remains high at about a gram of trans fat per day. In some jurisdictions such as New York and other cities, many private manufacturers and food chains have already banned the use of trans fats in commercial baking. Phasing out by other cities of use of trans fats in food production could prevent an estimated 20,000 heart attacks and 7,000 deaths each year. The US Food and Drug Administration announced that trans fats would be banned in the US by 2018. Removing artificial trans fats from the food supply with no adverse effects on food quality, is an important measure in reducing coronary heart disease. In 2015, the European Commission concluded that a legal limit for industrial TFA content would be effective in limiting use their use along with voluntary changes being implemented by food producers, restaurants and food chains.

Annual smoking-attributable economic costs in the United States, including direct medical costs and lost productivity, are estimated to exceed $289 billion. US-estimated annual costs for CVD and stroke for 2011 were $320.1 billion, including $195.6 billion in direct costs (hospital services, physicians and other professionals, prescribed medications, home health care, and other medical durables) and $124.5 billion in indirect costs from lost future productivity due to premature deaths from CVD and stroke. Direct and indirect CVD costs are greater than the costs attributable to any other diagnostic group.

Tobacco smoking is a major risk factor in cardiovascular disease. Significant successes have been achieved in reducing smoking mainly in high income countries. This has involved Health Promotion, legislation and legal action seeking damages from cigarette producers. Legislation limiting tobacco smoking requires combating the vested interests of powerful forces including the cigarette companies as well as organizations representing tobacco growers. Economic interests include governments who reap high incomes from tax surcharges on sales of tobacco products and their new alternatives. This struggle remains especially difficult in low-income countries. The 2005 WHO Framework Convention on Tobacco Control (WHO FCTC) has helped by internationalizing the legal and moral struggles to assist all countries to combat the global smoking epidemic.

CONCLUSION

The pioneering epidemiologic research from the 1950s onward such as the cutting-edge Framingham, North Karelia, MONICA, CINDI, and countless other studies provided the vital insights into CVD risk factors and community-intervention insights. These produced professional and public awareness and resulted in dramatic reductions in heart disease and stroke morbidity and mortality in high-income countries since the 1960s and 1970s, which are still continuing.

The early findings of the Framingham study demonstrated that there were many considerations in the causation of cardiovascular disease. This study still in process with a third generation of the study population defined a crucial new epidemiological concept of "multiple risk factors". This was in contrast to the classical single causation concept of disease as taught to generations of medical students based on the Germ Theory which has proved to be so highly successful in control and in some cases even eradication of infectious diseases. North Karelia and other studies showed the efficacy of interventions to address the multiple risk factors through national and community health promotion activities. The resulting reduction of CVD mortality throughout the industrialized countries demonstrated the efficacy of addressing the epidemiologic findings of these crucial studies.

Despite dramatic progress in declining mortality rates in most high-income countries, the burden of disease remains high with coronary heart disease the leading cause of mortality in high-, medium-, and low-income countries and stroke the third or fourth leading cause of death globally. Untreated hypertension, smoking, poor diet, lack of exercise, obesity, and control of hypertension are key risk factors that remain potent causes of morbidity and mortality. Poverty, inequality, unemployment, and social distress are also key factors.

Medical care to find and treat hypertension, along with cholesterol and lipids reduction by promoting dietary change, smoking cessation and regular exercise, preventive treatment of hypertension by routine daily use of low dose aspirin and statins to lower cholesterol levels prevent blood clots in coronary and cerebral arteries preventing heart attacks and strokes. Statins and in some cases anti-clotting therapy are recommended for people with risk factors for CVD to help reduce low density lipids. Increasing healthy high-density lipids is best achieved through exercise and diet. Rapid treatment of emergency cardiac events is also vital to minimizing heart and brain damage and preventing death but prevention remains our most successful set of tools for reducing the toll and costs of CVD. Public health and clinical care are mutually supportive measures for primary and secondary prevention. These are capable of preventing disease from occurring or when found early with effective intervention stopping or delaying progression to serious consequences providing many more years of relatively healthy living.

Public health offers population-based approaches and opportunities to manage hypertension and the burden of risk for cerebrovascular and coronary heart events with active community-based screening and education. The costs of population-based strategies are low and affect common beliefs and practices such as in smoking, exercise, and dietary habits. Even modest reduction in borderline elevated blood pressure levels can reduce overall mortality and morbidity, but this requires changes in perception and more than medical treatment alone. The role of smoking reduction, physical exercise, and diet are crucial. A healthy "Mediterranean diet" is crucial with high intake of fruit and vegetables which are rich in antioxidants, such as beans, berries and nuts, and contribute to delaying progress of arterial plaques and their closure by thrombosis, as well as olive oil and fish, and low meat consumption to reduce unhealthy fats that promote plaque formation in coronary and cerebral arteries.

Medical care also plays a crucial role in prevention and treatment of life-threatening conditions with multi-factorial causation such as coronary heart disease and stroke and has led to lower mortality rates in most OECD countries. The widespread use of aspirin, antihypertensive and anti-lipid statin medications for people with high risk profiles for cardiac or cerebrovascular tragic events especially for people with family or personal history of cardiac events or are hypertensive. All of this contributes to the control of the CVD pandemic.

Mortality rates following hospital admissions for heart attack fell by some 30 percent between 2003 and 2013 and for stroke by about 20 percent. The OECD in 2015 recommended that this highly encouraging progress can be used more widely emphasizing preventive interventions in low- and medium-income countries. This means adopting best practices to address the high prevalence of these conditions with primary, secondary, and tertiary prevention and above all with health promotion to prevent and reduce mortality from acute coronary events and strokes.

Despite dramatic progress in control, coronary heart disease and stroke are still the "big killers" as the first and third (or fourth) leading cause of death in virtually all high-, medium-, and low-income countries. With populations aging, CVD will increase numerically even as mortality rates decline, and thus prevalence of CVD and costs of care are expected to increase significantly. CVD is perhaps the most important global public health and health-promotion challenge in the 21st century.

New approaches to health promotion to increase awareness and management of CVD risk factors will in the future benefit from the use of health advocates (e.g., community health advocates, guides, or *promatores*) to help those at risk (perhaps in groups) to address their needs for appropriate changes in lifestyle and to prevent avoidable CVD disease and deaths. The US Preventive Services Task Force in 2017 reported on studies that suggest that community health workers (CHWs) can be deployed to improve use of health care services to reduce morbidity and mortality related to CVD. These interventions can be especially effective in improving health and reducing health disparities for minority and medically underserved groups.

WHO calls for a new global emphasis on prevention of cardiovascular diseases responsible in 2015 for 17.7 million deaths annually, including 7.4 million due to coronary heart disease and 6.7 million due to stroke. Over three quarters of all CVD deaths occur in low- and middle-income countries. WHO recognizes that most cardiovascular diseases are preventable by population-wide strategies addressing the major behavioral risk factors (tobacco use, unhealthy diet and obesity, physical inactivity and use of alcohol). The population approach to reducing these risk factors requires engagement through national health policy, with strong community and health system participation. Reaching out to deprived urban and rural sectors in high-, medium- and low-income populations includes: comprehensive tobacco control policies; regulation and taxation to reduce smoking and intake of foods that are high in fat, sugar and salt; building walking and cycle paths to increase physical activity; strategies to reduce harmful use of alcohol and providing healthy school meals to children. WHOs Global action plan for non-communicable disease control, mainly CVD, calls for increased access to medical treatment with drug therapy and counselling (including glycemic control) for secondary prevention of heart attacks and strokes. Access to quality management in hospital for acute coronary and stroke events is also vital for reducing avoidable mortality. Prevention of heart attacks and strokes through a total cardiovascular risk approach is the most effective element of a CVD reduction initiative.

Cardiovascular diseases are still the big killers globally and require the full attention of health planners, medical providers, and public health agencies. The outstanding contribution of the Framingham and North Karelia projects and other epidemiologic and intervention projects played vital, even critical roles in the remarkable reductions in mortality seen in recent decades, by defining the risk factors and health promotion interventions for individuals and for populations. This has advanced public health globally but much more needs to be done to continue the progress and to reduce inequalities due to socioeconomic and access to quality medical care.

The contribution of the Framingham study was the breakthrough to understanding CVD epidemiology. The North Karelia Project brought the concept of risk factors to apply at regional and community levels to address those factors in a high risk population setting. These studies were supported by many other studies which strengthened the case for action and continue to do so. Millions of lives are being saved and economies growing as a result of increasing longevity being seen globally at different rates country by country. This is what public health can achieve.

RECOMMENDATIONS

1. Based on the WHO guidelines for global control of NCDs including cardiovascular disease, the following goals are endorsed and promoted by national and global public health and clinical professional organizations:
    a. Reduction in mortality from CVDs, along with cancer, diabetes, and chronic respiratory diseases;
    b. Reduction in 1.7 million deaths which are attributed to excess salt intake by reducing salt intake from 10 grams/day to less than five grams/day;
    c. Redefining hypertension as blood pressure of over 120/80 and working to find cases by medical practitioners and other outreach workers for screening and follow-up.
    d. Targeting reduction in the prevalence of untreated hypertension by 25 percent as hypertension is associated with over nine million deaths per year globally and seven percent of the total burden of disease.
2. National and local governments, civil society organizations, donors, and global development institutions all need to participate in the process using this information to enhance open and transparent review and action. This should include priority to reducing risk factors in children and youth as well as adults and elderly with primary prevention cost-effective health goals.
3. Promote heart-healthy lifestyle education in kindergartens, primary, secondary, and higher education facilities and institutional settings.
4. Promote physical activity and exercise as part of the daily routine for all age and disability groups.
5. Promote cooperation with professional organizations in all health disciplines for promotion of hypertension awareness, definition, case finding, and management according to best practices standards and guidelines.
6. Promote availability of defibrillation equipment with training of first responders and the general public.
7. Promote, tax and regulate the food industry (agriculture, manufacturers, retail food stores, catering and restaurants) on food standards to reduce sodium, trans fats, total fat and sugar content.

8. Promote the role of healthy nutrition as a key measure for individual- and population-based strategies for cardiovascular disease prevention through:
   a. Increased daily consumption of fruit and vegetables;
   b. Reduced red meat consumption and promote, fish and poultry and lentils as healthy alternatives;
   c. Nutrient content of food labeling should be adapted for populations;
   d. Promote healthy diets at home and those offered by schools, hospitals, colleges, military services, and other institutional settings;
   e. Promote limits on sodium content of food to less than 140 mgm per serving.
   f. Promote wide use of whole grain flour and brown rice in place of unhealthful white flour and white rice.
9. Wide use of health-promotion measures to reduce smoking, increase management of high blood pressure, and promote healthful diets and physical activity in minority and other underserved population groups.
10. Use of community health workers as public health extenders to expand health promotion to reach the many high-risk groups reinforcing medical and public health care for CVDs before and following acute cardiac or stroke events.
11. Health education for healthful diets and physical activity should be promoted for children and adults in the work setting and in institutional and general community settings.
12. Support and promote participation of health care providers in community as well as individual health promotion especially in education for smoking reduction, hypertension identification and management.

STUDENT REVIEW QUESTIONS

1. What are the main findings and contributions of the Framingham study?
2. What are the main findings and contributions of the North Karelia project?
3. What have been the trends in cardiovascular diseases in high-income countries?
4. What have been the trends in cardiovascular diseases in low-income countries?
5. What elements of policy would you recommend to promote continued reduction in morbidity and mortality from cardiovascular diseases?
6. What would you recommend to international and national governments as well as voluntary agencies and donors in order to reduce and control the global pandemic of cardiovascular disease?
7. What are the basic and key prevention factors in controlling cardiovascular diseases?
8. How would you recommend achievement of healthy diet and moderate physical activity and exercise for all ages and especially for disadvantaged populations and for the mobility impaired?

RECOMMENDED READINGS

1. American Heart Association. Processed foods: where is all that salt coming from? Updated December 2015. Available at: http://www.heart.org/HEARTORG/Conditions/ HighBloodPressure/PreventionTreatmentofHighBloodPressure/Processed-Foods-Where-is-all-that-salt-coming-from_UCM_426950_Article.jsp#.Vm4ZZkorJix. (accessed 30 March 2017).
2. American Public Health Association. APHA commends FDA for removing transfat from nation's food supply, June 16, 2015. George Benjamin, Executive Director. Available at: https://www.apha.org/news-and-media/news-releases/apha-news-releases/fda-removes-trans-fat (accessed 30 March 2017).
3. Beaglehole R, Bonita R, Horton R, Adams C, Alleyne G, Assaria P, et al. Priority actions for the non-communicable disease crisis. Lancet. 2011;377:1438–1447. Available at: http://www.thelancet.com/pdfs/journals/lancet/PIIS0140-6736(11)60393-0.pdf (accessed 30 March 2017).
4. Benjamin EJ, Blaha MJ, Chiuve SE, Cushman M, Das SR, Deo R, et al. Heart disease and stroke statistics—2017 update: a report from the American Heart Association. Circulation. 2017;135. 00–00. Available at: http://circ.ahajournals.org/content/circulationaha/early/2017/01/25/CIR.0000000000000485.full.pdf (accessed 6 April 2017).
5. Bochud M, Marques-Vidal P, Burnier M, Paccaud F. Dietary salt intake and cardiovascular disease: summarizing the eidence. Public Health Review. 2011;33:BF03391649. doi:10.1007/BF03391649. Available at: https://publichealthreviews.biomedcentral.com/articles/10.1007/BF03391649 (accessed 20 July 2017).
6. Bovet P, Paccaud F. Cardiovascular disease and the changing face of global public health: a focus on low and middle income countries. Public Health Review. 2011;33:BF03391643. doi:10.1007/BF03391643. Available at: http://publichealthreviews.biomedcentral.com/articles/10.1007/BF03391643 (accessed 20 July 2017).
7. Bovet P, Paccaud F. Cardiovascular disease and the changing face of global public health: a focus on low and middle income countries. Public Health Review. 2012;33(2):397–415. Available at: http://www.publichealthreviews.eu/upload/pdf_files/10/00_Bovet.pdf (accessed 30 March 2017).
8. Capewell S, Ford ES, Croft JB, Critchley JA, Greenlund KJ, Labarthe DR. Cardiovascular risk factor trends and potential for reducing coronary heart disease mortality in the United States of America. Bull World Health Organ. 2010;88:120–130. Available at: http://www.who.int/bulletin/volumes/88/2/08-057885.pdf (accessed 30 March 2017).
9. Centers for Disease Control and Prevention. Prevalence of leading cardiovascular disease risk factors, United States 2005–2012. MMWR Morb Mortal Wly Rep. 2014;63(21):452–457. Available at: http://www.cdc.gov/mmwr/preview/mmwrhtml/mm6321a3.htm (accessed 30 March 2017).
10. Centers for Disease Control and Prevention. Achievements in public health, 1900–1999: decline in deaths from heart disease and stroke -- United States, 1900–1999. MMWR Morb Mortal Wkly Rep. 1999;48(30):649–656. Available at: http://www.cdc.gov/mmwr/preview/mmwrhtml/mm4830a1.htm (accessed 30 March 2017).
11. Centers for Disease Control and Prevention. Vital Signs: avoidable deaths from heart disease, stroke, and hypertensive disease — United States, 2001–2010. MMWR Morb Mort Wkly Rep. 2013;62(35):721–727.
12. Centers for Disease Control and Prevention. Office of Disease Prevention and Health Promotion. Healthy People. April 2017. Available at: https://www.healthypeople.gov/ (accessed 3 April 2017).

13. Centers for Disease Control and Prevention. Chronic diseases: the leading causes of death and disability in the United States. Updated 23 February 2016. Available at: http://www.cdc.gov/chronicdisease/overview/index.htm (accessed 30 March 2017).

14. Centers for Disease Control and Prevention. Heart disease facts: America's heart disease burden, Updated August 2015. Available at: http://www.cdc.gov/HeartDisease/facts.htm (accessed 30 March 2017).

15. Centers for Disease Control and Prevention. Get the facts: sodium's role in processed food. Available at: http://www.cdc.gov/salt/pdfs/sodium_role_processed.pdf (accessed 30 March 2017).

16. Centers for Disease Control and Prevention. The community guide: systematic review: cardiovascular disease: interventions engaging community health workers. Available at: http://www.thecommunityguide.org/cvd/CHW.html (accessed 30 March 2017).

17. Centers for Disease Control and Prevention. High blood pressure. Updated 3 March 2017. Available at: http://www.cdc.gov/bloodpressure/ (accessed 30 March 2017).

18. Dawber TR, Moore FE, Mann GV. Coronary heart disease in the Framingham Study. Am J Public. Health Nations Health. 1957;47:4−24. Available at: https://www.ncbi.nlm.nih.gov/pmc/articles/PMC1550985/ (accessed 30 March 2017).

19. Dawber TR, Moore FE, Mann II GV. Coronary heart disease in the Framingham Study. Am J Public Health Nations Health. 1957;47(4 Pt 2):4−24. Available at: https://www.ncbi.nlm.nih.gov/pmc/articles/PMC1550985/pdf/amjphnation01096-0007.pdf (accessed 1 August 2017).

20. Dawber TR. The Framingham Study. The epidemiology of atherosclerotic disease. Cambridge, MA: Harvard University Press, 1980.

21. Djousse L, Arnett DK, Coon H, Province MA, Moore LL, Ellison RC. Fruit and vegetable consumption and LDL cholesterol: the National Heart, Lung and Blood Institute Family Heart Study. Am J Clin Nutr. 2004;79(2):13−217. Available at: http://ajcn.nutrition.org/content/79/2/213.full (accessed 30 March 2017).

22. Doll R, Hill AB. The mortality of doctors in relation to their smoking habits. BMJ. 1954;1(4877):1451−1455. Available at: https://www.ncbi.nlm.nih.gov/pmc/articles/PMC437141/pdf/bmj32801529.pdf (accessed 1 April 2017).

23. Eyal N, Cancedda C, Kyamanywa P, Hurst SA. Non-physician clinicians in sub-Saharan Africa and the evolving role of physicians. Int J Health Policy Manag. 2016;5(3):149−153. http://dx.doi.org.10.15171/ijhpm.2015.215. Available at: https://www.ncbi.nlm.nih.gov/pmc/articles/PMC4770920/ (accessed 30 March 2017).

24. Framingham Heart Study. Available at: http://www.framinghamheartstudy.org/ and available at: http://www.framinghamheartstudy.org/about-fhs/history.php (accessed 30. A project of the National Heart. Lung and Blood Institute and Boston University, March 2017

25. Hales CM, Carroll MD, Simon PA, Kuo T, Ogden CL. Hypertension prevalence, awareness, treatment, and control among adults aged ≥ 18 years—Los Angeles County, 1999−2006 and 2007−2014. MMWR Morb Mortal Wkly Rep. 2017;66:846−849. doi:10.15585/mmwr.mm6632a3. Available at: https://www.cdc.gov/mmwr/volumes/66/wr/mm6632a3.htm?s_cid = mm6632a3_e#suggestedcitation 9 (accessed 17 August 2017).

26. Halprin HA, Morales-Suárez-Varela, Martin-Moreno J. Chronic disease prevention and the new public health. Public Health Review. 2010;32:BF03391595. doi:10.1007/BF03391595. Available at: https://publichealthreviews.biomedcentral.com/articles/10.1007/BF03391595 (accessed 2 June 2017).

27. Hurtado M, Spinner JR, Yang M, Evenson C, Windham A, Ortiz G, et al. Knowledge and behavioral effects in cardiovascular heath: community health worker disparity initiative 2007−2010. Prevent Chronic Disease. 2014;11:1. Available at: http://www.cdc.gov/pcd/issues/2014/13_0250.htm (30 March 2017).

28. Institute of Medicine. A population based policy and systems change approach to prevent and control hypertension. Washington, DC: National Academes Press, 2010. Available at: http://www.ncbi.nlm.nih.gov/books/NBK220087/pdf/Bookshelf_NBK220087.pdf (accessed 30 March 2017).

29. James PA, Oparil S, Carter BL, Cushman WC, Dennison-Himmelfarb C, Handler J, et al. Evidence-based guideline for the management of high blood pressure in adults: Report from the panel members appointed to the Eighth Joint National Committee (JNC8). JAMA. 2014;311(5):507–520. http://dx.doi.org10.1001/jama.2013.284427 Available at: http://jama.jamanetwork.com/article.aspx?articleid = 1791497 (accessed 30 March 2017).

30. John JH, Ziebland S, Yudkin P, Roe LS, Neill HA, (xford fruit and vegetable study group). Effects of fruit and vegetable consumption on plasma antioxidant concentrations and blood pressure: a randomized controlled trial. Lancet. 2002;359(9322):1969–1974. Available at: http://www.ncbi.nlm.nih.gov/pubmed/12076551 (accessed 30 March 2017).

31. Kannel WB. Clinical misconceptions dispelled by epidemiological research, the Ancel Keys lecture. Circulation. 1995;92:3350–3360. Available at: http://circ.ahajournals.org/content/92/11/3350 (accessed 1 August 2017).

32. Krantz MJ, Coronel SM, Whitley EM, Dale R, Yost MD J, Estacio RO. Effectiveness of a community health worker cardiovascular risk reduction program in public health and health care settings. Am J Public Health. 2013 January;103(1):e19–e27. Available at: https://www.ncbi.nlm.nih.gov/pmc/articles/PMC3518330/ (accessed 12 April 2017).

33. Kung H.-C., Xu J. Report: Hypertension-related mortality in the United States, 2000–2013. NCHS Data Brief No. 183, March 2015. Available at: http://www.cdc.gov/nchs/data/databriefs/db193.pdf (accessed 30 March 2017).

34. Lackland DT, Roccella EJ, Deutsch AF, Fornage M, George MC, Howard G, et al. Factors influencing the decline in stroke mortality: a statement from the American Heart Association/American Stroke Association. Stroke. 2014;45:315–353. Available at: http://stroke.ahajournals.org/content/45/1/315.full (accessed 30 March 2017).

35. Lang T, Lepage B, Schieber A-C, Lamy S, Kelly-Irving M. Social determinants of cardio-vascular diseases. Public Health Review. 2011;33:BF03391652. doi:10.1007/BF03391652. Available at: https://publichealthreviews.biomedcentral.com/articles/10.1007/BF03391652 (accessed 20 July 2017).

36. Lang T, Lepage B, Schieber Lamy S, Kelly-Irving MK. Determinants of cardiovascular diseases. Public Health Reviews. 2012;33(2):601–629. Available at: https://www.research-gate.net/publication/266597009_Social_Determinants_of_Cardiovascular_Diseases (accessed 30 March 2017).

37. Lonn EM, Bosch J, Lopez-Jaramillo P, et al. Blood-pressure lowering in intermediate risk persons without cardiovascular disease. N Engl J Med. 2016. http://dx.doi.org/10.1056/NEJMoa1600175. http://www.nejm.org/doi/full/10.1056/NEJMoa1600175#t=article (accessed 30 March 2017).

38. Lovasi GS, Grady S, Rundle A. Steps forward: review and recommendations for research on walkability, physical activity and cardiovascular health. Public Health Review. 2011;33: BF03391647. doi:10.1007/BF03391647. Available at: https://publichealthreviews.biomed-central.com/articles/10.1007/BF03391647 (accessed 20 July 2017).

39. Luepker RV. WHO MONICA Project: What have we learned and where to go from here? Public Health Review. 2011;33(2):373–396.

40. Luepker RV. WHO MONICA Project: What have we learned and where to go from here? Public Health Review. 2011;33:BF03391642. doi:10.1007/BF03391642 (accessed 20 July 2017).

41. Mahmood SS, Levy D, Vasan RS, Wang TJ. The Framingham Heart Study and the epidemiology of cardiovascular diseases: a historical perspective. Lancet. 2014;383 (9921):999–1008. doi:10.1016/S0140-6736(13)61752-3. Available at: https://www.ncbi. nlm.nih.gov/pmc/articles/PMC4159698/pdf/nihms588573.pdf (accessed 30 July 2017).

42. Marmot MG, Rose G, Shipley M, Hamilton PJS. Employment grade and coronary heart disease in British civil servants. J Epidemiol Community Health. 1978;32:244–249. Available at: https://www.ncbi.nlm.nih.gov/pmc/articles/PMC1060958/ (accessed 2 April 2017).

43. Miedema MD, Petrone A, Shikany JM, Greenland P, Lewis CE, Pletcher MJ, et al. The association of fruit and vegetable consumption during early adulthood with the prevalence of coronary artery calcium after 20 years of follow-up: the coronary artery risk development in young adults (CARDIA) study. Circulation. 2015;132(21):1990–1998. Available at: http://circ.ahajournals.org/content/132/21/1990.long (accessed 30 March 2017).

44. Mozaffarian D, Benjamin EJ, Go AS, Arnett DK, Blaha MJ, Cushman M, et al. Heart disease and stroke statistics—2015 update: a report from the American Heart Association. Circulation. 2015;131(4):e29–e322. Available at: http://circ.ahajournals.org/content/131/4/ e29#sec-1 (accessed 30 March 2017).

45. National Heart Lung Blood Institute. The Framingham heart study (FHS). Project period 1948–2015. Available at: https://www.nhlbi.nih.gov/research/resources/obesity/population/ framingham.htm (accessed 30 March 2017).

46. National Heart Lung and Blood Institute. Disease Statistics. Available at: https://www. nhlbi.nih.gov/about/documents/factbook/2012/chapter4#4_5 (accessed 3 April 2017).

47. National Institutes of Health. Office of the Director–August 23, 2011. Remembering Dr. William Kannel, Framingham heart study pioneer. Available at: https://www.nhlbi.nih.gov/ about/directorscorner/messages/remembering-dr-william-kannel-framingham-heart-study- pioneer (accessed 30 July 2017).

48. Nikogosian H, da Costa e Silva VL. WHO's first global health treaty: ten years in force. Bull World Health Organ. 2015;93:211. http://dx.doi.org/10.247/BLT.15.154823. Available at: http://www.who.int/bulletin/volumes/93/4/15-154823.pdf (accessed 30 March 2017).

49. OECD. Available at: http://www.oecd.org/els/health-systems/hcqi-cardiovascular-disease- and-diabetes.htm (accessed 30 .Health care quality indicators - cardiovascular disease and diabetes: policies for better health system performance. Paris: OECD Publishing, March 2017

50. OECD. Health at a glance 2015 Available at: http://dx.doi.org/10.1787/health_glance-2015- en (accessed 30 .OECD indicators. Paris: OECD Publishing, March 2017

51. Office of Disease Prevention and Health Promotion. Healthy people. Available at: https:// www.healthypeople.gov/ (accessed 3 April 2017).

52. Oppenheimer GM, Blackburn H, Puska P. From Framingham to North Karelia to U.S. community-based prevention programs: negotiating research agenda for coronary heart disease in the second half of the 20th century. Public Health Review. 2012;33:450–483. Available at: https://publichealthreviews.biomedcentral.com/articles/10.1007/BF03391646 (accessed 23 September 2017).

53. Pajak A, Kozela M. Cardiovascular disease in central and east Europe. Public Health Review. 2011;33:BF03391644. doi:10.1007/BF03391644. Available at: https://publicheal- threviews.biomedcentral.com/articles/10.1007/BF03391644 (accessed 20 July 2017).

54. Pajak A, Kozela M. Cardiovascular disease in Central and East Europe. Public Health Review. 2012;33:416–435. Available at: https://www.researchgate.net/publication/26531 3595_Cardiovascular_Disease_in_Central_and_East_Europe (accessed 30 March 2017).

55. Pearson TA. Recent advances in preventive cardiology and lifestyle medicine: public policy approaches to the prevention of heart disease and stroke. Circulation. 2011;124:2560–2571. Available at: http://circ.ahajournals.org/content/124/23/2560.full (accessed 30 March 2017).

56. Perry HB, Zulliger R, Rogers MM. Community health workers in low-, middle-, and high-income countries: an overview of their history: recent evolution, and current effectiveness. Annu Rev Public Health. 2014;35:399–421. Abstract available at: http://www.ncbi.nlm.nih.gov/pubmed/24387091 (accessed 30 March 2017).

57. Petrukhin IS, Lunina EY. Cardiovascular disease risk factors and mortality in Russia: challenges and barriers. Public Health Review. 2011;33:BF03391645. doi:10.1007/BF03391645. Available at: https://publichealthreviews.biomedcentral.com/articles/10.1007/BF03391645 (accessed 20 July 2017).

58. Pothineni NV, Delongchamp R, Vallurupalli S, Zufeng S, Dai Y, et al. Impact of hepatitis C seropositivity on the risk of coronary heart disease events. Am J Cardiol. 2014;114:1841–1845. Available at: https://www.ncbi.nlm.nih.gov/pmc/articles/PMC4372470/ (accessed 30 March 2017).

59. Puska P. Successful prevention of non-communicable diseases: 25 year experiences with North Karelia Project in Finland. Public Health Med. 2002;4(1):5–7. Available at: http://www.who.int/chp/media/en/north_karelia_successful_ncd_prevention.pdf (accessed 30 March 2017).

60. Puska P, Vartiainen E, Tuomilehto J, Salomaa V, Nissinen A. Changes in premature deaths in Finland: successful long-term prevention of cardiovascular diseases. Bull World Health Org. 1998;76(4):419–425. Available at: https://www.ncbi.nlm.nih.gov/pmc/articles/PMC2305767/pdf/bullwho00004-0101.pdf (accessed 15 August 2017).

61. Puska P. The North Karelia project: 30 years successfully preventing chronic diseases. Diabetes Voice. 2008;53:26–29. Available at: https://www.idf.org/sites/default/files/attachments/article_593_en.pdf (accessed 30 March 2017).

62. Qaseem A, Wilt TJ, Rich R, Humphrey LL, Frost J, Forciea MA, et al. Pharmacologic treatment of hypertension in adults aged 60 years or older to higher versus lower blood pressure targets: a clinical practice guideline from the American College of Physicians and the American Academy of Family Physicians. Ann Intern Med. 2017;166:430–437. http://dx.doi.org/10.7326/M16-1785 Available at: http://annals.org/aim/article/2598413/pharmacologic-treatment-hypertension-adults-aged-60-years-older-higher-versus (accessed 12 April 2017).

63. Rose G, Marmot MG. Social class and coronary heart disease. Br Heart J. 1981 Jan;45(1):13–19. Available at: https://www.ncbi.nlm.nih.gov/pmc/articles/PMC482483/pdf/brheartj00179-0021.pdf (accessed 2 April 2017).

64. Rahimi K, MacMahon S. Blood pressure management in the 21st century maximizing gains and minimizing waste. Circulation. 2013;128:2283–2285. Available at: http://circ.ahajournals.org/content/128/21/2283.full.pdf (accessed 30 March 2017).

65. SPRINT Research Group. A randomized trial of intensive versus standard blood-pressure control. NEJM. 2015;373(22):2103–2116. Available at: https://doi.org/10.1056/NEJMoa1511939. Available at: https://www.ncbi.nlm.nih.gov/pmc/articles/PMC4689591/ (accessed 18 December 2017).

66. Steinberg D. An interpretive history of the cholesterol controversy: part II: the early evidence linking hypercholesterolemia to coronary disease in humans. J Lipid Res. 2005;46(2):179–190. First Published on November 16, 2004, http://dx.doi.org/10.1194/jlr.R400012-JLR20. Available at: http://www.jlr.org/content/46/2/179.full.pdf+html (accessed 2 April 2017).

67. The Victoria Declaration on Heart Health. Declaration of the Advisory Board, International health conference, 1992. Ottawa, CA: Health and Welfare, Canada; 1992. Available at: http://www.internationalhearthealth.org/Publications/victoria_eng_1992.pdf (accessed 30 March 2017).

68. Tulchinsky TH, Varavikova EA. What is the "New Public Health". Public Health Review. 2010;32:BF03391592. doi:10.1007/BF03391592. Available at: http://publichealthreviews. biomedcentral.com/articles/10.1007/BF03391592 (accessed 20 July 2017).

69. Tunstall-Pedoe H, Connaghan J, Woodward M, Tolonen H, Kuulasmaa K. Pattern of declining blood pressure across replicate population surveys of the WHO MONICA project, mid-1980s to mid-1990s, and the role of medication. BMJ. 2006;332(7542):629−635. Available at: http://www.bmj.com/content/332/7542/629 (accessed 30 March 2017).

70. Tuomilehto J, Geboers J, Salonen JT, Nissinen A, Kuulasmaa K, Puska P. Decline in cardiovascular mortality in North Karelia and other parts of Finland. BMJ (Clin Res Ed). 1986 Oct 25;293(6554):1068−1071. Available at: http://www.ncbi.nlm.nih.gov/pmc/articles/PMC1341917/ (accessed 30 March 2017).

71. Tuomilehto J, Ryynanen O-P, Koistinen A, Rastenyte D, Nissinen A, Puska P. Low diastolic blood pressure and mortality in a population-based cohort of 16913 hypertensive patients in North Karelia, Finland. J Hypertens. 1998;16(9):1235−1242. Available at: http://www.ncbi.nlm.nih.gov/pubmed/9746108 (accessed 30 March 2017).

72. University of Minnesota. A history of cardiovascular disease epidemiology, 2012. http://www.epi.umn.edu/cvdepi/history-gallery/formal-studies-begin/ (accessed 30 March 2017).

73. USA.gov The Community Guide. Engaging community health workers recommended to prevent cardiovascular disease. Available at: https://www.thecommunityguide.org/content/engaging-community-health-workers-recommended-prevent-cardiovascular-disease (accessed 3 April 2017).

74. US Surgeon General's Report on Smoking and Health. Washington DC, US DHHS, 1964. Available at: https://profiles.nlm.nih.gov/ps/retrieve/Narrative/NN/p-nid/60 (accessed 30 March 2017).

75. US Department of Health and Human Services. Heart disease and stroke: HDS-2: Reduce coronary heart disease deaths. Healthy People 2020. (updated 14 December 2015) Washington, DC: US Department of Health and Human Services. Available at: http://www.cdc.gov/nchs/healthy_people/hp2020.htm (accessed 30 March 2017).

76. Vartiainen E, Laatikainen T, Peltonen M, Juolevi A, Männistö S, et al. Thirty-five year trends in cardiovascular risk factors in Finland. Int J Epidemiol. 2010;39(2):504−518. Available at: http://ije.oxfordjournals.org/content/39/2/504.long (accessed 30 March 2017).

77. Wald NJ, Morris JK. Quantifying the health benefits of chronic disease prevention: A fresh approach using cardiovascular disease as an example. Eur J Epidemiol. 2014;29:605−612. Available at: https://www.ncbi.nlm.nih.gov/pmc/articles/PMC4160564/ (accessed 12 April 2017).

78. Whelton PK, Carey RM, Aronow WS, Casey Jr DE, Collins KJ, Dennison Himmelfarb C, et al. 2017. ACC/AHA/AAPA/ABC/ACPM/AGS/APhA/ASH/ASPC/NMA/PCNA Guideline for the prevention, detection, evaluation, and management of high blood pressure in adults J Am Coll Cardiol. 2017;70(24):3074−3075. Available at: https://doi.org/10.1016/j.jac Epub ahead of print. Available at: http://www.onlinejacc.org/content/early/2017/11/04/j.jacc.2017.11.006?_ga = 2.250190786.513112374.1513965722-1419480967.1513965722 (accessed 18 December 2017).

79. Wong ND, Levy D. Legacy of the Framingham heart study: rationale, design, initial findings and implications. Global Heart. 2013;8(1):3–9. Available at: http://www.globalheart-journal.com/article/S2211-8160(12)00261-X/abstract (accessed 31 March 2017).

80. World Health Organization. WHO Framework Convention on Tobacco Control, 2003. Available at: http://www.who.int/fctc/text_download/en/ (accessed 30 July 2017).

81. World Health Organization. WHO global report on trends in tobacco smoking 2000–2025. Available at: http://www.who.int/tobacco/publications/surveillance/reportontrendstobaccos-moking/en/ (accessed 24 September 2017).

82. World Health Organization. European Region. Prevention and control of noncommunicable diseases: European Region: a progress report. Copenhagen: World Health Organization. 2014. Available at: http://www.euro.who.int/__data/assets/pdf_file/0004/235975/Prevention-and-control-of-noncommunicable-diseases-in-the-European-Region-A-progress-report-Eng.pdf (accessed 30 March 2017).

83. World Health Organization. European Health for All Database. July 2016. Available at: http://www.euro.who.int/en/data-and-evidence/databases/european-health-for-all-database-hfa-db (accessed 30 March 2017).

84. World Health Organization. Noncommunicable disease. Fact sheet. Updated September 2016. Available at: http://www.who.int/mediacentre/factsheets/fs317/en/ (accessed 30 March 2017).

85. World Health Organization. Cardiovascular disease (CVD) fact sheet. Updated May 2017. Available at: http://www.who.int/mediacentre/factsheets/fs317/en/ (accessed October 2017).

86. World Health Organization. Global status report on noncommunicable diseases 2014. (chapters 1 and 6). Available at: http://apps.who.int/iris/bitstream/10665/148114/1/9789241564854_eng.pdf (accessed 30 March 2017).

87. World Health Organization. Framework Convention on Tobacco Control; an overview, 2015. Available at: http://www.who.int/fctc/WHO_FCTC_summary_January2015_EN.pdf?ua=1 (accessed 30 March 2017).

88. World Health Organization. Media Center. Cardiovascular diseases (CVDs) fact sheet updated May 2017. Available at: http://www.who.int/mediacentre/factsheets/fs317/en/ (accessed 23 September 2017).

89. World Health Organization. Chronic diseases and health promotion. Integrated chronic disease prevention and control: community-based programmes. Available at: http://www.who.int/chp/about/integrated_cd/index2.html (accessed 2 April 2017).

90. World Heart Federation. Cardiovascular disease risk factors, 2017. Available at: http://www.world-heart-federation.org/cardiovascular-health/cardiovascular-disease-risk-factors/ (accessed 30 March 2017).

Chapter 15

Milton Roemer, Hospital Bed Supply and Economics of Health

ABSTRACT

Public policy for health systems of necessity faces working with distribution of resources between competing interests as a constant challenge. New science and technologies continuously emerge with high expectations that these innovations be available to all. The 1946 US "Hill Burton Act" provided federal funds to states and local government to upgrade hospitals that had suffered from underfunding during the Great Depression. This Act set upper limits to the hospital bed supply in a given region so as to limit the pressure of costs in the health system. Milton Roemer was a leading analyst of health systems in the United States and globally who articulated what came to be called "Roemer's Law" which stated that greater numbers of hospital beds result in increased utilization and costs of the health system when there is insurance for health services. This became widely accepted as a major factor in US health policy. It was also influential in most high-income countries which, since the 1960s, have adopted policies of reducing acute care hospital bed ratios. Major efficiencies in health care were evolving that enabled fewer admissions and shorter length of stay in acute care hospitals and resource shift to ambulatory and preventive care along with health promotion. Laparoscopic surgery, cures for chronic peptic ulcer disease, vaccines for rotaviruses and pneumonia and short stays for acute coronary event, all improving patient results, contributed to reduced utilization of hospital beds. In the 1970s changes in United States payment systems from per diem rates to Diagnosis Related Groups (DRGs) promoted rapid diagnosis, treatment, and shorter hospital stays. Roemer's Law became a basic foundation for health policy globally with growing emphasis on integration of hospital and community care, ambulatory care, long term care for the elderly, and health promotion programs to reduce morbidity from preventable diseases by addressing lifestyle challenges and health promotion.

Case Studies in Public Health. DOI: http://dx.doi.org/10.1016/B978-0-12-804571-8.00024-X

357

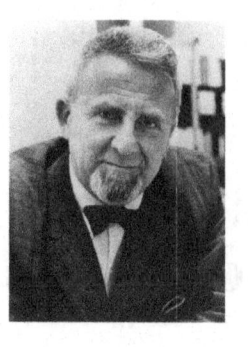

Milton Roemer, M.D. (1916–2001). American professor of health systems; originator of the concept that the more hospital beds are provided in a community, the more days of hospital care will be utilized if insured, recognized as Roemer's Law. *Source: Photo received from John Roemer (son of Milton Roemer)*

BACKGROUND

One of the key issues in health policy has been, and continues to be, how to provide universal access to health care—a significant and fundamental political dilemma. Countries which have achieved universal coverage through health insurance or health service systems, face the challenge of rising health costs and seek ways to control those costs, while keeping up with new innovations, emerging infectious diseases, aging populations, and lifestyle-related, noncommunicable diseases such as diabetes and obesity. Those countries which do not have universal health insurance, but wish to provide access for the entire population must find ways to finance it, and control costs while meeting rising health needs. With increasing coverage of health insurance and rising health care costs, the question of appropriate supply and use of services is raised. The use of hospital beds is one of the most important factors in health costs. Health policy needs to be based on an understanding of a complex range of inter-related ethical, political, social, organization, utilization, management and resource allocation, and funding for establishing priorities (see Chapter 8).

Milton Roemer MD (1916–2001), a pioneering health services researcher, teacher, and professional in the US and internationally, identified the excess and economic predominance of hospitals in health financing as an important issue in health policy. His research on hospital beds was so significant that it became known as Roemer's Law. His contributions to health policy in the United States and globally were vital in many countries' adaptation of health policy and financing with development of more comprehensive approaches, which are still an issue. His many notable achievements include studies showing that in an insured population, "a hospital bed built is a bed filled, especially if there is health insurance", —a finding that contributed to enactment in the US at the state level Certificate of Need (CON) in legislation and comprehensive health planning. CON requirements placed the onus of proof of need on hospitals and other health facilities to build or expand or acquire facilities with or without government financial help.

Roemer's vision was integrating hospital and community medical care centers focusing on prevention-oriented health systems. The American Public Health Association (APHA) honored Roemer with the Sedgwick Memorial Medal for distinguished service in public health.

Roemer earned his Doctor of Medicine (MD) from New York University in 1940, followed by a master's degree in sociology from Cornell University, and a master's in public health from the University of Michigan. In 1946, he played an important role in assisting the Canadian Province of Saskatchewan to successfully implement North America's first universal coverage hospital insurance program. In 1951, Roemer was appointed head of the Social and Occupational Health Section in the newly established World Health Organization (WHO) in Geneva, Switzerland. In 1953, as he was caught up in the McCarthy hysteria, he was forced to leave his work as an international civil servant when the US government withdrew approval of his WHO appointment.

Roemer's 60-year career included studies of all levels of health administration—county, state, national, and international. A world-renowned scholar, he consulted in 71 countries, published 32 books, and 430 articles on the social aspects of health services, public health, international health, primary care, and rural health, specializing in health-care organization. Together with colleagues, Roemer carried out studies in Upper New York State on the supply of hospital beds and hospital utilization. Their hypothesis, later known as Roemer's Law, was: the more hospital beds are provided in a community, the more days of hospital care will be utilized if insured. This proved to be a powerful concept which led the US and many other countries to gradually downsize the hospital sector of their health systems. This trend was further supported by growing efficiencies in prevention and medical care.

The US health system is highly decentralized with private medical practice, private hospitals, laboratories, and private insurance providers with strong political opposition to single payer governmental systems, despite Medicare for the elderly, Medicaid for the poor and other public systems for care of veterans and Indians. US health policy has traditionally believed in market forces as the means by which consumers could, in principle, seek the lowest price or best quality of goods or services from competing providers. However, in health care, there are many factors which must be considered as modifiers of the market theory in health economics. Planners, policy makers, and health systems managers need to understand these modifiers as part of their preparation and orientation (see Table 15.1). Roemer's Law introduced a new perspective in which regulatory mechanisms on hospital bed supply were crucial to developing a comprehensive approach to health care, to seek cost control, and to recognize the rapidly advancing efficiencies and effectiveness of medical care and public health. Roemer's Law as an approach, with or without attribution, became highly influential, as countries providing various forms of health insurance or service systems to all, or parts, of their

TABLE 15.1 National Health Expenditures, United States, Percent
Distribution, Selected Years, 1960–2015

	1960	1980	2000	2015
Per capita national health expenditures	$146	1,108	4,857	9,990
National health expenditures as percent GDP	5.0%	8.9	13.3	17.8
Total national health expenditures	100%	100	100	100
Investment, capital	6.7%	5.7	4.2	3.4
Research	2.6%	2.1	1.9	1.5
Administration government	0.2%	1.1	1.2	1.3
Net cost of health insurance	3.7%	3.6	4.7	6.6
Public health (government)	1.4%	2.5	3.1	2.5
Personal health care services	85.5%	85.0	84.8	84.8
Hospital care	33.0%	39.4	30.3	32.3
Physician, other clinical services	21.8%	20.1	23.8	22.5
Dental care	7.3%	5.2	4.5	3.7
Other personal care, residential care	1.6%	3.3	4.7	5.1
Nursing care, retirement homes	3.0%	6.0	6.2	4.9
Home health care	0.2%	0.9	2.4	2.8
Retail prescription drugs, medical products	18.5%	10.1	13.0	13.5

Source: National Center for Health Statistics. Health, United States, 2016: with chart book on
long-term trends in health. Hyattsville, MD. 2017, Tables 93, 94, pp. 314–317. Available at:
https://www.cdc.gov/nchs/data/hus/hus16.pdf (accessed 25 January 2018).

population faced a rapid increase in health costs and popular demand for
improved health care. The application of Roemer's Law in health system
planning strengthened modifications of market forces including regulation of
supply of, for example, hospital bed ratios, supported by changes in payment
systems incentives which has greatly affected health system management
since the latter third of the 20th century.

The US health system is described as entrepreneurial and competition-
based, primarily funded through private voluntary insurance, mostly through
labor union negotiated health insurance benefits. However there are major
public health insurance programs. In 1965, President Lyndon Johnson introduced publicly funded health insurance systems with Medicare for the
elderly (over age 65) and Medicaid for the poor- both provisions expanding
the 1935 Social Security Act. Public insurance was extended to millions of
children under the 1997 Children's Health Insurance Plan (CHIP), and

millions more under the Affordable Care Act (Obamacare) in 2010. Longstanding Indian and Veterans health service systems and other public health oriented direct service systems for maternity care, nutrition support, and others such as school lunch programs, expanded public health in the US. In contrast, health systems in Western Europe are socially oriented universal national health programs, provided by public programs or regulated by government with insurance companies administering the financing of most health care. Other national health systems operate as public service systems, as for example, public education systems.

Canada's mandatory system is based on universal coverage—a comprehensive, publicly administered, single-payer system operated by the provincial government with federal standards and fiscal support, without private insurance agencies. European systems are universal coverage public systems of insurance, or direct services administered by various levels of government as in Nordic systems or Sick Funds as in Germany and other countries. National health service systems such as that in the UK (the "Beveridge system") provide and administer comprehensive hospital and medical services for the total population financed through taxation. Universal health insurance under social security (the "Bismarckian system") is also common in many European countries with national- and state oversight. Health systems in countries of the former Soviet Union have a state-operated health socialist organizational structure, which now coexist with mandatory health insurance in a bi-modal system. Health system arrangements are influenced by a country's economic conditions and societal values (see Chapter 8).

In 1945, US President Harry Truman was strongly committed to a single, universal, comprehensive health insurance plan, and attempted to promote a law for a universal health insurance program which did not pass the US Congress. As an alternative approach to improving health care in the US, the federal Hill Burton Act was established as a funding system to financially assist states, municipalities and private not-for-profit organizations to raise the quality of hospitals, and later long-term care and community health facilities across the US which had suffered due to a lack of resources during the Great Depression and World War II and needed renovation or replacement. The Hill Burton Act set upper limits on hospital bed supplies per region to 4/1000 population (4.5 in rural areas). This plan also set standards for providing emergency care for all, and banned racial segregation, an important precedent for the Civil Rights movement a generation later. This Act included restriction on the hospital bed supply as part of federal funding to upgrade the hospitals. During this period the National Institute of Health (NIH) evolved from the US Public Health Service, with mandates to promote federal funding for research in academic medical centers across the US.

Studies by Roemer and his colleagues influenced the development of Health Maintenance Organizations (HMOs) and the subsequent introduction of reform in payment systems for hospital care, promotion of HMOs for linking insurance with service systems, and more recent formats of integrated health care such as Accountable Care Organizations (ACAs) under the US Affordable Care Act. Promoting ambulatory and preventive care as part of policies for national health insurance for the total population in the US has faced political opposition, but has played an increasing role in US health policy. The ACA increased insurance coverage while promoting widened preventive health orientation, along with rapid improvements in medical care, standards of living and population health.

Funding for hospitals has its origin in religious, municipal, and charitable organizations dating back hundreds of years. In modern times, hospitals have been funded through various approaches based on a country's prevailing value system. The most costly component of a health service is acute-care (short-term) hospitals. There are various methods of hospital service payments including historical, per diem, fee-for-service, normative, and Diagnosis Related Groups (DRGs).

Funding Models for Hospitals

Per Diem

Traditionally, a per diem (or flat rate per patient-day) rate based on daily operating costs divided by the number of beds was used to pay hospitals. The per diem rate is calculated through actual costs or by national, state, or regional averages, which at times is adjusted for teaching or research functions. The per diem method of payment encourages long lengths of stay, which results in hospitals retaining out dated technology and methods. Per diem rates based on national or regional averages may penalize hospitals with high levels of staffing and technology, such as academic hospitals. Moreover, when service is insured, there is less financial incentive for shortening a patient's hospital stay. Admissions to a hospital for diagnostic tests or prolonging a patient's stay for additional testing or care which could be provided through less costly ways, such as an out-patient alternative, is associated with inefficient use of facilities. Per diem payment provides the incentive to hospitalize and prolong care for a relatively healthy patient, while infirm patients and teaching or research activities represent financial liability—unless these are funded separately based on actual costs per patient in specific hospital units, such as intensive care. This system lacks incentives to improve efficiency by developing alternative ambulatory or day care services, while penalizing more efficient hospitals which reduce length-of-stay or occupancy rates.

Historical

Historically, funding is based on the previous year's budget, adjusted for inflation and the cost of approved new service programs. The budget may be reviewed by the paying authority with funding being approved on a global—or block budget—basis which allows the hospital to make internal adjustments within the overall allotment. Payment can include a separate capital fund for renovation. This method is often used when a hospital is funded directly by a country's department of health. The historical method should, theoretically, provide some incentive to reduce length-of-stay and to search for efficiency in the use of hospital resources. However, the hospital may use resources to establish other programs which are not approved by the paying authority and often lead to hospital budget deficits.

Fee-for-Service

The fee-for-service method is based on a payment structure for each service offered in a hospital. This system provides an incentive to over-service, without promoting cost savings by reducing admissions or length of stay. It favors unnecessary marginal care, high admission rates, and the provision of duplicate or unnecessary services. The patient's invoice for their hospital stay is submitted to the insurer with the patient being responsible for non-approved claims. This method was common in the US with its multiple insurance systems, but has been increasingly replaced by Diagnosis Related Groups (DRG) payments instead of per diem and fee-for-service payments.

DRGs

The DRG payment system was developed in the 1960s at Yale University in the US due to concerns about high costs and the search for alternative methods of payment. The DRG system was officially adopted in 1983 by the US Health Care Financing Administration (HCFA) as the basis for payment for hospitalization of Medicare patients. The DRG system has been the basis for paying for hospital care in the US since 1999 by most health insurers, and has been adopted by other industrialized countries—e.g., the United Kingdom and Israel—and some low- and middle-income countries, including the Philippines, and countries in eastern Europe, including nine countries in transition from the Soviet system.

In the DRG system, hospitals are funded based on a predefined payment rate for diagnoses or procedures in 495 classifications. This incentivizes the appropriate use of services with a reduction in length-of-stay, efficient use of diagnostic and treatment procedures, and reduces overall bed capacity. Implementation of the DRG system in the 1990s in the US led to a rapid decrease in admissions and an increase of outpatient services while bed occupancy rates and per capita hospital bed supply declined steadily. The DRG system, however, encouraged the falsification of diagnoses or reported severity of case definitions in order to increase revenues, which became known as "DRG creep."

Prospective payment systems, such as DRGs, support rational use of hospital care as an effective way to achieve a balanced health service system and must be associated with quality assurance mechanisms. A regional approach for hospital budgeting as part of a comprehensive network helps to achieve equity and provides incentives for increasing health in the population.

Normative

Hospital payment by norms entails financing based on national fixed standards for hospital capacity—beds, staffing, and other measures as set by the Ministry of Finance. This method—as practiced in the Soviet health system model—provided national incentives for hospitals to maintain high bed to population ratios and long lengths-of-stay, with little investment in improving ambulatory care, generally low quality of care, and low salaries. Reform in all post-Soviet countries required rejecting the norms method of payment, and adopting funding models which reduce hospital bed capacity and the adoption of incentives to increase efficiency in health care focused on ambulatory and health promotion programs.

Managing Hospital Bed Supply

In industrialized countries, measures to control hospital bed supply and utilization are vital elements of health system policy and planning. In settings with high levels of hospital bed supply, an excessively large share of health care expenditure goes to hospital care, while alternative services are deprived of resources. In such cases, financial incentives can be used to shift the balance between hospital and community care. For example, the Hill Burton Act approach may be used to promote "down-sizing and up-grading" in a health system that has overdeveloped institutional care with less emphasis on long-term care or primary care. Moreover, a system of incentives for integrated care arrangements can redirect funding for other services, including community and capital programs—e.g., to reduce total bed capacity and to promote the integration of maternity, mental health, geriatric, and tuberculosis departments into general hospitals.

An example of this method is the following: In a district with a population of 250,000, the current number of 2,500 acute-care hospital beds—or 10 beds per 1,000 people—is downscaled to 1,250 beds—five beds per 1,000—over a three-year period. A conditional grant to downsize and upgrade would provide a transition to an approved program of facilities and renovation to modernize hospital services. The grant would encourage the local authority to apply and match part of the funding to meet national criteria and guidelines for this process.

Roemer's Law became influential as increasing numbers of studies in the US showed wide variation in the use of health services, relating utilization to bed supply, with no relation to health status or mortality indicators. Similar

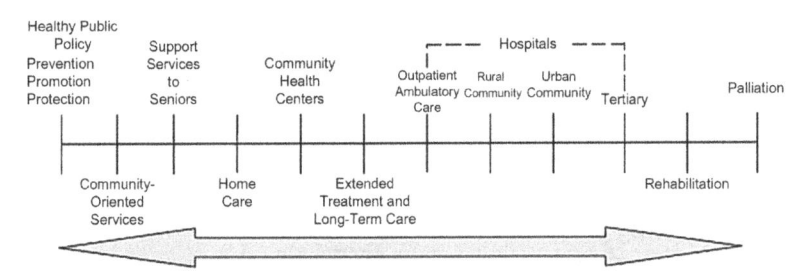

FIGURE 15.1   The continuum of health services. *Source: Tulchinsky TH, Varavikova EA. The New Public Health., 3rd edition, 2014. Chapter 10, p. 537.*

studies showed that utilization of surgical procedures was directly related to the supply of surgeons per capita, with large variations between the US and Canada, and even more so with the UK.

Experience with Health Maintenance Organizations (HMOs) in the US—the best known being the Kaiser Permanente system developed from the 1940s onward—showed lower rates of hospital utilization, compared with rates for insured persons with fee-for-service health plans. HMOs with emphasis on primary care and health promotion show a containment in costs of care consistent with good standards of care.

During the 1970s, payment for hospital care in the US for Medicare patients increasingly moved from per diem payment to DRGs. This shifted hospitals' incentives from maximization of utilization and average length-of-stay (LOS) to maximizing admissions while reducing LOS and increasing alternate forms of care such as outpatient day surgery.

A healthy public policy approach is a continuum of health services including adding promotion, protection, and prevention to the program. Development of the concept of a progressive patient care model (Figure 15.1) gained attention with the rapid development of home-based care, improved ambulatory care, and a growing emphasis on aggressive investigation, diagnosis, and treatment with rapid discharge rates and rehabilitation services. Increasingly, surgical and medical procedures were done on an outpatient basis with positive results and fewer complications, such as hospital-acquired infections. Health care planners and providers increasingly accepted the premise of Roemer's Law by recognizing the central importance of hospital bed supply in determining health economics and policy.

Integration of Hospitals with Community Services

Over time, reducing hospital bed supply and utilization led to linking hospital care to community health services, and also to hospital mergers or integration by rationalizing size and function. Figures 15.2 and 15.3 indicate different forms of hospital integration. Figure 15.2 shows a lateral model

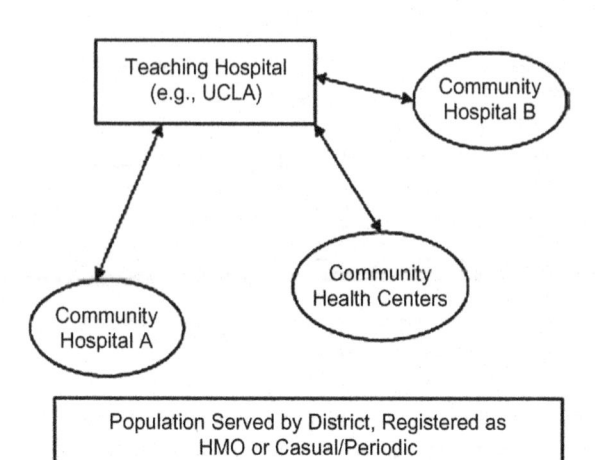

FIGURE 15.2 Integration of health services, University of California, Los Angeles (UCLA) Medical Center. Note: *HMO*, health maintenance organization. *Source: Tulchinsky TH, Varavikova E. The New Public Health, 3rd edition, 2014. Chapter 10, p. 565.*

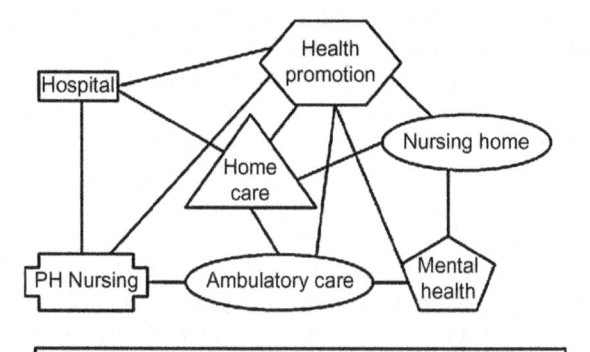

FIGURE 15.3 Vertical integration of health services. Note: *PH*, public health. *Source: Tulchinsky TH, Varavikova E. The New Public Health, 3rd edition, 2014. Chapter 10, p. 565.*

that links different hospitals within a common administrative format, such as that used for hotel chains. Figure 15.3 shows a vertical, more comprehensive form of integration, formed to promote efficiency, name recognition, and shared support services. This form of hospital integration was promoted by the Accountable Care Act of 2010 (Obamacare). Linking hospitals to community-based medical services, prevention, and health promotion can be enhanced through comprehensive payment systems to achieve greater effectiveness in the management of health services. The effectiveness of prevention in reducing hospitalization has been demonstrated in numerous studies on the effects of new vaccines—such as for influenza, pneumococcal pneumonia, and rotavirus—as well as more effective treatment modalities than were available in previous decades. Reorganization to shift emphasis from inpatient care to primary care has many examples. The Los Angeles Department of Health Services operating four large public hospitals reduced hospital care by increasing access to its large network outpatient and primary care. Enrollment in Obamacare benefited many uninsured persons, including homeless people, who used free public hospital emergency departments, thus reducing inpatient care costs by quality primary care.

Certificate of Need (CON)

Capital cost—i.e., the cost to build or renovate a health facility—is based on long-term considerations, but also has an impact on operating costs. The capital cost is pro-rated over the estimated life-time of the building and calculated into the annual operating budget. In some cases, the cost of operating a new health care facility may equal the capital cost of two to three years. Capital costs may be financed by public or private donations, risk-capital investment, or government-guaranteed loans.

State governments regulate capital projects for the construction or equipment of a hospital under CON legislation and procedures. CONs use regulatory powers over capital investments in hospitals and other health facilities to prevent over-development of institutional care as a driver of health financing and costs to public programs such as Medicare and Medicaid. This includes oversight of capital costs being included in operating costs. Regulation occurred both in the US—under the Hill-Burton Act—and in Canada—under the national health insurance system (Medicare). Hospitals operated independently from the government, could borrow or raise money privately through long-term bonds or low-interest loans, but could not build, expand, or amalgamate without CON approval, including the repayment of capital cost amortization built into operating costs over several years.

CON procedures and government assistance with capital costs, allows for greater regulatory control over the direction, distribution, and supply of health facilities. Government norms could also be used to set upper limits or provide incentives to reduce bed supply. Based on Roemer's Law, a common element of cost-containment strategies in most industrialized countries is the reduction in hospital bed supply and development of alternative, appropriate service programs without harming the quality of care. Hospital bed reduction is offset by the transfer of long-stay patients to rehabilitation centers, home-based care programs, or to nursing homes with lower capital and operating costs. Overall, maintaining quality of care is not compatible with policies that support a high ratio of beds to population, because of the excessive resources required to sustain, staff, and service these beds. In other words, hospital beds in excess of actual need are at the expense of other, more fundamental health needs in a community.

Health expenditures in the US by category of services for the period 1960–2014 are seen in Table 15.1. In general, per capita expenditures on health in proportion to Gross Domestic Product (GDP) have increased steeply over the years, while proportions have shifted primarily among hospitals, nursing homes, nursing and home-based care. In 1980, hospital care accounted for 39.4 percent of total health expenditures and declined to 32 percent in 2014 largely due to reduced bed capacity. Home-based care increased from 0.2 percent in 1960 to 2.7 percent in 2014. Between 1960 and 2014, physician and other clinical services have been relatively stable, involving around 21–23 percent of total expenditure. Expenditure on nursing homes increased, reflecting a policy to increase the availability of these facilities. Governmental and private health insurance administration grew from 3.9 percent to 7.7 percent of health costs between 1980 and 2014.

The OECD 2015 data report shows that the US spent far more per capita on health care than any other developed country—i.e., $9,451 per person, compared to $4,003 in the UK, $4,608 in Canada, and in Sweden $5,218 with the OECD average being $3,814. According to the World Bank, in 2015 the US spent 16.9 percent of its GDP on health compared to an average of 10.6 percent for other OECD countries.

Hospital Supply, Utilization and Costs

The hospital beds per 1,000 population in the US declined from 3.5 beds in 2000 to 2.9 beds/1,000 in 2013, while the hospital bed supply for OECD countries declined from 5.6/1,000 in 2000 to 4.8/1,000 population in 2013. However, Japan and Korea maintain high hospital bed capacity partially explained by higher proportions of aged population, yet operate efficient health services. The ratio of acute-care hospital beds to population in the US increased between 1940 and 1980, and declined thereafter. The role of hospital beds, ambulatory, and community-oriented care, is changing as a result of rising economic pressures for cost containment as well as the increasing effectiveness of community care. In the US, hospital utilization, average length-of-stay (ALS) and occupancy rates have shown a decline over the past few decades. Hospital staff per 1,000 patient days increased rather steeply since the 1960s, reflecting increased support, technical services, and greater severity of illness of patients hospitalized. Increased staffing, technological innovations, and expensive medications increased the cost of patient care in hospitals. Table 15.2 shows the trend in hospital bed supply and percentage occupancy in acute care nonfederal general hospitals in the US from 1980 to 2013.

Table 15.2 shows the decline in hospital beds and length of stay as an outcome of the policy changes resulting from application of Roemer's Law. The trend in the US has thus been to decrease hospital bed supply and utilization.

TABLE 15.2 Acute Care Hospital Bed Supply and Utilization, USA, 1970–2013

Facilities	1970	1980	1990	2000	2010	2013
Beds per 1,000 population	4.3	4.5	3.7	2.9	2.6	2.5
Discharges per 1,000 population	NA	175	125	113	116	NA
Average length of stay	NA	7.6	7.2	5.8	5.4	5.4
Total days of care per 1,000 population	NA	1303	819	558	554	NA
Percent occupancy	77	75	67	64	65	63
Outpatient surgeries % of total surgeries	NA	16.3	50.5	62.7	63.6	65.6

Note: Includes Acute care community hospitals; does not include federal hospitals. NA, data not available.
Figures rounded
Source: National Center for Health Statistics. Health, United States, 2015, Tables 89, 90, 91, 92, 93. Available at: https://www.cdc.gov/nchs/data/hus/hus15.pdf.

Despite population ageing, this resulted from a multitude of developments, including changing patterns of morbidity, ambulatory services, and inpatient care. Adoption of the DRG system of payment, greater stress on health economics, and cost containment, with enhanced efficiency in care, as well as advances in medical care, greater health consciousness in the general population, and primary prevention are features of current policy strategies to improve population health.

Governments can directly and indirectly implement regulatory factors that can affect both the supply of hospital beds, access to services, and the amount and method of payment. Other measures or incentives affect the need for care as well as the quality and efficiency of services provided. In health care, market mechanisms are modified by regulations, incentives and other factors used to promote a balance of preventive, curative, and rehabilitative services, as well as health promotion activities to improve health and selecting the most appropriate care for individual patients.

During the 1980s especially, many countries in Europe began reducing their hospital bed supply as a measure to constrain rates of increase in costs of health services and to shift emphasis to primary and preventive care. As seen in Figure 15.4, acute care hospital bed to population ratios declined from the 1980s to 2015 in the Russian Federation by 39 percent, in Germany by 26 percent, France by 24 percent, and in Israel by 37 percent. This represents a decline in Western Europe as a whole by 26 percent. Russia has relatively low total health expenditures per capita and high levels of hospital bed ratios, which have been reduced since 1990 and created the opportunity for

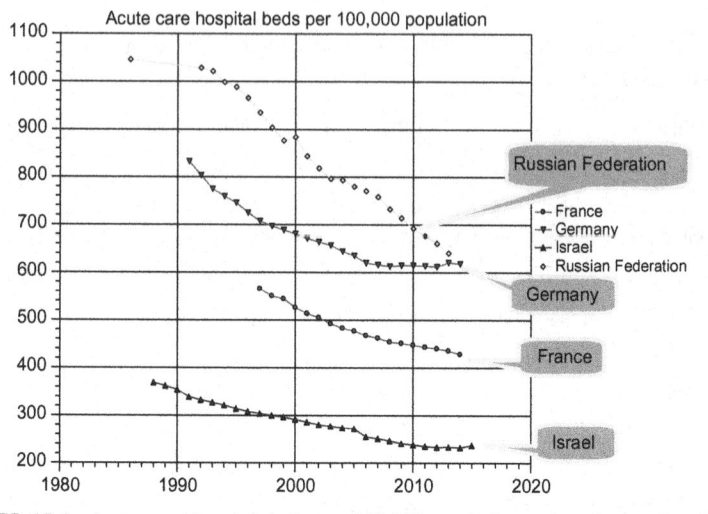

FIGURE 15.4 Acute care hospital beds per 100,000 population, selected countries, WHO European Region, 1985–2014. *Source: World Health Organization, European Region. Health for All Database, 2016. Available at: http://data.euro.who.int/hfadb/ (19 April 2017).*

BOX 15.1 Managing Excess Hospital Bed Capacity

- Convert to long-term care (LTC) facility—extended care, rehabilitation, chronic care, or elderly people's housing.
- Close maternity homes—replace with maternity units in district general hospitals.
- Develop acute psychiatric units in general hospitals—conversion of excess acute-care beds, closure of long-term psychiatric beds, development of community services and group residential facilities.
- Develop acute geriatric units in general hospitals—short-term care, with home and LTC facilities.
- Develop tuberculosis (TB) units in general hospitals—short-term investigation and therapy, with closure of long-term beds in TB hospitals and strengthening community care systems.
- Develop detoxification units for alcohol- and drug abuse—general hospitals with community facilities support.
- Convert to special needs shelters—refugees, homeless people, abuse- or rape survivors.

Source: Tulchinsky TH, Varavikova EA. The New Public Health. 3rd edition, 2014. Chapter 11, Box 11.11, p. 604.

---

reallocating staff and resources to other programs in support of population health. Israel maintains a low hospital bed to population ratio and moderate health expenditure as a percent of GDP while having high life expectancy.

Managing excess hospital facilities can be addressed in many ways (see Box 15.1). Integration of hospitals for efficiency, administration, and other functions is a major method of downsizing the hospital system. Hospitals can be integrated with community-based primary care, long-term care, health promotion, and preventive care. Services in obsolescent facilities—such as maternity homes—can be integrated into general hospitals to increase safety and reduce costs. Mental health units can be developed in general hospitals for short-term assessment and treatment. Similarly, geriatric and hospice units can be developed for short-term assessment. Tuberculosis short-term treatment can be incorporated into general hospitals and followed up with Directly Observed Therapy, short course (DOTs) by community-based health workers. Short-term detoxification units for alcohol- and drug abuse can be integrated with associated community-based follow-up systems and residential rehabilitation facilities. Obsolete facilities can be closed, demolished, or converted for other purposes.

Market Forces in Health

Market forces are those factors which encourage buyers to acquire the best product at the lowest cost compared with competing products, or in the case of health care, competing service providers. In health care, classic market forces include dedicated taxation or social security, out-of-pocket costs, insurance coverage, regulation of supply and demand, quality competition in costs, and the macro-efficiency of the system as a whole. Moreover, integration of similar, or complementary, facilities—also known as vertical and lateral integration of the system and incentives in its payment systems, availability of services, reputation, accessibility, and the existence of complementary programs, such as primary- and home-based care, play an important role, as does the efficiency of activities in health promotion, prevention, and care. More beds - more hospitalizations had corollary "laws" such as "more surgeons - more surgery" where excess supply resulted in higher, and often harmful, utilization. Major competitors and market factors in health care are included in Box 15.2.

In health systems there are modifying factors that have major effects on market forces. Understanding these factors, as summarized in Table 15.3, is an important part to prepare a strategic role for a manager, provider, and policy planner in health systems. The supply of hospital beds is one example of a modifier by governmental regulatory factors. Other factors are related to access to services, price and method of payment, along with others that affect need for care, as well as the quality and efficiency of a service modified by governmental regulatory factors.

Market mechanisms are modified by regulations and incentives, among others, that are used to promote a balance of preventive, curative, and rehabilitative services. These also include health promotion to improve general health while helping the individual seek, and find, the most appropriate care at any point in time. The factors that regulate markets are

BOX 15.2 Classical Market Forces in Health Systems

- Dedicated taxation/social security.
- Cost of out-of-pocket payments.
- Coverage and cost of insurance.
- Hospital bed supply regulation - acute and long term care
- Demand for services.
- Availability of services.
- Competition in cost and quality.
- System macro-efficiency.
- Vertical integration—amalgamation of similar facilities.
- Lateral integration—amalgamation of complementary facilities.
- System micro-efficiency.
- Incentives of payment systems.
- Disincentives of payment systems.
- Reputation.
- Accessibility.
- Complementary programs—primary care and home-based care.
- Efficiency of health promotion, prevention, and medical care.

Source: Adapted from Tulchinsky TH, Vatravikova EA. The New Public Health, 3rd edition, 2014. Chapter 11, Box 11.12, p. 604.

summarized in Box 15.3. The regulation of supply, which includes the restriction of hospital bed ratios by national policy, entails the application of Roemer's Law. This has been adopted in most industrialized countries as a cornerstone of health systems' adaptation to the need for cost containment. Greater efficiency in prevention and rapid diagnosis and treatment of many conditions, result in the avoidance of hospitalization or shortening length-of-stay. Dramatic reductions in gastric surgery resulted from the discovery of the readily curable bacterial cause of peptic ulcers (see Chapter 22). Cardiovascular surgery was also dramatically changed by efficient cardiac catheterization and stent insertion, resulting in reduced incidence of coronary events and coronary artery bypass surgery. Greater use of vaccines such as pneumomococcal pneumonia, influenza and rotavirus have similar effects in reducing hospitalizations and lengths of stay.

Funding system changes from hospital payments on a per diem basis to diagnosis-related groups (DRGs) have altered financial incentives by reducing length-of-stay and promoting greater efficiency, leading DRGs to become the standard method in the US and many other countries. Some countries require user fees, or insurance deductible limits, to provide disincentive for inappropriate hospitalization or length-of-stay. However, this usually tends to discriminate against the poor and those in greatest need, and is therefore not considered fair or effective and may deter people from seeking

TABLE 15.3 Market Forces and Modifying Factors in the Economics of Health

Determinants of Demand	Modifiers of Demand	Examples
Classical market factors	Supply Demand Competition in cost Competition in quality System macro-efficiency Vertical integration Lateral integration System micro-efficiency Incentives, disincentives Reputation Method of payment Satisfaction	Hospital beds per 1000; providers combine to restrict supply Prepayment increases effective demand Providers combine to restrict supply Managed care versus fee-for-service plans District health systems and HMOs Multiservice systems for defined populations Multihospital networks for efficiency Quality improvement, computerization, staff attitudes, scheduling, and service hours Budget, block, per diem, DRG Consumer, community, provider, staff
Regulatory factors	Regulate supply Regulate demand Regulate price Regulate method of payment Health promotion issues	Reduce acute care hospital beds/1,000 Gatekeeper functions User fees Fee control, income capping, salary, or capitation payment for doctors DRGs, block budgets for hospitals Food enrichment, immunization, smoking cessation, seat belts
Health and societal factors	Differing population needs Social inequities Improve infrastructure to reduce needs Socioeconomic improvements Public social policies Health as a national and local priority Health promotion Improve KABP (knowledge, attitudes, beliefs, and practices)	Demographic and epidemiologic transitions Reduce social gaps, universal access, risk groups Sewage, water treatment, road safety National and family incomes Social security, pensions, compensation Health system reform Involve community and providers in prevention Providers, beneficiaries, consumers rights, needs, responsibilities
System determinants	Shift in resource allocation Technological innovations Substitution Total Quality Management	Balance of institutional and community care New vaccines, drugs, diagnostics, oral rehydration therapy (ORT) community health workers Home care, generic drugs, nurse practitioners External accreditation, internal review systems patient choice, continuous quality improvement

Note: *HMO*, health maintenance organization; *DRG*, diagnosis-related group; *ORS*, oral rehydration salts.
Source: Tulchinsky TH, Varavikova EA. The New Public Health, 3rd edition, 2014. Chapter 11, p. 605.

BOX 15.3 **Regulatory Factors**

- Regulate supply.
- Regulate method of payment; substitute DRGs for per diem payment.
- Regulate demand—gatekeeper, user fees.
- Regulate price.
- Regulate benefits.
- Health promotion issues such as regulation of tobacco and seat belt usage.
- Accreditation of providers.

Source: *Tulchinsky TH, Varavikova EA. The New Public Health, 3rd edition, 2014. Chapter 11, p. 604.*

necessary clinical- and hospital care, and immunization. A balance of prevention (including health promotion), curative, and rehabilitation programs improves the health of a population and enables people to have the most appropriate care. Pay-for-Performance systems have been implemented in the UK, the US (e.g., California), and elsewhere as incentive programs meant to increase the quality of health care. However, they remain controversial with the concern being the validity in measuring improvement. This system, therefore, requires more documented experience.

Another important feature in terms of cost containment in health systems is the gatekeeper function of physicians and emergency departments. It is important for family physicians and hospital-based doctors to carefully assess the justification for hospitalization. Most physicians are aware of the importance of cost control and are in a position to deal with anxious families pressing for hospitalization which may, ultimately, do more harm than good. Quality monitoring and standard guidelines for hospitals is a growing method of promoting safety, efficiency in diagnosis and care with improved attention to outpatient care following discharge.

Of great importance is the concept of a health system as a continuum of programs and services (see Figure 15.1) with a balance in resource allocation for health promotion in funding systems. This places emphasis on the need to fill in the gaps in the range of services and programs in order to meet population health needs.

ETHICAL ISSUES

Rationing as a method of cost control is controversial and seems counter intuitive. The rationale has been to emphasize provision of a balance of publicly funded services while limiting overgrowth of some elements of a health system in order to develop other services required to meet needs of age, gender, underserved, and other relatively deprived risk groups. This is especially important for developing countries seeking universal coverage while underserved populations need proactive outreach services to address the heavier burden of disease. High numbers of hospitals—often founded by well meaning donors—are located in urban areas and if unconstrained by regulation, result in a focus of public expenditures on middle-class population centers. Research on the issues of hospital supply found a significant positive association between hospital bed availability and hospital utilization rates, and that historical development of major hospital centers dominate public funding for health.

Improvements in medical care and prevention have greatly contributed to the acceptance of Roemer's Law. Innovations such as laparoscopic surgery, early diagnosis and cure of chronic peptic ulcer disease, vaccinations such as pneumococcal pneumonia, influenza, and rotavirus, and vastly improving treatment of acute coronary incidents, HIV, and hepatitis C, among other examples, have shifted the emphasis to ambulatory medical care with a more cautious approach to hospitalization as the dominant element of health economics. Most cancer and chronic disease care is provided in outpatient departments.

Health care facility infections are of increasing concern due to harm they do to patients and prolonging hospital stays with attendant costs. They also occur in long term care facilities and in community care. Prevention of nosocomial infections has been increasingly worrisome as they are often caused by multidrug resistant organisms transferred to patients by common procedures such as drawing blood samples, catheters, and the many complex intrusive procedures of modern medical care. Hand washing and immunization of staff for common preventable conditions are important in hospital management and awareness of potential risks of hospitalization among the public (see Chapter Four).

Issues of inequality in health are important even in countries with advanced national health systems intended to provide health care for all, such as the UK's NHS. The original focus on hospital and medical and hospital services insurance in many health systems has been influenced by Roemer's Law, but a similar focus has to also develop in outreach care for economically and otherwise relatively deprived population groups at risk for a high burden of for a noncommunicable and communicable diseases.

ECONOMIC ISSUES

The practice of modeling health systems, such as applying Roemer's Law—and the experience derived from its many applications over the past 60 years—shows there is much to learn from market economics based on competition and the conversion to a more complex model. Regulation of supply of services and incentive payment systems are vital in any health system to balance the priorities between preventive and comprehensive treatment services.

Health systems have much to learn from operations research (OR), which was initiated in Britain in the 19th century to resolve practical problems such as sorting and delivering within the public mail system. Later, it was applied during World War I and II. In World War II, military planning—e.g., for the Battle of the Atlantic—evolved with interdisciplinary thinking and mathematical modeling producing innovative applications of increasing resources, training and new technology which were highly effective in overcoming the initial calamitous success of the Nazi submarines. Together they helped to increase the safety of convoys crossing the Atlantic from North America to Britain and to Murmansk, in order to sustain the war effort. In more recent iterations of OR, modeling became important in infectious disease control. Eleven Nobel Prizes have been awarded in Economics on Game Theory including for applications in health systems. Game Theory is used to develop alternative strategies and predict possible outcomes, with application in predicting epidemics or economics of managing health systems.

The financing of health services, the economics of health care, and the allocation of resources, whether in terms of money, work force, or fixed assets are a central issue in the New Public Health. Resource allocation decisions with incentives and disincentives are crucial to management of healthcare systems, as in other industries. Cost-effectiveness analysis has become essential in analysis of existing and new diagnostics, drugs, vaccines, and for priority determination in health policy. This approach has taken on the broad view of health promotion, health protection, preventative, curative, and long-term care services. The balance and interdependence are influenced by financing systems and options in alternative ways of expending, and sustaining, resources. Economic analysis, like epidemiologic assessment, is a vital tool in health planning and management, particularly in evaluating the allocation of resources within a health system. Failure to carry out such assessments results in inefficiency in health planning as economic analysis is essential to modern health system management.

The World Bank in 1993 underwent a radical self-appraisal and change regarding health expenditures that were previously seen as a liability for a developing economy. A new concept emerged that recognized investment in health is a positive contributor to economic development, just as education is in the development of people and society. This led to investment in health in developing countries by the International Monetary Fund (IMF) and World Bank, as well as by bilateral and nongovernmental organizations and donors, which are all essential for economic—as well as health—development.

CONCLUSION

Roemer's Law was an important contribution to the theory and practice of managing health systems. Since the 1970s, most high-income countries adopted this concept and reduced acute care hospital bed supplies as a major method to control health costs and improve efficiency in health care. While initially controversial, this approach became standard practice, even in countries with the Semashko Soviet system. Most postsocialist countries—including the Russian Federation during its transition—have adopted the Roemer approach since the 1990s.

For low- and medium-income countries (LMICs), the importance of, and lesson learned from Roemer's Law is to avoid the past mistakes of high income-countries which maintained high levels of hospital bed supply in the mid-20th century. Stress on development of the organization and trained workforce for public health will reap far greater rewards in improving health status than following outdated models of organization and financing systems.

This approach has contributed to a new direction of amalgamating hospitals with lateral integration for improved efficiency and downsizing shared functions. Vertical integration of hospitals with other services in the community creates shared functions in primary care, health promotion, mental health, and health of the elderly and handicapped and vulnerable high-risk groups. In the US, Accountable Care Organizations fostered by the Accountable Care Act (Obamacare) since 2010 characterized this approach. This act adopted some principles and practices of preceding organizations such as Health Maintenance Organizations and precedents like the Kaiser Permanente health care organization and the prepaid group practice model promoted by the labor movement since the 1920s. European countries have adopted variations of these principles and reduced hospital bed capacity while creating many links between hospitals and other community health services.

Challenges remain in all health systems when it comes to sustaining or developing universal coverage, addressing cost control, aging of the population, increasing obesity and diabetes, and emerging infectious diseases. Nonetheless, even in these cases, there are grounds for optimism that preventive and health promotion aspects of public health will gain support and implementation to improve efficiency and appropriate care.

RECOMMENDATIONS

Universal access to health care is a fundamental right recognized by international standards, and should, therefore, be effectively considered in the policy development of all political jurisdictions.

1. National policy should establish standards of licensing, payment- and incentive- systems, in order to maintain a strong balance between institutional care, such as hospitalization, in balance and linkage with ambulatory and primary care, as well as health promotion, health protection, and safety for all citizens.

2. Responsible management of public health systems should include the adoption of policies that ensure hospital regulation, including number of beds, staffing, and support services in order to provide for population needs

in equilibrium with the application of successful measures of health promotion and disease prevention.

3. Integrating hospitals to offer the full range of community-based medical and health promotion services should be fostered by state policy and financial payment systems, in order to achieve effective management of health services, avoid unnecessary duplication of services, and prevent medical errors in a cost-effective manner. Under the Obamacare plan, Accountable Care Organizations voluntarily integrated organization and service provision, and were encouraged with incentives to improve and coordinate better care for beneficiaries under Medicaid and Medicare programs. Links between service organizations to provide care lead to cost savings and redirection of resources (money and staff) from reduced hospitalization to close patient care follow-up and home-based care, compared with the care available to patients in traditionally separate service systems.

4. Roemer's Law was an outstanding concept which deeply affected heath policy and planning worldwide. The lesson is still being absorbed into policy making to achieve comprehensive health for all with limited resources to be used as effectively as possible.

STUDENT REVIEW QUESTIONS

1. Explain the importance of the Hill Burton Act (1946) in health economics and planning in the US.
2. How does the Hill Burton model of inter-government transfer of funds for health provide a model for developing countries?
3. What was the importance of Roemer's Law?
4. What was the impact of health insurance, private or governmental, on demand for hospital care in the US?
5. What innovations in methods of payment were introduced to reduce hospital bed utilization?
6. What other key factors in health helped to change need and demand for hospital care in the US and other countries?
7. What are the trends in acute-care hospital bed supply in the US and other high income countries since the 1970s?
8. How is Roemer's Law important for medium- and low-income countries?
9. What are the alternatives to hospital care?
10. What preventive prevention and health promotion measures reduce the burden of hospitalization?

RECOMMENDED READINGS

1. Bay KS, Nestman LJ. The use of bed distribution and service population indexes for hospital bed allocation. Health Serv Res. 1984;19(2):141–160. Available at: https://www.ncbi.nlm.nih.gov/pubmed/6547418 (accessed 17 April 2017).

2. Bobadilla JL, Cowley P, Musgrove P, Saxenian H. Design, content and financing of an essential national package of health services. Bull World Health Organ. 1994;72:653−662. Available at: https://www.ncbi.nlm.nih.gov/pubmed/7923544 (accessed 17 April 2017).

3. Bunker JP. Surgical manpower: a comparison of operations and surgeons in the United States and in England and Wales. New Engl J Med. 1970;282(3):135−144. Available at: https://www.ncbi.nlm.nih.gov/pubmed/5409538 (accessed 17 April 2017).

4. Centers for Disease Control. A framework for assessing the effectiveness of disease and injury prevention. MMWR Recomm Rep. 1992;41 RR-3:1−12. Available at: https://www.cdc.gov/mmwr/preview/mmwrhtml/00016403.htm (accessed 17 April 2017).

5. Centers for Disease Control and Prevention. Assessing the effectiveness of disease and injury prevention programs: costs and consequences. MMWR Recomm Rep. 1995;44 RR-10:1−10. Available at: https://www.cdc.gov/mmwr/pdf/rr/rr4410.pdf (accessed 17 April 2017).

6. Centers for Medicare & Medicaid Services. Accountable Care Organizations (ACO), 2015. Available at: https://www.cms.gov/Medicare/Medicare-Fee-for-Service-Payment/ACO/index.html (accessed 05 March 2017).

7. Centers for Disease Control and Prevention. Health, United States, 2015. Available at: https://www.cdc.gov/nchs/data/hus/hus15.pdf (accessed 21 April 2017).

8. Chassin MR, Kosecoff J, Park RE, Winslow CM, Kahn KL, Merrick NJ. Does inappropriate use explain geographic variations in the use of health services? JAMA. 1987;258(18):2533−2537. Available at: https://www.ncbi.nlm.nih.gov/pubmed/3312655 (accessed 17 April 2017).

9. Delamater PL, Messina JP, Grady SC, Winkler Prins V, Shortridge AM. Do more hospital beds lead to higher hospitalization rates? a spatial examination of Roemer's Law. PLoS One. 2013;8(2):e54900. Available at: http://journals.plos.org/plosone/article/file?id = 10.1371/journal.pone.0054900&type = printable (accessed 10 January 2017).

10. Dielman JL, Baral R, Birger M, Bui AL, Chapin A, Bulchis A, et al. US spending on personal health care and public health, 1996−2013. JAMA. 2016;316(24):2627−2646. Available at: http://jamanetwork.com/journals/jama/fullarticle/2594716 (accessed 10 January 2017).

11. Ferrier G, Leleu H, Valdmanis V. The impact of CON regulation on hospital efficiency. Health Care Manag Sci. 2010;13:84−100. Available at: https://www.ncbi.nlm.nih.gov/pubmed/20402285 (accessed 17 April 2017).

12. Fielding JE, Teutsch S, Breslow L. A framework for public health in the United States. Public Health Rev. 2010;32(1):174−189. Available at: https://www.researchgate.net/publication/45432987_A_Framework_for_Public_Health_in the_United_States (accessed 5 April 2017).

13. Health Resources and Services Administration. Hill-Burton free and reduced-cost health care. US Department of Health and Human Development, 2016. Available at: https://www.hrsa.gov/gethealthcare/affordable/hillburton/ (accessed 26 December 2016).

14. Institute of Medicine. Crossing the quality chasm: a new health system for the 21st century. Washington, DC: National Academies Press, 2007. Available at: https://www.nap.edu/catalog/10027/crossing-the-quality-chasm-a-new-health-system-for-the (accessed 17 April 2017).

15. Institute of Medicine. Crossing the quality chasm: a new health system for the 21st century. Washington, DC: National Academies Press, 2001. Available at: https://www.nap.edu/read/10027/chapter/2#2 (accessed 10 January 2017).

16. Kaiser Family Foundation. Health care costs: a primer. Technical Rep. 2009. 7670−02. Available at: http://kff.org/report-section/health-care-costs-a-primer-2012-report/ (accessed 17 April 2017).

17. Kelley JE, Burrus RG, Burns RP, Graham LD, Chandler KE. Safety, efficacy, cost and morbidity of laparoscopic versus open cholecystectomy; a prospective analysis of 228 consecutive patients. Am Surg. 1993;59:23–27. Available at: https://www.ncbi.nlm.nih.gov/pubmed/8480927 (accessed 17 April 2017).

18. Kleczkowski BM, Roemer MI, Van Der Wertt A. National health systems and their re-orientation towards health. Geneva: World Health Organization, 1984. Available at: http://apps.who.int/iris/bitstream/10665/41638/1/WHO_PHP_77.pdf (accessed 5 April 2017).

19. Koehlmoos TL. The US healthcare system and the Roemer model. Available at: http://www.powershow.com/view/8400f-ZjA4Y/The_US_Healthcare_System_and_the_Roemer_Model_powerpoint_ppt_presentation (accessed 12 April 2017).

20. Kuttner R. Market-based failure-a second opinion on U.S. health care costs. New Engl J Med. 2007;358:549–551. Available at: http://www.nejm.org/doi/full/10.1056/NEJMp0800265#t=article (accessed 17 April 2017).

21. Mathauer I, Wittenbecher F. Hospital payment systems based on diagnosis-related groups: experiences in low- and middle-income countries. Bull World Health Org. 2013;91:746–756A. Available at: http://www.who.int/bulletin/volumes/91/10/12-115931/en/ (accessed 10 January 2017).

22. McGlynn E, Asch M, Adams J, Keesey J, Hicks J, DeCristoforo A, et al. The quality of health care delivered to adults in the United States. New Engl J Med. 2003;348:2635–2645. Available at: http://www.nejm.org/doi/full/10.1056/NEJMsa022615#t=article (accessed 17 April 2017).

23. Medicare. Health, United States spotlight health care expenditures & payers, September 2016. Available at: https://www.cdc.gov/nchs/data/hus/hus_spotlight_sept16.pdf (accessed 10 January 2017).

24. Mitchell JB. Physician DRG's. New Engl J Med. 1985;313:670–675. Available at: http://www.nejm.org/doi/full/10.1056/NEJM198509123131106 (accessed 19 April 2017).

25. Mulley AG. Inconvenient truths about supplier induced demand and unwarranted variation in medical practice. BMJ. 2009;339:b4073. Available at: http://www.bmj.com/content/339/bmj.b4073.long (accessed 19 April 2017).

26. Murray CJL, Govindaraj R, Musgrove P. National health expenditures: a global analysis. Bull World Health Org. 1994;72:623–637. Available at: http://apps.who.int/iris/bitstream/10665/53378/1/bulletin_1994_72(4)_623-637.pdf (accessed 19 April 2017).

27. National Center for Health Statistics. Health, United States, 2015: with special feature on racial and ethnic health disparities. Hyattsville, MD. 2015. Available at: https://www.cdc.gov/nchs/data/hus/hus15.pdf (accessed 10 January 2017).

28. National Conference of State Legislatures: CON-certificate of need state laws. 2016. Available at: http://www.ncsl.org/research/health/con-certificate-of-need-state-laws.aspx (accessed 19 April 2017).

29. Nobel Prize for Economics. Robert J. Aumann-Facts. Nobelprize.org. Nobel Media AB 2014. Web. 23 Apr 2017. http://www.nobelprize.org/nobel_prizes/economic-sciences/laureates/2005/aumann-facts.html (accessed 21 April 2017).

30. OECD. Health Data. 2014. How does the United States compare. Available at: http://www.oecd.org/unitedstates/Briefing-Note-UNITED-STATES-2014.pdf (accessed 10 January 2017).

31. OECD. Fiscal sustainability of health systems: bridging health and finance perspectives. Paris: OECD Publishing, 2015. Available at: DOI: http://dx.doi.org/10.1787/9789264233386-en (accessed 19 April 2017).

32. OECD. Health at a Glance 2015. OECD Indicators. Available at: http://www.keepeek. com/Digital-Asset-Management/oecd/social-issues-migration-health/health-at-a-glance-2015_health_glance-2015-en#page106 (accessed 19 April 2017).
33. Parnaby J, Towill D. Enabling innovation in health-care delivery. Health Serv Manage Res. 2008;21:141−154. Available at: https://www.ncbi.nlm.nih.gov/pubmed/18647942 (accessed 10 January 2017).
34. Pasley BH, Lagoe RJ, Marshall NO. Excess acute care bed capacity and its causes: the experience of New York State. Health Serv Res. 1995;30:115−131. Available at: https://www.ncbi.nlm.nih.gov/pmc/articles/PMC1070353/ (accessed 19 April 2017).
35. Rechel B, Wright S, Barlow J, McKee M. Hospital capacity planning: from measuring stocks to modeling flows. Bull World Health Org. 2010;88:632−636. Available at: http://www.who.int/bulletin/volumes/88/8/09-073361/en/ (accessed 10 January 2017).
36. Rittenhouse DR, Robinson JC. Improving quality in Medicaid: the use of care management processes for chronic illness and preventive care. Med Care. 2006;44(1):47−54. Available at: https://www.ncbi.nlm.nih.gov/pubmed/16365612 (accessed 19 April 2017).
37. Rivers PA, Fottler MD, Younis MZ. Does certificate of need really contain hospital costs in the United States? Health Educ J. 2007;66(3):229−244. Available at: http://journals.sagepub.com/doi/pdf/10.1177/0017896907080127 (accessed 19 April 2017).
38. Robinson R. Cost-benefit analysis. BMJ. 1993;307:924−926. Available at: http://www.bmj.com/content/bmj/307/6909/924.full.pdf (accessed 19 April 2017).
39. Roemer MI. National health systems throughout the world. Annu Rev Publ Health. 1993;14:335−353. Available at: http://www.annualreviews.org/doi/pdf/10.1146/annurev.pu.14.050193.002003. (accessed 15 April 2017).
40. Schroeder SA. We can do better-improving the health of the American people. New Engl J Med. 2007;357:1221−1228. Available at: http://www.nejm.org/doi/full/10.1056/NEJMsa073350#t = article (accessed 19 April 2017).
41. Shain M, Roemer MI. Hospital costs relate to the supply of beds. Mod Hosp. 1959;92(4):71−73.
42. Smith C, Cowan C, Heffler S, Shortell SM, Gillies R, Wu F. United States innovations in healthcare delivery. Public Health Rev. 2010;32:190−212.
43. Steen J. The Dartmouth atlas on Roemer's Law, 2008. Available at: http://ahpanet.org/files/TheDartmouthAtlasonRoemer'sLaw%20b.pdf (accessed 10 January 2017).
44. Thomasson M. Health insurance in the United States. Available at: https://eh.net/encyclopedia/health-insurance-in-the-united-states/ (accessed 17 April 2017).
45. Tulchinsky TH, Varavikova EA. The new public health. 3rd edition. San Diego: Academic Press/Elsevier, 2014. Chapter 11, p. 575−611. Available at: http://www.sciencedirect.com/science/book/9780124157668 (accessed 19 April 2017).
46. University of California Los Angeles. Milton I. Roemer, pioneering UCLA health services professor dies, January 08, 2001. Available at: http://newsroom.ucla.edu/releases/Milton-I-Roemer-Pioneering-UCLA-2053 (accessed 10 January 2017).
47. US Department Health and Human Services Health Services and Resources Administration. Hill-Burton free and reduced-cost health care, updated April 2017. Available at: https://www.hrsa.gov/get-health-care/affordable/hill-burton/index.html (accessed 28 December 2017).
48. US Federal Trade Commission and US Department of Justice: Improving health care: a dose of competition. Washington, DC: Tech. rep., US, Government Printing Office, 2004. Available at: https://www.ftc.gov/reports/improving-health-care-dose-competition-report-federal-trade-commission-department-justice (accessed 18 April 2017).

49. Vayda E. A comparison of surgical rates in Canada and in England and Wales. New Engl J Med. 1973;289(23):1224–1229. Available at: http://www.nejm.org/doi/full/10.1056/NEJM197312062892305 (accessed 19 April 2017).

50. Welch HG, Sharp SM, Gottlieb DJ, Skinner JS, Wennberg JE. Geographic variation in diagnosis frequency and risk of death among medicare beneficiaries. JAMA. 2011;305 (11):1113–1118. Available at: http://jamanetwork.com/journals/jama/fullarticle/646152 (accessed 19 April 2017).

51. Welch WP, Miller ME, Welch HG, Fisher ES, Wennberg JE. Geographic variation in expenditures for physicians' services in the United States. New Engl J Med. 1993;328 (9):621–627. Available at: http://www.nejm.org/doi/full/10.1056/NEJM199303043280906 (accessed 19 April 2017).

52. Wennberg JE. Outcomes research, cost containment, and the fear of health care rationing. The New Engl J Med. 1990;323:1202–1204. Available at: http://www.nejm.org/doi/full/10.1056/NEJM199010253231710 (accessed 19 April 2017).

53. World Bank. World development review, 1993: investing in health. New York, NY: Oxford University Press, 1993. Available at: https://openknowledge.worldbank.org/handle/10986/5976 (accessed 19 April 2017).

54. World Health Organization, Regional Office for Europe. European health care reforms: analysis of current strategies, Summary. Copenhagen: WHO, 1996. Available at: http://www.euro.who.int/__data/assets/pdf_file/0005/111011/sumhecareform.pdf (accessed 19 April 2017).

55. World Health Organization. Global Health Observatory (GHO) data 2016. Accessible at: http://www.who.int/gho/en/ (accessed 10 January 2017).

56. World Health Organization. European Region. Heath for All Data Base, 2016. Available at: http://www.euro.who.int/en/data-and-evidence (accessed 17 April 2017).

Chapter 16

John Enders, Jonas Salk, Albert Sabin and Eradication of Poliomyelitis

ABSTRACT

Poliomyelitis has been one of the most feared infectious diseases because of its crippling effects and its presence in high- and medium-income countries especially during the 1920s to 1950s. The development of effective inactivated (killed) Salk (IPV) vaccine and live attenuated Sabin vaccine (OPV) in the 1950s and 1960s led to immunization programs which vastly reduced the disease and led the World Health Organization (WHO) in 1988 to call for eradication of polio following the successful eradication of smallpox. Enormous global effort has led to final stages of eradication but with some worrying problems in the "end stage" strategies. In most of the world, Sabin OPV has been used to provide herd and personal immunity, but rarely converts to active vaccine-associated paralytic poliomyelitis (VAPP) which can cause local outbreaks of clinical polio. For this reason, the United States and most industrialized countries adopted policies of Salk IPV alone which is not prone to cause clinical polio but can allow the silent spread of wild poliomyelitis virus (WPV).

In 2014, the WHO recommended adding IPV to the widely used OPV along with removing type 2 so that OPV becomes a bivalent vaccine. The addition of IPV will enhance antibody development and protect against rare but worrying conversion of OPV to wild virus activity as vaccine-associated paralytic poliomyelitis (VAPP). Inclusion of IPV will strengthen routine immunization coverage and reduce the need for frequent massive supplementary immunization activities (SIAs). Adding OPV to immunization schedules in IPV-only countries would protect against inadvertent silent entry of wild poliovirus (WPV) by travelers or refugees from countries where WPV may still circulate. The combination of OPV (bivalent instead of trivalent) and IPV is the logical safest and least costly choice for the end game of polio eradication. In 2013–14, WPV silently entered and spread in Israel but without causing clinical cases. As of Sepember 2017, WPV cases are known in only two countries (Pakistan 4 cases and 6 cases in Afghanistan). The end-game strategy for global eradication is still in process with hope for eradication by 2024.

Case Studies in Public Health. DOI: http://dx.doi.org/10.1016/B978-0-12-804571-8.00014-7
383

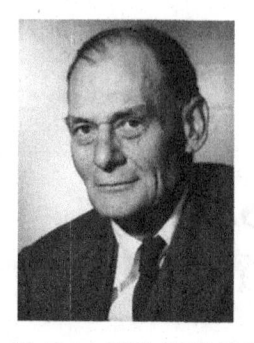

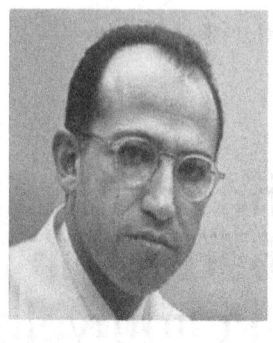

John Franklin Enders (1897–1985), Nobel Prize 1954 in Medicine for discovery of polio virus. *Courtesy: Harvard University, Portrait Collection, Francis A Countway Library of Medicine, Dept. of Rare Books and Special Collections, C-CL02, Box 43, f. 2. (photo credit Walter R Fleischer).*

Jonas Salk (1914–1995), developed and field tested the inactivated polio vaccine (IPV) 1954, known as Salk vaccine and used worldwide. *Courtesy of the Jonas Salk Polio Vaccine Collection, 1917–2005, UA.90.F89, University Archives, Archives & Special Collections, University of Pittsburgh Library System.*

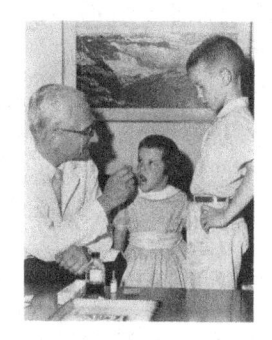

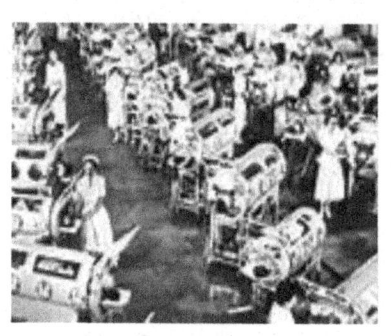

Albert Sabin (1906–1993), developed and field tested the attenuated live polio vaccine (OPV), licenced in 1961, known as Sabin vaccine and used worldwide as the basis for global eradication of polio. *Courtesy of the Hauck Center for the Albert B. Sabin Archives, Henry R. Winkler Center for the History of the Health Professions, University of Cincinnati Libraries.*

Patients with bulbar poliomyelitis in iron lungs during the 1940s and 1950s epidemics. *Source: WHO Global polio eradication initative. Available at: http://www.polioeradication.org/.*

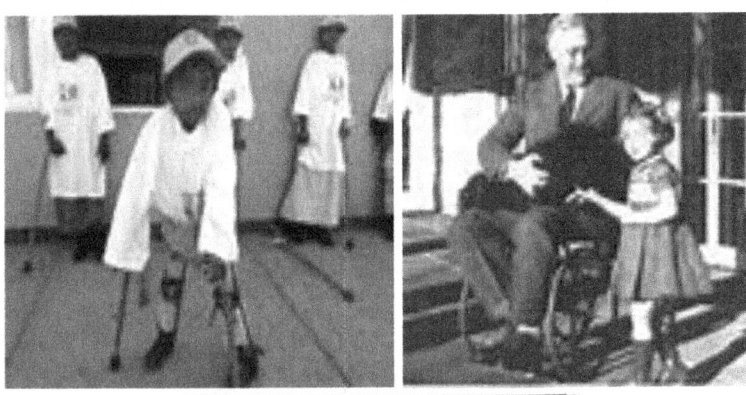

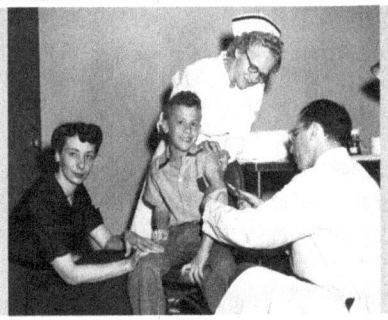

Peter Salk receiving the still experimental inactivated poliovirus vaccine from his father, Jonas Salk. Salk also injected himself, his wife, and his two other sons. Victims of crippling polio including US President Franklin Roosevelt. *Courtesy: March of Dimes.*

BACKGROUND

Poliomyelitis was first described by British pediatrician Michael Underwood in 1789. The first epidemic in the United States was reported in 1843, but the disease was sporadic until the 20th century when improved sanitation changed the epidemiology of the widespread distribution, onset age and severity of poliovirus infection and clinical poliomyelitis. In the early part of the 20th century polio epidemics struck every few years in the summer months paralyzing hundreds of thousands of children and adults every year, including those in rich and poor countries striking terror in parents of temporary or lifelong paralysis of their children, although death was infrequent.

Poliovirus infection may be asymptomatic or cause an acute nonspecific mild febrile illness. It may reach more severe forms of aseptic meningitis and acute flaccid paralysis (AFP) with long-term residual paralysis or death during the acute phase. Poliovirus has strains 1, 2, and 3. Poliomyelitis is transmitted by oral-fecal contamination by direct person-to-person contact, but also via environmental contamination from sewage. Large-scale

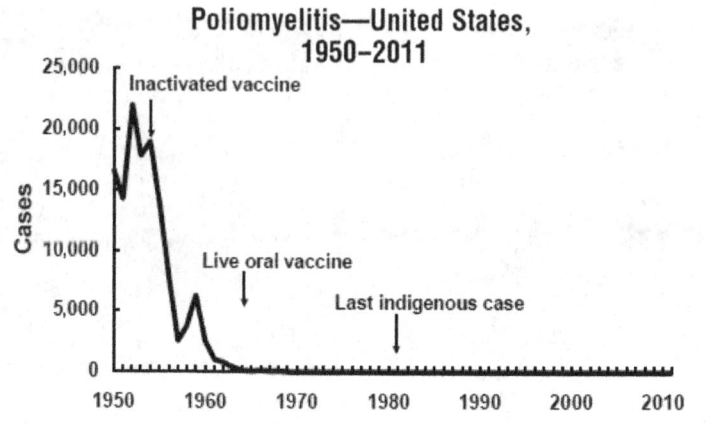

FIGURE 16.1   Poliomyelitis, cases and impact of vaccines, United States 1950–2010. *Source: CDC. Poliomyelitis. 13th edition, 2015. Available at: http://www.cdc.gov/vaccines/pubs/pink-book/polio.html.*

epidemics of disease, with attendant paralysis and death, occurred in industrialized countries in the 1940s and 1950s, engendering widespread fear and panic with thousands of clinical cases of what was commonly called "infantile paralysis"

The principle pioneers in the poliomyelitis eradication process were John Enders, Jonas Salk, and Albert Sabin each of whom benefited from working with dedicated colleagues to lay the foundation for polio control and ultimate eradication. John Enders was born in West Hartford, CT in 1897. His father was a banker. After high school he went to Yale University in 1916, but in 1917 he joined the US Army Air Corps as an Ensign pilot. After the war he returned to Yale to finish undergraduate studies to become a language teacher. He moved to Harvard in 1920 studying biology achieving his PhD in 1930 working with virus immunity such as for mumps. At the Boston Children's Medical Center, he worked with colleagues TH Weller and FC Robbins on the polio virus which they were able to isolate and grow in the laboratory. For this the three members of this team were awarded the Nobel Prize in Medicine in 1954. In 1952, more than 21,000 paralytic cases of the disease were reported in the United States (Figure 16.1).

Growth of the poliovirus in tissue culture by Enders and colleagues in 1949 led to development and wide-scale testing of the first inactivated (killed) polio vaccine (IPV) by Jonas Salk in the mid-1950s. Jonas Salk was born in 1914 in a poor Jewish immigrant family in New York City where his father worked in the garment industry. Jonas flourished in studies and attended New York City College for his BA then medical school at New York University graduating in 1939. He moved to the University of Michigan to work on influenza viruses and in 1947 he moved to the

University of Pittsburgh to work on research on polio, then known as infantile paralysis. By 1951, Salk and colleagues developed an inactivated killed virus vaccine for all three seroypes of the disease. Testing of the polio vaccine began in 1952 and expanded over the next 2 years, to become one of the largest and most highly publicized clinical trials including prior testing the experimental vaccine on himself, his wife and sons. The inactivated Salk vaccine was used in the United States and many other countries successfully reducing polio cases drastically. Salk's achievement following the largest clinical trial ever conducted involving 1.8 million children in the United States, Canada, and Finland with some 300,000 volunteers to carry it out stirred great public interest and hope worldwide. With the outstanding success of an international field trial in the control of this much feared disease Salk became a national and global folk hero.

In 1955, the "Cutter incident" occurred, in which an inadequately inactivated Salk vaccine containing live virulent polio virus was used to immunize 200,000 persons, of whom 70,000 became ill, 200 permanently paralyzed and 10 died. This incident led to the cessation of use of Salk vaccine and its replacement with Sabin attenuated vaccine. A federal National Vaccine Injury Compensation Program introduced in 1986 provided a compensation system to prevent manufacturers from withdrawing from vaccine production due to litigation.

In the 1990's, Salk vaccine was reintroduced initially along with Sabin vaccine in the US with more stringent monitoring, enhanced safety and immunogenicity to prevent the eight − ten vaccine associated polio cases per year arising from genetic mutations from the attenuated oral vaccine. Later IPV was used alone in the US and adopted in most high income countries while OPV was the staple method used in medium and low income countries.

Albert Sabin was born in 1906 in Poland, and in 1919 his Jewish family left Bialystock to escape pogroms to emigrate to the United States arriving in 1922 at age 16 moving to New Jersey where his father worked in the clothing industry. Albert, with very little English initially, succeeded to excel in high school and he entered New York University medical faculty obtaining his medical degree in 1931. As a first year medical student he worked nights in the hospital laboratory and while working at the laboratory, he gained recognition as a researcher by developing a way to dramatically speed up the typing of pneumococci bacteria so that it took only a fraction of the previous time required to conduct the tests. He trained in Bellevue Hospital 1931−33, spent a year (1934) studying virology at the Lister Institute for Preventive Medicine (London) then returned to the Rockefeller Institute in New York working on a variety of infectious diseases including poliomyelitis, later moving to Cincinnati to concentrate on poliomyelitis research. In 1941 Sabin and colleagues in Cincinnati proved that the polio virus was transmitted via the alimentary tract, an important breakthrough. During

World War II, Sabin served as a lieutenant colonel in the US Army Medical Corps, where he studied diseases affecting American troops such as sandfly fever and Japanese encephalitis. After the war, Sabin returned to Cincinnati to focus on poliomyelitis and with other scientists for all three strains of polio virus. He believed that a live attenuated oral vaccine was essential to control polio and could interrupt the chain of transmission of the virus and allowed for the possibility that polio might be eradicated. Sabin developed his live attenuated vaccine which was approved for testing by the FDA in 1955. The live vaccine given orally was encouraged by WHO and accepted for testing in many countries outside the US. Between 1955 and 1961, OPV was tested on at least 100 million people in the Soviet Union, Eastern Europe, Singapore, Mexico, and the Netherlands. After massive testing abroad, in 1960 Sabin conducted an OPV campaign in 200,000 children in the Cincinnati region in its first public distribution in the United States. OPV was licensed for testing in the US in 1960, recommended for general use by the American Medical Association in 1961 and adopted as the standard polio vaccine in the US in 1963 and continued as such until 2006. As early as 1961, Sabin had begun agitating for eradication: *"In oral poliovirus vaccine, we now have a simple tool with which we may attempt to rid large parts of the world of both paralytic poliomyelitis and the virulent viruses that cause it. I hope that public health authorities everywhere will now provide the necessary leadership for its use and show us the extent to which poliomyelitis can really be eradicated and stay eradicated"*. The mass immunization techniques that Sabin pioneered with his associates effectively eradicated polio in the most parts of the world. Sabin became an internationally prominent public figure advocating expanded access to vaccines globally. He stressed the need for recognition of relationships between poverty and poor health, i.e., the social determinants of health. Sabin was elected to the National Academy of Sciences in 1951. He was the recipient of over 40 honorary degrees and numerous prestigious awards worldwide, an active member of dozens of scientific societies, and author of over 350 scientific articles. Sabin's OPV was the goal for global eradication of poliomyelitis. Sabin died in 1993 at age 87. He was honored internationally and in the US. *"The world has lost a giant, but the fruits of his labor will continue to benefit future generations"* (James Grant, UNICEF in Jimenez, National Academy of Science, 2014). In 1986, President Ronald Reagan awarded Sabin the Presidential Medal of Freedom, and in the same year the Soviet Union honored him with its highest civilian honor.

Albert Sabin's development of the live attenuated oral poliomyelitis vaccine (OPV), licensed in 1960, added a major new dimension to poliomyelitis control due to its effect on producing intestinal and humoral immunity to the live virus, OPV was outstanding in the global community because of its effectiveness in the gut, low cost, and ease of administration. Sabin successfully promoted global vaccination interrupting the chain of transmission of WPV providing the basis for global eradication. The two vaccines in their more modern forms, enhanced strength inactivated polio vaccine (eIPV) and triple oral polio vaccine (tOPV), have been used in different settings with great success. But each of the two vaccines has important limitations: IPV provides high levels of humoral antibodies but fails to provide immunity of cells of the intestinal lining so that the wild poliovirus (WPV) may not cause clinical disease but can grow in the gut and be spread in environmental contamination. Use of eIPV produces early and high levels of circulating antibodies, as well as protection against the vaccine-associated disease. IPV is also costlier than OPV, in short supply, and cannot be given by a non-health professional, so its total replacement of OPV is not a practical alternative for the endgame of polio eradication.

OPV induces both humoral and cellular (including intestinal) immunity but rarely converts to wild status and can then spread in local outbreaks of clinical paralytic poliomyelitis. OPV can spread in sewage and by excreta of immunized infants in the sewage gives a booster effect in the community. Immunization using OPV, in both routine and on National Immunization Days (NIDs), has proven effective in dramatically reducing poliomyelitis and circulation of the wild virus worldwide.

OPV is an extremely safe and effective tool for immunizing children in the global struggle to eradicate polio. WHO in 2015 reported that over the previous decade, more than 10 billion doses of OPV were administered to some 2.5 billion children worldwide, preventing more than 10 million polio cases. OPV is made with live attenuated (weakened) polioviruses but can very rarely undergo genetic change in the gut of an immunized person and result in a case of vaccine-associated paralytic polio (VAPP). On rare occasions, VAPP spreads in local outbreaks as vaccine-derived poliovirus (VDPV) in approximately one in 2.7 million doses of OPV among unimmunized persons. This risk led the US Advisory Committee on Immunization Practices (ACIP) to recommend a revised schedule including two doses of IPV followed by two doses of OPV. VAPP occurred less frequently with this schedule, and in 2000 ACIP recommended switching to IPV alone. OPV is no longer produced or available in the US (CDC). In countries with less than 90 percent coverage in routine immunization, OPV remains the better choice due to its spread environmentally to reinforce immunization and herd immunity and fending off wild polio virus (WPV) that may enter the gut because of its better intestinal immunity. The combination of OPV as the basis with IPV added since 2016 gives greater potential for completion of eradication than IPV alone could provide. Approximately eight–ten cases of VAPP occurred annually in the United States during the 1990s following the elimination of natural transmission. The CDC changed recommendations to use in 1997 a combination of OPV and IPV but then switched to IPV alone in 1999 due to concern that VAPP risk would outweigh risk of local wild polio from imported cases. Most high-income countries have followed suit. While this

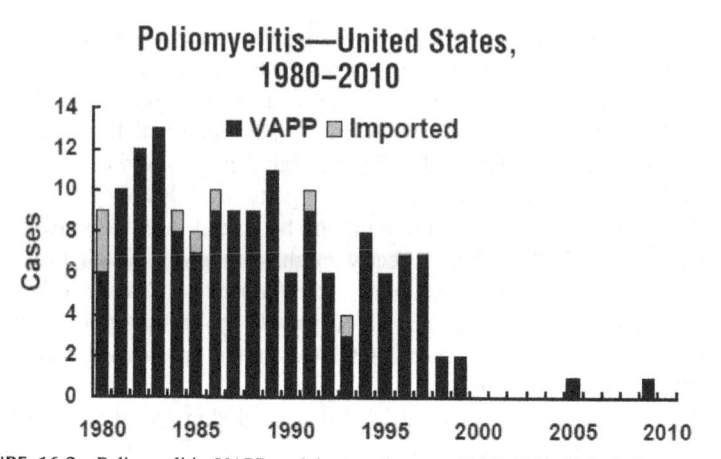

FIGURE 16.2   Poliomyelitis VAPP and imported cases, 1980–2011 United States. *Source: Centers for Disease Control and Prevention. Poliomyelitis. 13th edition, 2015. Available at: http://www.cdc.gov/vaccines/pubs/pinkbook/polio.html (accessed 3 January 2018).*

eliminates risk for VAPP, concerns remain that herd immunity may be reduced due to lower intestinal immunity as noted with IPV use (Figure 16.2).

Global Eradication

As early as 1961, Albert Sabin was promoting global eradication of polio, stating: *"In oral poliovirus vaccine we now have a simple tool with which we may attempt to rid large parts of the world of both paralytic poliomyelitis and the virulent viruses that cause it. I hope that public health authorities everywhere will now provide the necessary leadership for its use and show us the extent to which poliomyelitis can really be eradicated and stay eradicated."*

In 1988, the global polio eradication initiative was launched by WHO as the Global Polio Eradication Initiative (GPEI), and progress has been impressive. In 2016, 85 percent of infants around the world received three doses of polio vaccine as reported by WHO compared to 76 percent in 1990. African region coverage with three doses of OPV was 55 percent in 1990, increasing to 72 percent in 2000, and 73% in 2016 (WHO, 2017). India's coverage with three doses of OPV increased from 66 percent in 1990 to 86 percent in 2015, with many special immunization activities (SIAs) and no reported cases of polio since 2011. Six countries (India, Nigeria, Pakistan, Indonesia, Ethiopia, and the Democratic Republic of the Congo) have accounted for more than half the world's population of unvaccinated children for the past 19 years. National immunization days (NIDs) are conducted in many countries throughout the world, achieving coverage of over 400 million children annually. Mop-up programs to reinforce coverage of children in still-endemic areas are proceeding, along with increased emphasis on acute flaccid paralysis (AFP) monitoring.

Following the success of smallpox's eradication, the WHO in 1988 targeted eradication of poliomyelitis. Although polio epidemics continue, endemic largely in countries with limited access to public health services, the global burden of polio has been greatly reduced. At the initiation of the polio eradication campaign, 350,000 cases of childhood paralysis were attributed to polio in 125 countries. By 2009, this number was reduced to 1,604 cases. Thus, since 1988, the number of polio cases has fallen by over 99 percent. In 2016, only 2 countries, Afghanistan and Pakistan, have never achieved WPV interruption, and remain endemic for polio, down from more than 125 countries in 1988. However, despite the enormous effort and massive reduction in cases, the danger still exists that *"as long as a single child remains infected, children in all countries are at risk of contracting polio. Failure to eradicate polio from these last remaining strongholds could result in as many as 200,000 new cases every year, within 10 years, all over the world."* (WHO).

In most countries, the global effort has expanded capacities to tackle infectious diseases by building effective surveillance and immunization systems. With continued national and international emphasis and support of the WHO, Rotary International, UNICEF, GAVI, and bilateral donor countries, there is the real possibility of a world without polio. India and Nigeria have had no polio cases since 2011 and 2014, respectively, while Pakistan and Afghanistan continue to have decreasing numbers of endemic WPV cases. After two years without polio cases, in 2016 Nigeria reported three laboratory confirmed cases of WPV1. In addition, there was one laboratory finding of circulating VDPV type2, which may have been circulating for two years without prior detection. These findings raised concerns that countries declared polio free can still experience reentry of WPV and also VAPP.

However, in 2009–10, among polio-free countries, 23 countries were reinfected (including Angola, Chad, and Democratic Republic of the Congo). Many WHO member countries and international organizations and agencies such as UNICEF and GAVI along with donors such as the Bill and Melinda Gates Foundation and Rotary International, are providing important financial and organizational help, which has promoted wide-scale increases in immunization coverage throughout the world. The global polio eradication process uses OPV as part of routine infant immunization during NIDs. This strategy has been successful in the Americas, Europe, and China, but several countries remain problematic. India had its last WPV case in January 2011 in contrast to the 42 cases in 2010 as a result of a massive commitment to SIAs (supplementary immunization activities) and slow improvement in basic immunization coverage in key problematic states where poliomyelitis remained endemic at low levels. In 2012 India was no longer listed as a polio endemic country and certified as polio-free in 2014 by the WHO.

Eradication of wild poliomyelitis will require flexibility in vaccination strategies and necessitate the combined approach using both OPV and eIPV as adopted in the United States between 1997 and 2000 to address concerns that OPV can generate VAPP cases associated rarely with local outbreaks of poliomyelitis. The United States then switched to an IPV-only vaccination policy, which has been adopted by most industrialized countries, but is impractical for developing nations because of high costs and limited supply for the less than adequate immunization coverage in many countries which is needed for herd immunity.

IPV-only policies have also been adopted since 2000 in many industrialized countries where interruption of WPV was deemed to have occurred, but this provides the risk of less intestinal immunity and risk for imported WPV though travelers or refugees. The combination of OPV and IPV may be needed where enteric disease is common and leads to interference in OPV uptake, especially in tropical areas where endemic poliovirus and diarrheal diseases are still found. In 2004–05, polio resurged in Nigeria and in a number of countries previously thought to be under control. The use of OPV has been put in doubt by recent recommendations and decisions of the WHO for the end-game strategy based on the US experience with IPV-only. Developing countries will need to rely on OPV in the coming years because of high cost and limited supply of IPV as well as human resource issues. The US STOP (stop transmission of polio) program provides much needed technical support for polio eradication in many countries. The program trains volunteers and focuses on capacity building and training of local community health workers in host countries.

CURRENT RELEVANCE

Controversy regarding the relative advantages of each vaccine continues and the momentum to eradicate poliomyelitis is building. The OPV program of mass repeated vaccination for control of poliomyelitis in the Americas established the primacy of OPV in public health practice. OPV requires multiple doses to achieve protective antibody levels. Where there are many enteroviruses in the environment, interference in the uptake of OPV may result in cases of VAPP and circulating vaccine-derived polio (cVDPV) among those who have received three or even four doses of OPV. Use of IPV as initial protection eliminates this problem of VAPP.

During the 1970s and 1980s, a combined approach bolstering IPV immunity with OPV boosters showed promise in Gaza and Israel, where natural poliovirus was eradicated. Although sequential use of IPV and OPV was adopted in the routine infant immunization program in the United States in 1997, since 2000 the OPV was discontinued and current programs use

IPV-only. This policy for IPV has been adopted as the exclusive polio vaccine in most industrialized countries, while developing countries continue to rely on the less costly and easier to administer OPV.

Mass campaigns of SIAs going door to door and to public places to give OPV to all children now mainly use monovalent OPV (type 1) in still-endemic areas such as specific regions of Afghanistan and Pakistan as well as in other countries with still inadequate routine immunization and poor sanitation such as India and Nigeria. But even today polio can still reoccur in many low-income countries and spread to neighboring or even distant countries. There are concerns that exclusive use of either vaccine alone will not lead to the desired goal of eradication of poliomyelitis.

In 2012 the World Health Assembly declared a "programmatic emergency" for global public health and the world eradication program with the Director General referring to application of international health regulations to stop the spread of WPV from endemic to neighboring countries. In 2014, WHO recommended that all OPV using countries switch to bOPV (i.e. with strains 1 and 3 only) along with routine use of IPV, even as fractionated dosages, which have proved effective in raising antibody levels, due to shortage of supply and high prices and then to cease use of OPV at all, using IPV as the mainstay of the end-game strategy.

Great reliance is placed on acute flaccid paralysis (AFP) surveillance with polio cases rate varying from 1:100 to 1:1000 but asymptomatic infections may be higher in vaccinated populations. Polio transmission may not be detected for many months, and thus environmental surveillance has become much more important. An effective program of environmental monitoring of sewage and wastewater signaled the presence of imported polio virus in Israel in 2013. This was also the experience in India, which led to success in 2012. Environmental surveillance is important for ongoing surveillance with the post-eradication phase of polio and is being adopted in many European and sub-Saharan African countries.

Over the past 10 years, more than 10 billion doses of OPV have been administered to over 2.5 billion children worldwide, preventing more than 10 million polio cases during that period, nearly halting transmission of the polio virus. OPV provides protection to the individual and herd immunity for the community in contrast to IPV, which protects only the individual. However, rarely the vaccine strains undergo changes and become more like the wild virus and can cause VAPP. Addition of one dose of IPV in OPV using countries is expected to reduce this phenomenon, but OPV is still the indispensable basis for polio eradication. VAPP occurs at a rate of approximately one in 2.7 million doses of OPV but varies by the dose, being less for second and third doses and occuring more in poor hygienic situations. VAPP is limited to individual cases and does not spread to cause outbreaks.

Even more rarely, a vaccine strain can undergo conversion to vaccine-derived poliovirus (VDPV) in which the virus is genetically changed from the original strain of the OPV in under-immunized populations and cause paralysis in humans and also the capacity for sustained person-to-person circulation, which is known as cVDPV. It may persist and circulate in the environment as "persistent cVDPV" for more than six months. Only 24 cVDPV outbreaks have been recorded in 21 countries, almost all due to type 2 strain, resulting in more than 750 recorded cases of paralytic polio. However, the last case or finding of type 2 polio virus strain was reported in 1999, and the strain was declared eradicated in 2015. In 2016 type 2 was removed from the tOPV to become bivalent OPV to reduce the risk of vaccine derived and circulating virus capable of causing disease and spreading.

Since the 1988 global polio eradication initiative was launched, progress has been impressive. Global coverage of infants with three doses of OPV reached 86 percent in 2014 as compared to 83 percent in 1995 (UNICEF). During this period, OPV coverage increased in the African Region from 51 percent in 2000 to 77 percent. NIDs are conducted in many countries throughout the world, achieving coverage of over 400 million children annually. Mop-up operations to reinforce coverage of children in still-endemic areas are proceeding, along with increased emphasis on AFP monitoring. Worldwide clinical cases from WPV have been reduced to 359 per year in 2014.

By the end of 2006 four countries remained endemic for polio: India (676 cases); Pakistan (40 cases); Afghanistan (31 cases); and Nigeria (1125 cases); another 13 countries in Africa, the Middle East, and South-East Asia reported clinical cases of poliomyelitis due to active transmission in 2006. Pakistan (306 cases) and Afghanistan (28 cases) remain endemic for polio in 2014 with eight countries vulnerable to polio. The number of global polio cases has been reduced by more than 99 percent from 1988 to 2015, including the prevention of five million cases of paralysis and more than 250,000 deaths. In 2014, all cases of paralytic polio due to WPV were caused by type one WPV.

With continued national and international emphasis, and support of the WHO, Rotary International, UNICEF, GAVI, and donor countries, eradication of polio is possible. India was certified polio-free in 2014 and Nigeria polio-free in 2015. Pakistan (80% of total cases) and Afghanistan continue to have endemic WPV cases. In 2014 there were 359 cases globally as compared to 223 in 2012 and 650 in 2011. Endemic countries had 341, 217, and 340 of the total cases in 2011, 2012, and 2014, respectively. In nonendemic countries there were 309 in 2011, six cases in 2014, and 19 in 2012, respectively.

Global eradication programs mobilized, trained, and deployed volunteers in large numbers in many countries. SIAs are mass vaccination campaigns that aim to administer additional doses of oral poliovirus vaccine to children under five years of age regardless of their vaccination history. SIAs are meant to augment the limited ability of routine immunization services to reach at-risk children with the number of OPV doses required to generate immunity, and to reduce the spread of WPV or VAPP in high risk areas.

Since 2012, the murder of polio workers by radical Islamic Taliban fighters primarily in Pakistan has cast a shadow over immunization programs. But due to strengthened initiatives and increasing numbers of volunteers, government polio programs continue and will succeed in achieving polio elimination and at the same time educate a generation of mothers and fathers of the importance of immunization. Improved quality SIAs preventing the spread of polio exportation to polio-free countries and improvement in surveillance for AFP, outbreak preparedness, and a focus on high-risk areas would help stop transmission of polio virus.

Surveillance for AFP along with fecal samples and environmental monitoring to identify cVDPV are critical elements of a polio control and elimination strategy. Global eradication of type 2 WPV was declared in 2015, and type 3 WPV has not been found since 2012.

The successful end of polio is in sight, but great care must be taken in the end-stage strategy of continued vaccination incorporating both OPV and IPV along with strong surveillance and monitoring systems. The potential for reappearance of both WPV and VAPP are issues for policymakers that affect strategies and ultimately outcomes.

In 2000, the polio eradication campaign seemed to be nearing its end. Wild type 2 poliovirus had been stamped out worldwide the previous year, while poliovirus types 1 and 3 were confined to a few hundred cases. Although cases of cVDPV paralysis had been known for many years, they were extremely rare. However, it was alarming that in several situations VDPV had spread in a mode similar to a wild virus, causing an outbreak with 21 children in Hispaniola (Dominican Republic and Haiti) who became paralyzed, two of whom died before the mass vaccination stopped the outbreak. This raised concerns that OPV, the most widely used vaccine globally, could itself lead to new polio outbreaks. Such outbreaks have occurred in 16 countries since the Hispaniola outbreak, but are extremely rare, given that globally at least 10 billion doses of OPV have been administered to more than two billion children. However, the WHO eradication program faced a new challenge. As a result of these concerns, most high-income countries switched from OPV to reliance on IPV, which could not induce VDPV.

In 2013, a "natural experiment" occurred that would provide evidence of the need for use of both OPV and IPV in the final stages of polio eradication. A comparison of the effectiveness of combined OPV/IPV versus IPV-alone polio immunization programs is important in understanding measures limiting the spread of imported type 1 WPV, which entered highly immunized Israel and Palestinian territories from Egypt.

During the late 1970s Gaza and the West Bank experienced high levels of clinical poliomyelitis with many cases occurring among children immunized with multiple doses of OPV. This was attributed to findings of other studies that showed that OPV produced lower levels of protective antibodies in nonindustrialized than in industrialized countries, due to interference in uptake of the tOPV by other enteroviruses. In 1970, the immunization policy for Gaza and the West Bank was changed to use of a combination of both live OPV and inactivated IPV vaccine, which within a short period, eliminated polio in both jurisdictions.

Israel has used OPV since the 1960s, but in two districts IPV-only was used for a 10-year period. In 1988, an outbreak of 15 cases of poliomyelitis occurred in Hadera, one of the IPV districts. Israel then adopted the combined OPV/IPV control strategy, with no further cases occurring, and also implemented a routine sewage-monitoring system for polioviruses for Israel, the West Bank, and Gaza leading to adoption of an OPV and IPV combined program. In 2004 Israel followed recommendations from the WHO to convert to IPV-only, and adopted this policy in keeping with practices adopted in European and North American countries, which considered VAPP cases a greater threat than WPV itself. In cooperation between the Israeli and Palestinian Ministries of Health, the Israel Central Virus Laboratory routine monitoring of sewage samples for polioviruses from Israel, Gaza, and the West Bank has been in place since 1998.

In 2013, routine monitoring tests showed type 1 WPV in sewage in southern and later central Israel. In consultation with international experts, increased surveillance showed that findings of WPV were widespread in Southern and Central Israel during 2013 and early 2014. A mass campaign of OPV was conducted for children up to age 10 in early 2014. The positive sewage findings were primarily in Israel, initially mainly among Bedouin communities, but later spreading to mixed communities in Central Israel. Increased sampling in the West Bank and Gaza showed few positives, but the Palestinian Authority conducted a two-dose OPV booster campaign as well. No cases of poliomyelitis occurred in either Israel or the Palestinian territories.

This "natural experiment" compares the effectiveness of the combined (sequential) use of both IPV and OPV as compared to an IPV-only program in protecting against silent entry and spread of WPV into areas with high immunization coverage. Both policies protect against clinical polio, but the combined OPV/IPV program induced greater protection against the silent spread of imported WPV. In 2012 the WHO made a decision, which was reaffirmed in 2014, to recommend one dose of IPV in countries using OPV in their routine immunization program and SIAs for mass population coverage. As of January 2014, for the first time, the WHO is formally recommending adding at least one dose of IPV in OPV-using countries.

ETHICAL ISSUES

Adoption of IPV in the high-income countries since 2000 leaves medium- and low-income countries to use OPV, which the WHO concluded has the potential for causing rare outbreaks of the Sabin vaccine converting to a wild form. This raises both epidemiologic and ethical questions. Further concern was raised when evidence appeared in 2013 that WPV can enter and spread among populations using IPV alone since little or no enteric immunity allows vaccine-protected persons to become carriers who grow and spread the virus without become clinically ill. As a result, the WHO is recommending at least one dose of IPV along with three doses of OPV to gain both humoral and enteric immunity.

Modification of the WHO's strong recommendation for early cancellation of OPV has been modified by adopting recommendations to add at least one dose of IPV in countries still using OPV as the basis of their polio-eradication programs. Advocates for the use of both OPV and IVP as an alternative were not acknowledged in the debates of a combined policy seen to be highly successful in eradication of both WPV and VDPV polio cases, and the WHO actually called for a policy of stopping the use of OPV, the mainstay vaccine in most countries. But costs and supply of IPV may hinder development of the late-stage combined IPV/OPV policy.

Eradication of important diseases is a worthy goal of the world health movement, following the success of smallpox eradication and the hope for successful eradication of poliomyelitis in the coming years. The incidence and complications of many viral diseases such as tetanus, measles, rubella, and mumps have been vastly reduced by the achievements of vaccination, yet some of these diseases are coming back due to incomplete vaccination and refusal by countries to keep up with proven effective vaccines as needed. There are many candidate diseases for control and elimination as public health problems but they require governmental policies, strategies, commitment, awareness, promotion, and resource allocation as well as public support and participation. Many "neglected tropical diseases" are being vastly reduced by vector control and mass periodic treatment of vulnerable populations.

Public apathy or hostility to vaccination (antivaccinationism) is still a widespread problem that public health has to address in order to fulfill its mission of improved health of the world's population. This position is often fostered by erroneous information spread on the Internet and other media by ideologically motivated opponents to vaccination. Fabricated data used by a UK study group led by Andrew Wakefield was published in Lancet in 1998, and only withdrawn 12 years later after media coverage and investigation led to withdrawal of Wakefield's medical license by the UK General Medical Council. After the data were proven fraudulent in late March 2016, an anti-vaccination movie was featured at a film festival based on fraudulent and disproven allegations that autism is associated with important and safe vaccines, but was later withdrawn. However, apathy and opposition are still major public health issues as seen recently with parental refusal to immunize children against measles during outbreaks in California during 2014 continuing up to 2017 especially among unimmunized groups including adults, despite increased immunization coverage to over 95 percent of children.

Diseases such as malaria and tuberculosis, still present despite progress in their control, are mass killers. While they are, in principle, diseases that can be eliminated as public health problems given strong support and use of proven systems such as vector control, along with new technologies for rapid diagnosis and improved treatments becoming available, resistance to available therapy is a serious global public health issue. Disease control and elimination of local and regional prevalence are important steps toward eradication. Long-hoped-for vaccines for malaria, hepatitis C, HIV, Zika West Nile Fever, and dengue viruses and others will open the way to more rapid control. But effective modes of health promotion and environmental and social modalities can make enormous contributions to these preliminary stages and ultimate elimination as public health problems as are being seen for HIV, and even in 2014–15 for the ebola epidemic in West Africa and even for neglected tropical diseases such as leprosy, dracunculiasis, onchocerciasis, and filariasis. The coming decade will hopefully bring forth effective, safe, and inexpensive vaccines for many diseases that are still great public health threats and others that may yet appear.

ECONOMIC ISSUES

Adoption of a combination of OPV and IPV will allow transition from repeated SIAs, which in many countries result in large numbers of children receiving multiple doses of OPV without protection of IPV. This also will help focus limited public health resources on one disease. Successful polio eradication will allow the focus to shift to consolidating the public health infrastructure and manpower to refocus on basic child immunization coverage.

Governments and their partners have invested some US $9 billion in 25 years into polio eradication efforts. The economic gain from polio eradication is expected to be very high, according to the Global Polio Eradication Initiative, but the world is only expected to realize a return on this investment—estimated at a minimum direct savings of US $40–50 billion by 2035, in low- middle-, and high-income countries—if the last remaining endemic countries eliminate the disease.

Continued surveillance of AFP and other suspect cases of poliomyelitis will be needed for many years to come along with maintenance of adequate emergency stores of both IPV and OPV to meet potential challenges of resurgence of WPV and its silent spread in IPV-vaccinated countries. As long as routine vaccination coverage in sub-Saharan Africa, India and Middle East countries is below 80 percent and sanitation is poor for large population groups the potential for return of poliomyelitis is a real risk especially if IPV alone is adopted with abandonment of OPV as recommended by the WHO. Investment in sustained polio prevention will be a justified economic burden well into the 2030s.

An in-depth economic analysis by Tebbens et al. (Vaccine, 2011) found high strong economic justification of the global polio eradication initiative (GPEI) especially when including additional benefits due to vitamin A supplements distributed during SIAs helping to reduce child mortality. Eradication of diseases such as smallpox and poliomyelitis requires not only funds but human resources to carry out the program. Eradication of a specific vaccine-preventable disease is carried out in phases mainly by routine immunization programs, the foundations of public health control on infectious diseases. Supplementary SIAs complement routine immunization reaching out to the community to increase coverage for the needed herd immunity. The GPEI is overseen by WHO's Strategic Advisory Group of Experts on immunization (SAGE) with support of the Global vaccine alliance (GAVI) with financial support of the Bill and Melinda Gates Foundation, the Rotary Club, the US CDC and many other supporters. When eradication is achieved, the huge investment in SIAs will be phased out with very large cost savings. These resources can be switched to strengthening routine immunization and to expanding the vaccines used to reduce the total burden of diseases especially of children.

CONCLUSION

Following the successful eradication of smallpox, the WHO adopted a polio eradication policy, which has come close to achieving the goal of eradicating the disease. Polio is not a big killer but a major cause of crippling of children that is spread readily through the environment. The global polio eradication program has reduced the number of cases by 99 percent since 1988 and is nearing completion, which has freed up major resources in manpower and money to apply to strengthening public health infrastructures and routine immunizations and providing new vaccines badly needed in low- and medium-income countries. Global consensus activities will benefit from programs that eliminate congenital rubella syndrome, measles, mumps, pneumonia, cancer of the cervix and other vaccine preventable diseases, along with neglected tropical diseases.

Ultimate success in eradication of polio will be a civilizational achievement no less important than walking on the moon. Hopefully it will increase public awareness and support for vaccine research, development, and utilization. Eradication of polio will also open opportunities due to redeployment of financial and human resources to reduce non-communicable diseases (NCDs) and nutritional deficiency conditions.

In April 2016, the WHO stated that *"failure to implement strategic approaches, however, leads to ongoing transmission of the virus. Endemic transmission is continuing in Pakistan and Afghanistan. Failure to stop polio in these last remaining areas could result in as many as 200,000 new cases every year, within 10 years, all over the world. In most countries, the global effort has expanded capacities to tackle other infectious diseases by building effective surveillance and immunization systems."*

The WHO's Strategic Advisory Committee has recommended cessation of use of OPV and continuing use of IPV only following global certification of eradication. This policy may be revised in the light of concern over potential silent circulation of WPV in IPV immunized populations, as occurred in Israel in 2013. Post-eradication policy will need to be adapted according to epidemiologic information including AFP and laboratory monitoring of sewage sites in as many locations as possible. Other factors include the supply and cost of IPV and the extent of immunization coverage of children and young adults. Discontinuing polio immunization after global certification of eradication depends on: a recommended IPV schedule (doses, timing, formulation) after OPV withdrawal; criteria when countries could stop polio vaccination depending on supply, cost, and price of the vaccine; and national and local routine immunization coverage. Post-eradication policy must include sewage sampling, laboratory testing and monitoring of acute flaccid paralysis (AFP) cases for a significant number of years.

In 2017 fewer polio cases were being reported in Pakistan and Afghanistan. In 2016, 85 percent of infants around the world received three doses of polio vaccine, whereas over 90 percent is considered the minimum safe requirement. IPV (one dose) has been added added by WHO recommendations in most countries since 2016. Some countries considered polio-free have been infected by imported WPV and VAPP viruses. All countries, particularly with conflict and instability, remain at risk until polio is fully eradicated. It's not over yet but the end is within reach and the post-endgame "two-pronged" strategy for polio eradication is combining OPV and IPV as the most promising policy for success.

Lessons learned from polio eradication and from previous success in smallpox eradication (see Chapter 2) are important for eradication efforts for other diseases and global health generally. Key issues include mobilizing national and international political and public support, strategic planning and policy development, public-private management and donor coordination, program operations and tactics, with monitoring, oversight and response to epidemiologic evidence (Cochi et al., 2014). National efforts to strengthen routine immunization systems are fundamental to global public health for control as well as for eradication of important diseases such as measles, rubella, rotavirus (See Chapters 3, 12, and 19) as well as neglected tropical diseases where great progress is already being made. New generations of public health workers will have many worthy challenges to address in coming decades.

RECOMMENDATIONS

1. Polio monitoring is essential for the endgame and post-endgame period and for the foreseeable future.
2. AFP surveillance is an essential component of polio monitoring.

3. Systematic sewage testing for poliovirus is a vital aspect of polio monitoring and early detection of poliovirus and polio eradication activities.

4. Adding IPV in OPV-only countries will together reduce the risk of VAPP as well as boost humoral and intestinal immunity decreasing potential silent spread of imported WPV. This policy has already been adopted by the WHO.

5. IPV-only countries should reevaluate their risk of silent WPV importation and maintain OPV stocks if importation or environmental detection occur.

6. A combined/sequential schedule using both OPV and IPV should be considered in IPV-only countries to reduce risk of WPV introduction and circulation.

7. Silent transmission of WPV should be considered an international health risk in the coming years.

8. When switching from mass immunization programs, international donors and national governments should devote resources to strengthening routine immunization.

9. Resources of funds and human resources released from polio eradication should be transferred to the addition of new vaccines vital for reducing mortality and morbidity such as a second dose of MMR, haemophilus influenza b, human papilloma virus, rotavirus and pneumonia vaccines.

10. Development of the public health organization and infrastructure of management and field-service providers is essential to reach out to underserved populations in rural areas, urban slums, and migrant populations.

STUDENT REVIEW QUESTIONS

1. What are the advantages and disadvantages of oral (Sabin) polio vaccine?

2. What are the advantages and disadvantages of inactivated (Salk) polio vaccine?

3. Why was poliomyelitis eradication given top priority after success in eradicating smallpox?

4. Describe the strategies and components for a disease control and eradication program such as for polio.

5. Do mass immunization activities disrupt or hinder development of routine immunization programs in low-income countries?

6. What are the risks and benefits of stopping polio immunization after eradication is achieved?

7. What kind of environmental monitoring will be needed after polio eradication is achieved?

8. What other diseases would you recommend to prorititize for a disease eradication policy?

RECOMMENDED READINGS

1. Adams P. Ending polio, one type at a time. Bull World Health Organ. 2012;90:482−483. Available at: http://www.who.int/bulletin/volumes/90/7/BLT.12.020712.pdf?ua = 1 (accessed 14 September 2017).

2. Anis E, Kopel E, Singer SR, Kaliner E, Moerman L, Moran-Gilad J, et al. Insidious rein-troduction of wild poliovirus into Israel, 2013. Euro Surveill. 2013;18(38):pii = 20586. Available at: http://www.eurosurveillance.org/ViewArticle.aspx?ArticleId = 20586 (accessed 6 September 2017).

3. Aylward B, Hennessey KA, Zagaria N, Olivé J-M, Cochi S. When is a disease eradicable? 100 years of lessons learned. Am J Public Health. 2000;90:1515−1520. Available at: http://ajph.aphapublications.org/doi/pdf/10.2105/AJPH.90.10.1515 (accessed 6 September 2017).

4. Aylward B, Tangermann R. The global polio eradication initiative: lessons learned and prospects for success. Vaccine. 2011;29(Suppl 4):D80−D85. Available at: http://www.sciencedirect.com/science/article/pii/S0264410X11015994 (accessed 6 September 2017).

5. Aylward B, Yamada T. The polio endgame. N Engl J Med. 2011;364(24):2273−2275. Available at: http://www.ncbi.nlm.nih.gov/pubmed/21675884 (accessed 6 September 2017).

6. Centers for Disease Control and Prevention, Immunization Systems Management Group of the Global Polio Eradication Initiative. Introduction of inactivated poliovirus vaccine and switch from trivalent to bivalent oral poliovirus vaccine—worldwide, 2013−2016. MMWR Morb Mortal Wkly Rep. 2015;64(25):699−702. Available at: http://www.cdc.gov/mmwr/preview/mmwrhtml/mm6425a4.htm (accessed 10 September 2017).

7. Centers for Disease Control and Prevention. Poliomyelitis, Ch 18. In: Hamborsky J, Kroger A, Wolfe S, editors. Epidemiology and prevention of vaccine preventable diseases (pink book). 13th ed. Washington, DC: Public Health Foundation, 2015297−310. Available at: http://www.cdc.gov/vaccines/pubs/pinkbook/index.html (accessed 10 September 2017).

8. Centers for Disease Control and Prevention. Progress toward eradication of polio—world-wide January 2011−March 2013. MMWR Morb Mortal Wkly Rep. 2013;62(17):335−338. Available at: http://www.cdc.gov/mmwr/preview/mmwrhtml/mm6217a4.htm (accessed 10 September 2017).

9. Centers for Disease Control and Prevention. The global polio eradication initiative: stop transmission of polio (STOP) program1999−2013. MMWR Morb Mortal Wkly Rep. 2013;62(24):501−503. Available at: http://www.cdc.gov/mmwr/preview/mmwrhtml/mm6224a5.htm (accessed 10 September 2017).

10. Cochi SL, Freeman A, Guirguis S, Jafari H, Aylward B. Global polio eradication initiative: lessons learned and legacy. J Infect Dis. 2014;210(S1):S540−S546. Available at: http://polioeradication.org/wp-content/uploads/2016/07/LessonsLearnedLegacy-1.pdf (accessed 10 September 2017).

11. College of Physicians of Philadelphia. History of vaccines. Available at: http://www.historyofvaccines.org/content/articles/history-polio-poliomyelitis (accessed 10 September 2017).

12. Dowdle WR. The principles of disease elimination and eradication. MMWR Morb Mortal Wkly Rep. 1999;48(SU01):23−27. Available at: http://www.cdc.gov/mmwr/preview/mmwrhtml/su48a7.htm (accessed 10 September 2017).

13. Duintjer Tebbens RJ, Pallansch MA, Cochi SL, Wassilak SGF, Linkins J, Sutter RW, et al. Economic analysis of the global polio eradication initiative. Vaccine. 2011;29(2):334−343.

Available at: http://www.who.int/immunization/sage/10_eonomic_analysis_gpei_Duintjer
Tebbens_Vaccine_2010_10_26_apr_2011.pdf (accessed 10 September 2017).

14. Encyclopedia of world biography, http://www.notablebiographies.com/Ro-Sc/Sabin-Albert.
html; Sabin Vaccine Institute, http://www.sabin.org/legacy-albert-b-sabin (accessed 17
September 2017).

15. Fitzpatrick M. Book Review: Offit P. The Cutter Incident: how America's first polio vaccine led to a growing vaccine crisis. J R Soc Med. 2006;99(3):156. Available at: https://
www.ncbi.nlm.nih.gov/pmc/articles/PMC1383764/ (accessed 20 September 2017).

16. Flahault A, Orenstein W, Garon J, Kew O, Bickford J, Tulchinsky T. Commentary: comparing Israeli and Palestinian polio vaccination policies and the challenges of silent entry
of wild polio virus in 2013−14: a "Natural Experiment". Int J Public Health. 2015;60
(7):765−766. Abstract available at: https://link.springer.com/article/10.1007%2Fs00038-
015-0700-0 (accessed 14 September 2017).

17. Global Polio Eradication Initiative. Vaccine-associated paralytic polio (VAPP) and vaccine-derived poliovirus (VDPV). Fact sheet February 2015. Available at: http://www.
who.int/immunization/diseases/poliomyelitis/endgame_objective2/oral_polio_vaccine/
VAPPandcVDPVFactSheet-Feb2015.pdf?ua = 1 (accessed 10 September 2017).

18. Goldblum N, Gerichter CB, Tulchinsky TH, Melnick JL. Poliomyelitis control in Israel,
the West Bank and Gaza strip: changing strategies with the goal of eradication in an
endemic area. Bull World Health Organ. 1994;72(5):783−796. Available at: https://www.
ncbi.nlm.nih.gov/pmc/articles/PMC2486552/pdf/bullwho00416-0089.pdf   (accessed   12
September 2017).

19. Goodman RA, Foster KL, Trowbridge FL, Figueroa JP. Global disease elimination and
eradication as public health strategies. MMWR Morb Mortal Wkly Rep. 1999;48
(Suppl):1−216. Available at: http://www.cdc.gov/mmwr/pdf/other/mm48su01.pdf (accessed
14 September 2017).

20. Hagan JF, Wassilak SGF, Craig AS, Tangermann RF, Diop OM, et al. Progress towards
polio eradication worldwide, 2014−2015. Wkly Epidemiol Rec. 2015;90:253−260.
Available at: http://www.who.int/wer/2015/wer9021.pdf?ua = 1 (accessed 12 September 2017).

21. Helleringer S, Frimpong JA, Abdelwahab J, Asuming P, Touré H, Awoonor-Williams JK,
et al. Supplementary polio immunization activities and prior use of routine immunization
services in non-polio-endemic sub-Saharan Africa. Bull WHO. 2012;90:495−503.
doi:10.2471/BLT.11.092494. Available at: http://www.who.int/bulletin/volumes/90/7/11-
092494/en/ (accessed 12 September 2017).

22. Jimenez MR, Albert B. Sabin 1906−1993: a biographical memoir. Washington DC:
National Academy of Sciences, 2014. Available at: http://www.nasonline.org/publications/
biographical-memoirs/memoir-pdfs/sabin-albert.pdf (accessed 20 September 2017).

23. Juskewitch JE, Tapia CJ, Windebank AJ. Lessons from the Salk polio vaccine: methods for
and risks of rapid translation. Clin Translat Sci. 2010;3(4):182−185. http://dx.doi.org/
10.1111/j.1752-8062.2010.00205.x. Available at: https://www.ncbi.nlm.nih.gov/pmc/
articles/PMC2928990/ (accessed 16 September 2017).

24. Lahariya C. Global eradication of polio: the case for "finishing the job". Bull WHO.
2007;85(6):421−500. Available at: http://www.who.int/bulletin/volumes/85/6/06-037457/
en/ (accessed 23 August 2017).

25. Mangal TD, Aylward RB, Grassly NC. The potential impact of routine immunization with
inactivated poliovirus vaccine on wild-type or vaccine-derived poliovirus outbreaks in a
posteradication setting. Am J Epidemiol. 2013;178(10):1579−1587. Available at: http://
www.ncbi.nlm.nih.gov/pubmed/24100955 (accessed 10 September 2017).

26. Manor Y, Shulman LM, Kaliner E, Hindiyeh M, Ram D, Sofer D, et al. Intensified environmental surveillance supporting the response to wild poliovirus type 1 silent circulation in Israel, 2013. Euro Surveill. 2014;19(7):1−10. Available at: http://www.eurosurveillance. org/ViewArticle.aspx?ArticleId = 20708 (accessed 10 September 2017).

27. Martinez-Bakker M, King AA, Rohani P. Unraveling the transmission ecology of polio. PLoS Biol. 2015;3(6):e1002172. Available at: http://journals.plos.org/plosbiology/article? id = 10.1371/journal.pbio.1002172 (accessed 14 September 2017).

28. Moturi EK, Porter KA, Wassilak SG, Tangermann RH, Diop OM, Burns CC, et al. Progress toward polio eradication—worldwide, 2013−2014. MMWR Morb Mortal Wkly Rep. 2014;63(21):468−472. Available at: www.cdc.gov/mmwr/preview/mmwrhtml/ mm6321a4.htm (accessed 14 September 2017).

29. Mundel T, Orenstein WA. No country is safe without global eradication of poliomyelitis. N Engl J Med. 2013;369:2045−2046. Available at: http://www.nejm.org/doi/full/10.1056/ NEJMe1311591 (accessed 14 September 2017).

30. Nathanson N, Kew OM. From emergence to eradication: the epidemiology of poliomyelitis deconstructed. Am J Epidemiol. 2010;172(11):1213−1229. Available at: https://www.ncbi. nlm.nih.gov/pmc/articles/PMC2991634/ (accessed 14 September 2017).

31. Nkowane BM, Wassilak SGF, Orenstein WA, Bart KJ, Schonberger LB, Hinman AR, et al. Vaccine-associated paralytic poliomyelitis United States: 1973 through 1984. JAMA. 1987;257(10):1335−1340. doi:10.1001/jama.1987.03390100073029. Abstract available at: https://jamanetwork.com/journals/jama/article-abstract/364942?redirect=true (accessed 20 September 2017).

32. Nobel Prize in Physiology or Medicine 1954. John F. Enders, Thomas H. Weller, Frederick C. Robbins. Nobelprize.org. John Enders Biographical. Available at: https:// www.nobelprize.org/nobel_prizes/medicine/laureates/1954/enders-bio.html (accessed 16 September 2017).

33. Orenstein WA. Eradicating polio: how the world's pediatricians can help stop this crippling illness forever. Pediatrics. 2014;135(1):197−202. Available at: http://pediatrics.aappublications.org/content/pediatrics/135/1/196.full.pdf (accessed 14 September 2017).

34. Patriarca PA, Wright PF, John TJ. Factors affecting the immunogenicity of oral poliovirus vaccine in developing countries: review. Rev Infect Dis. 1991;13(5):926−939. Abstract available at: http://cid.oxfordjournals.org/content/13/5/926.abstract (accessed).

35. Plotkin SA, Orenstein WA, Offit PA, editors. Vaccines. *6th edition*. Philadelphia, PA: Saunders, 2012.

36. Schmeck HM. Obituary. Albert Sabin. New York Times, 4 March 1993. Available at: http://www.nytimes.com/learning/general/onthisday/bday/0826.html (accessed 20 September 2017).

37. Routh JA, Oberste MS, Manisha PM. Manual for the surveillance of vaccine-preventable diseases, chapter 12 poliomyelitis. 1. Available at https://www.cdc.gov/vaccines/pubs/surv-manual/chpt12-polio.html (accessed 4 January 2018).

38. Sabin AB. Oral poliovirus vaccine: history of its development and prospects for eradication of poliomyelitis JAMA. 1965;194(8):872−876. Abstract Available at: https://jamanetwork. com/journals/jama/article-abstract/657114?redirect = true (accessed 23 December 2017).

39. Sabin AB. My last will and testament on rapid elimination and ultimate global eradication of poliomyelitis and measles Pediatrics. 1992;90(1):162−169. Abstract Available at: http://pediatrics.aappublications.org/content/90/1/162?download = true (accessed 20 September 2017).

40. Slater P, Costin C, Yarrow A, Morag A, Avni A, Handsher R, et al. Poliomyelitis outbreak in Israel in 1988: a report with two commentaries. Lancet. 1990;335(8699):1192−1195. Abstract available at: http://www.ncbi.nlm.nih.gov/pubmed/1971043 (accessed 14 September 2017).

41. Subalya S, Dumolard P, Lydon P, Garcic-Dobo M, Eggers R, Conklin L. Global routine vaccination coverage, 2014. MMWR Morb Mortal Wkly Rep. 2015;64(44):1252−1255. Available at: http://www.cdc.gov/mmwr/preview/mmwrhtml/mm6444a5.htm (accessed).

42. Sutter RW, John TJ, Jain H, Agarkhedkar S, Ramanan PV, Verma H, et al. Immunogenicity of bivalent types 1 and 3 oral poliovirus vaccine: a randomised, double-blind, controlled trial. Lancet. 2010;376(9753):1682−1688. Available at: http://www.ncbi.nlm.nih.gov/pubmed/20980048 (accessed 7 February 2016).

43. Tebbens RJD, Pallansch MA, Cochi SL, Wassilak SGF, Linkins J, Sutter RW, et al. Economic analysis of the global polio eradication initiative. Vaccine. 2011;29:334−343. Available at: http://cdrwww.who.int/immunization/sage/10_eonomic_analysis_gpei_DuintjerTebbens_Vaccine_2010_10_26_apr_2011.pdf (accessed 14 September 2017).

44. Thompson KM, Tebbens RJ. Eradication versus control for poliomyelitis: an economic analysis. Lancet. 2007;369(9570):1363−1371. Available at: http://www.thelancet.com/journals/lancet/article/PIIS0140-6736(07)60532-7/abstract (accessed 7 February 2016).

45. Tulchinsky TH, Abed A, Shaheen S, Toubassi N, Sever Y, Schoenbaum M, et al. A ten year experience in control of poliomyelitis through a combination of live and killed vaccines in two developing areas. Am J Public Health. 1989;79:1648−1655. Available at: http://www.ncbi.nlm.nih.gov/pmc/articles/PMC1349770/pdf/amjph00238-0062.pdf (accessed 14 September 2017).

46. Tulchinsky TH. Letter to Editor: Polio eradication: end stage challenges. Bull World Health Organ. 2005;83(2):160. Available at: http://www.who.int/bulletin/volumes/83/2/160.pdf (accessed 14 September 2017).

47. Tulchinsky TH, Ramlawi A, Abdeen Z, Grotto I, Flahault A. Polio lessons 2013: Israel, the West Bank, and Gaza. Lancet. 2013;382(9905):1611−1612. Abstract available at: http://www.thelancet.com/pdfs/journals/lancet/PIIS0140-6736(13)62331-4.pdf (accessed 14 September 2017).

48. World Health Organization. Polio vaccines: WHO position paper, January, 2014. Wkly Epidemiol Rec. 2014;89(9):73−92. Available at: http://www.who.int/wer/2014/wer8909.pdf (accessed 14 September 2017).

49. World Health Organization. Polio eradication and endgame strategic plan 2013−2018. Global Polio Eradication Initiative. Available at: http://www.polioeradication.org/resourcelibrary/strategyandwork.aspx (accessed 12 September 2017).

50. World Health Organization. WHO vaccine-preventable diseases monitoring system: global summary 2017, Last updated 06-Sep-2017. Available at: http://apps.who.int/immunization_monitoring/globalsummary/countries?countrycriteria%5Bcountry%5D%5B%5D = NGA (accessed 12 September 2017).

51. World Health Organization. Vaccine-associated paralytic polio (VAPP) and vaccine-derived poliovirus (VDPV). EPI fact sheet, February 2015. Available at: http://www.who.int/immunization/diseases/poliomyelitis/endgame_objective2/oral_polio_vaccine/VAPPand cVDPVFactSheet-Feb2015.pdf?ua = 1 (accessed 12 September 2017).

52. World Health Organization. IPV recommended for countries to mitigate risks and consequences associated with OPV2 withdrawal. SAGE, November 2012. Available at: http://www.who.int/immunization/sage/meetings/2012/november/news_sage_ipv_opv_nov2012/en/ (accessed 14 September 2017).

53. World Health Organization. Poliomyelitis fact sheet No. 114, updated April 2017. Available at: http://www.who.int/mediacentre/factsheets/fs114/en/ (accessed 14 September 2017).

54. World Health Organization, CDC, UNICEF. Polio Eradication & Endgame Strategic Plan 2013–2018. Available at: http://polioeradication.org/wp-content/uploads/2016/07/PEESP_EN_A4.pdf (accessed 14 September 2017).

55. World Health Organization. Strategic Advisory Committee October 2015, Polio eradication. Wkly Epidemiolog Rec. 2016;91:265–284. Available at: http://www.who.int/wer/2016/wer9121.pdf?ua = 1 (accessed 14 September 2017).

56. World Health Organization. Media Center. Immunization coverage fact sheet updated July 2017. Available at: http://www.who.int/mediacentre/factsheets/fs378/en/ (accessed 15 September 2017).

57. World Health Organization. Expanded program of immunization. Global Eradication Initiative. Vaccine-associated paralytic polio (VAPP) and vaccine-derived poliovirus (VDPV). Available at: http://www.who.int/immunization/diseases/poliomyelitis/endgame_objective2/oral_polio_vaccine/VAPPandcVDPVFactSheet-Feb2015.pdf (accessed 15 September 2017).

Chapter 17

Preventing Vitamin K Deficiency Bleeding in Newborns

ABSTRACT

Vitamin K administration at birth is a widely implemented procedure to prevent a potentially lethal condition, formerly called hemorrhagic disease of the newborn (HDN), now vitamin K deficiency bleeding (VKDB), a bleeding disorder of infants in which poor coagulation can cause serious or lethal bleeding in infancy, but which is prevented by vitamin K supplementation. The American Academy of Pediatrics recommended routine intramuscular injection of vitamin K for all newborns since 1961 and repeatedly renewed this recommendation since. In 1987 it was mandatory in only five states in the United States. In New York State, a review of infant deaths and hospitalizations over a decade attributed to HDN and other neonatal hemorrhagic conditions revealed that in 65 percent of the 34 deaths identified and reviewed, vitamin K was not documented as given or given only after the onset of hemorrhage; vitamin K was not included in standing orders in any of 22 hospitals contacted. This review led to vitamin K being made a mandatory newborn care procedure in the New York State Public Health Code.

Subsequently, in all 50 states, adoption of mandatory or standard practice of vitamin K for newborns virtually eradicated VKDB for causes of death in the United States. In 2013, VKDB returned to the US scene with reports from Tennessee of five cases with death and brain damage among neonates where parental refusal of vitamin K had occurred.

Globally, prevention of VKDB is increasingly recognized as essential for all newborns, but practice varies widely. In 2012, the World Health Organization (WHO) recommended vitamin K prophylaxis with all newborns given 1 mg of vitamin K intramuscularly after birth.

Implementation is nearly universal in the United States and other high-income countries, but still not widely adopted in practice in many low-income countries with high neonatal mortality. Conflicting recommendations between intramuscular and oral vitamin K in Europe raise problems of compliance with multiple oral doses and failure of protection from late VKDB. Recent reports in the United States of parental refusal of vitamin K injections leading to serious intracranial and intestinal bleeding raise concerns that this preventable disorder may increase in the future. Vitamin K by injection for all newborns should be given high priority globally to reduce preventable morbidity or death among neonates.

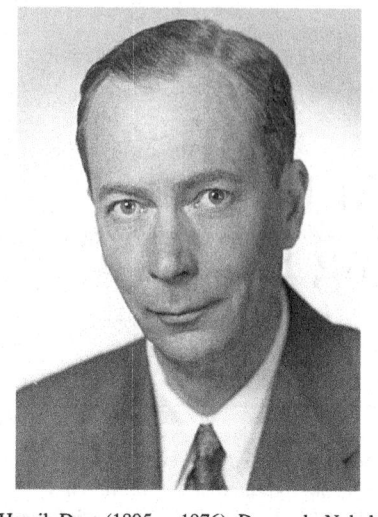

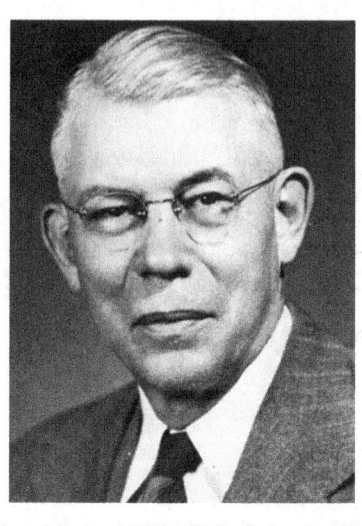

Henrik Dam (1895 – 1976), Denmark, Nobel Prize 1943 "for discovery of vitamin K." *Courtesy of The Royal Danish Academy of Sciences and Letters at www.royalacademy.dk. (accessed 7 September 2017).*

Edward Doisy (1893–1986), St Louis, USA, Nobel Prize 1943 "for discovery of the chemical nature of vitamin K." *Courtesy of Saint Louis University Libraries Digital Collections, Dr. Edward A. Doisy. SLU Photo Collection - Archives. Saint Louis University, Saint Louis, Missouri. Available at: http:// cdm.slu.edu/cdm/singleitem/collection/photos/ id/1130/rec/1. (accessed 7 September 2017).*

BACKGROUND

Charles Townsend was the first to describe "hemorrhagic disease of the newborn" (HDN) in 1894 in Boston with 50 cases occurring during their first few weeks of life. In 1929, vitamin K was isolated from alfalfa by Henrik Dam (Denmark) and Edward Doisy (United States), with clinical trials showing vitamin K protects against the condition later named vitamin K deficiency bleeding (VKDB). Dam and Doisy were jointly awarded the Nobel Prize in Medicine in 1943 for their work on vitamin K.

Prophylactic use of vitamin K has been recommended for all newborns since 1961 by the American Academy of Pediatrics (AAP) and the American College of Obstetricians and Gynecologists (ACOG), with repeated affirmation since and referenced in major neonatology, pediatrics, and hematology textbooks.

VKDB is a condition in which diffuse hemorrhage results from low levels of prothrombin and other vitamin K-dependent clotting factors caused by vitamin K deficiency. Low levels of vitamin K cause a physiologic deficiency of clotting factors and have been shown to occur in more than 20 percent of cord bloods in normal newborns in the first few days of life. Solely breastfed children are at higher risk for vitamin K deficiency as vitamin K is not sufficient in breast milk, as are babies with liver or enteric diseases that affect vitamin K absorption, or babies of mothers on antiepileptic medications. Without vitamin K prophylaxis, the Centers for Disease Control (CDC) reported in 2013 incidence of early and classical VKDB ranges from 0.25 percent to 1.7 percent of births. Incidence of late VKDB in the absence of vitamin K injection ranges from 4.4 to 7.2 per 100,000 infants with clinically significant and life threatening bleeding. In 2014 the CDC reported that VKDB fell from 4.4−7.2 cases per 100,000 births to 1.4−6.4 cases per 100,000 births in Asia and Europe after regimens for vitamin K prophylaxis were instituted.

Common clinical manifestations associated with low levels of prothrombin common in newborns breastfed and not given vitamin K prophylaxis include bleeding in the gastrointestinal tract, the umbilical stump, the scalp, or the urinary tract and intracranially. VKDB presents in various stages of infancy up to 6 months of age as:

- **Early VKDB** may appear as early as 0−24 hours after birth. It occurs mainly in newborns of mothers taking antiepileptic (phenobarbitone, phenytoin) or antituberculosis therapy (isoniazid and rifampicin). It may lead to serious bleeding and death.
- **Classic VKDB** is the most common form occurring between 1 and 7 days after birth in infants not given vitamin K prophylaxis, usually as bruising and umbilical cord bleeding but can go on to intracranial hemorrhages, gastrointestinal bleeding, and/or death.
- **Late VKDB** usually occurs between 2 and 12 weeks after birth but may occur up to 6 months in solely breastfed babies not receiving vitamin K prophylaxis with gastrointestinal and intracranial hemorrhage occurring in 30−60 percent of cases according to various reports. This can also occur in infants with other diseases such as bile-duct atresia or liver disease as contributory factors. Late VKDB is responsible for nearly all mortality and long-term sequelae due to this condition.

In the 1980s the New York State Department of Health conducted a review of infant mortality during the previous decade which revealed 32 infant deaths identified from vital records and hospital discharges, which were attributed to HDN and other neonatal hemorrhagic conditions. The search of vital records of infant deaths for the period 1980−86 included primary cause of death for the International Classification of Disease (ICD 9) codes for what was then called: hemorrhagic disease of the newborn (HDN), Disseminated Intravascular Coagulation (DIC) and unspecified hematological disorders specific to fetus or newborn).

Hospital records were reviewed for those infants whose deaths were attributed to these diagnoses. Each chart was reviewed by two graduate students in nursing to determine whether and when vitamin K was given, and the nature and timing of onset of bleeding. In cases where there was no documentation of vitamin K, the chart was reviewed with a senior consultant nurse.

A second review of vital records for infant deaths that included primary and up to four secondary causes of death (available for 1982−88 only) from what was then called Hemorrhagic Disease of the Newborn (HDN) and other hemorrhagic conditions of the newborn was carried out for the period 1981 through 1990. The database was searched for HDN and DIC. Since intraventricular hemorrhage is also a common feature of late VKDB, the search was extended to include it and subdural or cerebral (i.e. intracranial) hemorrhage (ICH).

Hospital discharge information from the statewide reporting system covering all hospitals providing maternity and newborn care in the state was analyzed for 1981−90 for these diseases, again including primary and four secondary diagnoses. In 1987, vitamin K was not included in standing medical orders in any of the 18 New York hospitals visited for case reviews, nor in four other hospitals consulted, thus the procedure required a written medical order for each newborn. In the vital records review, 44 infant deaths were identified throughout New York due to HDN and DIC.

Hospitals records were located and reviewed for 34 of these cases. Of these, 6 (18%) received no vitamin K at all, 16 (47%) received it after the onset of bleeding, and 12 (35%) had been given the vitamin K before the clinical presentation of hemorrhage. The documented clinical and laboratory differentiation between HDN and DIC was not always clear; some cases lacked confirmatory hematologic laboratory findings.

Data from the second review included primary along with second, third, and fourth listed diagnoses as contributory causes of death and hospitalization including HDN, DIC, and ICH. Multiple causes of death in the vital records review produced more cases than were found using primary diagnosis alone. During 1981−90, 163 hospitalizations were attributed to HDN alone, totaling 1,286 days of care. Of these, 5 had HDN as the principal diagnosis, but 158 additional cases were found when the search included four secondary diagnoses.

Vitamin K was thought to be standard practice in New York State during the 1980s. However, this study showed that standard policies for vitamin K were not consistently followed as this condition still occurred in this time period. Among neonatal deaths reviewed, in two-thirds of neonatal deaths vitamin K was not given, or was given after bleeding commenced. None of the 22 hospitals visited or consulted had standing orders for vitamin K administration (Tulchinsky et al., 1993).

Vitamin K deficiency may contribute to neonatal morbidity and mortality appearing under other diagnoses, such as DIC or intracerebral hemorrhage (ICH). The pathophysiologic process of DIC may include deficiency of vitamin K. ICH is a known entity but not always considered as a manifestation of HDN. They both commonly affect high-risk groups such as solely breast fed premature infants with respiratory distress syndrome (RDS) and/or sepsis.

The diagnosis of DIC may not take the possibility of vitamin K deficiency into account if it is made in the absence of hematological data, as in some of the cases reviewed. While these deaths could not be attributed to lack of vitamin K, late administration or nonuse of vitamin K in a bleeding neonate is of concern. Absence of documentation of giving vitamin K was interpreted to mean that it was not given. Lack of uniform policy in this procedure also resulted in the injection being given at various times following birth, including after onset of bleeding and in some cases, not being given at all.

Mandating preventive practices for some procedures in care of newborns, as well as school immunization, is accepted in the United States. However, at that time only 5 states in the US had mandated Vitamin K injections for all newborns. Findings of the review led the Commissioner of Health to recommend to the New York State Public Health Council to mandate use of vitamin K as a preventive measure within 6 hours of birth in the New York State Sanitary Code. Administration of vitamin K to newborns became a mandatory procedure in New York State and subsequently mandatory practice in all other states of the United States and elsewhere. A policy of mandatory vitamin K for newborns is especially important in developing countries and those in transition from the former Soviet system, as well as in Western countries, such as Germany, the Netherlands, and the UK where controversy reigns over oral versus intramuscular use of vitamin K.

During the 1990s Golding et al. reported that injected vitamin K was associated with an increased risk of lymphomas in children. A number of studies and reviews by Victora, Klebanoff, Zipursky, and others in different countries refuted this. Fear et al. in a large study in the UK reported finding no evidence of an association between intramuscular (IM) vitamin K and childhood cancer in general, or leukaemia. In Denmark Ekelund et al. reported no increased risk of cancer after IM administration of vitamin K as compared with that following oral administration. A systematic Cochrane-method literature review published in 2000 confirmed no relationship between vitamin K and cancer or leukemia. A United Kingdom Childhood Cancer Study in 2003 also concluded that there is no evidence that neonatal vitamin K given by injection or orally influences the risk of children developing leukaemia or any other cancer. A study in Italy points to confusion in policy and lack of clear guidelines harming neonatal care in rural areas, calling for standardized procedures adoption by national health authorities.

CURRENT RELEVANCE

Although vitamin K prophylaxis is widely accepted for routine care of newborns, there is great variance in practice. Reports from various parts of the world, including the UK and Europe, Japan, the United States, Canada, Australasia, and the Middle East, indicate the problem of VKDB is still important in the 21st century where vitamin K is not routinely used, or where its use may be waning due to parental resistance and professional confusion. Because prematurity, low birth weight, and breastfeeding are important risk factors for vitamin K deficiency this subject is of great importance in developing countries. Late VKDB is still an important cause of intracranial morbidity and mortality in developing countries where vitamin K prophylaxis is not routinely practiced, with intracranial hemorrhage a common mode of presentation.

In 2013, the CDC reported four cases of late VKDB with one death and three cases of intracranial bleeding reported as intraventricular bleeding with long-term brain damage in a hospital in Tennessee due to parental refusal of vitamin K injection. A 2014 review of cases in a teaching hospital in Nashville, by Schulte et al., reported seven cases of late VKDB of which four had intracranial hemorrhage of which two required urgent neurosurgical intervention. The reason for failure to give vitamin K was parental refusal and omission at homebirth or in birthing centers.

Globally the practice of vitamin K for newborns is highly variable. Extensive reviews of the literature such as that conducted by Victora in a UNICEF consultation report (1998) on cumulative reports from many high-income and developing countries describe the range of variation in VKDB and urge recognition of its significance as a global public health problem. Both India and China have been slow in adopting an effective program for administering vitamin K injections to newborns to prevent VKDB-related morbidity and mortality.

India and China together account for almost 37 percent of the world's population and thus were crucial for attaining Millennium Development Goal 4 (MDG 4)—to reduce two-thirds of the under-five mortality rate (U5MR) between 1990 and 2015. According to 2014 UN estimates, India's U5MR declined from 126/1,000 live births in 1990 to 53/1,000 live births in 2013 as compared to the target of 42/1,000 live births by 2015. In the same period, China achieved the MDG target with a 2013 U5MR of 13/1,000 live births. Neonatal deaths, however, remain a daunting challenge in both India and China, accounting for 61 percent and 55 percent, respectively, deaths of those age under-five. India's approximately 760,000 neonatal deaths annually, a neonatal mortality rate (NMR) of 29/1,000 live births, compares poorly with that of China at 8/1,000 live births.

WHO guidelines for neonatal care include 0.5–1.0 mg of vitamin K by injection for all newborns but this is not consistently included in all documents related to meeting the MDGs, and follow-up Sustainable Development Goals (SDGs). Promotion of breastfeeding, while worthy and necessary, is an added risk factor for vitamin K deficiency and an important reason to actively promote mandatory vitamin K injection for newborns especially in low- and medium-income countries, but is not currently a high-priority issue in low-income countries. This may be due to continuing controversy in European literature on oral versus intramuscular vitamin K as well as a growing community of mothers, and some care givers, who refuse or discourage vitamin K injections, as well as immunizations, for newborns and infants.

ETHICAL ISSUES

The American Academy of Pediatrics (AAP) in 2003 renewed its recommendation that all infants should receive vitamin K within 6 hours of birth by injection and reaffirmed this recommendation in 2014. This recommendation was also adopted by Canadian, Australian, New Zealand, and other pediatric associations. The WHO in 2012 issued a strong recommendation: *"All newborns should be given 1 mg of vitamin K intramuscularly after birth."* The UK recommendations were to adopt either oral or intramuscular vitamin K, although the oral dose requires multiple doses and has a record of poor compliance and efficacy.

Parental refusal is a growing issue. A study reported by Clayton et al. in Nashville hospitals following the six cases of VKDB in 2013 identified 2.7 percent of surveyed mothers in Nashville hospitals refusing vitamin K, and 28 percent of mothers at five birthing centers refusing; 65 percent of refusers also rejected other preventive measures including hepatitis B vaccination and routine antibiotic eye treatment to prevent gonorrheal eye infection, in the past a common cause of blindness. Refusal of vitamin K is also an indicator of refusal of routine infant immunizations, a growing problem in the United States and elsewhere (see Chapter 3).

In a population-based study in Canada Sahni et al. showed that planned home deliveries by midwives were eight times more likely to have mother refusal of vitamin K prophylaxis as compared to hospital deliveries. A report by Schulte et al. characterized parents who are likely to decline vitamin K for their infants and whose children are also likely to be unimmunized. Early identification of high-risk parents may provide strategies to increase uptake of both vitamin K and childhood immunizations. Deliveries at home or at private maternity homes have high rates of non-implementation of vitamin K prophylaxis.

Promoting routine vitamin K by injection is vital for global child survival and health. However, there are new reports of parental refusal along with rejection of some vaccines. As a result children are suffering from VKDB with serious intracranial damage and even death. The effect of parental refusal places children at risk of serious debility or death. Libertarian views suggest that the parent has the right of refusal, while a public health response is that the child is being placed at serious risk.

Globally vitamin K injection at birth is confounded by debate over use of oral vitamin K, which is not widely available and requires at least four doses to prevent early and late VKDB, and thus compliance is prejudiced especially where primary care services are weak or nonexistent. Thus vitamin K by injection is the feasible alternative in most situations, but this is debated or unclear and left to local professional decision. Oral vitamin K is used more commonly in Europe than in North America. Globally, VKDB is reported, but consistent and population-based incidence data are lacking.

China and India have both placed this condition on their maternal child health (MCH) priority lists in recent years, but implementation is highly variable. WHO had recommended vitamin K be added to neonatal care in recent years, but many international health agencies such as UNICEF and major donors such as the Bill and Melinda Gates Foundation and the World Bank do not clearly include this in their priorities. Theme issues of leading journals such as *Lancet* have only recently noted VKDB as an important health issue to promote neonatal survival.

Policy failure to adopt vitamin K to prevent VKDB by leading international organizations such as UNICEF or by major donors such as the Gates Foundation leaves the issue aside in most settings in low-income countries and in doubt in medium- and high-income countries.

ECONOMIC ISSUES

Use of vitamin K as prophylaxis is cost-effective compared to the burden of ongoing care and long-term disability for infants with permanent sequelae. The type of personnel used to administer the prophylaxis is an additional cost. The cost per injection is less than US$1 per dose excluding staff and facility costs. At a unit cost of US$ 1.00 per injectable dose, Victora estimated that saving one disability-adjusted life year would cost US$ 52 and US$ 133 in high- and intermediate-incidence scenarios, respectively. The World Bank classifies interventions costing under $100 per disability-adjusted life year as cost-effective, thus IM vitamin K prophylaxis are cost-effective in high-incidence medium- and low-income countries (Sankar et al. 2016). WHO and UNICEF have concluded that this is an economically justifiable recommendation especially because of strong recommendation of exclusive breast feeding, a risk factor for VKDB. In middle-income countries, most births take place in hospitals and Vitamin K injection may easily be added. In industrialized countries, vitamin K prophylaxis is certainly justified for mandatory vitamin K by injection, as a professional and ethical issue. The economic cost of an individual case of death or intracranial hemorrhage due to VKDB is a burden for health systems and bears severe emotional and economic consequences for the family involved (CDC).

CONCLUSION

Vitamin K prophylaxis is a well-established, safe, and cost-effective intervention for the prevention of VKDB in newborns in developed countries, yet the incidence and implications of vitamin K deficiency in developing countries have received little attention. The examples of India and China indicate that although China has had greater success in reducing U5MR at a faster rate than India, the proportion of neonatal deaths to under-five deaths remains a challenge to the Chinese public health system. While no reliable data are publicly available, the issue of VKDB is at last receiving attention by the Chinese public health system as well as by the Indian government.

VKDB is increasingly recognized as a public health problem in low- and middle-income countries, where primary prevention is not part of common preventive care of newborns. It is also still a significant concern in industrialized countries due to mixed messages of policy between oral vitamin K, which requires multiple doses, versus a single dose of intramuscular vitamin K with a long and safe track record of prevention. Lack of proper laboratory test facilities to diagnose VKDB, particularly in developing countries, and the failure to diagnose neonatal deaths may distort statistics as late VKDB is often sudden in onset and the infant may die before reaching a hospital.

However, vitamin K by injection as a safe, inexpensive, and effective intervention should be given to all newborns as a high priority in the public health policy of governments and international donor organizations. Even in high-income countries, parental refusal of recommended vitamin K injection at birth is resulting in a return of this preventable condition with serious morbidity and fatal results. In some high-income countries choice of oral vitamin K administration is also a factor in the return of VKDB. But especially for low- and middle-income countries mandatory vitamin K injection following birth would be an effective addition to recommended interventions for global initiatives and agencies to help reduce preventable neonatal mortality and morbidity.

Public and professional confusion remain in many countries between intramuscular and oral vitamin K despite the clear advantage of the intramuscular single dose versus the multiple oral doses required for full protection. In global health, the issue is important for the achievement of reducing infant mortality. In high-income countries continual education efforts for health care providers and families and government officials along with renewed and concerted leadership by governments are required to improve the adverse impacts of vitamin K deficiency in infants and improvement toward attaining the UN Sustainable Development Goals for maternal and child health.

RECOMMENDATIONS

1. Vitamin K should be given as a 1 mg intramuscular injection to all newborns within 6 hours of birth as standing orders by hospitals, birthing centers, physicians, midwives, and in health promotion of maternity and newborn care.

2. Prevention of VKDB by routine vitamin K injections should be promoted as policy and funding by international agencies and donors as a funding

priority for routine newborn care in high-, medium-, and low-income countries.

3. Concerted action by all international, national, and global health agencies and donors is needed to implement strategies for vitamin K prophylaxis and treatment on a global basis with an emphasis on developing countries.
4. In low- and middle-income countries where home deliveries are common, midwives, traditional birth attendants (TBAs), or community health workers (CHWs) should be trained and supplied with vitamin K for routine postpartum administration.
5. In high-income counties, birthing centers outside of hospitals and providers of home deliveries should be trained and held responsible and monitored for giving vitamin K for the safety and well-being of all newborns.

STUDENT REVIEW QUESTIONS

1. HDN or VKDB have been known for well over a century. So why is their prevention not part of recommended global health preventive measures?
2. Is the administration of vitamin K for prophylaxis of hemorrhagic disease of the newborn an accepted procedure or mandatory for neonatal care in your country?
3. How can this issue be investigated in your country?
4. How should international practice guidelines be adopted for routine vitamin K intramuscular injection, and how should they be promoted in your country?
5. Why should a relatively uncommon condition such as VKDB be of priority concern to health systems and policymakers?
6. What possible public health action could be implemented to improve and change the situation of preventing VKBD to increase awareness by medical workers and to promote and implement regulation or legislation?
7. Why has VKDB recurred after years without cases in the United States? What should be done to protect newborns from VKDB?
8. Why are VKDB mortality data not available and reported by international disease studies?

RECOMMENDED READINGS

1. Adame N, Carpenter SL. Closing the loophole: midwives and the administration of vitamin K in neonates. J Pediatr. 2009;154(5):769–771. doi:10.1016/j.jpeds.2008.11.038. Abstract available at: http://www.ncbi.nlm.nih.gov/pubmed/19364563 (accessed 26 August 2017).
2. Alpan G, Avital A, Peleg O, Dgani Y. Late presentation of hemorrhagic disease of the newborn. Arch Dis Child. 1984;59:482–483. Available at: https://www.ncbi.nlm.nih.gov/pmc/articles/PMC1628491/pdf/archdisch00734-0100.pdf (accessed 1 September 2017).
3. American Academy of Pediatrics, American College of Obstetricians and Gynecologists. Care of the newborn. In: Riley LE, Stark AR, editors. Guidelines for perinatal care. 7th ed. Elk Grove Village, IL: American Academy of Pediatrics and American College of Obstetricians, 2012.

4. American Academy of Pediatrics Committee on Fetus and Newborn. Controversies concerning vitamin K and the newborn. Pediatrics. 2003;112(1):191−192. Available at: http://pediatrics.aappublications.org/content/112/1/191.full; (accessed 25 August 2017).
5. Bang AT, Bang RA, Baitule SB, Reddy MH, Deshmukh MD. Effect of home based neonatal care and management of sepsis on neonatal mortality: field trial in rural India. Lancet. 1999;354(9194):1955−1961. Abstract available at: http://www.thelancet.com/journals/lancet/article/PIIS0140-6736(99)03046-9/abstract (accessed 25 August 2017).
6. Behrmann BA, Chan WK, Finer NN. Resurgence of hemorrhagic disease of the newborn: a report of three cases. CMA J. 1985;133(9):884−885. Abstract available at: http://www.ncbi.nlm.nih.gov/pmc/articles/PMC1346300/pdf/canmedaj00272-0053.pdf (accessed 25 August 2017).
7. Bhutta ZA, Das JK, Bahl R, Lawn JE, Salam RA, Paul VK, et al. Can available interventions end preventable deaths in mothers, newborn babies, and stillbirths, and at what cost? Lancet. 2014;384(9940):347−370. Abstract available at: http://www.thelancet.com/journals/lancet/article/PIIS0140-6736(14)60792-3/fulltext (accessed 25 August 2017).
8. Busfield A, McNinch A, Tripp J. Neonatal vitamin K prophylaxis in Great Britain and Ireland: the impact of perceived risk and product licensing on effectiveness. Arch Dis Child. 2007;92:754−758. Abstract available at: http://adc.bmj.com/content/92/9/754 (accessed 25 August 2017).
9. Canadian Pediatric Society. Position statement: routine administration of vitamin K to newborns. Posted: Dec 1 1997. Paediatr Child Health. 1997;2(6):429−431. Available at: http://www.cps.ca/en/documents/position/administration-vitamin-K-newborns (accessed 25 May 2017).
10. Canadian Agency for Drugs and Technologies in Health. Neonatal vitamin K administration for the prevention of Hemorrhagic Disease: a review of the clinical effectiveness, comparative effectiveness, and guidelines, 28 May 2015. Available at: https://www.ncbi.nlm.nih.gov/pubmedhealth/PMH0078451/pdf/PubMedHealth_PMH0078451.pdf (accessed 14 August 2017).
11. Canfield LM, Hopkinson JM, Lima AF, Silva B, Garza C. Vitamin K in colostrum and mature human milk over the lactation period: a cross-sectional study. Am J Clin Nutr. 1991;53:730−735. Abstract available at: http://www.ncbi.nlm.nih.gov/pubmed/2000828 (accessed 25 August 2017).
12. Caravella SJ, Clark DA, Dweck HS. Health codes for newborn care. Pediatrics. 1987;80 (1).1−5. Abstract available at: http://www.ncbi.nlm.nih.gov/pubmed/3601503 (accessed 25 August 2017).
13. Centers for Disease Control and Prevention. Late vitamin K deficiency bleeding in infants whose parents declined vitamin K prophylaxis—Tennessee, 2013. MMWR Morb Mort Wkly Rep. 2013;62(45):901−902. Available at http://www.cdc.gov/mmwr/preview/mmwrhtml/mm6245a4.htm (accessed 25 August 2017).
14. Centers for Disease Control and Prevention. Facts about vitamin K deficiency bleeding, updated 15 September 2017. Available at: https://www.cdc.gov/ncbddd/vitamink/facts.html (accessed 14 December 2017).
15. Chaou W, Chou M, Eitzman D. Intracranial hemorrhage and vitamin K deficiency in early infancy. J Pediatrics. 1984;105:880−884. Abstract available at: http://www.jpeds.com/article/S0022-3476(84)80070-0/abstract (accessed 25 August 2017).

16. Clayton J., Marcewicz L., Traylor J., Grant A.M., Jones T.F., Dunn J. et al. Vitamin K refusal rates and parental attitudes—Tennessee, 2013. Presentation at 2014 CSTE conference, Nashville Tennessee, 2014. Abstract available at: https://cste.confex.com/cste/2014/webprogram/Paper3680.html (accessed 15 February 2017).

17. Committee of Nutrition, America Academy of Pediatrics. Vitamin K compounds and the water-soluble analogues: use in therapy and prophylaxis in pediatrics. Pediatrics. 1961;28:501−506. Available at: http://pediatrics.aappublications.org/content/28/3/501.full.pdf (accessed 25 August 2017).

18. Crowther C, Crosby DD, Henderson-Smart DJ. Vitamin K prior to preterm birth for preventing neonatal periventricular hemorrhage. Cochrane Database Syst Rev. 2010;1: CD000229. Abstract available at: http://onlinelibrary.wiley.com/doi/10.1002/14651858. CD000229.pub2/abstract;jsessionid = F03FB0C7451D66F2505DF35AD625DAE0.f04t02 (accessed 25 August 2017).

19. Danielsson N, Hoa DP, Thang NV, Vos T, Loughnan PM. Intracranial haemorrhage due to late onset vitamin K deficiency bleeding in Hanoi province, Vietnam. Arch Dis Child Fetal Neonatal Ed. 2004;89(6):F546−F550. Available at: https://www.ncbi.nlm.nih.gov/pmc/articles/PMC1721780/pdf/v089p0F546.pdf (accessed 25 August 2017).

20. Darmstadt GL, Bhutta ZA, Cousens S, Adam T, Walker N, de Bernis L, et al. Evidence-based, cost-effective interventions: how many newborn babies can we save? Lancet. 2005;365(9463):977−988. Available at: http://www.ncbi.nlm.nih.gov/pubmed/15767001 (accessed 25 August 2017).

21. Ekelund H, Finnström O, Gunnarskog J, Källén B, Larsson Y. Administration of vitamin K to newborn infants and childhood cancer. BMJ. 1993;307(6896):89−91. Available at: https://www.ncbi.nlm.nih.gov/pmc/articles/PMC1693492/pdf/bmj00029-0017.pdf (accessed 25 August 2017).

22. Eventov-Friedman S, Vinograd O, Ben-Haim M, Penso S, Bar-Oz B, Zisk-Rony RY. Parents' knowledge and perceptions regarding vitamin K prophylaxis in newborns. J Pediatr Hematol Oncol. 2013;35:409−413. Abstract available at: http://www.ncbi.nlm.nih.gov/pubmed/23242324 (accessed 25 August 2017).

23. Fear NT, Roman E, Ansell E, Simpson J, Day N, Eden OB. Vitamin K and childhood cancer: a report from the United Kingdom Childhood Cancer Study. Br J Cancer. 2003;89:1228−1231. Available at: http://www.ncbi.nlm.nih.gov/pmc/articles/PMC2394315/ (accessed 25 August 2017).

24. Forbes D. Delayed presentation of hemorrhagic disease of the newborn. Med J Aust. 1983;2:136−138. Abstract available at: http://europepmc.org/abstract/med/6877145 (accessed 25 August 2017).

25. Guala A, Guarino R, Zaffaroni M, Martano C, Fabris C, Pastore G, et al. The impact of national and international guidelines on newborn care in the nurseries of Piedmont and Aosta Valley, Italy. BMC Pediatr. 2005;5:45. Available: https://www.ncbi.nlm.nih.gov/pmc/articles/PMC1315318/pdf/1471-2431-5-45.pdf (accessed 14 May 2017).

26. Golding J, Greenwood R, Birmingham K, Mott M. Childhood cancer, intramuscular vitamin K, and pethidine given during labour. BMJ. 1992;305(6849):341−346. Available at: https://www.ncbi.nlm.nih.gov/pmc/articles/PMC1883000/pdf/bmj00086-0023.pdf (accessed 25 August 2017).

27. Hanawa Y, Maki M, Murata B, Matsuyama E, Yamamoto Y. The second nation-wide survey in Japan of vitamin K deficiency in infancy. Eur J Pediatr. 1988;147:472−477. Abstract available at: http://www.ncbi.nlm.nih.gov/pubmed/3409922 (accessed 25 August 2017).

28. Handel J, Tripp JH. Vitamin K prophylaxis against haemorrhagic disease of the newborn in the United Kingdom. BMJ. 1991;303:1109. Available at: http://www.bmj.com/content/303/6810/1109 (accessed 25 August 2017).

29. Haelle T. More parents nixing anti-bleeding shots for their newborns. Scientific American, August 2014. Available at: https://www.scientificamerican.com/article/more-parents-nixing-anti-bleeding-shots-for-their-newborns/ (accessed 15 February 2017).

31. Klebanoff MA, Read JS, Mills JL, Shiono PH. The risk of childhood cancer after neonatal exposure to vitamin K. N Engl J Med. 1993;329(13):905−908. Available at: http://www.nejm.org/doi/full/10.1056/NEJM199309233291301 (access 26 August 2017).

32. Lane PA, Hathaway WE. Vitamin K in infancy. J Pediatr. 1985;106:351−359. Available at: http://www.sciencedirect.com/science/article/pii/S0022347685806569 (accessed 25 August 2017).

34. Lee ACW, Li CH, So KT. Vitamin K deficiency bleeding revisited. Hong Kong J Pediatr. 2002;7:157−161. English available at: http://www.hkjpaed.org/pdf/2002;7;157-161.pdf (accessed 26 May 2017).

35. Lippi G, Franchini M. Vitamin K in neonates: facts and myths. Blood Transfus. 2011; 9(1):4−9. doi:10.2450/2010.0034-10. Available at: http://www.ncbi.nlm.nih.gov/pmc/articles/PMC3021393/ (accessed 25 August 2017).

36. Liu L, Oza S, Hogan D, Perin J, Rudan I, Lawn JE, et al. Global, regional, and national causes of child mortality in 2000−13, with projections to inform post-2015 priorities: an updated systematic analysis. Lancet. 2015;385(9966):430−440. Available at: http://www.thelancet.com/journals/lancet/article/PIIS0140-6736(14)61698-6/fulltext (accessed 25 August 2017).

37. Martín-López JE, Carlos-Gil AM, Rodríguez-López R, Villegas-Portero R, Luque-Romero L. Prophylactic vitamin K for vitamin K deficiency bleeding of the newborn. Farm Hosp. 2011;35(3):148−155. Available at: http://www.aulamedica.es/fh/pdf/ING/343.pdf (accessed 25 August 2017).

38. McNinch A. Vitamin K deficiency bleeding: early history and recent trends in the United Kingdom. Early Hum Dev. 2010;86(Suppl. 1):63−65. doi:10.1016/j.earlhumdev.2010.01.017. Abstract available at: https://www.ncbi.nlm.nih.gov/pubmed/20167443 (accessed 25 August 2017).

39. McNinch AW, Tripp JH. Haemorrhagic disease of the newborn in the British Isles: two year prospective study. BMJ. 1991;303:1105−1109. Available at: https://www.ncbi.nlm.nih.gov/pmc/articles/PMC2549009/pdf/bmj00583-0026.pdf (accessed 25 August 2017).

40. Motohara KEF, Matsuda I. Effect of vitamin K administration on Acarboxy Prothrombin (PIVKA-II) levels in newborns. Lancet. 1985;2(8449):242−244. Abstract available at: http://www.sciencedirect.com/science/article/pii/S0140673685902910 (accessed 25 August 2017).

41. Nimavat DJ, Sherman MP, Itani O, Windle ML, Clark DA, Wagner CL, et al. Hemorrhagic disease of the newborn. Medscape. 2014. Available at: http://emedicine.medscape.com/article/974489-overview#showall (accessed 25 August 2017).

42. Nobel Prize in Physiology or Medicine 1943. Nobelprize.org. Nobel Media AB 2014. Web. 27 May 2015. Available at: http://www.nobelprize.org/nobel_prizes/medicine/laureates/1943/index.html (accessed 15 May 2017).

43. Osrin D, Prost A. Perinatal interventions and survival in resource-poor settings: which work, which don't, which have the jury out? Arch Dis Child. 2010;95(12):1039−1046. doi:10.1136/adc.2009.179366. Available at: http://www.ncbi.nlm.nih.gov/pmc/articles/PMC3428881/ (accessed 25 August 2017).

44. Pooni PA, Singh D, Singh H, Jain BK. Intracranial hemorrhage in late hemorrhagic disease of the newborn. Indian Pediatr. 2003;40(3):243–248. Abstract available at: http://www.ncbi.nlm.nih.gov/pubmed/12657759 (accessed 25 August).

45. Puckett R, Offringa M. Prophylactic vitamin K for vitamin K deficiency bleeding in neonates. Cochrane Database Syst Rev. 2000;4:CD002776. Abstract available at: http://www.cochrane.org/CD002776/NEONATAL_prophylactic-vitamin-k-for-vitamin-k-deficiency-bleeding-in-neonates (accessed 25 August 2017).

46. Rai RK, Jing L, Tulchinsky TH. Vitamin K supplementation to prevent haemorrhagic morbidity and mortality in newborns: focus on India and China. World J Pediatr. 2017 Feb;13(1):15-19. doi: 10.1007/s12519-016-0062-6. Epub 2016 Nov 15. Abstract available at: https://www.ncbi.nlm.nih.gov/pubmed/27878777 (accessed 14 August 2017).

47. Roman E, Fear NT, Ansell P, Bull D, Draper G, Mc Kinney P. Vitamin K and childhood cancer: analysis of individual patient data from six case-control studies. Br J Cancer. 2002;86:63–69. Available at: http://www.nature.com/bjc/journal/v86/n1/full/6600007a.html (accessed 25 August 2017).

48. Sahni V, Lai FY, MacDonald SE. Neonatal vitamin K refusal and nonimmunization. Pediatrics. 2014;134(3):497–503. Available at: http://pediatrics.aappublications.org/content/134/3/497.long (accessed 25 August 2017).

49. Sankar MJ, Chandrasekaran A, Kumar P, Thukral A, Agarwal R, Paul VK. Vitamin K prophylaxis for prevention of vitamin K deficiency bleeding: a systematic review. J Perinatol. 2016;36(Suppl. 1):S29–S35. doi:10.1038/jp.2016.30. Available at: https://www.ncbi.nlm.nih.gov/pmc/articles/PMC4862383/ (accessed 25 August 2017).

50. Schulte R, Jordan LC, Morad A, Naftel RP, Wellons III JC, Sidonio R. Rise in late onset vitamin K deficiency bleeding in young infants because of omission or refusal of prophylaxis at birth. Pediatr Neurol. 2014;50(6):564–568. Available at: http://www.pedneur.com/article/S0887-8994(14)00141-6/pdf (accessed 25 August 2017).

51. Shapiro AD, Jacobson LJ, Armon ME, Manco-Johnson MJ, Lane PA. Vitamin K deficiency in the newborn infant: prevalence and perinatal risk factors. J Pediatr. 1986;109 (4):675–680. Abstract available at: http://www.ncbi.nlm.nih.gov/pubmed/3761086 (accessed 25 August 2017).

52. Shearer MJ, Fu X, Booth SL. Vitamin K nutrition, metabolism, and requirements: current concepts and future research. Adv Nutr. 2012;3(2):182–195. Available at: http://advances.nutrition.org/content/3/2/182.full (accessed 25 August 2017).

53. Shearer MJ. Vitamin K deficiency bleeding (VKDB) in early infancy. Blood Rev. 2009;23 (2):49–59. Available at: http://www.ncbi.nlm.nih.gov/pubmed/18804903 (accessed 25 August 2017).

54. Sutor AH, Dagres N, Niederhoff H. Late form of vitamin K deficiency bleeding in Germany. Klin Padiatr. 1995;207(3):89–97. Abstract available at: https://www.ncbi.nlm.nih.gov/pubmed/7623433 (accessed 4 September 2017).

55. Tulchinsky TH, Patton MM, Randolph LA, Meyer MR, Linden JV. Mandating vitamin K prophylaxis for newborns in New York State. Am J Public Health. 1993;83(8):1166–1168. Available at: https://www.ncbi.nlm.nih.gov/pmc/articles/PMC1695173/pdf/amjph00532-0096.pdf (accessed 25 August 2017).

56. UNICEF United Nations Children's Fund. Level and trends in child mortality, report 2014. New York: United Nations Children's Fund, 2014. Available at: http://www.unicef.org/media/files/Levels_and_Trends_in_Child_Mortality_2014.pdf (accessed 25 August 2017).

57. Victora C. Vitamin K deficiency and haemorrhagic disease of the newborn: a public health problem in less developed countries? New York: UNICEF, 1997. Available at: http://www.

unicef.org/french/evaldatabase/files/Global_1997_Vitamin_K.pdf (accessed 25 August 2017).

58. Victora CG, Van Heake P. Vitamin K prophylaxis in less developed countries: policy issues and relevance to breast-feeding promotion. Am J Public Health. 1998;88:203−209. Available at: http://www.ncbi.nlm.nih.gov/pmc/articles/PMC1508196/pdf/amjph00014-0031.pdf (accessed 25 May 2017).

59. von Kries R, Göbel U. Vitamin K prophylaxis: oral or parenteral. Am J Dis Child. 1988;142:14−15. Abstract available at: http://jamanetwork.com/journals/jamapediatrics/article-abstract/513826 (accessed 25 August 2017).

60. Weddle M, Empey A, Crossen E, Green A, Green J, Philippi CA. Are pediatricians complicit in Vitamin K Deficiency Bleeding? Pediatrics. 2015;136(4):753−757. Abstract available DOI: 10.1542/peds.2014-2293" at: http://pediatrics.aappublications.org/content/early/2015/09/08/peds.2014-2293 (accessed 25 August 2017).

61. Wefring K. Hemorrhage in the newborn and vitamin K prophylaxis. J Pediatr. 1962;61:663−666. Abstract available at: http://countdown2030.org/ (accessed 25 August 2017).

62. World Health Organization. Recommendations for management of common childhood conditions: evidence for technical update of pocket book recommendations: newborn conditions, dysentery, pneumonia, oxygen use and delivery, common causes of fever, severe acute malnutrition and supportive care. Geneva, Switzerland: WHO, 2012. Available at: http://apps.who.int/iris/bitstream/10665/44774/1/9789241502825_eng.pdf?ua = 1&ua = 1 (accessed 2 April 2017).

63. World Health Organization. Countdown to 2030. Maternal, newborn and child survival. Geneva, Switzerland: WHO, 2014. Available at: http://countdown2030.org/ (accessed 25 May 2017).

64. World Health Organization. Guidelines on maternal, newborn, child and adolescent health approved by the Who Guidelines Review Committee. Recommendations on newborn health. Geneva, Switzerland: WHO, 2012. Available at: http://www.who.int/maternal_child_adolescent/documents/guidelines-recommendations-newborn-health.pdf (accessed 26 May 2017).

65. World Health Organization. Maternal, newborn, child and adolescent health: newborn care at birth. Geneva, Switzerland: WHO, 2015. Available at: http://www.who.int/maternal_child_adolescent/topics/newborn/care_at_birth/en/ (accessed 26 May 2017).

66. Zhang H, Wang W. Analysis of 3 970 cases of late vitamin K deficiency bleeding in infancy. China J Child Healthcare. 2004;12(1):31−32 (Chinese) English abstract available at: http://en.cnki.com.cn/Article_en/CJFDTOTAL-ERTO200401014.htm (accessed 26 May 2017).

67. Zipurski A. Prevention of vitamin K deficiency in newborns. Br J Haematol. 1999;104:430−437. doi:10.1046/j.1365-2141.1999.01104.x. Available at: http://www.ncbi.nlm.nih.gov/pubmed/10086774 (accessed 25 August 2017).

Chapter 18

Eliminating Beta Thalassemia Major and Other Congenital Blood Disorders

ABSTRACT

Thalassemia was first described as a hemolytic anemia by Cooley and Lee in 1925 in several Italian-American children with severe anemia, enlarged spleen and liver, discoloration of the skin, and bone changes. The disorder was first named Cooley's anemia and later thalassemia from the term "thalassa anemia" or Mediterranean anemia due to its association with the Mediterranean Sea and throughout the Middle East region. Originally, thalassemia was thought to be a disease mainly among Greek, Arab, Southern Italian and Turkish populations. However, as early as the 1930s there were case reports among Asians as well. Thalassemia in its various forms as the most common genetic disorder of public health significance in the World Health Organization (WHO) Southeast Asia, Indian subcontinent and sub-Saharan Africa as well as countries with immigration of population from affected regions. Sickle Cell Disease is a milder but clinically important hemoglobin disorder primarily among people of African origin. Estimates suggest that between 300,000 and 400,000 babies are born with serious hemoglobin disorders annually, the vast majority in low- or middle-income countries. Preventive efforts, genomics and developments in bone marrow technology along with treatment with blood transfusions and chelating agents are extending the life of those afflicted. Experience with community health promotion measures for prevention of new cases of Beta thalassemia major in Cyprus, a high prevalence country, became a model for preventing genetic disorders. This came well before the genome era with important lessons for genetic disease control in many countries with much more potential for wider application in low and medium income countries.

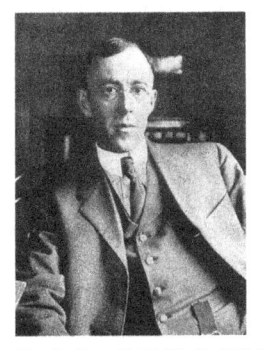

Thomas Benton Cooley (1871−1945), first described anemia in 1925 later called Cooley's anemia, then Mediterranean anemia, and finally Beta thalassemia major; Professor of Pediatrics, Hematology and Hygiene, University of Michigan, USA. *Original Source: History of the University of Michigan, 1906, by Burke Hinsdale; Current Source: available at: https://commons.wikimedia.org/wiki/File:Thomas_Benton_Cooley.jpg#file.*

Case Studies in Public Health. DOI: http://dx.doi.org/10.1016/B978-0-12-804571-8.00004-4

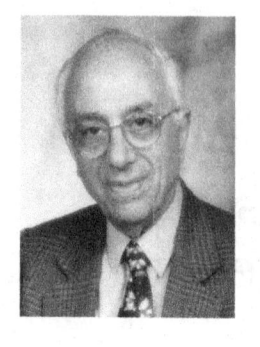

Dr Minas Hadjiminas; MD at the University of Birmingham with pediatric training in London and Edinburgh. He returned to Cyprus to lead the Paediatric Clinic of the Nicosia General Hospital. In 1971 he initiated an innovative and successful program for control of the disease; a goal achieved famously within a decade. *Source: Courtesy of National Population Laboratory - Reference Laboratory for Haemoglobinopathies, Public Health Services, Archbishop Makarios III Hospital, Ministry of Health, Nikosia, Cyprus.*

BACKGROUND

Thalassemia was first described in 1925 by Dr. Thomas Benton Cooley, Professor of Pediatrics at Wayne State University in Michigan as cases of severe anemia with an enlarged spleen, bone deformities, and fatigue in Italian immigrant children. Later recognized as a common condition among people from the Mediterranean Sea region, it was termed Mediterranean anemia, the name thalassemia from the Greek word for sea. It became a treatable condition by blood transfusions and medication to remove excess iron from the body. In countries with a high prevalence of the disease, such as Cyprus, later Sardinia and across the Mediterranean populations, methods of screening of married carriers of the recessive gene and community supported education, screening, and genetic counseling were tried.

Successful prevention of beta thalassemia showed how to overcome some genetic disorders of newborns. This case study reviews the incidence and long-term management of thalassemia and thus improved prognosis for those afflicted. Newborn screening for a wide range of birth disorders including phenylketonuria (PKU), congenital hypothyroidism (CH), sickle-cell disease (SCD), hearing deficit, and many other conditions indicates the importance of early diagnosis and initiation of supportive care needed to sustain quality and duration of life, including for groups at risk for beta thalassemia major (BTM). Nutritional interventions such as folic acid taken before pregnancy and ideally in fortified basic foods along with iodine in salt, iron, and other trace elements in improved maternal nutrition as well as avoidance of smoking, alcohol, and nonprescription drug use provide great hope for improved neonatal outcomes and lifelong health (See Chapter 20).

In 1973, a program of public education, population screening, genetic counseling, and for those with the defective gene present in both mother and father, antenatal diagnosis for beta thalassemia began in Cyprus. In 1981, Angastiniotis and Hadjiminas reported on the successful program of prevention of thalassemia in Cyprus. Initiated in 1976, the rate of births of BTM cases based on pre-program experience which was one per 135 births, the number of cases fell from 23 (of an expected 71 cases) in 1978 to 18 (of an expected 77 cases) in 1979, (i.e. inherited the defective gene from both mother and father). A similar program was successful in Sardinia. Since that time, many countries in the Mediterranean region and other countries to which people from that region migrated have instituted education, screening, and clinical management programs with considerable success in reducing the number of births with BTM. The principles learned from these experiences have been applied to other ethnic groups subject to serious genetic diseases.

Thalassemia is the name of a group of recessive genetic disorders of the blood that includes alpha- and beta thalassemia, each affecting different proteins in hemoglobin, with different variations in each group. Alpha thalassemia is commonly found in Africa, the Middle East, India, Southeast Asia, southern China, and occasionally the Mediterranean region. It is generally mild, although it includes several variations that are life threatening to the affected fetus.

Thomas Benton Cooley was born in Michigan to a family of distinguished lawyers. After completing medical school at the University of Michigan in 1895, he took specialized training in hygiene and contagious diseases at Boston City Hospital and in Germany. As medical director of the Babies' Milk Fund in Detroit, Cooley made a big contribution to a dramatic reduction of infant deaths. During World War I he worked with the American Red Cross in France leading projects to ensure the health of children, for which in 1924 he was awarded the Legion of Honour. On returning from France in 1921, Cooley became head of pediatrics at the Children's Hospital of Michigan and investigated a form of childhood anemia with bone changes in children of Italian and Greek heritage. In 1925 he presented his findings to the American Pediatric Society, naming this disorder erythroblastic anemia; it became known as Cooley's anemia. His contributions to hematology laid the groundwork for thalassemia research and treatment in the following decades. (Cooley's Anemia Foundation, 2017).

BTM originally known as Cooley's or Mediterranean anemia is a severe recessive genetic disorder of hemoglobin structure with hemolysis or rapid breakdown of red blood cells resulting in anemia and iron overload in the heart, liver and other organs. When the gene is inherited from both parents, the child will have BTM. The carrier or heterozygous state, beta thalassemia minor, is usually without clinical significance but when two carriers marry, each pregnancy has a 25 percent chance of becoming BTM, and others have chance of carrier status.

Beta thalassemia major (BTM) is widespread throughout the Middle East, southern Europe, North Africa, and across southern India and Southeast Asia. Prevalence rates for carrier status vary. In the Arab countries, carrier rates are around three percent; in Azerbaijan and Iran (4−10 percent); and in Greece, eight percent. It is ultimately fatal for those afflicted, but with current standards of treatment, including blood infusions and chelating agents (i.e., iron binding for excretion) to reduce iron overload and hemochromatosis (i.e., overload of iron in the blood so that iron deposits damage many organs), well-managed patients can now survive into their thirties.

According to the World Health Organization (WHO) there have been 240,000 deaths and over 300,000 new cases of severe hemoglobinopathies, and approximately five percent of the world population are carriers of the genes for thalassemia and sickle cell disease (SCD). Currently, worldwide annual total incidence of individuals with symptoms is about 1:100,000, with incidence in the European Union estimated at 1:10,000.

Congenital disorders of hemoglobin are widespread; originally identified in the Mediterranean areas, they are now recognized in Southeast Asia (i.e., thalassemia) and in sub-Saharan Africa (especially SCD). Because of population migration, these disorders are now spread worldwide, with 10 percent of the population at risk in the United States, especially in states with high immigration of peoples with South Asian, Chinese, Mediterranean, and Arab ethnicity. With large scale migration from South East Asia new variants of the genetic makeup of thalassemia are becoming more prominent in the US and other western countries. Asia, India, and the Middle East will account for 95 percent of births with Beta Thalassemia Major in the coming years. In 2010, the 63rd World Health Assembly of WHO adopted a resolution calling for world wide efforts for the prevention and management of birth defects, specifically emphasizing thalassemia and sickle cell disease.

Dr Minas Hadjiminas was born in the village of Agios Amvrosios of the Kyrenia District of Cyprus. He obtained his medical degree at the University of Birmingham and worked in hospitals in London and Edinburgh, including Great Ormond Street Hospital for Sick Children in London. He returned to Cyprus as a qualified paediatrician to lead the Paediatric Clinic of the Nicosia General Hospital in 1960. In 1971 as Director of the Thalaessaemia Centre he initiated an innovative program for control of the disease. This goal was achieved within a decade, completing his life dream 'that no child with thalassaemia should ever be born in Cyprus'. An active pioneer and leader, Dr Hadjiminas contributed to the development of the Cyprus National Programme for Management of Hepatitis B and AIDS, and by his personal initiative the Cyprus Paediatric Society was established.

In 1973 the Cypriot government, acting on Dr Hadjiminas' proposal and a recommendation from the WHO, established a policy of compulsory pre-marital carrier screening and counseling with active support by community and political leaders as well as by the Greek Orthodox Church of Cyprus. In Cyprus, some 14 percent of the population were carriers of BTM, and the affected gene was present in one percent of the population with one in 158 births having BTM. Due to intervention programs, only rarely are new cases of BTM reported in Cyprus and other Mediterranean locations such as Sardinia (rate decline from 1:250 live births to 1:4,000) and Greece. Reports of the prevalence of the beta thalassemia genotype vary widely even in Cyprus with greater prevalence in the south and lesser in the north with the effects of centuries of migration of peoples of different origins in countries such as Macedonia.

This reduction was achieved by a nationwide, long-term preventive program with a combination of public education, active screening for carriers, and individual counseling. Marriage between carriers was reduced as a result of a community education program, and counseling when such marriages occurred, but the major effect is in careful screening of all pregnancies and termination of affected pregnancies all of which have led to a reduction in the number of thalassemia major births. Similarly, screening and education and case management programs in Sardinia reduced the rate of new cases from one in 250 births in the 1970s to one in 4,000 births in the 1990s. Figure 18.1 indicates the expected versus actual birth of new cases of BTM in Cyprus from 1974 to 2015 showing a dramatic reduction in cases attributable to the innovative community-based screening and prevention program implemented.

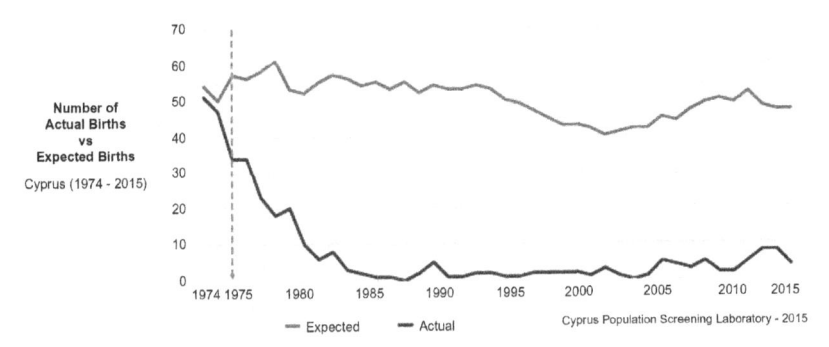

FIGURE 18.1   Number of Expected and Actual Births with Beta Thalassemia Major, Cyprus, 1974–2015. *Courtesy of National Population Laboratory-Reference Laboratory for Haemoglobinopathies, Public Health Services, Arch. Makarios III Hospital, Ministry of Health Cyprus.*

The success of the Cyprus program provides a model of elimination of a genetic disorder with a combination of health education, screening, and community support. Similar approaches have developed in Nigeria, Bahrain, Cuba, Brazil, Iran, Saudi Arabia, Tunisia, and Pakistan. Prevention of beta thalassemia is now a key part of genetic public health. Preventive approaches to this disorder over the past two decades have produced dramatic results in reducing the number and rate of new cases of BTM in its natural locations such as Sardinia, Cyprus, and Greece, but also in the United Kingdom, Canada, and other locations where this disease has come along with immigration from endemic countries, especially from Mediterranean, Arabian, and South Asian countries.

Public education, premarital screening, health education in schools, and access to prenatal screening are all part of a program to reduce new cases of this disorder. The WHO (Fact sheet N 308) stresses the public health importance of BTM and recommends adoption of demonstrably successful preventive approaches to member states with this problem. Estimates of annual births of BTM cases for the world are new cases 40,618, and deaths 22,522; and for leading regions, South East region new cases 20,420; eastern Mediterranean 9,914; Western Pacific 7,538.

Screening for congenital anemia should take place at birth and at school age, because clinical cases may not appear until several years after birth. Gene carriers need to know at an age when they can understand the limitations this may place on them in terms of partner selection. When two carriers do marry, the chance of a homozygous fetus is 25 percent in each case, so each pregnancy should be assessed by chorionic villus of the placenta sampling early in the pregnancy to determine if the fetus is affected. Termination of the pregnancy will allow the couple to have other pregnancies. Abortion is currently recommended if the fetus is affected with BTM, but bone marrow transplantation is showing promise in the treatment of new cases. The success of primary prevention in reducing new cases of thalassemia provides a model for application to other disorders affecting other population groups, such as sickle cell disease, Tay Sachs disease, and many others.

CURRENT RELEVANCE

With globalization and mass migration of populations, previously localized diseases can occur worldwide. BTM patients have a lifespan of $5-10$ years without treatment. About 80 percent of affected children are born in low- and middle-income countries, which have a low human development index and low per capita health expenditures. Malaria-endemic countries (formerly or currently) have a higher prevalence of thalassemia. With mass migration from high carrier rate countries including South East Asia, a more complex challenge faces health systems for prevention. In homogeneous community oriented populations, community solidarity and consciousness of the problem makes health promotion, screening and genetic counseling feasible in populations such as Cyprus, Sardinia, Greece and southern Italy more than in heterogeneous urban populations in North America or Western Europe.

BTM can be treated successfully by blood transfusions and iron-chelating agents to reduce the effects of iron overload affecting many organ systems. Bone marrow transplants are also used but not readily available in many settings. Recent advances in human stem cell gene therapy are showing promise of success with BTM. But the most effective measure is the prevention program pioneered in Cyprus and other Mediterranean populations.

With such genetic risk of specific diseases, preventive programs previously located in high-risk areas for thalassemia such as Cyprus, Sardinia, Greece, southern Italy, the Middle East, India, and Southeast Asia also need to be applied in countries to which people from these areas migrate. This means ethnic-focused educational and screening programs. Such an approach has been successfully applied in the United States and Israel with Tay-Sachs disease among Ashkenazi Jews and in Canada and the United Kingdom for thalassemia among Greek and Italian immigrants in particular. The same lessons need to be considered in addressing the more widespread sickle cell disease common among African Americans and in sub-Saharan Africa. With immigration of Asians to the United States in the past several decades, cases of thalassemia have appeared among the Laotian, Chinese, and Cambodian immigrant groups. A report from California shows prevalence of BTM in Caucasians (including Italians and Greeks) is 1/276,723 births, significantly lower than the prevalence in Southeast Asians (1/9,580), Middle Easterners (1/7,226), and Asians (1/26,182) births.

In Germany, the prevalence of BTM has increased in recent decades due to Turkish immigration and studies among the immigrant groups showed low levels of awareness of the problem. Screening programs were not successful in this population and remains of concern in the population at risk. In India, BTM is a public health problem with estimates of 30 million carriers, a mean prevalence of 3.3 percent, 65,000−67,000 β-thalassemia patients and 9,000−10,000 new cases added yearly (Indian Pediatrics 2007). A review of studies conducted in mainland China between 1981 to 2015 of prevalence of thalassemia carrier status shows the overall prevalence of α-thalassemia and β-thalassemia were 7.9 and 2.2 percent respectively. Rates in southern provinces are high for beta thalassemia with higher risk of births of a severe form of thalassemia than in other regions of China (Lai, 2017). Recently reported studies of thalassemia carrier status in countries such as Iran and Cambodia show high carrier rates for thalassemia justifying development of national programs of prevention.

In the United States screening, education and counseling programs are located in state health departments with partnerships between public and private systems. Advocacy organizations including the Cooley's Anemia Foundation promote community awareness, and advances in screening and treatment technologies, research, and policy development, but oversight is the responsibility of the state.

Control programs are promoted by nongovernmental organizations such as the International Thalassemia Federation. The major priorities are premarital screening of people in reproductive age groups, along with education and counseling. For pregnancy care, screening is done in the first trimester of pregnancy to determine carrier status of the husband/partner; if positive, determination of whether the pregnancy is affected is done by chorionic villus sampling and amniocentesis after 16 weeks. Chorionic villus testing is now the method of choice because it allows time for termination of affected pregnancies during the first trimester.

Prevention programs vary in different countries due to cultural and political differences, available resources, and priority given to the subject. The issue of mandatory premarital screening raises concerns in many societies, but the history of public health has included such screening in the past. The effectiveness of screening in deterring marriages between carriers seems problematic, but the coupling of screening with follow-up and care in pregnancy can reduce the rate of birth of new cases. The value of screening can also be seen in reassurance of couples from at-risk populations that they will be assured safety from this danger if only one partner is a carrier.

Success in screening and prevention strategies for genetic diseases has led to the search for applications to other genetic conditions. In 1993, a workshop sponsored by the US Centers for Disease Control (CDC) and the Cystic Fibrosis Foundation reviewed the benefits and risks associated with newborn screening for cystic fibrosis (CF), the most common genetic disorder in the United States. This report describes new research findings and presents recommendations. The peer-reviewed evidence presented at the workshop supports the clinical utility of newborn screening for CF. Demonstrated long-term benefits from early nutritional treatment include improved growth and, in one study, cognitive development. Other benefits might include reduced hospitalizations and improved survival. Newborn screening in the United States is associated with a diagnosis of CF a median of one year earlier than symptomatic detection, which may reduce the expense and anxiety associated with medical assessment for cases of failure to thrive (see Chapter 20).

A premarital screening program for reducing the incidence of BTM was started under the auspices of the Regional Health Administration in 1995 in the capital city of one region in Turkey. After four years, all couples who applied for marriage procedures were screened for the beta thalassemia trait. Couples at risk were counseled and offered prenatal diagnosis and termination of pregnancy in the case of an affected fetus. From 1995 to 1999, a total of 9,902 couples were screened, with prevalence of the beta thalassemia trait of 2.6 percent and 0.11 percent with the sickle cell trait. In 15 of the 9,902 couples, both partners were found to be carriers of the beta thalassemia trait, but after genetic counseling, only two of the 15 planned carrier marriages were canceled, and seven couples were not ready to have children. Prenatal diagnosis was sought by six couples; one fetus was normal, four had thalassemia minor, and one had thalassemia major (the pregnancy was terminated by elective abortion). This study indicated that premarital screening is a very useful tool for detecting carrier couples and an effective way of controlling thalassemia major.

Psychological and social risks for carrier children and their families (e.g., anxiety and misunderstanding) are associated with newborn screening, and exposure of affected infants to other children may result in person-to-person spread of respiratory infective organisms. Newborn screening is a well-established procedure in many states in the United States. The CDC, and the American College of Medical Genetics with the support of the March of Dimes, a national nongovernmental agency long supportive of newborn care, have determined that it is cost effective to screen for SCD but screening for beta thalassemia is not mandatory. They recommend a uniform panel of diseases for screening of all infants born in every state. An evidence-based review process was developed for adding other conditions in the future. Implementation throughout the country meant all babies born would be screened by a uniform screening program, which was codified in 2008, based on the federal Newborn Screening Saves Lives Act of 2007.

Mandatory newborn screening for a variety of diseases including PKU, CH, and sickle cell disease plus many other inborn errors of metabolism such as maple syrup disease are included since 2006 in all 50 states in the United States (see Chapter 20). The benefits of addressing PKU by screening at birth along with CH, thalasssemia, sickle cell disease and others have proven to be effective in early diagnosis of treatable if not curable conditions such as PKU and CH. Premarital and prenatal screening coupled with advocacy group promotion, community support, education and genetic counselling have proven capable of preventing serious genetic birth conditions including thalassemia, Tay Sachs and Gaucher's disease. These successes enhanced by advances in screening tests technology and genetic sciences are beyond doubt as these diseases are treatable and without treatment the affected child suffers from serious brain damage and mental retardation. The extent to which screening for other diseases of the newborn is beneficial is still open for research and demonstration programs. Sickle cell disease (SCD), while sharing some characteristics with thalassemia, is generally far less severe. But SCD affecting an estimated 70,000–100,000 Americans, affects a large population globally and has significant health consequences and requires special preventive measures during childhood and beyond to promote health and longevity. The US Sickle Cell Anemia Control Act in 1972 indicated federal interest in the SCDs and other hemoglobinopathies, but only since 2006 have all states required and provided universal newborn screening for SCD.

The UK National Screening Committee in 2014 announced expansion of routine screening of all newborns for PKU, CH, thalassemia, SCD, and additional genetic disorders to allow early treatment and prevent death or severe disability. All pregnant women in England are offered a blood test for carrier status of the gene for thalasemia; those at high risk of being a sickle cell carrier are offered a test for SCD.

Societies will need to address the potential for early discovery of genetic disorders before they happen and if after to develop effective treatments to prolong life and health. With the rapid increase in knowledge and science associated with the Human Genome Project, the potential in this field will become increasingly significant. There are social and ethical issues associated with screening and the ethnic focus of educational programs, but the success of thalassemia control is a great achievement of public health in the 20th century and its application in the 21st century may be even more important with increased knowledge of genetic factors in cancer, cardiovascular disease, and other common conditions. This will raise many ethical and political issues that must also be addressed in the context of different settings, religious beliefs, and cultural norms.

An essential element of newborn care includes screening for congenital anemia at birth and followed up at school age, as clinical cases may not appear until several years after birth. Gene carriers need to know at an age when they can understand the limitations this may place on them. In each pregnancy when both parents are carriers, chorionic villus sampling or amniocentesis should be carried out to determine if the fetus is affected. Abortion is currently recommended if the fetus is affected with thalassemia major. Long-term management by blood transfusions and chelating agents to reduce body iron load are successful in prolonging life well into the thirties. Bone marrow transplantation is showing promise in the treatment of new cases. The success of primary prevention in reducing new cases of thalassemia provides a model for application to disorders affecting other population groups, such as those with sickle cell disease.

ETHICAL ISSUES

Newborn screening now covering metabolic and genetic disorders includes many inborn errors of metabolism including thalassemia and sickle cell disease. Ethical issues include genetic screening, pregnancy termination, clinical care improvements, legal and research issues, informed consent, and respect of family choices. Health service providers should have basic knowledge of thalassemia, a fertile field for research and future prevention including health promotion activities. With rapidly increasing knowledge and science associated with the Human Genome Project, the potential in this field will become increasingly large. There are social and ethical issues associated with screening and educational programs which often focus on ethnicity.

The problem of hemoglobinopathies is global. In closed communities such as the island of Cyprus, where there are two main population groups, Greek and Turkish, both have high rates of carrier status of beta thalassemia. A common program of community education, premarital and pregnancy screening was accepted by the population because of a high level of awareness of the tragedy associated with birth of affected children especially when treatment was unavailable or very invasive.

In the case of Tay-Sachs and Gaucher's diseases, even more horrendous diseases than thalassemia, the occurrence in relatively closed communities of ultra Orthodox Ashkenazi Jews, community consensus and support of religious leasers led to a rapid decline in affected cases and virtual extinction of the diseases. When mass migration of affected Greek, Arab and Turkish populations to western Europe and the Americas occurred, the disease presented itself clinically. Advocacy groups have a key role in promoting public policy and community support for preventive measures as had been successfully employed in in Cyprus, Greece, Italy, Sardinia and other locations. In western urban societies, advocacy functions are vital for thalassemia and for wide-spread sickle cell disease. Over time migrants to western countries may be less likely to exclusively marry in the same ethnicity or in consanguineous marriages as in their home countries, so that carrier marrying carrier would become less common.

ECONOMIC ISSUES

Beta thalassemia major is a disease causing early breakdown of fragile red blood cells and requires continuous lifesaving treatment with blood transfusions, which over time causes iron excess deposition in many organs of the body including heart, liver, spleen, and bones, causes gall stones and leg ulcers, and interferes with normal growth of children. Untreated, the iron deposition in vital organs leads to early death, but treatment with medications called chelating agents removes and excretes deposited iron. This treatment successfully prolongs life.

Costs of prevention of hemoglobinopathies compared with costs of treatment show a high benefit-to-cost ratio in many studies. A US retrospective study using a large US health insurance claims database spanning January 1997–December 2004 and representing 40 million members of plans (Delea et al., 2007) examined costs of treating patients diagnosed with thalassemia or SCD (n = 145 total, 106 SCD, 39 thalassemia) including a treatment mean of 12 transfusions (whole blood or red blood cells) per year and one or more treatments with chelating agents. The mean total medical costs were US $59,233 per year including US $10,899 for the chelating agent and US $8,722 for administration of chelation therapy.

A UK study (Weidlich et al., 2016) calculated total health care expenditures attributable to managing beta thalassemia major (BTM) was estimated to be US $720,201 at 2013–14 prices over 50 years. The probability for survival to age 50 was 0.53 with two thirds of survivors living with complications, but costs and suffering could be reduced by bone marrow transplantation. A study in India where some 10,000 BTM cases are born annually showed that Kolkota (Calcutta, India) families of patients spent up to 20% of their income on transfusions and chelating agents for survival (Mallik et al., 2010).

A study by Koren et al., of BTM in Northern Israel reported lifetime costs of patients for care with transfusions and chelating agents and additional costs to the national health insurance system. The cost of treating a BTM patient for 50 years was calculated at $1,971,380 (annual cost of USD $39,427), not including expenses for treatment of deteriorating patients due to poor compliance with chelation therapy, heart failure, endocrine workup and replacement therapy, diagnosis and treatment of osteoporosis, and treatment of blood-related acquired infections. The cost of preventing one affected newborn was US $63,660. Screening and termination of some affected fetuses reduced the number of births from an expected 70 to 30 cases in 2011. Prevention of 45 affected newborns over a ten-year period represented a net savings of US $88.5 million to the health budget.

Patients in low-income countries such as Thailand may not have access to adequate therapy with transfusions and chelating agents. The screening and counseling approach based on community health promotion is a more cost-effective approach, which should specifically be advocated by international organizations and donors. The public health approach is the only viable option in such circumstances.

Irrespective of the costs of prevention of cases and case management, the costs will be less than the direct costs of treatment. Study results in the Province of Quebec, Canada confirmed the benefits of a comprehensive program compared to the cost of sole reliance on treatment. Cost-effectiveness studies are a component of service provision including health technology assessment. A centrally controlled information management system is necessary for purposes of policy and program planning, research, and program evaluation and within recognized standards of ideally an integrated program.

CONCLUSION

Prevention of thalassemia is one of the success stories of genetic public health with elimination of new cases in Cyprus and many countries of the Mediterranean area, but the disorder is still a major public health problem in other regions of the world. Preventive approaches since the 1970s have produced dramatic results in reducing the number and rate of new cases of BTM in Sardinia, Cyprus, Greece, the United Kingdom, Canada, and other locations where it has been endemic among peoples of the Mediterranean region. Premarital screening, health education in schools, and access to prenatal screening are all part of a program to reduce new cases of this disease. The WHO stresses the public health importance of this disorder and recommends adoption of demonstrably successful preventive approaches to member states with this problem but notes that policies for treatment and prevention are still needed in 162 countries. Thus leadership is needed at government levels to include thalassemia in policy and program initiatives.

Newborn screening is practiced in most high-income countries, but is still needed in medium- and low-income countries to reduce family and societal burden as well as pain and suffering of thalassemia and other hemoglobinopathies. The WHO recognizes the importance of inherited disorders of hemoglobin, but very little international action has been taken toward the development of services for the control and management of these conditions. Cyprus had a high prevalence of thalassaemia and pioneered a national and community program of population-wide prevention based on education and premarital screening, community awareness, education, pregnancy screening, genetic counseling, and prenatal diagnosis. The WHO estimates that some 300,000 infants are born with major haemoglobinopathies and recommends measures to reduce the burden of this group of diseases based on the successful management in Cyprus and many other countries.

Genomics is revolutionizing diagnosis and treatment of many conditions especially birth defects, which affect some seven million newborns each year according to the WHO. Of these, 90 percent are born in developing countries that are still unable to utilize routine screening and care. The advent of nutritional fortification of basic foods with key micronutrients such as folic acid, iodine, iron, zinc, selenium, and others can, however, be applied to prevent birth defects along with nutritional care of women in the age of fertility and especially during pregnancy. The eradication of beta thalassemia in many countries provides hope for wider accomplishments in the field of improving child health.

Prevention of birth defects and low birth weight requires attention to nutritional security for women of child-bearing age including during pregnancy. These are essential elements of public health including prevention of low birth weight and specific birth defects such as neural tube defects, iodine deficiency, anemia, and other trace-element deficiencies causing poor growth and development. Newborn screening should also incorporate testing of hearing and for congenital heart disease.

Epidemiological analysis of laboratory data can show high-risk population concentrations of birth prevalence of SCD and sickle cell trait (SCT), which can be valuable in focusing community-based health education and genetic counseling to prevent/avoid births of children with BTM. The Cyprus model worked brilliantly, and has been replicated widely in Mediterranean and other countries to which vulnerable populations have migrated. In low-income countries access to treatment of BTM by blood transfusions and chelating agents is not widely available. Health promotion is the only realistic model to address the global problems of BTM and SCD. The Cyprus experience paved the way for prevention of BTM with methods applicable to SCD and other genetic disorders.

RECOMMENDATIONS

1. Countries should identify the policy importance of nutritional security programming for women, multivitamin supplements, and close attention to prenatal and delivery care followed by screening for newborn health.
2. Screening newlyweds, pregnant women and newborns for congenital anemia such as beta thalassemia and SCD especially in high-risk population groups and highly endemic areas is an essential public health activity at birth and at school age, as clinical cases may not appear until several years after birth.

3. Other diseases that have been eliminated by screening and education include Tay Sachs and Gaucher's disease, improve prevention and care for SCD and CF. Advances in genetic and other fields of medical research will provide new advances for widespread application and improved health.
4. Applications of currently available technology should be incorporated into public health programs in developing countries with the support of international donors, as is being achieved by immunization in many countries.
5. Research priorities and areas of inter-country cooperation and support for an interdisciplinary workforce have great potential for improving and strengthening thalassemia services.
6. Advocacy groups have a vital role to play in providing support for affected families, in promoting proactive public health policies to reduce the burden of disease through community awareness, screening and genetic counselling as achieved such success in Cyprus.
7. Newborn screening program development in medium- and low-income countries should be promoted in national and donor programs in keeping with WHO recommendations for routine child care.

STUDENT REVIEW QUESTIONS

1. Define dominant and recessive gene defects.
2. When both parents are carriers of a gene defect, what is the risk in each pregnancy of the fetus inheriting the disease?
3. Why was thalassemia called Cooley's anemia or Mediterranean anemia?
4. When and why did Cyprus begin its preventive program for beta thalassemia major (BTM)?
5. What were the key components of the Cyprus program?
6. What were the results of the Cyprus program?
7. What other genetic disorders have been successfully eliminated by a community-based intervention program?
8. Where is sickle cell disease (SCD) important and what can be adopted from the Cyprus approach to prevent this disease?
9. Why is prevention of BTM, SCD, Tay Sachs disease, and Gaucher's disease prevention important for public health where appropriate globally?
10. Why should low and medium income countries adopt the Cyprus approach to the prevention of hemoglobinopathies and other amenable genetic conditions?

RECOMMENDED READINGS

1. Agency for Healthcare Research and Quality. Screening for hemoglobinopathies in newborns. Reaffirmation update for US preventive services task force, 2007. Available at: http://www.uspreventiveservicestaskforce.org/BrowseRec/ReferredTopic/230 (accessed 25 August 2017).

2. American College of Obstetricians and Gynecologists. Carrier screening for genetic conditions. Committee Opinion No. 691. Obstet Gynecol. 19 March 2017;129:e41–55. Available at: https://www.acog.org/Resources-And-Publications/Committee-Opinions/Committee-on-Genetics/Carrier-Screening-for-Genetic-Conditions (accessed 31 August 2017).

3. American Society for Hematology. ASH priorities for sickle cell disease and sickle cell trait. Available at: http://www.hematology.org/Research/Recommendations/Sickle-Cell/ (accessed 10 August 2017).

4. Angastiniotis M, Eleftheriou A, Galanello R, et al. In: Old J, editor. Prevention of thalassaemias and other haemoglobin disorders: volume 1: principles [Internet]. 2nd edition. Nicosia, Cyprus: Thalassaemia International Federation, 2013. Available at: http://www.ncbi.nlm.nih.gov/books/NBK190485/ (accessed 30 August 2017).

5. Angastiniotis M, Modell B, Engelzos P, Boulyjenkov V. Prevention and control of haemoglobinopathies. Bull World Health Organ. 1995;73(3):375–386. Available at: https://www.ncbi.nlm.nih.gov/pmc/articles/PMC2486673/pdf/bullwho00407-0102.pdf (accessed 10 August 2017).

6. Angastiniotis MA, Hadjiminas MG. Prevention of thalassaemia in Cyprus. Lancet. 1981; 14(1):369–371. Abstract available at: http://www.ncbi.nlm.nih.gov/pubmed/6109998 (accessed 30 August 2017).

7. Angastiniotis M, Vives Corrons J-L, Soteriades ES, Eleftheriou A. The impact of migrations on the health services for rare diseases in Europe: the example of haemoglobin disorders. Sci World J. 2013:727905. https://www.ncbi.nlm.nih.gov/pmc/articles/PMC3614063/pdf/TSWJ2013-727905.pdf (accessed 14 December 2017).

8. Ashiotis T, Zachariadis Z, Sofroniadou K, Loukopoulos D. Thalassaemia Jn Cyprus. Br Med J. 1973;2(5857):38–42. Available at: https://www.ncbi.nlm.nih.gov/pmc/articles/PMC3614063/pdf/TSWJ2013-727905.pdf (accessed 29 December 2017).

9. Baer K. Cooley's Anemia Foundation in Cooperation with CDC. 2013. Living with thalassemia, 2013. Available at: http://www.cooleysanemia.org/updates/pdf/GuideToLivingWithThalassemia.pdf (accessed 26 May 2017).

10. Benson JM, Therrell Jr. BL. History and current status of newborn screening for hemoglobinopathies. Semin Perinatol. 2010;34:134–144. Abstract available at: http://www.ncbi.nlm.nih.gov/pubmed/20207263 (accessed 30 August 2017).

11. Boletini E, Svobodova M, Divoky V, Baysal E, Curuk MA, Dimovski AJ. Sickle cell anemia, sickle cell beta thalassemia, and thalassemia major in Albania: characterization of mutations. Hum Genet. 1994;93(2):182–187. Available at: http://www.ncbi.nlm.nih.gov/pubmed/8112743 (accessed 30 August 2017).

12. Borgna-Pignatti C. The life of patients with thalassemia major. Hematologica. 2010;95(3):345–348. Available at: https://www.ncbi.nlm.nih.gov/pmc/articles/PMC2833059/pdf/0950345.pdf (accessed 30 August 2017).

13. Cao A, Rosatelli MC, Galanello R. Control of beta thalassaemia by carrier screening, genetic counselling and prenatal diagnosis: the Sardinian experience. Ciba Found Symp. 1996;197:137–151. discussion 151–555. Abstract available at: https://www.ncbi.nlm.nih.gov/pubmed/8827372 (accessed 29 August 2017).

14. Cao A. Carrier screening and genetic counselling in beta thalassemia. Int J Hematol. 2002;76(Suppl 2):105–113. Abstract available at: http://www.ncbi.nlm.nih.gov/pubmed/12430909 (accessed 30 August 2017).

15. Centers for Disease Control and Prevention. Public health genomics: state public health genomics programs: measuring outcomes. Available at: http://www.cdc.gov/genomics/ (accessed 30 August 2017).

16. Centers for Disease Control and Prevention. Sickle cell disease (SCD): 5 facts you should know about SCD, last updated 4 October 2017. Available at: http://www.cdc.gov/ncbddd/sicklecell/index.html (accessed 30 December 2017).

17. Centers for Disease Control and Prevention. 2014. National Center on Birth Defects and Developmental Disabilities (NCBDDD), last revised 5 January 2018. Available at: http://www.cdc.gov/ncbddd/ (accessed 13 January 2018).

18. Centers for Disease Control and Prevention. Last update 1 November 2017. Available at: http://www.cdc.gov/ncbddd/thalassemia/index.html (accessed 30 December 2017).

19. Cheevra A.C., Bleibel S.A., Jones-Crawford J.L., Kutlar A., Leonard A.J., Raj A.B. 2014. Alpha thalassemia. Medscape. Last updated 7 November 2017. Available at: http://emedicine.medscape.com/article/955496-overview#showall (accessed 30 December 2017).

20. Christianson A, Howson CP, Modell B. March of Dimes global report on birth defects. New York, NY: March of Dimes Foundation, 2006. http://www.marchofdimes.org/materials/global-report-on-birth-defects-the-hidden-toll-of-dying-and-disabled-children-executive-summary.pdf (accessed 30 August 2017).

21. Christopher SA, Collins JL, Farrell MH. Effort required to contact primary care providers after newborn screening identifies sickle cell trait. J Natl Med Assoc. 2012;104:528−534. Available at: https://www.ncbi.nlm.nih.gov/pmc/articles/PMC3880776/pdf/nihms535784.pdf (accessed 30 December 2017).

22. Conte R, Ruggieri L, Gambino A, Bartoloni F, Baiardi P, Bonifazi D. The Italian multiregional thalassemia registry: centers characteristics, services, and patients' population. Haemoglobin. 2016;21(7): 515−424. http://www.tandfonline.com/doi/full/10.1080/10245332.2015.1101971 Abstract available at: http://www.tandfonline.com/doi/full/10.1080/10245332.2015.1101971?src = recsys (accessed 12 January 2018).

23. Cooley's Anemia Advocacy Forum Update. 2015. Advances in thalassemia reported at annual hematology meeting. Available at: http://www.thalassemia.org/caf-applauds-advances-in-thalassemia-reported-at-annual-hematology-meeting/ (accessed 30 August 2017).

24. Cooley's Anemia Foundation, 2014. Available at: http://www.thalassemia.org/learn-about-thalassemia/about-thalassemia/ (accessed 31 August 2017).

25. Cooley TB, Lee P. A series of cases of splenomegaly in children with anemia and peculiar bone changes. Trans Am Pediatr Soc. 1925;37:29. Available in Hematology: Landmark Papers of the Twentieth Century. Available at: https://www.sciencedirect.com/science/book/9780124485105 (accessed 30 December 2017).

26. Dehshal MH, Namini MT, Ahmadvand A, Manshadi M, Varnosfaderani S, Abolghasemi H. Evaluation of the national prevention program in Iran, 2007−2009: the accomplishments and challenges with reflections on the path ahead. Hemoglobin. 2014;38(3):179−187. Abstract available at: http://www.tandfonline.com/doi/abs/10.3109/03630269.2014.893530 (accessed 26 August 2017).

27. Delea TF, Hagiwara M, Thomas SK, Baladi J-F, Phatak PD, Coates TD. Outcomes, utilization, and costs among thalassemia and sickle cell disease patients receiving deferoxamine therapy in the United States. Am J Hematol. 2007;(October);263−270. https://doi.org/10.1002/ajh.21049. Available at: http://onlinelibrary.wiley.com/doi/10.1002/ajh.21049/full (accessed 14 January 2018).

28. Efremov GD. Dominantly Inherited beta Thalassemia. Hemoglobin. 2007;31(2):193−207. Abstract available at: https://www.ncbi.nlm.nih.gov/pubmed/17486503 (accessed 29 August 2017).

29. Galanello R, Origa R. Beta thalassemia. Orphanet J Rare Dis. 2010;5:11. http://dx.doi.org/
     10.1186/1750-1172-5-11. Available at: https://www.ncbi.nlm.nih.gov/pmc/articles/
     PMC2893117/pdf/1750-1172-5-11.pdf (accessed 26 December 2017).
30. Ghotbi N, Tsukatani T. An economic review of the national screening policy to prevent
     thalassemia major in Iran. Discussion paper. Kyoto Institute of Economic Research Kyoto
     University, 2002. Available at http://www.kier.kyoto-u.ac.jp/DP/DP562.pdf (accessed
     26 May 2017).
31. Giardina PJ, Forget BG. Thalassemia syndromes. In: Hoffman R, Benz EJ, Shattil SS,
     et al., editors. Hematology: basic principles and practice. 5th edition. Philadelphia, PA:
     Elsevier Churchill Livingstone, 2008. Chapter 41.
32. Ginsberg G, Tulchinsky T, Filon D, Goldfarb A, Abramov L, Rachmilevitz EA.
     Cost−benefit analysis of a national thalassemia prevention programme in Israel. J Med
     Screen. 1998;5(3):120−126. Abstract available at: https://www.ncbi.nlm.nih.gov/pubmed/
     9795870 (accessed 29 August 2017).
33. Hashemizadeh H, Noori R. Premarital screening of beta thalassemia minor in north-east of
     Iran. Iran J Ped Hematol Oncol. 2013;3(1):210−215. Available at: https://www.ncbi.nlm.
     nih.gov/pmc/articles/PMC3915444/pdf/ijpho-3-210.pdf (accessed 25 May 2017).
34. Heer N, Choy J, Vichinsky EP. The social impact of migration on disease. Cooley's ane-
     mia, thalassemia, and new Asian immigrants. Ann NY Acad Sci. 1998;850:509−511.
35. Hoedemaekers R, ten Have H. Geneticization: the Cyprus paradigm. Med Philos.
     1998;23(3):274−287. Available at: https://www.ncbi.nlm.nih.gov/pubmed/9736189
     (accessed 29 August 2017).
36. Hoppe CC. Newborn screening for hemoglobin disorders. Hemoglobin. 2011;35:556−564.
     Available at : http://www.tandfonline.com/. Available from: http://dx.doi.org/10.3109/
     03630269.2011.607905 (accessed 31 August 2017).
37. Iron Health Alliance. Epidemiology of thalassemia. Available at: http://www.
     ironhealthalliance.com/disease-states/thalassemia/epidemiology-and-pathophysiology.jsp
     (accessed 26 May 2015).
38. Kaye CI, Committee on Genetics. Introduction to the newborn screening fact sheets.
     Pediatrics. 2006;118(3):1304−1312. Reaffirmed AAP Publications Retired and Reaffirmed.
     Pediatrics. 2011;127(3):pe857. Available at: http://www.ncbi.nlm.nih.gov/pubmed/16960984;
     http://pediatrics.aappublications.org/content/127/3/e857.full (accessed 30 August 2015).
39. Koren A, Profeta L, Zalman L, Palmor H, Levin C, Bril Zamir R, et al. Prevention of β thalasse-
     mia in Northern Israel Prevention of β thalassemia in Northern Israel − a cost-benefit analysis.
     Mediterr J Hematol Infect Dis. 2014;6(1):e2014012. Published online 2014 Feb 17. Available
     at: https://www.ncbi.nlm.nih.gov/pmc/articles/PMC3965716/ (accessed 15 January 2018).
40. Kountouris P, Kousiappa I, Papasavva T, Christopoulos G, Pavlou E, Petrou M, et al. The
     molecular spectrum and distribution of haemoglobinopathies in Cyprus: a 20-year retro-
     spective study. Sci Rep. 2016;6:26371. https://doi.org/10.1038/srep26371. Available at:
     https://www.nature.com/articles/srep26371 (accessed 12 January 2018).
41. Kyrri AR, Kalogerou E, Loizidou D, Ioannou C, Makariou C, Kythreotis L. The changing
     epidemiology of β-thalassemia in the Greek-Cypriot population. Haemoglobin. 2013;37
     (5):435−443. Abstract available at:http://www.tandfonline.com/doi/citedby/10.3109/
     03630269.2013.801851?scroll = top&needAccess = true (accessed 12 January 2018).
42. Lai K, Huang G, Su L, He Y. The prevalence of thalassemia in mainland China: evidence
     from epidemiological surveys. Sci Rep. 2017;7(920):1−11. Available from: http://dx.doi.
     org/10.1038/s41598-017-00967-2. Available at: http://www.nature.com/articles/s41598-
     017-00967-2.pdf (accessed 26 August 2017).

43. Leung TY, Lao TT. Haematological disorders in pregnancy. Thalassemia in pregnancy. 2012. Best Pract Res Clin Obst Gynaecol. 2012;26(1):37–51. Available at: http://www.sciencedirect.com/science/article/pii/S1521693411001581 (accessed 29 August 2015).

44. Mallik S, Chatterjee C, Mandal PJ, Sardar JC, Ghosh P, Manna N. Expenditure to treat thalassemia: an experience at a tertiary care hospital in India. Iranian J Public Health. 2010;39(1):78–84. Available at: https://www.ncbi.nlm.nih.gov/pmc/articles/PMC3468966/ (accessed 14 January 2018).

45. Manitsa A, Theodoridou S, Stamna K, Alemayehou M. Incidence of heterozygous carriers of haemoglobinopathies among immigrants in Northern Greece. Haema. 2002;5:115–117. Available at: https://www.ncbi.nlm.nih.gov/pmc/articles/PMC4094755/pdf/1750-1172-9-97.pdf (accessed 25 December 2017).

46. Martinez PA, Angastiniotis M, Gulbis B, Pereira MDMM, Petrova-Benedict R, Corrons JLV. Haemoglobinopathies in Europe: health & migration policy perspectives. Orphanet J Rare Dis. 2014;9:97. Published online 2014 Jul 1. PMCID: PMC4094755. Available at: https://www.ncbi.nlm.nih.gov/pmc/articles/PMC4094755/ (accessed 13 August 2017).

47. Modell B, Benson A, Payling Wright CR. Incidence of Beta thalassaemia trait among Cypriots in London. BMJ. 1972;3:737–738. Available at: https://www.ncbi.nlm.nih.gov/pmc/articles/PMC1788629/pdf/brmedj02223-0033.pdf (accessed 29 May 2017).

48. Modell B, Darlison M, Birgens H, Cario H, Faustino P, Giordano PC, et al. Epidemiology of haemoglobin disorders in Europe: an overview. Scand J Clin Lab Invest. 2007;67(1):39–70. Available at: http://www.tandfonline.com/doi/full/10.1080/00365510601046557?scroll = top&needAccess=true (accessed 12 August 2017).

49. Modell B, Kuliev A. The history of community genetics: the contribution of the haemoglobin disorders. Community Genet. 1998;1(1):3–11. Available at: https://www.ncbi.nlm.nih.gov/pubmed/15178981 (accessed 31 August 2017).

50. Modell B, Harris R, Lane B, Khan M, Darlison M, Petrou M, et al. Informed choice in genetic screening for thalassaemia during pregnancy: audit from a national confidential inquiry. BMJ. 2000;320(7231):337–341. Abstract available at: https://www.ncbi.nlm.nih.gov/pmc/articles/PMC27278/pdf/337.pdf (accessed 29 August 2017).

51. Modell B, Darlison M. Global epidemiology of haemoglobin disorders and derived service indicators. Bull World Health Organ. 2008;86(6):417–496. Available at: http://www.who.int/bulletin/volumes/86/6/06-036673/en/ or http://www.ncbi.nlm.nih.gov/pmc/articles/PMC2647473/pdf/06-036673.pdf (accessed 26 May 2017).

52. Mohanty D, Colah RB, Gorakshakar AC, Patel RZ, Master DC, Mahanta J, et al. Prevalence of β-thalassemia and other haemoglobinopathies in six cities in India: a multicentre study. J Commun Genet. 2013;4(1):33–42. Available at: http://dx.doi.org/10.1007/s12687-012-0114-0 (accessed 30 August 2017).

53. Munkongdee T, Tanakulmas J, Butthep P, Winichagoon P, Main B, Yiannakis M, et al. Molecular epidemiology of hemoglobinopathies in Cambodia. Hemoglobin. 2016;40(3):163–167. Abstract available at: https://www.ncbi.nlm.nih.gov/pubmed/27117566 (accessed 26 August 2017).

54. New York Academy of Sciences. Cooley's anemia: ninth symposium, 2009. Available at: https://www.nyas.org/events/2009/ninth-cooleys-anemia-symposium/ (accessed 30 August 2017).

55. Obituary: Thomas Benton Cooley MD, 1871–1945. Am J Dis Child. 1946;71(1):77–79. Available at: http://dx.doi.org/10.1001/archpedi.1946.02020240084008 (accessed 29 August 2017). Abstract available at: http://jamanetwork.com/journals/jamapediatrics/article-abstract/1180201 (accessed 31 August 2017).

56. Ojodu J, Hulihan MM, Pope SN, Grant AM. Incidence of sickle cell trait—United States, 2010. Morb Mortal Wkly Rep. 2014;63(49):1155–1158. Available at: https://www.cdc. gov/mmwr/preview/mmwrhtml/mm6349a3.htm (accessed 31 August 2017).

57. Old J, Angastiniotis M, Eleftheriou A, Galanello R, Harteveld CL, Petrou M, et al. Prevention of thalassaemias and other haemoglobin disorders. Volume 1: Principles. Thalassemia International Federation. Second Edition. TIF Publication no. 18, 2013. Available at: http://ukts.org/pdfs/tifpubs/preventionv1.pdf (accessed 31 August 2017).

58. Ostrowsky JT, Lippman A, Scriver CR. Cost benefit analysis of thalassemia disease prevention program. Am J Public Health. 1985;75(7):732–736. Available at: http://ajph.aphapublications.org/ Available from: http://dx.doi.org/10.2105/AJPH.75.7.732 (accessed 30 August 2017).

59. Pederson C, Grosse SD, Oster MF, Olney RS, Cassell CH. Cost-effectiveness of routine screening for critical congenital heart disease in US newborns. Pediatrics. 2013;132(3): e595–e603. doi:10.1542/peds.2013-0332. Available at: http://pediatrics.aappublications. org/content/early/2013/07/31/peds.2013-0332.abstract (accessed 30 August 2017).

60. President's Page. Prevention of thalassemia in India. Ind Pediatrics 2007;44:647-648. Available at: http://www.indianpediatrics.net/sep2007/sep-647-648.htm (accessed 25 August 2017).

61. Public Health England. UK Screening Portal. UK National Screening Committee. UK NSC Meetings and Minutes. Available at: http://webarchive.nationalarchives.gov.uk/ 20150525133544/http://screening.nhs.uk/meetings (accessed 29 August 2017).

62. Riewpaiboon A, Nuchprayoon I, Torcharus K, Indaratna K, Thavorncharoensap M, Ubo B. Economic burden of beta-thalassemia/Hb E and beta-thalassemia major in Thai children. BMC Research Notes. 2010;3:29. Available at: http://www.biomedcentral.com/1756-0500/ 3/29 (accessed 14 January 2018).

63. Ryan K, Bain BJ, Worthington D, James J, Plews D, Mason A, et al. British Committee for Standards in Haematology. Significant haemoglobinopathies: guidelines for screening and diagnosis. Br J Haematol. 2010;149(1):35–49. Available at: http://www.ncbi.nlm.nih. gov/pubmed/20067565 (accessed 29 August 2017).

64. Tadmouri GO, Tüzmen B, Özçelik H, Özer A, Baig SM, Senga EB, et al. Molecular and population genetic analyses of beta thalassemia in Turkey. Am J Hematol. 1998;57: 215–220. Available at: https://www.ncbi.nlm.nih.gov/pubmed/9495372 (accessed 30 August 2017).

65. Thalassemia International Federation. Available at: http://www.thalassaemia.org.cy/ about-haemoglobin-disorders/beta thalassaemia/epidemiology.shtml (accessed 26 May 2017).

66. Verma IC, Saxena R, Kohli S. Past, present & future scenario of thalassaemic care & control in India. Ind J Med Res. 2011;134(4):507–521. Available at: https://www.ncbi.nlm. nih.gov/pmc/articles/PMC3237251/ (accessed 25 August 2017).

67. Vichinsky EP, MacKlin EA, Waye JS, Lorey F, Olivieri NF. Changes in the epidemiology of thalassemia in North America: a new minority disease. Pediatrics. 2005;116:818–825. Available at: http://pediatrics.aappublications.org/content/pediatrics/116/6/e818.full.pdf (accessed 31August 2017).

68. Waitzman NJ, Romano PS, Scheffler RM. Estimates of the economic costs of birth defects. Inquiry. 1994;31:188–205. Abstract available at: https://www.ncbi.nlm.nih.gov/pubmed/ 8021024 (accessed 30 August 2017).

69. Weidlich D, Kefalas P, Guest JF. Healthcare costs and outcomes of managing β-thalassemia major over 50 years in the United Kingdom. Transfusion. 2016;56(5):1038–1045.

Abstract available at: https://www.ncbi.nlm.nih.gov/pubmed/27041389 (accessed 14 January 2018).

70. Wilkinson J, Bass C, Diem S, Gravley A, Harvey L, Maciosek M, et al. Institute for Clinical Services Improvement: Preventive services for children and adolescents. Updated September 2013. Available at: https://www.icsi.org/_asset/x1mnv1/PrevServKids.pdf (accessed 26 May 2015).

71. Weatherall DJ. The inherited disorders of haemoglobin: an increasingly neglected global health burden. Indian J Med Res. 2011;134:493–497. Available at: http://icmr.nic.in/ijmr/2011/october/1014.pdf (accessed 26 May 2017).

72. World Health Organization. Genomic Resource Centre. Global applications of genomics in healthcare: Cyprus/Sardinia. Screening for thalassemias. Available at: http://www.who.int/genomics/professionals/cyprussardinia/en/ (accessed 25 May 2017).

73. World Health Organization. 63rd World Assembly: Report by the Secretariat. Birth defects, 2010. Available at: http://apps.who.int/gb/ebwha/pdf_files/WHA63/A63_10-en.pdfhttp://www.who.int/genomics/ (accessed 25 May 2017).

Chapter 19

Maurice Hilleman: Creator of Vaccines That Changed the World

ABSTRACT

Maurice Ralph Hilleman (1919–2005) was one of the greatest microbiologists/vaccinologists of all time. He played a key role in developing vaccines for Asian flu in 1957 and Hong Kong flu in 1968. Over six decades, most of which were spent at Merck & Company, his leadership and innovations blazed new trails in virology, epidemiology, immunology, cancer research, and vaccine development that were unmatched. His work resulted in current vaccines used for the prevention of measles, mumps, hepatitis A and B, chickenpox, meningitis, and pneumonia, which have saved millions of lives across the globe. The need for close cooperation between public and private agencies, including donors, to promote research in vaccinology is reemphasized by recent global health crises such as the Ebola and Zika viruses, as well as the annual influenza virus threats. Eradication of many diseases is feasible, but requires political support for resources, vaccine development and harmonization of vaccination policies, to be achievable. Hilleman worked with many collaborators in academic centers, in industrial management, with which he led his research and development team to produce world-changing achievements.

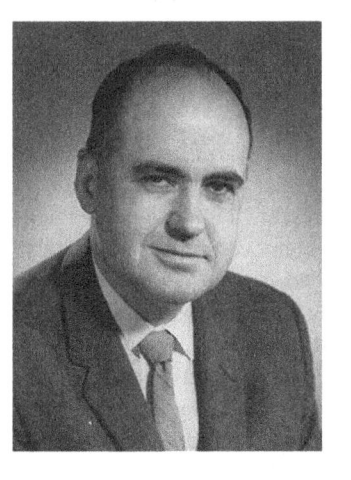

Maurice Ralph Hilleman (1919-2005). Creator at Merck Company of most vaccines used routinely in child care.
Courtesy: Mrs. Lorraine Hilleman.

Case Studies in Public Health. DOI: http://dx.doi.org/10.1016/B978-0-12-804571-8.00003-2

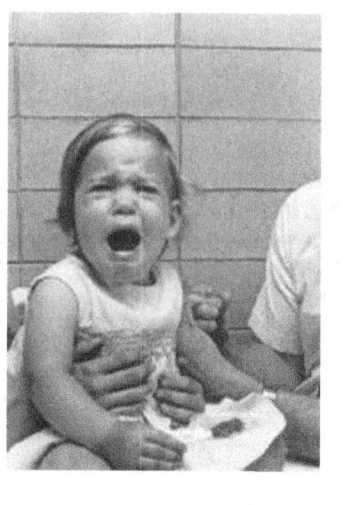

Vaccinating Hilleman's daughter, Kirsten, with the Jeryl Lynn Mumps strain Vaccine derived from her sister. *Courtesy, Mrs Lorraine Hilleman. Available at: http://www.historyofvaccines.org/content/articles/mumps (accessed 27 August 2016).*

BACKGROUND

Maurice R. Hilleman was born in 1919 in Miles City, Montana, United States, but tragically his mother died 2 days after his birth. Hilleman was raised by his uncle while his father struggled to cope with raising his eight children under harsh circumstances on their family farm. Hilleman graduated from high school in 1937 in the midst of the Great Depression. As a poor farm boy without prospects or means, he took jobs in local stores and worked very hard but had little opportunity to advance his education. Inspired by an older brother studying at a divinity school, Hilleman applied for, and won, a full scholarship to Montana State University where he graduated first in his class at the age of 21 with a joint degree in chemistry and microbiology. He was offered scholarships at ten universities, and chose the University of Chicago for graduate studies in microbiology where, despite scholarships, he lived under squalid conditions. He received his PhD in 1944 with an award-winning dissertation which was on Chlamydia.

After graduating, Hilleman elected to work in the pharmaceutical industry instead of accepting offers to continue in academia. He took a position in E.R. Squibb & Sons and immediately started researching vaccine development. Viruses and other infectious agents which can cause disease can also be used to stimulate the host—i.e., the vaccinated person—to produce antibodies that act to defend against the infecting agent. Producing vaccines requires introducing a weakened live- or dead agent—i.e., virus, bacteria, parasite, or other infective organism, or part of the organism—that can stimulate the production of protective antibodies. He developed a vaccine against Japanese B encephalitis, which was urgently needed to immunize troops at the Pacific front of World War II.

In 1948, Hilleman joined the Walter Reed Army Medical Center as chief of the Department of Respiratory Diseases, where he was assigned to study respiratory illnesses which had military significance, and to devise a science and strategy for dealing with influenza. He demonstrated that influenza A viruses underwent *"gradual and progressive minor antigenic characteristics called 'drift and shift,' which are the basis of modern influenza vaccine strategies"* (Olanski, Lancet 2005).

In 1957, at age 38, Hilleman was recruited by the pharmaceutical company Merck & Company at West Point, Pennsylvania, to lead its virus and vaccination research programs for the next 47 years, continuing to direct the Merck Institute for Vaccinology for another 20 years—after compulsory retirement from Merck Research Labs in 1984 at age 65—until his death at age 85. From the 1950s to the 1990s, Hilleman and his team created more than 40 experimental and licensed human and animal vaccines, including those in use currently offering protection against measles, mumps, chickenpox, rubella, hepatitis A, hepatitis B, pneumococcal pneumonia, meningitis, pandemic influenza, and chlamydia.

Hilleman led the development of the Asian flu vaccine in 1957 which was important in alleviating the world-wide pandemic. Influenza remained a yearly occurrence after the horrendous 1918 Swine Flu pandemic which killed tens of millions of people, primarily young men. But no new, virulent influenza type emerged until early 1957. In February 1957, a life-threatening wave of flu was spreading across China with reports of 20,000 cases in Hong Kong. Then still a microbiologist at Walter Reed Army Medical Center, Hilleman suspected this could become a pandemic threat and coined the term Asian flu. He obtained a sample of the virus from an ill US serviceman and determined that most people lacked antibody protection for this new influenza virus. He initiated vaccine production by sending virus samples to manufacturers and urging them to develop a vaccine within four months, producing 40 million doses of vaccine and so reducing the US epidemic, which caused an estimated 70,000 deaths in the United States. World-wide, from 1957 to 1958, some two million people died from Asian flu. Subsequently new influenza strains have continuously emerged in Asia.

In 1968, Hilleman was active in developing a vaccine for the Hong Kong influenza pandemic. Because of the continuing threat of annual flu epidemics, the World Health Organization (WHO) developed new pandemic guidelines in 2005 to upgrade pandemic-preparedness plans in cooperation with vaccine manufacturers and national public health agencies, especially addressing the need for quicker development and distribution of influenza vaccines (College of Physician of Philadelphia).

He worked with academic scientists, but was also responsible for the field work of collecting samples for vaccine development as well as administrative and scientific leadership, which resulted in field testing and the production of many new—or improved—vaccines. He characterized and isolated antigens, performed the basic- and process research as well as doing clinical studies, all the way through to the manufacturing process which resulted in fundamental breakthroughs in vaccine development. Table 19.1 shows the timeline of vaccines licensed in the United States.

Leonard Hayflick, born in Philadelphia, Pennsylvania in 1928, graduated with a bachelor's degree in microbiology at the University of Pennsylvania on a GI (US veterans) bill after completing his army service. He continued studying and received his master's degree in 1953, and was awarded full scholarship toward a PhD in medical microbiology and chemistry. Working at the University of Texas in Galveston from 1956 to 1958, Hayflick learned techniques of cell cultures producing large numbers of selected cells with long term survival and replication living in controlled conditions. Fetal cells were considered safer than other cell lines as the latter could be genetically abnormal, contain undetected viruses such as those of animal origin, or carry cancer genes. The famous HeLa cell line was the oldest and most commonly used human cell line derived from cervical cancer cells from Henrietta Lacks, a patient who died of her cancer in 1951. The cell line, extremely readily grown and survivable, was used extensively in scientific research including production of the inactivated Salk vaccine in 1954. Considerable controversy surrounds this even today because the sample was taken without the patient's permission and because of the possibility of its carrying cancer genetic material.

Lung cells from human fetal specimens developed by Hayflick from a legal abortion in Stockholm were considered promising, but controversial, due to ethical questions disputes over the source, ownership, and distribution rights. The Hayflick strain developed at the Wistar Institute in Philadelphia called WI-38 was widely accepted as an alternative to primary monkey kidney and HeLa cells. WI-38 provided a cell line from normal human embryonic tissues with a normal chromosomal constitution with no transfer of tumors in animal models. This cell strain was accepted in Europe where Hayflick's WI-38 cell line was approved for use in vaccines. Since the 1960s, WI-38 became the most widely used and highly characterized normal human cell population in the world. WI-38 was provided by Hayflick to Stanley Plotkin for use for the development of a new rubella virus growth and its resultant vaccine, licensed in 1970. WI-38 was also used in the production of the first oral polio vaccine made on a continuously propagated cell strain. Hayflick is renowned as a professor of gerontological studies at the University of California, San Francisco. His landmark studies are characterized as "Hayflick Limit" in cellular ageing and basic longevity studies. His contribution to vaccinology is the WI-38 cell line along with chick embryo cells which have been used for the manufacture of most human virus vaccines world-wide. Vaccines using WI-38 cells have immunized many hundreds of millions of people, include oral poliomyelitis (Sabin), measles, rubella, varicella, mumps, rabies, adenoviruses, and hepatitis A vaccines. Hilleman and his team using WI-38 cells developed the majority of the

TABLE 19.1 Selected Vaccine Development, Developer and Year of Licensure, 1798–2014

Vaccine	Developer	Year
Smallpox	Jenner	1798
Anthrax (animal)	Pasteur	1881
Rabies	Pasteur	1885
Cholera	Hafkine	1911
Diphtheria	von Behring	1913
Tetanus	Glenny	1924
Pertussis	Bordet and Gengou	1926
Tuberculosis (BCG)	Calmette and Guerin	1927
Diphtheria-pertussis-tetanus (DPT) combined[a]	Eldering, Gordon, Kendrick	1948
Japanese encephalitis	Hilleman	1944
Poliomyelitis, Salk inactivated vaccine[a]	Salk	1955
Hong Kong flu	Hilleman	1957
Poliomyelitis, Sabin attenuated vaccine	Sabin	1960
Measles	Hilleman	1963
Mumps	Hilleman	1967
Hong Kong flu pandemic	Hilleman	1968
Rubella	Hilleman	1969
MMR[a]	Hilleman	1969
Meningococcal polysaccharide	Hilleman	1974
Pneumococcal pneumonia[a]	Hilleman	1977
Hepatitis B subunit	Hilleman	1981
Varicella—Chicken pox[a]	Hilleman	1981
Hepatitis B recombinant[a]	Hilleman	1986
Conjugate Haemophilus influenza b (Hib)[a]	Robbins and Schneerson	1987
Hepatitis A[a]	Hilleman	1995
Diphtheria, tetanus toxoids and acellular pertussis vaccine adsorbed (DTaP)[a]	Commercial firms	2002
Rotavirus[a]	Clark, Plotkin, and Offit	2006
Human papilloma virus[a]	Frazer and Zhou	2006
Meningococcal group B	Pfizer	2014

[a]Vaccines recommended for routine use in US children. BCG vaccine is not used routinely in the United States, but selectively for persons considered to be at risk for TB. Smallpox routine vaccination ended in 1971. The United States discontinued routine usage of Sabin vaccine in 2000.
Source: Adapted from Centers for Disease Control and Prevention. Achievements in public health, 1900–1999: impact of vaccines universally recommended for children—United States, 1990–1998. MMWR Morb Mortal Wkly Rep. 1999;48(12):243–248. Available at: https://www.cdc.gov/mmwr/preview/mmwrhtml/00056803.htm (accessed 2 February 2018); Centers for Disease Control and Prevention. Vaccines and immunization: human papillomavirus. Available at: http://www.cdc.gov/vaccines/pubs/pinkbook/hpv.html#vaccines (accessed 29 April 2017); College of Physicians of Philadelphia. The history of vaccines: vaccine development and licensing of vaccines. Last updated 17 January 2018. Available at: https://www.historyofvaccines.org/content/articles/vaccine-development-licensing-events (accessed 1 February 2018).

14 vaccines currently recommended for childhood routine immunization and led in the development of other vaccines.

In 1968, Hilleman produced a more attenuated measles vaccine derived from the virus isolated by John Enders in 1962, which is still used today. The Hillman rubella vaccine was also more attenuated i.e., less likely to cause the disease but still induce antibodies in the vaccinated person than the 1962 vaccine and remains in use today. In 1963, Hilleman isolated the mumps virus from a throat swab from his five-year old daughter and developed a new vaccine, which was licensed in 1967, and was officially named "Jeryl Lynn" after her. Hilleman's iconic Measles, Mumps, Rubella (MMR) combination vaccine was licensed by the FDA in 1971, and is used worldwide. Hilleman also produced the 1967 Hong Kong A2 pandemic influenza vaccine and the meningococcal polysaccharide vaccine, which was licensed in 1974.

After many decades of searching for a pneumococcal pneumonia vaccine, in 1977 Merck licensed a polysaccharide vaccine i.e., long chains of sugar molecules that make up the cell wall of a bacteria, offering protection against 14 types of pneumococcal bacteria. In 1983, the vaccine was extended to include 23 types of pneumococcal bacteria based on the work of selection by Robert Austrian—University of Pennsylvania School of Medicine—who isolated cell lines from more than 90 types of pneumococcal bacteria as types most appropriate for the vaccine. Austrian provided this information to Hilleman who, with associates at Merck, then developed the vaccine from the polysaccharide outer coatings of the bacteria (College of Physicians of Philadelphia, Vaccine Timeline, 2016).

Hilleman's work was based on cooperation with leading scientists to translate scientific studies into safe and effective vaccines suitable for mass production. The measles vaccine went through a long process of development with many key players, including John Enders and Samuel L. Katz, who isolated measles virus in a blood sample from 13-year-old David Edmonston, subsequently called the "Edmonston strain." Working with other scientists, Enders and Katz turned this strain into a vaccine licensed in the United States in 1963. This was an attenuated i.e., using a live, but weakened, measles strain so that it would not cause the disease, but rather act as a vaccine by promoting the production of sufficient antibodies to protect against subsequent exposure to the natural measles virus. In 1968, Hilleman and colleagues developed and further improved the "Edmonston-Enders" strain, which remains the primary measles vaccine used in the United States. In 1981 Hilleman developed the first viral subunit vaccine based on the work of Baruch Blumberg and Wolf Szmuness on the Australian antigen, a cell membrane surface protein of the hepatitis B virus, rather than the entire virus, producing a vaccine licensed in 1986. Hepatitis B recombinant vaccine is inexpensive to produce and is used worldwide for newborns to prevent later development of chronic liver disease, cirrhosis, and liver cancer.

The recombinant hepatitis B vaccine is based on Hepatitis B surface antigen (HBsAg) gene inserted into yeast or cells free of any concerns associated with human blood products. This was a breakthrough in vaccinology as recombinant vector vaccines methods promised improvements in vaccine research, production, lower costs, temperature stability, and ease of administration. This also provided hope for faster vaccine response to emerging infectious agents. In 1987 Hilleman produced and the first US FDA licensed congugate vaccine based on fat from the bacterial cell wall attached to a protein to produce Hemophilus influenza type b (Hib) vaccine. This vaccine protects against this serious respiratory infection in babies aged 0–18 months with dramatic reductions in cases and deaths within a few years. Hilleman also developed varicella (chicken pox) and hepatitis A vaccines—both licensed in 1995—with important public health benefits.

Hilleman traveled the world as an advisor to the World Health Organization (WHO) and to many other public health and infectious disease groups. His outstanding scientific endeavors led to vaccines that saved millions of lives, extended human life expectancy, and improved the economies of numerous countries. While he received many professional awards for his lifetime achievements, he never received a much-deserved Nobel Prize, nor the level of public or professional recognition given to other great scientists in immunology such as Pasteur (for anthrax and rabies vaccines) and Salk or Sabin (for poliomyelitis vaccines). Hilleman's death in 2005 was reported in many scientific journals and major news media with laudatory obituaries.

CURRENT RELEVANCE

Hilleman's innovations advanced the filed of vaccinology providing a base for further progress in vaccine development to address many old devastating diseases including malaria, tuberculosis, and dengue, as well as meeting the challenges of relatively new diseases being transmitted to wider habitats becoming endemic, including spreading diseases of West Nile virus (WNV), Lassa fever, Rift Valley fever (RVF), Middle East respiratory syndrome coronavirus (MERS-CoV), chikungunya, and long-known diseases such as dengue and yellow fever which were spreading via travelers and vectors bringing these older diseases into new habitats. More recently, alarming epidemics of the Ebola virus in West Africa (2013-2016) killed over 11,000 people. The Zika virus, known since 1947, burst into an epidemic in Brazil in 2016, and spread widely to South American, Caribbean and southern US states. Both Ebola and Zika for which there are no vaccines, were declared global public health emergencies by WHO. With the emergence of these viral diseases, society has returned to the era of infectious diseases, the control of which depends on population support through education, hygiene, vector control and relentless, well-funded searches for safe and effective vaccines are developed (National Academies Press, 2016).

New scientific breakthroughs may also lead to improvements in current vaccines by lowering their cost and ease of administration with increasing global coverage rates, and with enhanced effectiveness and safety. The value and benefits of vaccines for disease control include prevention of infection, clinical or subclinical, (such as in poliomyelitis, hepatitis B), or cancer (e.g., cancer of the liver and cervix), and prevention or mitigation of disease severity, such as in pneumococcal pneumonia, and influenza. We now have proven capacity to eliminate, and even eradicate, a disease and its causative agents in nature, such as smallpox (1980), poliomyelitis and measles in the 2020s. Vaccination reduces mortality, morbidity, and complications by protecting individuals and also the community by reducing the spread of disease.

Vaccines protect the immunized individual, but when a sufficient percentage of a population are vaccinated this provides "herd immunity," in which a critical portion of the community—over 95 percent—is immunized resulting in protection for vulnerable individuals who may not have been immunized due to neglect or refusal, being in an age group that was underimmunized in childhood—e.g., by receiving only one dose of measles vaccine, being underage for immunization—e.g., in early infancy—or with an auto-immune disease—e.g., rheumatoid arthritis, systemic lupus erythematosus, or Crohn's disease— with a weakened immune system—e.g., HIV positive—or being medically immunosuppressed, e.g., under cancer treatment and after an organ transplant.

Immunization for individual and herd immunity is a vital factor in public health. Levels of immunization coverage required for herd immunity can vary for different disease organisms, but in the case of measles it requires over 95 percent immunization coverage over a long period of time by an adequate two-dose policy, with monitoring, funding, and quality assurance for immunization programs. Adequacy means coverage of the population at risk of the disease as groups with inadequate vaccination become unexpectedly vulnerable as, for example, in recent importation and spread of measles and mumps in the Americas where these diseases had previously been considered eliminated. New challenges emerge requiring increasing vaccination coverage including tetanus, diphtheria, pertussis, and influenza for pregnant women, and their family members and care givers to protect newborns who are vulnerable until their immunization can be completed. Herd immunity (i.e., immunity by vaccination among a high percentage of a population sufficient to reduce the risk of transmission by isolated cases which varies for different diseases) must be achieved and maintained to reduce the potential for transmission of a disease to vulnerable people such as people with immune deficiency due to infection with HIV, cancer chemotherapy, or immunodeficiency diseases. In other cases, giving rubella vaccine to boys as well as girls to reduce or eliminate circulation of the virus prevents infections during pregnancy, which can lead to congenital rubella syndrome in infants, a disease that can result in lifelong disability (see Chapters 3, 12, 16).

As vaccination programs reach a higher percentage of the vulnerable population, elimination of diseases locally can be achieved without global eradication of the causative microorganism. Global eradication of an infectious disease once seemed an impossible dream, but when achieved for smallpox demonstrated that human diseases with no animal host—such as smallpox, poliomyelitis, measles, mumps, and rubella—could also be eradicated. Efforts to eradicate poliomyelitis are coming close to success, while eradication of measles and rubella is targeted by WHO to be achieved by 2020.

Vaccination to prevent cancer is an important advance in public health with success of hepatitis B immunization (see Figure 19.1), which will prevent many cases of liver cirrhosis and liver cancer globally. The impact of Hilleman's hepatitis B virus (HBV) vaccine first issued in 1982 in the United States (Figure 19.1), is used in other high, medium and low-income countries. Incidence of HBV where vaccination with high coverage of newborns has declined dramatically. Chronic HBV infection produces high risk

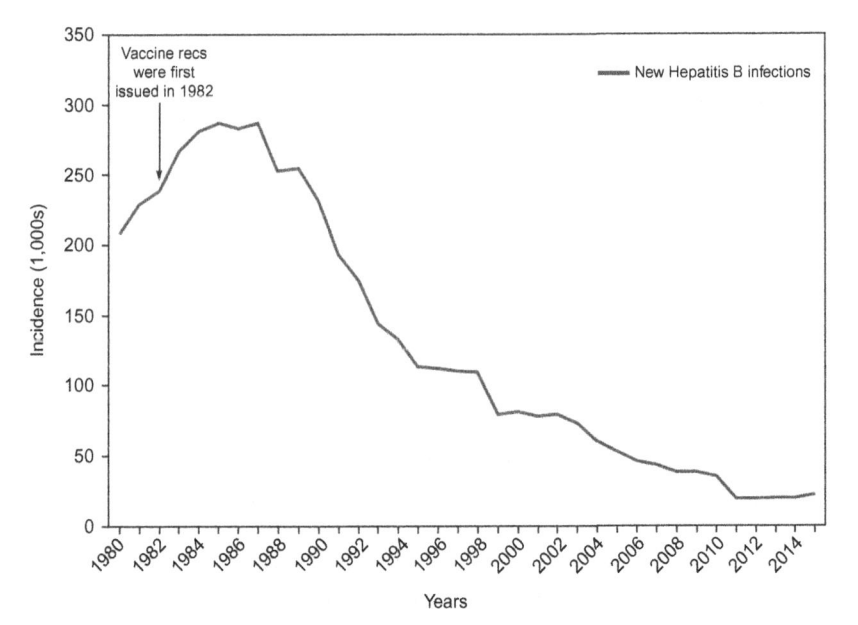

FIGURE 19.1 Incidence of hepatitis B virus infection, United States, 1980–2015. *Source: Schillie S, Vellozzi C, Reingold A, Harris A, Haber P, Ward JW, Nelson NP. Prevention of Hepatitis B virus infection in the United States: recommendations of the Advisory Committee on Immunization Practices. MMWR Recomm Rep 2018;67(No. RR-1):1–31. Available at: https:// www.cdc.gov/mmwr/volumes/67/rr/rr6701a1.htm (accessed 21 January 2018)*

for cirrhosis and liver cancer. The recommended practice is for HBV carrier status testing in pregnancy with universal hepatitis B vaccination of all newborns within 24 hours of birth. CDC recommends completion of the vaccination series in infants, vaccination of other children and adolescents who missed infancy coverage, as well as adults at risk for liver disease. Despite progress, HBV remains a major global problem. WHO reports that globally 84% of children born in 2015 received the three recommended doses of hepatitis B vaccine, but HBV mortality remained high in 2015 with 887,000 deaths globally mostly from cirrhosis and liver carcinoma. HBV is also an important occupational hazard for health workers.

More recently, slowly increasing use of Human papilloma virus (HPV) vaccination will prevent cervical cancer being reduced by Pap smear screening but ultimately the HPV vaccine will be the dominant factor in control of HPV infection causing cancer of the cervix. In addition, boys are also immunized to reduce spread of the virus by heterosexual intercourse, as well as reducing the increasing rates of oral and anal cancers from homosexual relations.

The search for vaccines against other cancers will benefit from the significant progress over recent decades in genetic, microbiologic, computer, and molecular sciences. The scientific and manufacturing advances led by Hilleman produced vaccines with economic and health sector benefits for many nations. Their increasing use for preventing pneumococcal pneumonia, meningitis, and measles reduces dependence on antibiotics for the complications of these diseases a factor in reducing antibiotic usage thus slowing the development of antibiotic resistance. Vaccines protect people with chronic medical conditions such as chronic lung-, heart- or kidney diseases as in the success of pneumococcal pneumonia and influenza vaccines reducing serious complications, hospitalizations, and avoidable deaths (see Figure 19.2).

Globally, it is estimated that 14.5 million episodes of serious pneumococcal disease occur annually. These include pneumonia, meningitis, and sepsis mainly in children aged under five years resulting in some 500,000 deaths, mostly in low- and middle-income countries. Pneumococcal conjugate vaccine (PCV), first licensed in 2000, provided protection against seven of the most common pneumococcal serotypes. In 2006, WHO recommended that this vaccine be included in all routine immunization programs, particularly in high incidence countries. In 2010, new PCV formulations protecting against 10 and 13 serotypes became available, providing better coverage for serotypes common in low- and middle-income countries. Pneumococcal polysaccharide vaccine for 23 serotypes of pneumococcal bacteria is now in use and recommended for adults 65 years or older, for children at high risk and increasingly for all older adults. More and more, this vaccine is recommended for all children, and adults, including pregnant women.

Hilleman demonstrated the value of combining vaccines such as in the enormously successful measles, mumps, rubella vaccine (MMR) and later

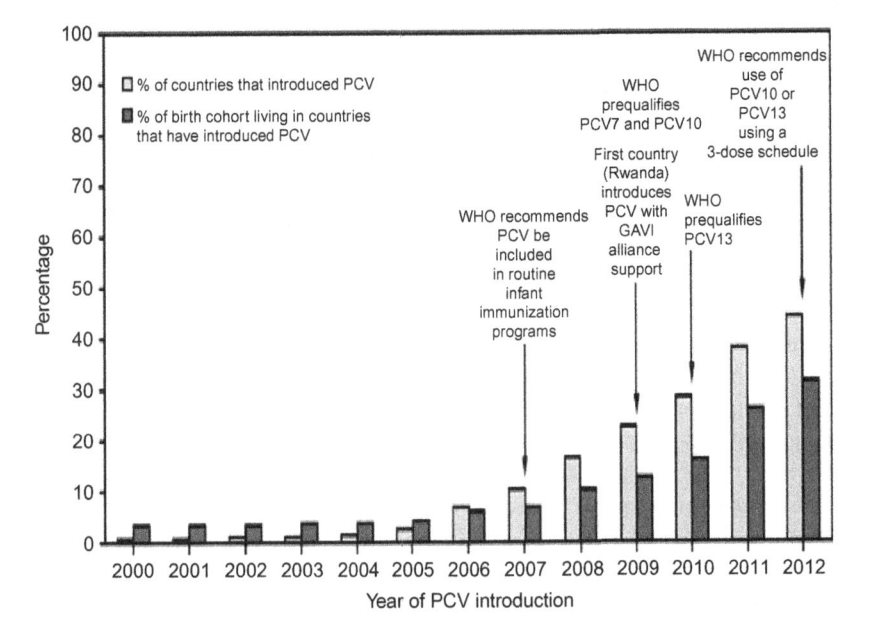

FIGURE 19.2 Progress in introduction of pneumococcal conjugate vaccine (PCV), world-wide, 2000–2012, by World Health Organization (WHO). Abbreviations: *PCV7*, 7-valent PCV; *PCV10*, 10-valent PCV; *PCV13*, 13-valent PCV. *Source: Centers for Disease Control and Prevention. Progress in introduction of pneumococcal conjugate vaccine world-wide 2000–2012. Morb Mort Wkly Rep. 2013;62(16):308–311. Available at: <https://www.cdc.gov/mmwr/preview/mmwrhtml/mm6216a4.htm> (accessed 4 September 2016).*

adding inactivated poliomyelitis vaccine (IPV) and varicella (chickenpox) vaccine. Standard vaccine combinations have been expanded with the addition of polio (IPV) along with hemophilus influenza (Hib) in the combination of diphtheria, pertussis, tetanus (DPT). This pentavalent vaccine can be given to infants simultaneously with rotavirus, meningitis B, and pneumococcal pneumonia vaccines without loss of effectiveness. The benefits include better compliance with improved coverage and injection safety, less cost and fewer visits to a medical service. Vaccination also provides protective safety from some potential biological forms of bioterrorism, such as smallpox, anthrax, and potential respiratory infectious agents.

A large-scale epidemic of measles spread across Europe between 2010 and 2017. Travelers spread measles to North and South America. In 2017, measles cases were registered in 14 European countries: Austria, Belgium, Bulgaria, the Czech Republic, Hungary, France, Germany, Iceland, Italy, Portugal, Romania, Spain, Switzerland, and Sweden with an estimated total of over 7,500 cases of measles, with Romania being the most affected country with 4,793 measles patients reported between January 2016 and

April 2017, according to the European Centers for Disease Prevention and Control (ECDC). In total, there have been 25 deaths in Europe, of which 22 occurred in Romania. Portugal, Switzerland, and Bulgaria also had measles fatalities. The ECDC is exploring national Immunization Information Systems to improve the monitoring of immunization coverage at local geographical levels, linking individual immunization histories with health outcome data for vaccine safety, effectiveness, as well as failures, and educational material for vaccine researchers, producers, providers, and recipients.

Imported and secondary measles cases appeared in California in 2015, a state that allowed personal beliefs exemptions to easily override laws requiring full immunization such as two doses of MMR vaccine for all children and young adults attending schools. This led to extremely low MMR vaccination rates at some schools, particularly private schools, with even zero coverage in some kindergartens. The outbreak led to 2016 changes in Californian law requiring parents to consult with the local public health office and requiring a medical certificate stating medical reasons for exemption. This process will make it more difficult for parents to deny this immunization to their children, which puts all unimmunized children at risk due to the highly infectious nature of measles. The new immunization requirement in California has resulted in increased coverage of MMR and other vaccines to over 95 percent.

The science behind vaccine development has increased its capacity markedly in recent years with genetics and immunology entering new spheres of research for vaccines to combat cancers and genetic diseases, which is expected to play a major role in clinical medicine and public health in the coming decades. The cases of measles and hepatitis B are prime examples of vaccines that have been developed in partnership with many contributing laboratories, manufacturers and public health leaders with shared information and scientific advances leading to reduced global mortality rates. Scientists and manufacturers worked together to create the HBV vaccine produced by using one element of the cellular wall of the virus instead of the whole virus, increasing the safety of the vaccine. Hilleman later developed the first immunizations with recombinant vaccines, contributing to the application of advances in genetic sciences for vaccinology in the future to provide low-cost and widely effective new approaches to vaccination.

ETHICAL ISSUES

Public trust in vaccines has become an important global health issue, with negative attitudes due to fears over false but highly publicized side-effects and hesitancy among some doctors. Italy and Germany are making vaccination mandatory after health officials warned that a fall-off in vaccination rates had triggered a measles epidemic. In 10 European countries, cases of measles doubled in number in the first two months of 2017 compared to 2016, as reported by the ECDC, with more than 2,000 cases in 2017, almost ten times the number in 2015. Notwithstanding the astonishing success of vaccines in saving millions of lives and promoting civil societies, vaccine development, production, and implementation have many ethical issues and controversies. These range from ideological anti-vaccinatonism, to professional jealousies and controversies, along with economic and legal disputes over cell lines for vaccine production, to allegations of vaccines causing diseases in children, slow adoption of life-saving vaccines, inadequate resource allocation in developing countries, lack of harmonization of vaccination policies, and others.

Anti-vaccinationism has been around since the days of Jenner's discovery of vaccination to prevent smallpox in the 18th century and continues to the present time (see Chapter 2). Recently, rates of parental refusals of vaccination have increased. This is due, in part, to increased public skepticism of public health professionals, policymakers, and the pharmaceutical industry. Reduced public health awareness is also due to the successful control and near-elimination of many once dreaded infectious diseases such as smallpox and poliomyelitis. Today, most parents, health care staff and doctors have never seen the diseases prevented by vaccines and do not understand their gravity.

Public anxiety surrounding vaccinations rose in the United Kingdom in the 1980s in response to concerns about the safety of the pertussis vaccine. This resulted in a decline of immunization coverage and the return of this once well controlled disease. In the mid - 1990s UK uptake of MMR vaccination fell from a peak of 92 percent at the age of two to 82 percent in 2003, with uptake falling below 75 percent in parts of London. This has serious implications for mutual protection of the population, i.e., herd immunity. In the US and elsewhere, recent outbreaks of pertussis and diphtheria, and spread of imported measles after decades of control raise the need to ensure immunization of pregnant women and their close family members to protect the fetus and newborns from serious preventable infections before the infants' immunization protection takes hold.

The harm created by publication of fraudulent and unethical research activities has had an adverse impact on professional and public perception of matters such as vaccines. In 1998, an article published in *Lancet* by Andrew Wakefield purported to show that the measles−mumps−rubella (MMR) vaccine caused autism. This created a storm of public concern and parental refusals of the MMR vaccine. Media investigation and professional studies proved the study was fabricated, and many reliable studies have since disproved its claims. Following an ethics investigation by the UK's General Medical Council, Wakefield's medical license was revoked in 2010, and the article partially retracted by *Lancet* in 2004 was fully withdrawn by the journal in 2010. However, despite the media coverage and retraction of the article, the credibility of vaccinations—specifically MMR vaccine—in the eyes of the public was damaged substantially. The allegation, although proven to have been fabricated, continues to be widely believed and spread via the internet and social media.

Popular resistance to vaccination is both a legal and ethical question as reflected in current controversies in the United States, where opting out of mandatory vaccination has contributed to measles outbreaks, a disease that was considered eradicated many years ago. Compulsory immunization is currently not politically acceptable due to concerns over parental rights of refusal and active lobbying on the internet and in public media against "government medicine." But state mandates requiring certification of complete immunization are well established in the United States. All 50 US states have legislation requiring specified vaccines for students. However, exemptions are allowed for medical reasons, and for reasons of religious beliefs and 18 states allow philosophical exemptions for those who object to immunizations because of personal, moral, or other beliefs (National Conference of State Legislatures, 2017).

Pediatricians in the United States are reporting increased refusal of parents to immunize their children, prompting the American Academy of Pediatrics (AAP), the American Medical Association (AMA) and the American College of Physicians to recommend the elimination of non-medical exemptions in state immunization laws. to call for State legislators to increase limitations on exemption clauses for philosophical reasons. Refusal of vaccination can be seen as posing a threat to other children, as well as a form of child neglect such as having a child in a car without an appropriate child car seat. In part, this action is stimulated by concern over increasing resistance of parents to vaccination along with return of previously controlled diseases. Failure to vaccinate is a form of child neglect.

Both the public and private sectors, including the pharmaceutical industry, have contributed greatly to increasing vaccine coverage rates, and public–private partnerships remain vital to vaccinology. As a senior staff member of Merck, responsible for vaccine development at a major pharmaceutical company, Hilleman conducted industry-funded research and his contribution led directly to manufacture of the majority of vaccines created in the latter half of the 20th century that have been, and remain, vital for public health in the US and globally. The role of the private pharmaceutical industry needs to be recognized as crucial for advances in this field, but is equally dependant on scientists at universities and public research institutions with their contribution to the knowledge base that enabled breakthroughs in vaccine production and distribution. In the period 2014–2016, large epidemics of two deadly "new" viruses, Ebola and Zika, were designated by WHO as a global health crises with justifiable concern that they could spread rapidly to many parts of the world. The Zika virus transmitted to a pregnant woman by Anopheles mosquitoes, or by sexual relations with a Zika infected partner may produce a mild illness. but has tragic effects on fetuses resulting in serious birth defects including small head size, i.e., microcephaly, and brain damage. The race to develop effective vaccines must involve public–private cooperation to achieve a working vaccine within several years. The media and WHO concern have reminded skeptics of the essential role of vaccine research with cooperation between governments, donors, academics and industrial scientists as promoted by Maurice Hilleman in his life's work.

The long time gap from availability and proof of vaccine success until it is adopted globally is an ethical issue for reducing global health inequities as well as a question of priorities and resource allocation in public health. Adoption and implementation of vaccination is slow to respond to important advances, especially in low-income countries where policy-makers have traditionally given health low priority in governmental financing. Delays in vaccine adoption lead to preventable infections, with high rates of illness, deaths, human misery, and slowing of economic progress.

Lack of harmonization of vaccination policies is a major professional, public policy, ethical issue and a limiting factor in achieving the full potential of proven successful and safe vaccines. Europe, and the European Union, still does not have a common harmonized immunization program, in some cases not even in the same country, which contributed to the massive measles epidemics since 2010.

ECONOMIC ISSUES

The benefits to society of vaccination are enormous, not only in saving lives and reducing morbidity, but also in reduced health care costs. Vaccines are life-saving and cost-effective, and they should be supported by national governments and international donor programs alongside the buildup of public health education and infrastructure development within recipient countries. Vaccines have been crucial in reducing child illness and birth defects —e.g., congenital rubella syndrome. Vaccines help men, women and especially children to have healthy lives without morbidity of many previously common childhood diseases (e.g., poliomyelitis). They also lessen infections among people with chronic medical and disabling conditions such as pneumococcal pneumonia and influenza vaccines. Reducing disease and high mortality rates promotes economic growth as supported by the World Bank and other economic analyses. Successful vaccination also increases equity in society by reducing diseases that were often more common among poorer populations.

Expansion of vaccine coverage during the "Decade of Vaccines" funded by the Bill and Melinda Gates Foundation in 2010 in the world's poorest countries from 2011 to 2020 is estimated to save more than US$5 billion in acute care costs and increased productivity value of at least US$151 billion (Stack et al., 2011). The CDC estimates savings from averted direct health care costs of US $402 billion USD and more than one trillion dollars in societal costs for the cohort of children born in the United States between 1994 and 2013 (Whitney et al., 2014). Since 1993, the World Bank and economic analysts have accepted that the economic benefit to low- and medium-income countries (LMICs) of reducing child mortality—mostly resulting from reduced morbidity and mortality from infectious diseases—is vital to their economic and social advancement.

Nearly universal use of hepatitis B vaccine for newborns has helped to prevent mother-to-child transmission and subsequent prevention of liver cirrhosis and liver cancer, which is of enormous economic value to health systems. The vaccine to prevent the spread of hepatitis A is available and used in many countries, but a vaccine for the more serious disease of Hepatitis C has regrettably not yet been developed. Although effective, life-saving treatments are available, these are costly and an effective vaccine would bring greater benefits and advances.

Vaccine coverage in low- and middle-income countries (LMICs) such as Brazil, Russian Federation, India, China, and South Africa (BRICS) varies widely. A review of cost effectiveness and economic benefit studies of vaccines in LMICs concluded that vaccination brings important economic benefits and recommends that policy-makers should consider vaccines to be an efficient investment. For example, the health, economic, and social benefits of vaccination with Hemophilus influenza b (Hib), pneumococcal pneumonia, and rotavirus vaccine coverage in BRICS countries have been estimated at more than US$15 billion annually (see Table 19.2).

Immunization averts an estimated two to three million deaths every year from diphtheria, tetanus, pertussis (whooping cough), and measles. However, an additional 1.5 million deaths could be prevented if global vaccination coverage improves from under 85 percent to 90 percent. GAVI, the Global Vaccine Alliance, is a major entity working to increase coverage in low-income countries. GAVI is a public—private global alliance for vaccine implementation supported by WHO, UNICEF, the World Bank, the Gates Foundation, pharmaceutical companies, and others. Since its founding in 2000, GAVI helps finance adoption of vaccines in low-income countries dependent on external support to finance vaccination. The percentage of low-income countries financing vaccines in their national budgets rose from 64 percent in 2000 to 75 percent in 2006, with a modest increase in national government share of routine immunization rising from 35 percent to 39 percent between 2000 and 2008.

A 2017 study reviewed publications from 27 countries which introduced rotavirus vaccine into their national routine immunization programs since 2006. Substantial reductions (30%–60%) were found in rotavirus and all-cause acute gastroenteritis (AGE) hospitalizations and AGE mortality among children under age one and age five years.

Measles is a highly contagious and potentially fatal disease which is a leading cause of death among young children (see Box 19.1). Efforts to control, eliminate, and ultimately eradicate measles are part of international organizations and WHO strategy. An economic analysis by Levin et al. in

TABLE 19.2 Estimated Annual Economic and Social Benefits from Increased Haemophilus Influenza Type b, Pneumoncoccal Conjugate Vaccine, and Rotavirus Vaccine Coverage in Brazil, the Russian Federation, India, China, and South Africa (BRICS)

Country	GDP per Capita 2012 (US$)	Life Expectancy at Birth (Years)	Estimated Annual No. of Averted Deaths				Estimated Annual Economic and Social Benefits (Million USD)
			Hib	SP	RV	Total	
Brazil	11,359	73.8	0	25	10	35	18.2
Russian Federation	14,302	67.9	373	474	31	878	559.7
India	1,501	66.3	52,709	54,429	29,612	136,820	9,084
China	6,071	75.2	9,538	10,079	1,170	20,787	5,796.8
South Africa	2,525	57.1	856	319	85	1,260	398.0

Note: *CDP,* gross domestic product; *Hib,* Haemophilus influenza type b; *RV,* rotavirus; *SP, Streptococcus pneumonia; US$,* United States dollars.
Source: Mirelman A, et al. The economic and social benefits of childhood vaccinations in BRICS. Bull World Health Organ. 2014;92:454–456.
Available at: http://www.who.int/bulletin/volumes/92/6/13/132597.pdf (accessed 29 April 2017).

BOX 19.1 Global Impact of Measles Vaccine

- Measles is a highly contagious, serious disease caused by a virus.
- In 1980, before widespread vaccination, measles caused an estimated 2.6 million deaths globally each year.
- Measles is still a leading global cause of death among young children even though a safe and cost-effective vaccine is available since the 1960s.
- Global measles deaths decreased by 84 percent world-wide from 550,100 deaths in 2000 to 89,780 in 2016.
- An estimated 20.4 million people were affected by measles in 2016, particularly in Africa and Asia.
- In 2015, about 85 percent of the world's children received one dose of measles vaccine by their first birthday through routine health services—an increase up from 73 percent in 2000.
- During 2000–2015, measles vaccination prevented an estimated 20.3 million deaths making measles vaccine one of the most cost-effective investments in public health.

Source: *World Health Organization. Measles fact sheet, reviewed March 2017. Available at: <http://www.who.int/mediacentre/factsheets/fs286/en/> (accessed 29 April 2017) and World Health Organization. Immunizations, vaccines, biologicals: measles. Last updated November 2017. Available at: http://www.who.int/immunization/diseases/measles/en/ (accessed 20 January 2018).*

2011, indicated that measles eradication by 2020 was the most cost-effective scenario in the six countries studied and globally. WHO's "Global Measles and Rubella Strategic Plan: 2012–2020" considers the economic benefits for promotion of public health and economic growth to be powerful justification for targeting measles and rubella for eradication as a high priority in LMIC. In recent years, many cost-effectiveness studies of vaccines for hepatitis B, rotavirus, human papilloma virus, and influenza have shown that vaccination is an effective economic tool with significant health benefits. Global targeting of rubella for eradication along with measles for achievement by 2020 will require new tactics in Europe, such as harmonization of immunization programs across the region, and certainly in the European Union where there is free border crossing between member states and large-scale refugee entry without evidence of past immunization. The tools exist in outstanding vaccine combinations, especially the MMR vaccine created by Hilleman. Measles and rubella control—and ultimately eradication—are within the capacity of well-led public health policy and resources (see Box 19.2).

The sciences of vaccinology depend on academic research and on the private sector of the limited number of vaccine producers in the world. With a drumbeat of public health emergencies in the 21st century with SARS, H1N1 influenza, Ebola and Zika virus epidemics indicate the problem. Long known diseases such as malaria, HIV, TB, dengue, West Nile fever and

BOX 19.2 Global Impact of Rubella Vaccine

- Rubella is a contagious, generally mild viral infection that occurs most often in children and young adults.
- There is no specific treatment for rubella, but the disease is preventable by vaccination.
- Rubella infection in pregnant women may cause fetal death or congenital defects known as congenital rubella syndrome (CRS).
- A rubella pandemic developed during 1962–1965 in the United States, with more than 20,000 babies born with congenital rubella syndrome.
- Children with CRS can suffer hearing impairments, eye- and heart defects and other lifelong disabilities, including autism, diabetes mellitus, and thyroid disorders.
- Worldwide, an estimated 100,000 babies are born with CRS every year.
- The recommendation of CDC and WHO is two doses of measles- and rubella-containing vaccine, preferably as MMR.
- WHO has set a target for the end of 2020, when the world should achieve measles- and rubella-elimination in at least five WHO regions.
- After the US licensed rubella vaccine in 1969 the number of reported cases of CRS declined dramatically to <one case per year or four cases in total during 2005–2011.
- In 2004, a panel of internationally recognized experts reviewed rubella epidemiology and unanimously agreed that rubella elimination (i.e., the absence of year-round endemic transmission) was achieved in the United States.

Sources: WHO. Rubella fact sheet, reviewed March 2017. Available at: <http://www.who.int/ mediacentre/factsheets/fs367/en/> (accessed 29 April 2017). Centers for Disease Control and Prevention. Vaccines and immunization. Chapters 14, 15. Rubella and congenital rubella syndrome, updated 1 April 2014. Available at: <http://www.cdc. gov/vaccines/pubs/surv-manual/chpt14-rubella.html and http://www.cdc.gov/vaccines/pubs/ surv-manual/chpt15-crs.html#> (accessed 29 April 2017).

others are also part of the urgent call for new vaccines challenging the research capacity of academia and private manufacturers. The process of discovery is only part of a long and costly process of initial testing of safety and efficacy. New institutional and funding arrangements will be needed to make the most of new technology and genetics in vaccine development for these and new challenges that may be expected to arise. We will also need "future Maurice Hillemans."

CONCLUSION

Vaccine development and distribution have saved millions of lives, and have the potential to save millions more as new vaccines emerge from public and private research centers, through the pioneering achievements of the next generations of Hilleman and colleagues. Science will continue to develop new tools, such as finding ways to produce vaccines using genetic techniques of adding key genes to simple microorganisms to produce protective antibodies and improving heat stability of vaccines to eliminate the cumbersome and costly "cold chain" (i.e., storing and transportation of vaccines within a specified temperature range). Policy-makers in public health systems will continue to improve vaccine delivery and to implement vaccination programs for reduced morbidity and mortality rates across the globe.

Vaccines are among the most efficient preventive measures available to both clinical medicine and public health. However gains from successful immunization campaigns are being rolled back as rates of vaccine refusal increase. Public support can be won or eroded by pro- and contra-advocacy groups. Public concerns over vaccine safety can become wildly exaggerated and has the effect of reducing vaccine acceptance. The support of medical practitioners and the media is vital to promote adoption and acceptance of newer vaccines by an often skeptical public.

Neither the science, nor the application of its advances, occur automatically. Instead, vaccine discovery, development and implementation coverage requires the skill and dedication of future "Hillemans", a well-trained public health workforce, and a strong organizational base for public health. Hilleman believed and demonstrated that academic and industry-based scientists could work in a complementary fashion in support of global public health goals for disease control and eradication, as vaccine development and distribution have a crucial role in population health. The prospects look favorable for scientific advances leading to new vaccines and to the potential for further disease control and eradication. This process requires long and expensive periods of basic sciences research and vaccine testing, and when proven effective and safe, the implementation of immunization programs. Academic/industry partnerships with government support should be encouraged to improve the efficiency of vaccine development.

In many countries, adoption of new vaccines in routine immunization programs has proven to be slow. A CDC publication, "Framework for Preventing Infectious Diseases, 2011", emphasizes: modernization of infectious disease surveillance; expanding the role of public health and laboratories for disease control and prevention; and advancing workforce development and training to sustain, and strengthen, public health practice, and above all the committed leadership role of national governments. Disease control depends on monitoring case reports including quantity, common factors such as time, location, risk factors, and available intervention that can be applied to control epidemic or endemic diseases. It is essential to reach out to especially vulnerable groups living in urban poverty areas as well as remote villages and those with particular risk factors for diseases. This is the context in which vaccines are of enormous social and economic benefit, as well as being critical to improve health, prevent disease, and avoidable mortality. A well-trained public workforce is required to meet these challenges. Ultimately, ensuring the development of these key preventive measures to reduce—and in some cases, eradicate—infectious diseases requires public health and governmental leadership. The public health system is responsible for total population health and must take the lead to finance, organize, monitor, and deliver needed services such as child vaccination. Public health widely suffers from low priority in national government budgets. Harmonization of immunization policies and public support are needed, as are resources. Strong support by national government policy and funding are key to the reduction in incidence, prevalence, and control of diseases which can be ameliorated by known, as well as yet-to-be discovered, vaccines.

The CDC considers vaccines to be *"one of the greatest achievements of biomedical science and public health"* (CDC 1999). The vast majority of vaccines used currently were developed in the 20th century on the basis of Louis Pasteur's work on anthrax and rabies in the 19th century and over 40 vaccines were developed by Maurice Hilleman with academic and industry colleagues at Merck (College of Physicians of Philadelphia, 2016). Hilleman was undoubtedly the leading vaccinologist of the 20th century, and perhaps of all time. In 1988, he was awarded the National Medal of Science, the highest scientific honor in the United States, and although he received many professional honors he never achieved the popular recognition or fame of other pioneers in vaccine development and implementation such as the developers and leaders in poliomyelitis vaccine, Jonas Salk and Albert Sabin.

In 1997 Hilleman was awarded the Albert Sabin Gold Medal Award. Dr. Anthony Fauci, Director of the US National Institute of Allergy and Infectious Diseases at the US National Institutes of Health, called Hilleman "one of the true giants of science, medicine and public health in the 20th century." When Hilleman died in 2005, after a truly magnificent scientific career of 60 years, Dr. Paul Offit, chief of infectious diseases at the Children's Hospital of Philadelphia, told the BMJ: *"His commitment was to make something useful and convert it to clinical use. Maurice's genius was in developing vaccines, reliably reproducing them, and he was in charge of all pharmaceutical facets from research to the marketplace."* The BMJ obituary for Hilleman stated: *"Almost all of Hilleman's career was in the pharmaceutical industry to develop, in cooperation with academic scientists, vaccines that brought science to the direct benefit of mankind saving millions of deaths especially of children."* Dr. Faucci, stated: *"Maurice was perhaps the single most influential public health figure of the twentieth century, if one considers the millions of lives saved and the countless people who were spared suffering because of his work. Over the course of his career, Maurice and his colleagues developed more than forty vaccines. Of the fourteen vaccines currently recommended in the United States, Maurice developed eight."*

Although largely unknown among the general public and even among public health practitioners and teachers, Maurice Hilleman was the outstanding scientist in the field of vaccinology in the 20th century who brought dynamism and creativity to develop vaccines saving countless lives and bringing the means and the hope for eradication of important diseases such as measles, congenital rubella syndrome, and hepatitis B. He introduced new approaches to vaccinology which others following his path can use help to control—or eliminate—important diseases now, and others that in the future may face humanity. Hopefully "new Hillemans" will emerge to advance the sciences of genetics and vaccinology to face existing and new challenges of science and population health.

RECOMMENDATIONS

1. Progress in vaccinology application relies on funding, prioritizing, monitoring, surveillance, routine immunization programs, and outbreak control as cornerstones of public health goals in disease control or its eradication.
2. Public health must improve its leadership responsibility and realize its important role in reaching out to at-risk, vulnerable segments of the population in outlying rural areas and urban dwellers.
3. Harmonization of vaccination policies is urgently needed in Europe and low-income countries to halt resurgence and achieve eradication of still significant diseases including measles, rubella, and other targeted vaccine-preventable disease in the coming years.
4. Public health should increase advocacy efforts in health promotion to extend vaccine development and to assure public support for measles control and eradication, as well as other vaccine-preventable diseases.
5. Resources for science advancement and for service delivery are equally important and must be accepted as a governmental responsibility in LMICs as well as in high-income countries.
6. Training of public health and community health workers is vital to meet old and new vaccine challenges of premature death, disease, and disability in aging populations, with severe climate and social inequality challenges.
7. Governments, academic research centers, vaccine manufacturers, and public health authorities require well-designed plans to respond to pandemic illnesses, especially in recognizing the global importance and urgency of the need for quicker development and distribution of the influenza vaccine, as well as for newly emerging infectious disease such as Ebola and Zika, among others.

STUDENT REVIEW QUESTIONS

1. What are the roles of public and private sector research in vaccine development?
2. Why was Maurice Hilleman so important in vaccinology?
3. Why are vaccines important in public health and modern societal development?
4. Why is it slow and costly to develop new vaccines and to adopt them in public health practice?
5. What mechanisms exist to help adoption of new vaccines by LMICs?
6. Which infectious diseases would you place on a priority list for vaccine development to save the maximum feasible number of people from disease and avoidable death?
7. Should vaccination be made mandatory for well-proven vaccines? Why, or why not?
8. Why has measles rebounded after being considered eliminated in Europe and the Americas?
9. Discuss factors that affect progress toward the eradication of infectious diseases such as measles?
10. What methods of public health are available to control diseases for which there is no vaccine?
11. What new methodologies are expected to become available to produce vaccines in less-costly and more easily-usable ways?
12. Why is vaccinology a crucial field in research and practice for cancer control?

RECOMMENDED READINGS

1. Altman LK. Maurice Hilleman: master in creating vaccines, dies at 85. NY Times. April 12, 2005. Available at: http://www.nytimes.com/2005/04/12/us/maurice-hilleman-master-in-creating-vaccines-dies-at-85.html?_r = 0 (accessed 31 May 2017).
2. Andre FE, Booy R, Bock HL, Clemens J, Datta SK, John TJ, et al. Vaccination greatly reduces disease, disability, death and inequity worldwide. Bull World Health Organ. 2008;86(2):140−146. Available at: http://www.who.int/bulletin/volumes/86/2/07-040089/en/ (accessed 29 April 2017).
3. Advisory Committee for Immunization Practices (ACIP). Vaccine recommendations, updated 26 January 2018. Available at: http://www.cdc.gov/vaccines/hcp/acip-recs/index.html (accessed 27 January 2018).
4. Azvolinsky A. Of cells and limits: Leonard Hayflick, The Scientist | March 1, 2015. Available at: http://www.the-scientist.com/?articles.view/articleNo/42256/title/Of-Cells-and-Limits/ (accessed 25 April 2017).
5. Bartlett Z. Leonard Hayflick (1928−). Embryo project encyclopedia, 20 July 2014. Arizona State University. School of Life Sciences. Center for Biology and Society. Available at: https://embryo.asu.edu/pages/leonard-hayflick-1928 (accessed 2 May 2017).

6. Burnett E, Jonesteller CL, Tate JE, Yen C, Parashar UD. Global impact of rotavirus vaccination on childhood hospitalizations and mortality From diarrhea. J Infect Dis. 2017. http://dx.doi.org/10.1093/infdis/jix186. Available at: https://academic.oup.com/jid/article/doi/10.1093/infdis/jix186/3738521/Global-Impact-of-Rotavirus-Vaccination-on (accessed 27 May 2017).

7. Carter Center. Summary of the twentieth meeting of the international task force for disease eradication (II) November 27, 2012. Available at: https://www.cartercenter.org/resources/pdfs/news/health_publications/itfde/itfde-summary-112712.pdf (accessed 29 April 2017).

8. Centers for Disease Control and Prevention. Achievements in public health, 1900–1999: impact of vaccines universally recommended for children—United States, 1990–1998. Morb Mortal Wkly Rep. 1999;48(12):243–248. Available at: http://www.cdc.gov/mmwr/preview/mmwrhtml/00056803.htm (accessed 24 April 2017).

9. Centers for Disease Control and Prevention. A CDC framework for preventing infectious diseases: sustaining the essentials and innovating for the future. Atlanta, Georgia: Centers for Disease Control, 2011 October. Available at: http://www.cdc.gov/oid/docs/ID-Framework.pdf (accessed 24 April 2017).

10. Centers for Disease Control and Prevention. Achievements in public health, 1900–1999: control of infectious diseases. Morb Mortal Wkly Rep. 1999;48:621. Available at: http://www.cdc.gov/mmwr/PDF/wk/mm4829.pdf (accessed 24 April 2017).

11. Centers for Disease Control and Prevention. Vaccines and immunization. Chapter 15. Congenital rubella syndrome, updated 1 April 2014. Available at: http://www.cdc.gov/vaccines/pubs/surv-manual/chpt15-crs.html# (accessed 24 April 2017).

12. Centers for Disease Control and Prevention. Measles history, 3 March 2017. Available at: http://www.cdc.gov/measles/about/history.html (accessed 29 April 2017).

13. Centers for Disease Control and Prevention. Measles—United States, January 4–April 2, 2015. Morb Mortal Wkly Rep. 2015;64(14):373–376. Available at: http://www.cdc.gov/mmwr/preview/mmwrhtml/mm6414a1.htm (accessed 27 April 2017).

14. Centers for Disease Control and Prevention. Influenza (Flu): types of influenza viruses, updated 27 September 2017. Available at: http://www.cdc.gov/flu/about/viruses/types.htm (accessed 22 December 2017).

15. Centers for Disease Control and Prevention. World immunization week, 24–30 April, 2017. Available at: http://www.who.int/campaigns/immunization-week/2017/en/ (accessed 27 April 2017).

16. College of Physicians of Philadelphia. The history of vaccines. Available at: http://www.historyofvaccines.org/content/timelines/hilleman (accessed 29 April 2017).

17. College of Physicians of Philadelphia. Vaccine development and licensing events. Philadelphia, PA. Available at: http://www.historyofvaccines.org/content/articles/vaccine-development-licensing-events (accessed 29 April 2017).

18. Encyclopedia of World Biography. Hilleman, Maurice Ralph, 2006. Available at: http://www.encyclopedia.com/doc/1G2-2550300079.html (accessed 24 April 2017).

19. Derrough T, Olsson K, Gianfredi V, Simondon F, Heijbel H, Danielsson N, et al. Immunization information systems—useful tools for monitoring vaccination programs in EU/EFA countries, 2016. Eurosurveillance. 2017;22(17). Available at: http://www.eurosurveillance.org/ViewArticle.aspx?ArticleId=22782 (accessed 28 April 2017).

20. Famousscientists.org. Maurice Hilleman, 1919–2005. Available at: http://www.famousscientists.org/maurice-hilleman/ (accessed 23 April 2017).

21. Ginsberg GM, Berger S, Shouval D. Cost–benefit analysis of a nationwide neonatal inoculation programme against hepatitis B in an area of intermediate endemicity. Bull World Health Organ. 1992;70(6):757–767. Available at: http://www.ncbi.nlm.nih.gov/pmc/articles/PMC2393399/pdf/bullwho00045-0070.pdf (accessed 29 April 2017).

22. Gerlich WH. Medical virology of hepatitis B: how it began and where we are now. Virol J. 2013;10:239. http://dx.doi.org/10.1186/1743-422X-10-239 Available at: http://www.virologyj.com/content/10/1/239 (accessed 29 April 2017).

23. Hayflick L, Moorhead PS. Exp Cell Res. 1961;25:585–621. Available at: http://cogforlife.org/Hayflick1961ExpCell.pdf (accessed 25 April 2017).

24. Hilleman MR. The roles of early alert and of adjuvant in the control of Hong Kong influenza by vaccines. Bull World Health Org. 1969;41:623–628. Available at: https://www.ncbi.nlm.nih.gov/pmc/articles/PMC2427699/pdf/bullwho00220-0275.pdf (accessed 24 April 2017).

25. Hilleman MR. Personal reflections on twentieth century vaccinology. Southeast Asian J Trop Med Public Health. 2003;34(2):244–248. Abstract available at: https://www.ncbi.nlm.nih.gov/pubmed/12971543 (accessed 26 May 2017).

26. Hilleman MR, Ellis R. Vaccines made from recombinant yeast cells. Vaccine. 1986;4 (2):75–76. Available at: https://www.ncbi.nlm.nih.gov/pubmed/3014772 (accessed 26 May 2017).

27. Hilleman MR, McLean AA, Vella PP, Weibel RE, Woodhour AF. Polyvalent pneumococcal polysaccharide vaccines. Bull World Health Organ. 1978;56(3):371–375. Abstract available at: https://www.ncbi.nlm.nih.gov/pmc/articles/PMC2395578/ (accessed 26 May 2017).

28. Hilleman MR. Newer directions in vaccine development and utilization. J Infect Dis. 1985;151(3):407–419. Abstract available: https://www.ncbi.nlm.nih.gov/pubmed/2982958 (accessed 27 May 2017).

29. Hilleman MR. Overview of the needs and realities for developing new and improved vaccines in the 21st century. Intervirology. 2002;45(4–6):199–211. Available at: https://www.ncbi.nlm.nih.gov/pubmed/12566702 (accessed 26 May 2017).

30. Hilleman MR. Overview: cause and prevention in biowarfare and bioterrorism. Vaccine. 2002;20(25–26):3055–3067. Abstract available at: https://www.ncbi.nlm.nih.gov/pubmed/12163257 (accessed 26 May 2017).

31. Hilleman MR. Recombinant vector vaccines in vaccinology. Dev Biol Stand. 1994;82:3–20. Abstract available at: https://www.ncbi.nlm.nih.gov/pubmed/7958480 (accessed 26 May 2017).

32. Hilleman MR. Vaccines in historic evolution and perspective: a narrative of vaccine discoveries. Vaccine. 2000;18(15):1436–1447. Abstract available at: https://www.ncbi.nlm.nih.gov/pubmed/10618541 (accessed 27 May 2017).

33. Jacobson Vann JC, Jacobson RM, Coyne-Beasley T, Asafu-Adjei JK, Szilagyi PG. Patient reminder and recall interventions to improve immunization rates. Cochrane Database Syst Rev. 2018;1(Art: CD003941). Available at: https://doi.org/10.1002/14651858.CD003941.pub3. Available at: http://onlinelibrary.wiley.com/doi/10.1002/14651858.CD003941.pub3/pdf/abstract (accessed 27 January 2018).

34. Kaiser Health News, 29 August 2016, Available at: http://khn.org/morning-breakout/pediatricians-push-back-against-rising-tide-of-vaccination-hesitancy/ (accessed 29 April 2017).

35. Kilbourne ED. Influenza pandemics of the 20th century. Emerg Infect Dis. 2006;12 (1):9–14. https://dx.doi.org/10.3201/eid1201.051254 Available at: https://wwwnc.cdc.gov/eid/article/12/1/05-1254_article (accessed 30 April 2017).

36. Kim JJ. The role of cost-effectiveness in U.S. vaccination policy. N Engl J Med. 2011;365:1760–1761. November 10, 2011 http://dx.doi.org/10.1056/NEJMp1110539. Available at: http://www.nejm.org/doi/full/10.1056/NEJMp1110539#t=article (accessed 29 April 2017).

37. Oransky I, Maurice R, Hilleman. Lancet. 2005;365(9472):1682. Available at: http://www.download.thelancet.com/journals/lancet/article/PIIS0140-6736(05)66536-1/fulltext (accessed 29 April 2017).

38. Levin A, Burgess C, Garrison LP, Bauch C, Babigumira J, Simmons E, et al. Global eradication of measles: an epidemiologic and economic evaluation. J Infect Dis. 2011;204 (suppl 1):S98–S106. Abstract available at: https://www.ncbi.nlm.nih.gov/pubmed/21666220 (accesseed 28 January 2018).

39. Lozano R, Naghavi M, Foreman K, Lim S, Shibuya K, Aboyans V, et al. Global and regional mortality from 235 causes of death for 20 age groups in 1990 and 2010: a systematic analysis for the Global Burden of Disease Study 2010. Lancet. 2012;380:2095–2128. Available at: http://ipa-world.org/society-resources/code/images/95b1494-Lozano%20Mortality%20GBD2010.pdf (accessed 24 August 2015).

40. Medscape. German kindergartens must report parents for refusing vaccine advice under new law. Available at: http://www.medscape.com/viewarticle/880700?src = wnl_edit_tpal&uac = 107534HX (accessed 31 May 2017).

41. Medscape. Vaccination gaps lead to dangerous measles outbreaks in Europe—ECDC—Medscape—April 24, 2017. Available at: http://www.medscape.com/viewarticle/878988? nlid=114455_2243&src=WNL_mdplsnews_170428_mscpedit_infd&uac=107534HX&spon=3&impID=1337601&faf=1 (accessed 28 April 2017).

42. Obituary Maurice Hilleman. BMJ. 2005;330(7498):1028. Available at: http://www.bmj.com/content/330/7498/1028 (accessed 12 May 2015).

43. Miller M, Barrett S, Henderson DA. Control and eradication, chapter 2. In: Jamison DT, Breman JG, Measham AR, et al., editors. Disease priorities in developing countries. Washington DC: World Bank, 2006. Available at: http://www.ncbi.nlm.nih.gov/books/NBK11763/ (accessed 29 April 2017).

44. Mirelman A, Ozawa S, Grewal S. The economic and social benefits of childhood vaccinations in BRICS. Bull World Health Organ. 2014;92:454–456. Available at: http://www.who.int/bulletin/volumes/92/6/13-132597.pdf (accessed 29 April 2017).

45. National Conference of State Legislatures. States with religious and philosophical exemptions from school immunization requirements, 20 December 2017. Available at: http://www.ncsl.org/research/health/school-immunization-exemption-state-laws.aspx (accessed 29 April 2017).

46. National Academies of Sciences, Engineering, and Medicine. Global health impacts of vector-borne diseases: workshop summary. Washington, DC: The National Academies Press, 2016. http://dx.doi.org/10.17226/21792. Available at: https://www.nap.edu/download/21792 (accessed 23 April 2017).

47. Newman L. Maurice Hilleman. BMJ. 2005 Apr 30;330(7498):1028. Available at: https://www.ncbi.nlm.nih.gov/pmc/articles/PMC557162/ (accessed 29 April 2017).

48. Ozawa S, Mirelman A, Stack ML, Walker DG, Levine OS. Cost-effectiveness and economic benefits of vaccines in low- and middle-income countries: a systematic review. Vaccine. 2012 December 17;31(1):96–108. http://dx.doi.org/10.1016/j.vaccine.2012.10.103. Epub 2012 November 8. Available at: http://www.sciencedirect.com/science/article/pii/S0264410X12015769 (accessed 29 April 2017).

49. College of Physicians of Philadelphia. History of vaccines. Maurice Hilleman. Available at: https://www.historyofvaccines.org/content/hilleman (accessed 29 April 2017).
50. Plotkin SA, Orenstein W, Edwards KM. Vaccines. 7th Edition. Philadelphia, PA: Sanders Co, 2013 6 June 2017. Available at: https://www.elsevier.com/books/plotkins-vaccines/plotkin/978-0-323-35761-6 (accessed 27 January 2018).
51. Schillie S, Vellozzi C, Reingold A, Harris A, Haber P, Ward JW, Nelson NP. Prevention of hepatitis B virus infection in the United States: recommendations of the advisory committee on immunization practices. MMWR Recomm Rep. 2018;67(RR-1):1−31. Available at: https://doi.org/10.15585/mmwr.rr6701a1. Available at: https://www.cdc.gov/mmwr/volumes/67/rr/rr6701a1.htm (accessed 21 January 2018.).
52. Sinha A, Levine O, Knoll MD, Muhib F, Lieu TA. Cost-effectiveness of pneumococcal conjugate vaccination in the prevention of child mortality: an international economic analysis. Lancet. 2007;369:389−396. Available at: http://www.thelancet.com/journals/lancet/article/PIIS0140-6736(07)60195-0/abstract (accessed 12 June 2015).
53. Stack ML, Ozawa S, Bisdhai DM, Mirelman A, Tam Y, Niessden L, et al. Estimated economic benefits during the "decade of vaccines" include treatment savings, gains in labor productivity. Health Aff (Millwood). 2011;30(6):10221−10228. Available at: https://www.healthaffairs.org/doi/full/10.1377/hlthaff.2011.0382 (accessed 27 January 2018).
54. Thomas SJ, L'Azou M, Barrett ADT, Jackson NAC. Fast-track Zika vaccine development—is it possible? N Engl J Med. 2016;375:1212−1216. September 29, 2016. http://dx.doi.org/10.1056/NEJMp1609300. Available at: http://www.nejm.org/doi/full/10.1056/NEJMp1609300#t=article (accessed 21 April 2017).
55. Wadman M. Medical research: Cell division. Nature. 2013;498:422−426. Available at: http://www.nature.com/news/medical-research-cell-division-1.13273 (accessed 25 April 2017).
56. Whitney CG, Zhou F, Singleton J, Schuchat A. Benefits from immunization during the Vaccines for Children program era—United States, 1994−2013. Morb Mortal Wkly Rep. 2014;63(16):352−355. Available at: http://www.cdc.gov/mmwr/preview/mmwrhtml/mm6316a4.htm (accessed 29 April 2017).
57. WHO, UNICEF, World Bank. State of the world's vaccines and immunization. 3rd edition. Geneva: World Health Organization, 2010. Available at: http://www.unicef.org/immunization/files/SOWVI_full_report_english_LR1.pdf (accessed 29 April 2017).
58. World Health Organization. Global measles and rubella strategic plan: 2012−2020. Geneva, Switzerland: WHO Geneva, 2012. Available at: http://www.unicef.org/immunization/files/Measles_Rubella_StrategicPlan_2012_2020.pdf (accessed 24 December 2017).
59. World Health Organization. Meeting of the international task force for disease eradication, April 2011. Wkly Epidemiol Rec. 2011;86(32):341−352. Available at: http://www.who.int/wer/2011/wer8632.pdf (accessed 29 April 2017).
60. World Health Organization. Meeting of the International Task Force for Disease Eradication, October 2017. Wkly Epidemiol Rec. 2018. 2018;93(4/5):33−44. Available at: https://outlook.live.com/owa/?id = 64855&path = /mail/inbox/rp (accessed 27 January 2018).
61. World Health Organization. Rubella fact sheet. Reviewed January 2018. Available at: http://www.who.int/mediacentre/factsheets/fs367/en/ (accessed 24 April 2017).
62. World Health Organization. Hepatitis B fact sheet. Reviewed July 2017. Available at: http://www.who.int/mediacentre/factsheets/fs204/en/ (accessed 24 April 2017).
63. World Health Organization. Measles fact sheet. Reviewed January 2018. Available at: http://www.who.int/mediacentre/factsheets/fs286/en/ (accessed 12 June 2016).

64. World Health Organization. Global hepatitis report, 2017. Available at: http://apps.who.int/iris/bitstream/10665/255016/1/9789241565455-eng.pdf (accessed 21 January 2018).
65. World Health Organization. Immunization, vaccines and biological: data, statistics and graphics, 17 October 2017. Available at: http://www.who.int/immunization/monitoring_surveillance/data/en/ (accessed 24 April 2017).
66. World Health Organization. BCG vaccine, 2016. Available at: http://www.who.int/biologicals/areas/vaccines/bcg/en/ (accessed 23 April 2017).
67. World Health Organization. Measles vaccine—WHO position paper April 2017. Wkly Epidem Rec. 2017;92(17):205–228. Available at: http://apps.who.int/iris/bitstream/10665/255149/1/WER9217.pdf?ua=1 (accessed 28 April 2017).

Chapter 20

Robert Guthrie and Nicholas Wald: Screening and Preventing Birth Defects

ABSTRACT

Birth defects affect about three percent of all babies born each year in the United States with highest prevalence among minority groups and are the leading cause (20%) of all infant deaths. The World Health Organization (WHO) estimates that globally some 3–6 percent of 131 million births per year are born with a serious birth defects, with higher rates in low income countries. European Region estimates 25 percent of neonatal deaths are due to congenital anomalies. Birth defects also cause long-term physical, physiologic or developmental disability to many more with severe medical, sociological and economic consequences for the affected children, their families, the health and welfare systems and the community. The most serious common defects are those of the heart, neural tube, Down syndrome, hemoglobin disorders and many inborn errors of metabolism.

Robert Guthrie pioneered neonatal screening in the 1960s by developing a screening test for phenylketonuria, a common cause of serious mental handicap. There are now as many as 60 birth conditions routinely screened in the United States but fewer in other countries. Newborn screening includes a growing number of conditions by simple, inexpensive methods for which treatment can save the child from serious intellectual/developmental disability and many birth defects. Early diagnosis and management of dietary, medical, and other therapeutic prevention and treatments can reduce the ill effects of infectious, nutritional deficiency conditions, blood disorders and complications of other birth defects.

Direct and indirect causes of birth defects include those due to genetic, infectious, nutritional, or environmental in origin. Some are now preventable by genetic counseling, good reproductive and pregnancy care, and public health measures such as nutritional policies including prevention of micronutrient deficiencies before and during pregnancy by food fortification and micronutrient supplements.

In 1991, Nicholas Wald completed studies proving that folic acid taken before and during pregnancy prevented 70 percent of neural tube defects (NTDs). Recommendations for women in the age of fertility to take folic acid tablets daily reached only one third of the target population. The United States, Canada, and Chile in 1998 adopted mandatory folic acid fortification of flour to reduce the prevalence of NTDs. This policy was adopted in over 80 countries by 2015, but none in Europe.

Implementing policies for preventive care for infectious and nutrition-related conditions, screening at birth, and accessible services are key to reducing the burden of birth

Case Studies in Public Health. DOI: http://dx.doi.org/10.1016/B978-0-12-804571-8.00009-3
471

defects. Care before and during pregnancy and at delivery are vital for prevention with a focus on early diagnosis and interventions to prevent irreversible health threats and long-term treatment. Prevention of birth defects is a major ongoing challenge of public health and clinical services with many successful interventions to reduce occurrence, severity, and long-term effects. Vaccination, essential mineral and vitamin supplements and micronutrient fortification of staple foods are effective, low-cost interventions. Advances in genetics, vaccinology, nutrition and other biological and social sciences will identify new interventions and standards of care to reduce the burden of birth defects and their long-term effects. The challenge to reduce birth defect occurrence and their consequences is a high priority for countries at all levels of development consistent with the Millennium and Sustainable Development Goals for child-population health.

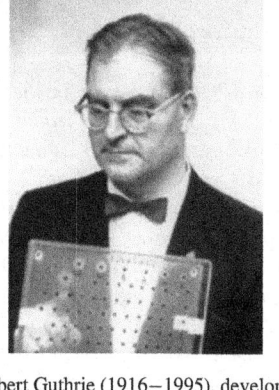
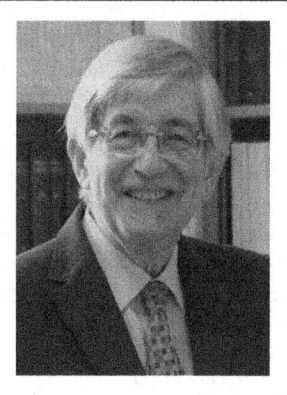

Dr. Robert Guthrie (1916−1995), developer of the Guthrie newborn screening test for phenyl-ketonuria (PKU) in 1961, and pioneering advocate for neonatal screening. *Source: Courtesy of Patricia S Guthrie on behalf of the Guthrie Family Foundation. Available at: http://www.robertguthriepku.org/.*

Nicholas Wald led the study published in 1991 establishing that folic acid taken before preg-nancy prevented most neural tube defects; Wolfson Institute of Preventive Medicine, Queen Mary University of London: *Courtesy of Sir Nicholas Wald FRCP,FRS.*

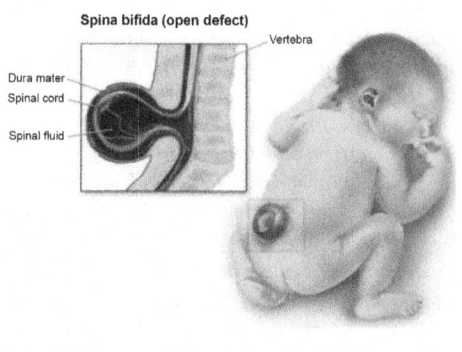
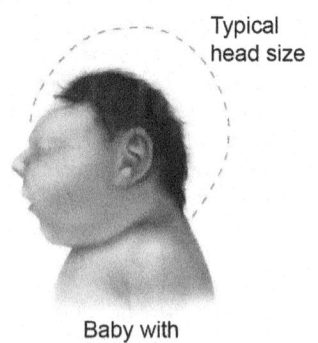

Spina bifida, neural tube defect. *Source: Centers for Disease Control and Prevention. Spina bifida basics, October 17, 2016. Available at: https://www.cdc.gov/ncbddd/spinabifida/facts.html (accessed 19 March 2016).*

Baby with microcephaly. *Source: Centers for Disease Control and Prevention. Facts about microcephaly, December 7, 2016. Available at: https://www.cdc.gov/ncbddd/birthdefects/micro-cephaly.html (accessed 19 March 2016).*

BACKGROUND

Dr. Ivar Asbjørn Følling (1888–1973), a Norwegian physician and biochemist, discovered the phenylketonuria (PKU) disorder in 1934 identifying patients in his own family and in institutions for the mentally retarded. This was a fundamentally important breakthrough for the fields of biochemistry, genetics, metabolism, and medicine (Gonzalez 2010). Dr. Richard Koch (1921–2011) a professor of pediatrics in Southern California became a pioneer and advocate for PKU. He advocated a "low protein diet for life" for PKU patients, which became the medical standard for this disorder. When early diagnosis and dietary management were proven successful, he became a major advocate for mandatory newborn screening for PKU of all newborns in California in 1966, and gradually in all US states and many countries abroad. Dr Horst Bickel (1918–2000) from Germany working with English colleagues in Birmingham led in developing in 1951 a nutritional formula preventing further mental deterioration which improved the quality of life for thousands of PKU patients, and if diagnosed early, to lead normal and healthy lives.

The World Health Organization (WHO) defines congenital anomalies or birth defects as "*structural or functional abnormalities, including metabolic disorders that are present from birth. Congenital anomalies are a diverse group of disorders of prenatal origin that can be caused by single gene defects, chromosomal disorders, multi-factorial inheritance, environmental teratogens or micronutrient malnutrition.*" This chapter discusses the damage present in a baby at birth including those caused by a genetic or nongenetic prenatal factors. Premature birth or low birth weight birth are the most common forms of birth damage affecting 15 million births globally of whom an estimated one million will die. WHO estimates that 7.9 million children are born annually with a serious birth defect of genetic or partially genetic origin, and that of these some 300,000 newborns die in the neonatal period of six weeks. Other birth anomalies are caused by the effects of many maternal causes including poverty and undernutrition, toxicity of smoking, alcohol and environment, or infections such as syphilis, rubella, and the newly recognized Zika virus.

In the United States, CDC reports that congenital birth defects affect one in every 33 babies (about 3 percent of all babies) born each year from 2004–2006 including a smaller range of categories than described here. They include 14 birth defects included in tracking programs to establish prevalence of birth defects in the United States (Parker et al., 2010). This includes 6,000 cases of Down syndrome (14.4 per 10,000 births), 6,136 congenital heart defects and 2,660 Neural Tube Defects. Birth defects are the leading cause of infant deaths in the US, accounting for 20 percent of all infant deaths.

In public health there are many causes of deleterious birth conditions that can be prevented or ameliorated. These include those that can be prevented by ensuring adequate intake of iron, iodine, vitamin D, C and B complex including folic acid and vitamin B12, preferably as multivitamin supplements with regulated content taken before and during pregnancy, and lactation. This should be supported by nationally mandated food fortification, as well as by screening and prevention of maternal infections, toxic exposures and others. In addition to identified specific causes, context is also important for understanding birth defects. Poverty, lack of maternal education, restrictive sociocultural influences, and consanguinity (close blood relation of the parents) all contribute to birth defects, and high rates of fetal and neonatal mortality, with low birth weight an important contributor to neonatal deaths. More than 90 percent of births < 2,500 grams die within a few days in low-income countries compared to less than 10 percent in high-income countries. The United States has about 517,000 preterm births annually and is among the 10 OECD countries with the highest rates of preterm births. Poverty and lack of access to and use of professionally provided or supervised antenatal, delivery and post natal care and primary care, widespread overt or subclinical malnutrition, youthful pregnancy, low educational levels, lack of birth control and spacing of pregnancies, high rates of parity (the number of pregnancies a woman brings to term), inadequate immunization, and exposure to sexually transmitted diseases (STDs) are all contributing factors that can be targets for prevention.

WHO reports that globally, 5.8 million children up to age five years died in 2015, a 53 percent decrease since 1990. Neonatal deaths and stillbirths fell at a slower pace (42.4%) between 1990 and 2015. Although this decline in annual child mortality from just over 12 million in 1990 to less than six million in 2015, represents clear improvement, it failed to reach the targeted annual decrease of a two-thirds reduction target set by the Millennium Development Goals (MDGs). The MDGs were replaced in 2015 with Sustainable Development Goals (SDGs), which continue to include maternal and child health improvement targets. During the MDG period (2000–15), total child deaths under age five years were reduced largely due to expanding control of communicable diseases by vaccination, along with nutritional and sanitary improvements.

However, neonatal conditions and birth defects continued to contribute to high levels of neonatal deaths. The relative rankings of congenital anomalies rose from 13th to 5th leading cause of child death from 2005 to 2015. In some countries (such as China, Iran, and Bhutan) large reductions in child death rates included decreases in congenital anomalies, a leading factor in under age five years mortality highlighting the importance of including active public health measures in national and local community measures for reducing congenital anomalies and birth defects.

Guthrie and Newborn Screening

During the 1960s, newborn screening to identify infants with conditions requiring early treatment to prevent irreparable health damage was initiated by the work of Robert Guthrie. Guthrie was born in a poor family in Marrionville, Missouri, located in the Ozark Mountains in 1916, and grew up in poverty during the Great Depression. Robert's father made a poor living selling sewing machines door to door during the Depression. Robert spent his school years in Minneapolis, and was accepted to the University of Minnesota Medical School under the "New Deal" National Youth Administration study and work program, which provided low-income students with federally subsidized jobs while attending state universities. Unsatisfied with medical school, he transferred to study bacteriology and biochemistry at the University of Maine, but later returned to complete his MD degree as well as obtaining a PhD degree in microbiology. Robert and his wife Margaret decided to raise their growing family near Buffalo, New York. Their second son of seven children suffered from mental disability and a niece with PKU giving Guthrie a strong lifelong interest in common causes of intellectual disability. This led him in 1960 at the University of Buffalo, in New York State to develop a drop of blood from the infant's heel a screening test for phenylketonuria (PKU), then a leading cause of severe mental disability. His bacterial inhibition assay PKU test later replaced by mass tandem spectrosopy which replaced separate assays needed for each possible metabolic disorder, in addition to tests for endocrine and hemoglobin disorders; the immunologic test is still known world wide as the Guthrie heel blood test for newborns.

Guthrie became world renowned and campaigned internationally at conferences on mental disability promoting newborn screening, and later developed similar blood spot tests for galactosemia and maple syrup urine disease (MSUD). His vigorous promotion of newborn screening stirred interest and was adopted in the United States and in the industrialized nations. He founded the field of routine newborn screening and early treatment of many birth defects of genetic origin in an expanding field of preventive early case-finding capacity and genetics.

The scope of Guthrie's work and outstanding leadership in this field is shown by the wide range of screening tests developed together with colleagues including EW Naylor, AP Orfanos, A Susi, WH Murphey, and others. The tests were mostly for use with blood spots on the Guthrie card for newborn heel blood samples for metabolic and hematologic disorders in newborns. These included (with year of publication): phenylketonuria (1963), galactokinase deficiency (1968), argininosuccinic aciduria, orotic aciduria, and other inherited enzyme deficiencies (1972), sickle cell anemia and other hemoglobinopathies (1973), arginase deficiency (1977), simple fluorometric assay of protoporphyrin in erythrocytes (EPP) as a screening test for lead poisoning (1977), adenosine deaminase deficiency (1978), maple syrup urine disease (1978), urinary pyrimidine bases and nucleoside (1979), beta-lipoprotein quantitation (cord blood 1980), arginase activity (1980), total glutathione (1980), argininosuccinic acid lyase deficiency and other urea cycle disorders (1982), alpha 1-antitrypsin (1982), alpha 1-antitrypsin (1987), galactose and galactose-1-phosphate (1986), delta-aminolevulinic acid, porphobilinogen and porphyrins related to heme biosynthesis by high-performance liquid chromatography

(1986), carnosinase (1987) (courtesy Brad Therrell, PhD, Director National Newborn Screening and Global Resource Center, February 2018). In 1975 Guthrie investigated lead levels in residents of mental disability institutions finding lead exposure cases and helped to initiate lead abatement and screening programs in California and in the United States generally.

The Guthrie test for PKU was the breakthrough pioneering effort leading to newborn screening (NBS) programs in the United States, Europe, and other countries. Over the following decades, technological advances allowed testing from a single blood spot on the Guthrie card using computerized tandem mass spectrometry. Many of the tests were originally developed by Guthrie and colleagues. Newborn screening programs expanded gradually to cover many conditions including rare disorders. Case finding of PKU and later congenital hypothyroidism allows for early intervention to improve quality and length of life. Over the years, preventive interventions have reduced important birth defects such as congenital rubella syndrome (CRS) by elimination of the rubella virus and thalasemia by education, screening, and counseling (See Chapters 12 and 18). For many birth defects, therapeutic measures have gradually developed to improve quality and duration of life even when fatal outcomes are inevitable. As genomic sciences evolve new measures for improving preventive and curative care will be gradually introduced stimulated by expanding capacity for early diagnosis by screening.

Prevention and management of birth defects/anomalies classified as genetic, infectious, nutritional, environmental, toxic, and multifactorial are a major public health concern, not only because of high prevalence in specific population groups, but also because of the financial, stress and social cost to the family and community. There are many contributory factors related to adverse birth conditions including consanguineous marriage (i.e., marriage between close blood relatives), parental age, parity (number of previous pregnancies), poverty, migration, parental status (e.g. lone parent, foster parent), maternal epilepsy, and Rhesus (Rh) blood type discrepancy between mother and child (Rh hemolytic disease of the newborn). Many birth defects are genetic, transmitted by abnormal chromosomes from one or both parents. Genetic and other birth disorders are increasingly treatable and preventable. New forms of screening tests, including genetic screening and family counseling, with community education and follow-up individual patient care are becoming even more important with the rapid development of gene therapy. Achievements in sequencing the human genome and genomics research in recent decades have raised scientific and popular expectations for translation from laboratory to population health benefits. Newborn screening has expanded to include many previously unknown or new rare conditions, which raise controversial social and difficult ethical questions. But the clinical and social care questions raised often lead to important health benefits to individual patients with advocacy groups promoting attention to their particular disease concern, such as for cystic fibrosis (CF) and sickle-cell disease.

Since introduction of the Guthrie test in the 1960s, newborn screening has become a key part of public health. By 1965, 32 US states had screening laws, all but five were mandatory. In 2000, 35 percent of US states screened for fewer than five conditions. In 2002, the federal Health Resources and Services Administration's Maternal and Child Health Bureau asked the American College of Medical Genetics (ACMG) to develop guidelines for newborn screenings. At that time, some states screened for as few as four conditions and others testing for as many as 50. The ACMG studied 81 potential conditions and placed 29 of them in a core screening panel, with another 50 conditions assigned to lower priority for screening due lack of available effective treatment. In 2003, all but four states screened for only six disorders. Since then, understanding of the importance of newborn screening has exploded and by 2011, all states were testing for at least 26 disorders. The federal Newborn Screening Saves Lives Act of 2008 led to federal guidelines and grants with expansion of screening in 2010 to every state and territory of the US screening for 21 conditions or more. Each state decides on tests to include; New York includes 58 conditions while Arkansas and Louisiana each include 33 tested conditions. The major diseases screened for are PKU, congenital hypothyroidism, sickle cell disease, thalassemia, cystic fibrosis, toxoplasmosis as well as rare conditions for inborn errors of metabolism and others. Prenatal tests for birth defects expanded screening to include Down syndrome and neural tube defects using ultrasound, genetic, and biochemical markers, and essential clinical tests for defects such as dislocated hips, newborn hearing loss and congenital heart disease.

By the mid-1970s, newborn screening for PKU had become routine in nearly every industrialized nation, and had even extended to many medium-income countries. In the European Union, newborn screening is available in many countries but with far fewer tests than in the United States, and is being extended with the introduction of improved technology e.g., tandem mass spectrometry. But each country has its own program of disorders included and organization of the programs. An EU survey conducted in 2009 showed wide variation in screening programs with; 37 conditions screened for in Spain, 25 in Portugal, 12 in the Czech Republic, seven in the UK, five in Sweden, three in France and one in Finland. Since 2013 many European (EU) countries are developing rare disease registries, specialized treatment centers, laboratories and increasing the range of conditions being tested but with wide national variation.

Birth defects and abnormalities can be categorized under a typology reflecting basic causative factors or a combination of factors. Many conditions are preventable if related to maternal abstinence from smoking and alcohol use, infection control by immunizations (influenza, pertussis, diphtheria, and pneumococcal pneumonia), and nutritional multivitamin supplements. Congenital anomalies, which can be determined by fetal and newborn screening for single-gene defects and chromosomal disorders, include hemoglobin disorders, Rh factor incompatibility, glucose-6-phosphate dehydrogenase deficiency (G6PD), Down syndrome, and PKU, which mostly occur in the first trimester. Other disorders can be due to metabolic, nutritional, infectious, toxic, environmental, and unknown conditions (see Table 20.1).

Genetic diseases are passed from one generation to the next and for each condition one or two genes are inherited. Dominant genes require only one copy to cause the genetic disorder in a heterozygote (i.e., a person who has one copy of the abnormal and one copy of the normal gene). For a dominant genetic disorder, a gene is inherited from the affected parent who carries the gene and each offspring has a 50 percent chance inheriting the disease. Recessive genetic diseases require the presence of the disease gene in both parents, e.g., thalassemia major, cystic fibrosis, Tay-Sachs disease. If both parents are carriers of the abnormal gene (i.e., both parents carry one normal and one abnormal gene), then each fetus has a 25 percent chance of being affected, a 50 percent chance of being a carrier, and a 25 percent chance of being unaffected. This allows for successful prevention of new cases by community education, premarital testing and genetic counseling as has been success in reducing new cases of thalassemia major (see Chapter 18) as well as Tay-Sachs and Gaucher's diseases in affected population groups. If only one parent is a carrier of the homozygous gene, the disorder is not passed on although the child has a 50 percent chance of being a carrier.

Prevention of complications due to birth defects, such as PKU and congenital hypothyroidism (CH), must be followed-up for confirmation of suspected cases with appropriate management of the disease. Other birth defects such as congenital hip dislocation, hearing deficits, cataracts and congenital heart disease are found by clinical examination of the newborn, with hearing tested within three months and appropriate follow-up care. Genetic or multifactorial conditions can be discovered during pregnancy by maternal blood test for fetal cell DNA, amniotic fluid or placental testing newborn screening and followed up with specialized care. Some conditions evident at birth identified as high risk, due to, for example, prematurity or low birth weight, can be given longer term follow-up screenings to identify problems and starting preventive care interventions early, such as in CF, thalassemia, and sickle-cell disease.

Maternal infections play a major role in birth defects; this includes sexually transmitted diseases (STDs) that can be passed on to the fetus, such as HIV, syphilis, gonorrhea, and cytomegalovirus, as well as other maternal infections causing severe birth consequences such as congenital rubella and Zika virus syndromes, congenital varicella syndrome (CVS, chickenpox), toxoplasmosis, and others. Pregnant women and their partners can be counseled in preventive measures to avoid infection and be screened for infections during pregnancy and treated.

Maternal nutrition is also a major contributor of damage to fetal development and birth defects including maternal protein energy levels and low birth

TABLE 20.1 Major Birth Defects and Intervention by Category of Cause

Cause	Defect	Interventions
Genetic defects	Down syndrome	Prenatal diagnosis, long-term care
	Phenylketonuria	Newborn screening, low alanine diet, long-term care
	Congenital hypothyroidism	Newborn screening, thyroxin replacement therapy, long-term care
	Beta thalassemia major	Premarital and newborn screening, genetic counselling, treatment, blood transfusion, chelating agents (see Chapter 18)
	Sickle cell anemia	Premarital screening, long-term care
	Cerebral palsy	Screening, long-term care
	Glucose—6 phosphatase deficiency	Screening, long-term care
	Tay-Sachs disease	Premarital screening, genetic counseling, community education
	Inborn errors of metabolism	Screening, genetic counselling, education, medical care
	Fragile X syndrome	Long-term care
	Cystic fibrosis	Screening, long term care
	Congenital dislocated hips	Long-term orthopedic care
	Congenital heart defects	Long-term care, cardiac surgery
	Cleft lip and palate	Long-term care, plastic surgery
	Familial Mediterranean fever	Long-term care
Nutritional deficiencies	Neural tube defects, spina bifida, anencephaly	Prenatal folic acid daily, mandatory fortification of flour
	Developmental delay due to deficiencies of iodine, iron, zinc, selenium; vitamin deficiencies (A, B complex, C, D, E)	Prepregnancy and pregnancy care Multivitamin supplements, fortification of basic foods (see Chapters 1, 9,10, 11)
	Low birth weight	Premarital and prenatal screening, nutrition, multivitamins supplements
	Ophthalmia neonatorum	Silver nitrate eye drops in newborn (see Chapter 4)
	Congenital Rubella syndrome (CRS)	Immunization MMR 2 doses; control and eradication, case follow-up (see Chapter 12)
	Varicella-zoster syndrome	Immunization (see Chapter 19)
	Cytomegalovirus (CMV)	Immunization

(Continued)

TABLE 20.1 (Continued)

Cause	Defect	Interventions
	Influenza	Immunization, treatment
	Toxoplasmosis	Treatment
	HIV, hepatitis B, hepatitis C	Screen and treat positives before and during pregnancy, screen all newborns, treat positives, hepatitis B vaccination of all newborns
	Zika virus	Vector control, mosquito protection, avoid travel to and delay pregnancy in risk areas; avoid sex with potentially infected partner
Physiological	Vitamin K deficiency bleeding disorder	Mandatory vitamin K injection at birth (see Chapter 17)
	Rh incompatibility	Rh testing and treatment
	Prematurity and low birth weight	Education, premarital testing, prepregnancy nutrition support and multivitamins
	Perinatal hypoxia, sepsis, hemorrhage	Delivery in a professional center
Unknown, poverty, deprivation, multiple causation	Prematurity, low birth weight	Adequate nutrition, micronutrients, social support, control/eradication of preventable diseases
	Developmental delay	Antenatal care
	Congenital heart defect	Folic acid supplements before and during pregnancy, long-term care
	Autism spectrum disorder	Symptoms appear at 12–18 months, early treatment
	Birth injury	Professional care for delivery
	Domestic child abuse	Screening
	Hearing deficit/deafness	Early diagnosis, education and management, cochlear implants
Toxic/trauma	Smoking	Education, stop maternal smoking, avoid environmental exposure
	Therapeutic drugs (e.g. thalidomide, antiepileptics)	Avoidance, regulation of pharmaceuticals
	Street drugs/abuse medications	Premarital and prenatal screening, treatment centers
	Alcohol, Fetal Alcohol Syndrome	Avoid alcohol completely during pregnancy; long term care
	X-rays, ionizing radiation	Prevent exposure to radiation prior to and during pregnancy
	Anesthesia	Avoid exposure and use

(Continued)

TABLE 20.1 (Continued)

Cause	Defect	Interventions
Contributory factors: culture, poverty, social-economic, religion, environment	Consanguinous marriage, maternal age, parity, poverty, migration, single parenthood, paternal age	Education, universal access to birth control, nutrition, reproductive care, community support, political action, social support

Source: Adapted from Tulchinsky TH, Varavikova EA. The new public health. 3rd edition. San Diego: Elsevier/Academic Press, 2014. Chapter 6, pp. 338–340.

weight. Maternal micronutrient deficiencies including folic acid, iodine, iron, and vitamins C, A, and D are important causes of birth defects. Food fortification and supplements before and during pregnancy and for the newborn are key to reducing these factors. Early or preterm births are the commonest birth defect when a baby is born before 37 weeks of pregnancy. The CDC reports that in 2015, preterm birth affected one of every 10 infants born in the United States including over 500,000 preterm babies born each year. WHO reports that an estimated 15 million babies are born globally each year and this number is rising. Worldwide complications of preterm birth are the leading cause of death among children under five years of age, and in 2015 responsible for nearly one million deaths. Survivors face a lifetime of disability, including learning disabilities, visual and hearing problems. The commonest causes are poverty, maternal malnutrition and toxic effects. Other causes of preterm birth include parental age, multiple pregnancies, infections, chronic maternal conditions such as diabetes and high blood pressure, but mostly no specific cause is identified, which may be due to a genetic influence.

Toxic effects of maternal smoking, alcohol consumption, drugs (prescription and illicit), air pollution (indoor and oudoor), pesticides, lead exposure, and household chemicals can all contribute to fetal damage with lifelong disability such as fetal alcohol syndrome disorder (FASD). Thalidomide was a classic case of a prescription teratogenic drug resulting in birth defects. Thalidomide was promoted and widely prescribed in the 1950s to 1960s in Europe, Canada and elsewhere for nausea and insomnia, but not allowed into the US by strict FDA regulators. It was inadequately tested for harmful effects and caused thousands of cases of serious physical deformities (i.e., short limbs, or phocomelia) in children. Pregnant women with tobacco, alcohol, and drug dependencies should receive appropriate help and counseling to encourage cessation. The use of prescription and over-the-counter (OTC) drugs during pregnancy should be carefully considered with input from the woman's health care provider.

Preventing Birth Defects

A number of studies in the United Kingdom by Smithells and others, and Czeizel in Hungary had indicated that dietary deficiency of folic acid was related to birth of children with neural tube defects (NTDs) and that supplements with folic acid with multivitamins showed a protective effect if taken before pregnancy.

The definitive multi-center study was carried out by Nicholas Wald (later Sir Nicholas) of the Wolfson Institute of Preventive Medicine, Queen Mary University of London. Wald's randomized double-blind trial showed that NTDs are a vitamin deficiency disorder which is largely preventable by folic acid taken daily before pregnancy and during early pregnancy preventing 70 to 80% of neural tube defects (NTDs).

Wald's parents were Jewish refugees who escaped in time from Nazi Germany to settle in England. Many of their family members were murdered in the Holocaust. Nicholas studied medicine at University College Hospital Medical School. Stimulated to enter epidemiology while working with Sir Richard Doll, Wald went on to a distinguished academic career focusing on birth defects, including development of alfa-fetoprotein tests of amniotic fluid and blood, prenatal tests and criteria for prenatal diagnosis of Down syndrome. He also worked on secondary smoking effects on cardiovascular disease, and other topics in public health. The crucial folic acid study, funded by the UK Medical Research Council became accepted as the definitive study that folic acid taken before pregnancy was preventive of 70−80 percent of NTDs.

This large randomized multi-center trial published in 1991 proved that adequate intake of folic acid and/or vitamin B12 before and during pregnancy can prevent most NTD cases. This discovery introduced a new era in prevention of birth defects from nutritional causes to join those due to genetic, infectious, and environmental causes. Recommending that women take folic acid for months before becoming pregnant was the first preventive approach tried, but it failed to cover more than one third of the target population leading to fortification of flour as the policy of choice.

Major Birth Defects

Neural tube defects (NTDs) are defects due to failure of closure of the central nervous system (brain and spinal cord) mainly in the spinal cord during the first few weeks of pregnancy. This group includes a range of abnormalities such as anencephaly, a severe malformation of the head and brain, which usually results in death within a few hours of birth. Less severe forms, but still a major birth defect, include spina bifida, a defective closure of the vertebral column. The major NTD types are: spina bifida occulta, meningocele, and myelomeningocele, occurring commonly in the lower back, but may also be in the middle back or neck. NTD impairment below the lesion results in lack of sensation, inability to walk and incontinence. Associated conditions include hydrocephalus, often require cerebrospinal fluid shunting. Other defects include vertebral column deformities, and genitourinary and gastrointestinal disorders. NTDs vary in degree of severity but many require extensive surgical and medical care. NTDs are a common, severe congenital malformation, affecting 0.5−2.0 per 1000 established pregnancies world wide. In many countries incidence is declining as a result of screening in pregnancy and primary prevention through folic acid supplements in pre- and early pregnancy. However, globally there are geographic variations such as in low-income countries. Screening for NTDs became possible in the early 1970s with amniocentesis and testing of amniotic fluid and later blood for alpha fetoproteins (AFP). Ultrasound can also detect NTDs. Prenatal diagnosis of NTDs and termination of pregnancies in Europe fails to reduce the NTD birth rates and is an unjustifiable method when effective folic acid fortification policies are available.

Czeizel et al. reported studies in Hungary which showed that folic acid in multivitamins taken before pregnancy prevented first pregnancy occurrence of NTDs and reduced the risk of recurrence by 3−25 percent in subsequent pregnancies. Wald's large multi-center study funded by the British Medical Research Council reported in 1991 definitively demonstrating that folic acid given before pregnancy greatly reduces the chance of NTD births by 70−80 percent. Since some 50 percent of pregnancies are unplanned, daily doses of folic acid consumption by all women in the age of fertility has been recommended since the 1990s with the US Food and Drug Administration (USFDA), recommending pre-pregnancy and pregnancy supplementation of folic acid, 400 mcg/day. However, in the United States, compliance with recommended folic acid supplementation is usually under 40 percent, so that mandatory fortification of flour with folic acid was implemented in the US, as well as Canada and Chile in 1998 followed by declining NTD birth rates.

In other high-income countries, studies by Khoshood et al. and McNulty et al. showed poor compliance with recommendations of folic acid supplements for women in the age of fertility in Europe. A Danish study (2012) reported that of 462 women being scanned for NTD only 10.4 percent had taken folic acid supplements at the recommended level. Voluntary compliance proved in many studies to be an inadequate partial solution, with variable national recommendations and with poor compliance usually well below one third in Europe, with no decrease in NTD prevalence as compared to experience in countries that adopted mandatory fortification of flour with folic acid. The European reviews of folic acid supplementation guideline and practices with non-adoption of folic acid fortification of flour are influenced by allegations that folic acid "excess" may result in elevated cancer risks. But this has been definitively rejected by a consensus of new studies. The reviews conclude that there is a policy failure of importance in Europe by current best practice standards. Thus, even in high-income settings, relying on voluntary folic acid supplementation is failing. In order to be effective folic acid supplementation must start before pregnancy and relatively few women are taking it prior to becoming pregnant. In medium- and low-income countries or among immigrant populations everywhere this is not a relevant solution and thus mandatory fortification of basic foods such as flour is required for effective prevention. NTDs, which are preventable, continue to occur where folic acid fortification of flour is not mandated. There may also be prenatal diagnosis followed by termination of the affected pregnancy, often later in pregnancy, a less desirable method than primary prevention by safe and inexpensive flour fortification.

Nutritional Deficiency Causes of Birth Defects

Normal weight before becoming pregnant and weight gain within the desirable range improve chances for a good outcome of the pregnancy. Excess weight gain has a risk for elevated blood pressure during pregnancy, toxemia of pregnancy (preeclampsia), gestational diabetes, caesarian section and premature childbirth. Supplements essential to protect the fetus include the following:

Iodine at a daily intake of 150−250 micrograms at least a month before the woman plans to conceive, and during the pregnancy and the entire period of breastfeeding. Iodine insufficiency remains a public health problem even where iodine enrichment of salt is in place for many years. This may be in part due to the levels of enrichment as well as reduced use of table salt as recommended for prevention of hypertension. Recommendations for use of iodized salt in baking and routine use of iodine-containing multivitamins before and during pregnancy and lactation are growing in the public health iodine-advocacy movement. Reports from the United Kingdom and Europe indicate that iodine insufficiency reduces IQ of newborns potential by up to 13 IQ points, even though gross forms of deficiency such as cretinism are rarely seen. Iodine deficiency has been found to be exacerbated by increasing use of desalinated seawater for community water supplies in Israel (see Chapter 10).

Vitamin D of 400 international units (equivalent to 10 micrograms) for the entire pregnancy and breastfeeding period. Vitamin D deficiency in women is common, so supplementation is needed during pregnancy and lactation. Vitamin D promotes absorption of calcium and regulates the concentration of calcium and phosphate in the serum to ensure a needed mineral content for bone health. This is essential for bone growth, ensuring lifelong skeletal strength, preventing fractures and spinal degeneration in aging. Vitamin D is also related to the function of the immune system and muscles and the reduction of infections. It protects the fetus from risk of rickets in stunting and rickets in infancy (see Chapter 11).

Folic acid During years of fertility, it is recommended that every woman consume 400 mcg (micrograms) of folic acid every day for at least one month before becoming pregnant. Consumption of folic acid is particularly important in the three months before pregnancy and throughout pregnancy, to reduce risk of neural tube defect (NTD), and to prevent macrocytic anemia in the woman. It is also recommended to consume foods rich in natural folic acid (folate) found in legumes, citrus fruits and green leafy vegetables. However natural folate does not meet the needs towards pregnancy and pregnancy, and therefore it is vital to have added folic acid.

Iron is needed as a supplement throughout pregnancy until at least six weeks after birth−30 mg every day, possibly combined with folic acid supplement. Women are more than likely to be in precarious iron adequacy due to loss from menstrual periods, and reluctance to include red meat in the diet for ideological and cardiovascular disease prevention reasons along with increasing popularity of vegetarianism. During pregnancy, extra iron is needed because of the increase in blood volume and to meet the needs of the growing fetus. Iron deficiency can cause anemia in the woman and symptoms such as fatigue, weakness, headaches, breathing difficulty and accelerated heart rate. In addition, during the pregnancy, fetal iron reserves are created that will be used during the first months of newborn life. In addition to taking the iron supplement, it is recommended to eat food rich in iron from animals (lean beef, dark turkey meat; plant foods with iron include beans, lentils, oatmeal, dried fruits, tahina, nuts, seeds and iron-fortified foods such as cereals without sugar. However, milk and milk products, coffee and tea interfere with the absorption of iron from various supplements and foods.

Vitamin C helps absorb the iron in fortified foods or supplements and to absorb iron from a plant source, so it is recommended to take the iron supplement along with foods rich in vitamin C including: citrus fruits, tomato, pepper, kiwi, melon and cabbage (see Chapter 1).

Foods with potential for transmission of infectious diseases can be dangerous during pregnancy. Some foods can contain substances potentially harmful to the fetus such as large sea fish with potential mercury contamination, although local pond or lake fish and canned tuna can be recommended. Fish that may contain mercury such as large fish like: shark, swordfish, king mackerel, tilefish, tuna steaks and white tuna (albacore tuna), should be avoided due to the possible presence of high mercury content. It is possible and desirable to consume a variety from among the other locally available fish, including pond fish and canned light tuna.

Neural tube defects Introducing mandatory fortification of flour with folic acid in both developed and developing countries will prevent many cases of NTDs. In 1996 the United States authorized mandatory fortification of flour with folic acid, which was implemented in 1998 along with Canada and Chile. The decline in prevalence of NTDs following mandatory flour fortification with folic acid fortification for 18 US screening programs between 1995 and 2011 is shown in Figure 20.1. NTD prevalence rates declined but remain high for Hispanics. The US data is for 18 US states and Puerto Rico birth defects surveillance programs, 1995–2011.

Since 1998, all countries in the Americas with a total of over 80 countries worldwide implemented mandatory fortification of flour with folic acid for primary prevention of this disorder. Resistance to folic acid fortification of flour is strong in Europe; many European countries have recommendations for folic acid supplements but none have adopted mandatory fortification of flour. A study of 28 European country surveillance of congenital anomalies registries covering approximately 12.5 million births in 19 countries between 1991 and 2011 showed that NTD rates have not declined in Europe. Figure 20.2 shows the decline in NTD prevalence in countries before and

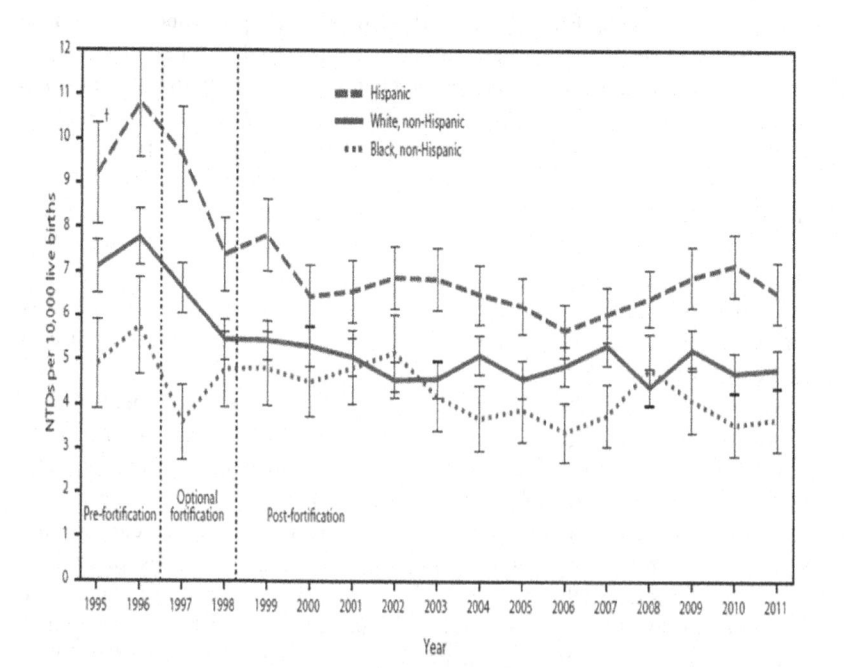

FIGURE 20.1 Prevalence of NTDs in US before and after mandatory folic acid fortification, population-based birth defects surveillance programs, 18 US states and Puerto Rico, 1995 to 2011. *Source: Williams J, Mai CT, Mulinare J, Isenburg J, Flood TJ, Ethen M, et al. Centers for Disease Control and Prevention. Updated estimates of neural tube defects prevented by mandatory folic acid fortification—United States, 1995–2011. MMWR Morb Mort Wkly Rep. 2015;64 (01);1–5. Available at: https://www.cdc.gov/mmwr/preview/mmwrhtml/mm6401a2.htm (accessed 3 June 2017).*

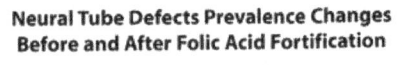

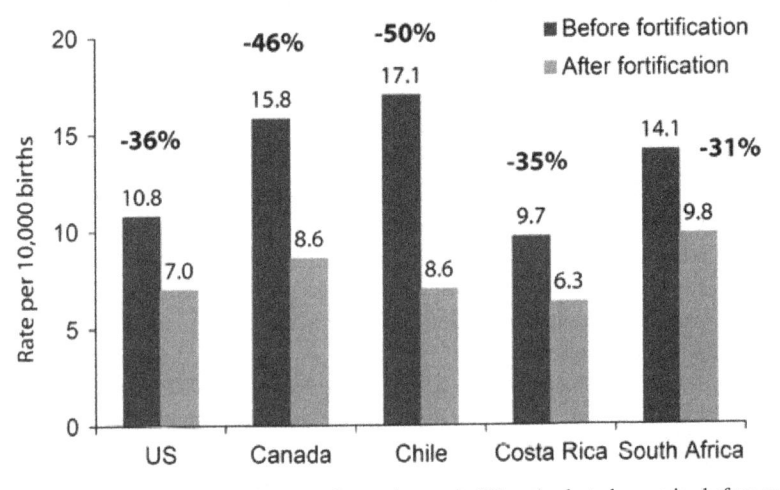

FIGURE 20.2   Neural tube defect prevalence changes in US and selected countries before and after folic acid fortification. *Source: Centers for Disease Control and Prevention. Folic acid: birth defects, last updated 1 February 2018. Available at: https://www.cdc.gov/ncbddd/birthdefectscount/data.html (accessed 12 February 2018).*

after adoption of mandatory flour fortification with folic acid (United States, Canada, Chile, Costa Rica, and South Africa).

Nutritional deficiencies include a lengthy list of essential vitamins and nutrients which are crucial to normal growth and development of the fetus and newborn. Iodine deficiency in the environment and food intake results in impaired synthesis of thyroid hormones during pregnancy in the mother and fetus. Insufficient levels of these hormones can lead to miscarriage, preterm birth, and mild to severe brain damage. Pregnant women, lactating mothers, and young infants are especially vulnerable to iodine deficiency and thus iodine fortification of salt or other common food source is successful and vital for newborn, child, and adult population health (see Chapter 10). Nutrition status before and during pregnancy is important for protection of the fetus from specific deficiency conditions at or following birth.

Birth Defects of Mixed Causation

Cerebral palsy (CP) is a group of neurological disorders occurring in about one per 400 births, causing motor disabilities. It may be associated with intellectual disability, seizure disorders, motor spasticity, or sensory problems. CP is related to low birth weight (<2500 g), and especially very low birth weight

(<1500 g), as well as intracranial hemorrhage, Rh incompatibility, intrauterine and birth trauma, maternal exposure to heavy metals such as mercury, and other unidentified factors. About 20 percent of CP cases are due to intrauterine fetal hypoxia. Preventive measures include smoking cessation during pregnancy, improving maternal nutrition, prenatal care and care in labor and delivery, giving vitamin K at birth, and reducing infant trauma. Use of professionally trained midwives reduces risk of CP. Prevention is limited by lack of identification of many causative factors.

Microcephaly is a condition of abnormal small size of the head associated with incomplete brain development. It can occur as a result of abnormal development of head size and brain development during pregnancy or from inadequate growth following birth. Microcephaly may be due to infections during pregnancy, nutritional deficiencies, toxic effects or environmental factors. Microcephaly ranges in prevalence in the United States from 2 to 12 per 10,000 live births. It can be an isolated condition and range in severity, occurring alone or in combination with other major birth defects. Microcephaly is associated with varying degrees of delayed development (e.g., sitting, standing, walking, speaking, problems with movement and balance and intellectual disability), seizures, and hearing and vision problems. Children with microcephaly need regular follow-up to monitor their growth and development and to respond to specific needs.

Genetic causes of microcephaly include single-gene disorders (syndromes), chromosomal abnormalities, and mutations. In utero infectious causes include toxoplasmosis, syphilis, or viruses such as rubella, (congenital rubella syndrome or CRS) cytomegalovirus (CMV), herpes, HIV, and Zika virus infection. Other causes include maternal alcohol consumption (fetal alcohol syndrome disorders FASD), nutritional deficiencies including folic acid and iodine, in utero ischemia/hypoxia (e.g., placental insufficiency), maternal smoking, teratogens (e.g., antiepileptic drugs), radiation, mercury (e.g., in fish and other seafood), and maternal conditions (e.g., poorly controlled diabetes).

Delayed intellectual development (intelligence quotient (IQ) of <50) occurs in between three and five per 1,000 newborns. This may be related to low birth weight, low oxygen supply at birth, maternal lack of iodine and other essential nutrients and is estimated to affect 15 million newborns globally. Prenatal factors that cause intellectual delay include smoking, alcohol and drug consumption as well as some infectious diseases as noted above, many infectious diseases can cause microcephaly and developmental delay. Nutritional causes include general maternal undernutrition or specific micronutrient deficiencies such as iodine, iron, and vitamin D. Pregnancy complications such as toxemia, urinary tract infections, and anemia can also cause intellectual delay. Intellectual impairment is often associated with other birth defects including PKU, CH, Down syndrome, CP, FAS, and others. A study published in 2018 reported a far higher prevalence of FASD (5%) among first-graders in four US communities compared to 1.1% previously reported. The American Academy of Pediatrics (AAP) estimates that more than one third of intellectual impairments are attributable to chromosomal abnormalities. Prenatal diagnosis, widespread use of amniocentesis in pregnant women over age 35, and termination of affected pregnancies have contributed to reduced rates of severe intellectual disability disorders. Prevention requires general prepregnancy health as well as well-organized and utilized prenatal, delivery, and perinatal and postnatal care.

Fetal alcohol spectrum disorder (FASD) Alcohol consumption during pregnancy causes a range of irreversible injuries to the fetus and infant. FASD is caused by the toxic influence of alcohol on the fetus via the placenta. FASD includes impaired fetal brain development, microcephaly, distorted facial features, growth disorders, mental disorders, and fetal and infant mortality. FASD leads to a wide range of lifelong health consequences. Individuals exposed to alcohol prenatally are at high risk of comorbid conditions and premature mortality. It is greatly under diagnosed, but the CDC estimates that US and European rates to be between 2% and 5% of school children. Costs of care of FASD cases are estimated at about $4 billion annually in the United States. FASD is completely preventable as it only occurs when the mother drinks alcohol during pregnancy. All pregnant women should be counseled on alcohol use and women with alcohol dependency should be offered treatment. Alcohol is conveyed directly to the fetus during pregnancy via the placenta, and to the infant during breast feeding.

Genetic Causes of Birth Defects

Familial Mediterranean Fever is a recessive hereditary condition found in Arabs, Armenians, Turks, Greeks, and Sephardic Jews with disabling periodic fevers and pains in the chest, abdomen, and joints. Control is by genetic counselling. Each genetic carrier parent has no signs of the condition but each pregnancy has a 25 percent chance of inheriting the disease. Treatment with colchicine prevents periodic attacks of abdominal pain and prevents long term complications.

Gaucher Disease is a rare genetic disorder that affects about one in 50,000- 100,000 Americans. People of Eastern and Central European (Ashkenazi (Jewish)) heritage are at higher risk of Gaucher disease. As an autosomal recessive disease, the gene must be passed on by both parents who are carriers but do not have the disease and so a child will develop the disease. A parent who carries an abnormal copy of the gene is called a silent carrier. This allows for prevention programs of screening at the time of marriage and genetic counselling if both husband and wife are carriers of the gene, which has been successfully carried out in Jewish population groups in the United States. The enzyme deficiency, which may manifest itself at any age can cause enlargement of the liver and spleen, delayed motor development, bleeding and bruising, as well as bone and lung complications, It increases the risk of certain cancers, Parkinson's disease, arthritis, and osteoporosis. Treatments with enzyme-replacement therapy have improved quality and length of life.

Phenylketonuria (PKU) is an inborn error of metabolism transmitted by a recessive gene. It occurs in approximately 1/12,000 births in North America, but prevalence rates vary from 1/5,000 to 1/300,000 births in different ethnic/racial groups. It involves a mutation in DNA (deoxyribonucleic acid) that causes inadequate production of an enzyme needed to metabolize phenylalanine, an amino acid present in most foods, whose accumulation causes irreversible brain damage to children. PKU can lead to severe intellectual disability, seizures, and behavior problems. However, individuals identified and treated early with a diet low in phenylalanine, including a specialized formula for infants, can go on to live a normal healthy life. In the United States and in many countries worldwide hospitals are required to screen for PKU for all newborns using the heel blood filter paper Guthrie test. Treatment involves the use of a special dietary formula for infants and a lifetime special diet of low-protein food that is high in fruit and vegetables, which is highly cost-effective in preventing severe brain damage and with good management enables a relatively normal life.

Congenital hypothyroidism (CH) is a relatively common congenital disorder occurring in about one per 2,000–3,000 live births in countries with neonatal screening. Deficient development of the thyroid may be confused with iodine deficiency disorders common in areas with deficient iodine in water and soil. Therapy with thyroid hormone (T4) replacement in CH and frequent case monitoring prevents the severe intellectual impairment that otherwise occurs. Screening within 48 hours of birth should uncover cases requiring lifelong follow-up and management and a second screening should be considered for preterm, low birth weight, and very low birth weight neonates as well as those admitted to neonatal intensive care units. Maternal iodine deficiency is a high risk factor for limiting intellectual development of children, providing an urgent reason for fortification of basic foods, salt and flour with iodine, and supplementation of women before, during pregnancy and lactation (see Chapter 10).

Fetal alcohol spectrum disorder (FASD) Alcohol, cigarettes and illicit drugs must be avoided during pregnancy to avoid harming the fetus. Alcohol consumption during pregnancy causes a range of irreversible injuries to the fetus and infant of impaired fetal brain development, small head, distorted facial features, growth disorders, mental disorders, and fetal and infant mortality. Alcohol is conveyed directly to the fetus during pregnancy via the placenta, and during nursing via breast milk. Fetal alcohol syndrome (FAS) is greatly under-diagnosed and leads to a wide range of lifelong health consequences. Individuals exposed to alcohol prenatally are at high risk of comorbid conditions and premature mortality.

Tay–Sachs disease is an inborn error of metabolism associated with progressive mental deterioration, loss of vision by 4–8 months of age, and death by age three–four years. In the past, Tay–Sachs affected 1/2,500 births among Jews of Eastern European origin, but awareness of the disorder, counseling, and screening risk groups before marriage, or early in pregnancy, have dramatically reduced births of new cases. Prenatal screening is done by amniocentesis or chorionic villus sampling (i.e., testing the fluid surrounding the fetus and tests of the placenta attaching the fetus to the mother's womb) to confirm whether the fetus is affected. In such cases termination of pregnancy may be requested while the next pregnancy has a 75 percent chance of being free of this dreadful disease.

Down syndrome is a relatively common genetic disorder, occurring in about 5,300 babies (1/800 live births) born in the United States each year, and approximately 250,000 people have the condition. The risk increases rapidly with advancing parental age; for mothers over age 40 it occurs in 1/40 births but overall the majority of cases are in younger women. It is the most common cause of mild to moderate intellectual and developmental disabilities in industrialized countries. In cases-at-risk, prenatal screening for detection of the chromosomal abnormality is done by amniocentesis, chorionic villus sampling, and fetal blood sampling, with optional parental choice of pregnancy termination. Even if the pregnancy is not terminated, there are high rates of miscarriage and stillbirths. Pregnant women over age 35 should be screened as early as possible in pregnancy. Biochemical and fetal DNA markers detected from maternal blood serum along with fetal measurements taken during routine ultrasound have helped to increase screening with less invasive procedures. The total incidence of Down syndrome birth cases fell by 50 percent between 1960 and 1978 in the United States, probably because of reduced fertility among older women, widespread use of birth control, and prenatal screening. Congenital heart disease as well as hypothyroidism are common comorbidities in Down syndrome.

Down syndrome babies have cranio-facial abnormalities and intellectual impairment, often with congenital cardiac defects and gastrointestinal obstruction. They are happy and pleasant members of families and society who now survive well into adulthood with an average lifespan of 60 years. Emphasis in care has increasingly moved to improving self-care and independent functioning in the community. Education and life skills training for Down syndrome children have been emphasized in recent years. With vocational training, many are able to live independently or in groups in the community and can be gainfully employed. Those who are integrated into the community often live longer and have a better quality of life than those in institutions.

Cystic fibrosis (CF) is due to a recessive gene present in five percent of the white population and two percent of African Americans in the United

States. Both parents must be CF carriers for the baby to have CF. The affected child has serious health issues due to production of abnormally thick mucus in the lungs, intestines, and other glands with chronic obstructive lung disease (COPD), repeated infections, and destruction of lung tissue requiring frequent hospitalization and finally causing death. Recent advances in multi-disciplinary care can be effective in prolonging life into the mid-to-late 30s on average and some into their 40s and 50s. It is the most common lethal genetic disease in the US white population, occurring in 1/2,000 live births (1/3,000 in a recent Canadian study) and a rate of 1/3,500 in Europe. Prenatal screening can be done with a small sample of amniotic fluid (i.e., amniocentesis) or sampling of the placenta at 10−13 weeks of pregnancy (i.e., chorionic villus sampling (CVS). There is a small chance of miscarriage (about 1 in every 300−500 procedures) with amniocentesis and CVS, but the risk is lower if performed by an experienced health care provider.

The incidence of CF in the European Union (EU) is similar to that in the United States, with 0.737/10,000 in 27 EU countries (except for Ireland, which was has a rate four times higher) and 0.797 in the United States. A Canadian study by Dupuis et al. reported CF birth rates to be stable from 1971 to 1987 (1/2,714), but after 1988 when newborn screening was becoming common, CF birth rates declined steadily to an estimated rate of 1/3,608 in 2000. CF birth rates since then have stabilized, but further decline may occur with implementation of carrier screening in the general population. As of 2008, national newborn screening programs to identify CF patients after birth were adopted in Europe, Australia, and Canada, in the hopes of improving CF outcomes, with benefits seen due to early identification of CF patients, including improved survival, better lung function and growth with less-intensive therapy, and reduced cost of therapy.

In the United States, all states have newborn screening programs with a minimum of 29 conditions tested, but the number of tests varies widely with Mississippi screening for 59 conditions, New York state for 56, and Kentucky for 52 conditions. Screening of pregnancies with a previous CF birth can prevent a second child with this condition. Early diagnosis as well as support and education of parents can significantly improve the duration and quality of life of the affected person. Treatment is complex and costly (e.g., average cost US $48,000 per person in 2006). Gene therapy techniques may be available in the next few years to improve case management. The Cystic Fibrosis Foundation in the United States is a highly effective advocacy group that promotes research and care of affected persons and families. Lung transplantation is increasingly common in high-income countries with improved life expectancy for CF patients. A study by Stephenson et al. found that Canadian CF patients have lower death rates, survive 10 years longer than US CF patients, and 10.3 percent have lung transplants as compared to 6.5 percent for US patients, mainly due to greater access to universal health insurance.

Hematologic Disorders

The WHO estimates that some five percent of the world's population carries genetic traits for hemoglobin disorders, mainly sickle-cell disease and thalassemia. These are genetic blood diseases due to inheritance of mutant hemoglobin genes from generally healthy parents who are both carriers of the affected gene. Over 300,000 babies with severe hemoglobin disorders are born globally each year. Early case finding makes it possible to better manage cases and to reduce disability and improve both quality and length of life. Because of migration, these diseases are now spread worldwide, with 10 percent of the population at risk in the United States.

Beta thalassemia is a recessive genetic disorder of hemoglobin structure. Beta thalassemia minor is usually without clinical significance but carries the gene. Beta thalassemia major, the homozygous state (two identical genes), is characterized by hemolytic anemia (i.e., early breakdown of red blood cells); also known as Cooley's anemia or Mediterranean anemia. It is widespread throughout the Middle East, southern Europe, across southern India, and Southeast Asia. It is ultimately fatal for those afflicted, but with current standards of treatment, including blood infusions and chelating agents (i.e., iron binding for excretion) to reduce iron overload and hemochromatosis, patients survive into their 30s.

Virtual eradication of thalassemia has been achieved in some formerly endemic areas. In Cyprus, 14 percent of the population carried the beta thalassemia gene and one percent of the Cyprus population (1 in 158 births) had the disease. Due to an intervention program, new cases of beta thalassemia major are rare in Cyprus and other Mediterranean locations such as Sardinia and Greece, as well as in countries where Greek migrants live such as Canada and the United Kingdom. This was achieved by a long-term preventive program consisting of public education, screening for carriers and genetic counseling. Marriage between carriers is reduced by a community education program, and when two genetic carriers do marry, careful screening of all pregnancies and termination of affected pregnancies reduces the number of thalassemia major cases born and the next pregnancy has a 75 percent chance of being free of the clinical disease. The success of this approach in Cyprus provides a model of elimination of a genetic disorder via a combination of health education, screening, and community support. Premarital screening, health education in schools, and access to prenatal screening are all part of a program to reduce new cases of this disease (see Chapter 18). The WHO stresses the public health importance of this disease and recommends adoption of demonstrably successful preventive approaches to member states having this problem.

Screening for congenital anemias, including thalassemia and sickle cell disease, should take place at birth and at school age, because clinical cases may not appear until several years after birth. Thalassemia and sickle cell gene carriers should be informed at an age when they can understand the implications and if marrying another carrier should be advised that each pregnancy has a 25 percent chance of being affected. In each pregnancy when both parents are carriers, testing should be carried out to determine if the fetus is affected. Primary prevention in reducing new cases of thalassemia provides a model for application to disorders affecting other population groups, such as sickle-cell anemia. Public knowledge and societal awareness are crucial factors and have shown success in both prevention and management of birth defects.

Sickle-cell disease is a group of disorders with an amino acid defect of red blood cells that affects one in every 400 African American newborns in the United States and is even more common in Africa, where it may have a protective effect against malarial parasites. The disease is caused by a recessive gene affecting hemoglobin structure, causing distortion of the shape and the fragility of red blood cells. The disease trait (gene from one parent only) is usually with a benign course in the carrier (heterozygous) state. But with inheritance of the gene from both parents the disease begins in infancy with fatigue, restlessness, jaundice, repeated infections and debilitating episodes of pain in legs, abdomen and back, due to small blood vessel blockage. Clinical symptoms appear in the second half of the first year of life. The individual develops moderately severe anemia, with an increased susceptibility to severe bacterial infections (meningitis, pneumonia, septicemia) and growth retardation. Identification of cases and carriers is important in order to assure prompt care in crises with preventive use of antibiotics, which reduce infection rates, and to ensure patients receive influenza, pneumococcal and all routine vaccines. Carriers should receive genetic counseling related to marriage and pregnancy.

Hemolytic disease of the newborn (HDN) is a serious condition of breakdown of red cells in the newborn due to an incompatibility between fetal and maternal blood. It occurs when the mother is Rh negative and the fetus is Rh positive (inherited from the father). Fetal red blood cells can mingle with the maternal blood during delivery causing the mother to produce antibodies to the fetal blood. This does not pose a risk in the first pregnancy, but may affect subsequent pregnancies causing hemolysis of fetal blood cells, producing anemia, jaundice, brain damage, or death. Rhesus hemolytic disease was the cause of many stillbirths and neonatal deaths until the development of exchange transfusions in newborns reduced the death rate. In the 1970s, an effective treatment with anti-D immunoglobulin was introduced. This is given to Rh-negative women following the birth of a Rh-positive baby to prevent the mother from developing antibodies that would affect the next pregnancy. Treatment with anti-D immunoglobulin should eliminate this disease, a major victory of preventive care.

Vitamin K deficiency bleeding (VKDB) occurs when a baby experiences severe intestinal or other, including intracranial bleeding, which can result in permanent brain damage or death. Vitamin K is required for blood clotting, but does not cross the placenta and at birth is not adequate in human breast milk nor produced by the immature fetal liver. As a result, infants have very little vitamin K and are not able to produce a key blood clotting factor (pro-thrombin) and thus are at risk for bleeding for up to six months after birth. An injection of vitamin K should be given at birth to prevent vitamin K bleeding disorder deficiency which has largely disappeared from industrialized countries. But due to parental refusals or non-use in home deliveries or in private delivery homes can occur with death or brain damage to affected infants. Lack of routine vitamin K by injection at birth in developing countries may be a larger factor in high rates of neonatal mortality than can be identified. Use of oral vitamin K requires compliance with repeated doses and is less effective in preventing late VKDB (see Chapter 17).

Glucose-6-phosphate dehydrogenase (G6PD) deficiency is a genetic disorder of an enzyme that causes red blood cells to break down prematurely (i.e., a hemolytic anemia). An estimated 400 million people worldwide have G6PD deficiency. This condition occurs most frequently in certain parts of Africa, Asia, and the Mediterranean. In the United States it affects mainly African American males, but also ethnic populations from Mediterranean countries, including Sephardic Jews of North African or Middle Eastern origin, Greeks, southern Italians, Southeast Asians, and southern Chinese. Episodes of hemolytic anemia (rapid breakdown of red cells of blood) occur after infections, reactions to certain foods (e.g., fava bean), or reactions to drugs such as sulfonamides, antipyretics, and antimalarial drugs. Identifying the condition helps the patient avoid exposure to hemolytic-inducing agents and enables treatment planning and prompt care in crises.

Infectious Diseases

Infectious diseases are important factors for screening and preventive care before and during pregnancy. These can include syphilis, gonorrhea, HIV, hepatitis B and C, and others. Screening during pregnancy can alert caregivers to undertake preventive care to reduce the danger of spread to the newborn. Immunization during pregnancy for diphtheria, pertussis, pneumonia, and influenza are now recommended to protect the newborn until the age of independent routine infant immunization. Babies that survive may be born with severe neurological problems. Treatment of pregnant women with HIV is successful in reducing transmission to the newborn.

HIV and sexually transmitted disease (STDs) can cause damage to newborns including transmission of the maternal infections. Sex with an infected person can cause STD from vaginal, anal or oral sex which is not always clinically apparent. About 19 million people get a STD each year in the

United States. STDs affecting the newborn can include: chlamydia, gonorrhea, hepatitis B, hepatitis C, human immunodeficiency virus (HIV), syphilis, bacterial vaginosis (BV), genital herpes, genital warts, trichomoniasis and Zika virus. Prenatal diagnosis can lead to treatment to prevent maternal-fetus transmission, as in syphilis, gonorhoea, HIV, and others. Untreated STDs can result in stillbirth, premature labor and transfer of the disease to the newborn e.g., HIV, syphilis, and Zika. HIV and Hepatitis CB and C are major issues in vertical transmission to newborns. These diseases are retransmitted sexually but may also be transmitted by needle sharing, accidental exposure to contaminated needles, or by blood transfusion in inadequate professional health care settings. Prevention of vertical transmission is by screening early in pregnancy, treating HIV, Hepatitis B and C positive pregnant women. Screening for hepatitis B and C is recommended during pregnancy. Hepatitis B vaccine is recommended for all newborns, but as of 2018 this is done in only half the countries in the Americas and European Regions and less than 20% of African nations (Xi et al., 2018; see Chapter 19). Hepatitis C screening of pregnant women should also be included with consideration of treatment as well. Testing of blood for transfusion is important in reducing possibilities of transmission of these diseases to mothers and newborns as well.

Toxoplasmosis is due to a parasite that can be acquired from cat feces, unwashed produce, raw or undercooked meat, and contaminated soil. Toxoplasmosis can lead to preterm birth and stillbirth. Babies infected with toxoplasmosis can be born with eye infections, enlarged liver and spleen, jaundice, and pneumonia. If untreated, they develop problems later in life, including intellectual disabilities, vision problems, cerebral palsy, seizures, and hearing loss.

Cytomegalovirus (CMV) is a herpes type virus that as congenital CMV can cause premature birth, microcephaly, hearing and vision loss, intellectual disability, muscle weakness, and seizures. The virus can be transmitted to the fetus via the placenta. The Centers for Disease Control and Prevention (CDC) reports that although CMV is common, almost half of pregnant women have had CMV infection previously. About one out of every 150 babies are born with congenital CMV infection, but only about one in five babies with congenital CMV infection are affected or will have long-term health problems.

Congenital rubella syndrome (CRS) is due to maternal infection with rubella virus and can include heart problems, microcephaly, vision problems, hearing problems, intellectual disability, bone and growth problems, and liver and spleen damage. It can also lead to miscarriage, stillbirth, and preterm birth. Routine vaccination is available for rubella (see Chapter 12).

Zika virus is a mosquito-born and sexually transmitted infection that can lead to severe birth defects, including microcephaly, severe neurological defects, eye problems, hearing loss, and impaired growth. Its appearance in

Brazil in 2016 on a large scale spread by Aedes aegypti mosquito created a global public health crisis. It spread via individual contact cases to many semi-tropical locations and via secondary spread infected visitors with further transmission by sexual contact.

Aedes mosquitos and Zika virus are both present in the US (Florida) and Puerto Rico—and in 2016 in 68 countries including Polynesia, Central and South America. Zika along with dengue and chikungunya are now spread across wide areas of the globe and are transmitted by the same Aedes mosquitoes. There is still no vaccine for any of these diseases (dengue, chikungunya and Zika virus). Of the three, only Zika causes birth defects but the others are dangerous to vulnerable populations including pregnant women. Zika has the added factor of sexual transmission. CDC reports that from January 2015 to July 2017 there were 5,381 symptomatic Zika virus disease cases reported in the US including 5,109 cases in travelers returning from affected areas, and 224 cases acquired through presumed local mosquito-borne transmission, with 48 cases acquired through other routes, mainly sexual transmission. Public health needs to focus on education and vector control to prevent infections. WHO has called Zika a global health crisis and this is appropriate. Public health leaders and funders need to focus on helping local authorities reduce the vector population. Scientists and funders need to seek vaccines with all possible speed.

Prevention of Birth Defects

The underlying principle goal of reducing the incidence of birth defect disorders is to enhance individual and community health and well-being and stresses the importance of involvement and control by the individual and the community. Thus the levels of prevention including health promotion, and primary, secondary, and tertiary prevention during the prepregnancy, pregnancy, and newborn periods are critical to protecting and advancing maternal and infant health during prepregnancy, pregnancy, and the newborn periods.

Individual prevention focuses on prepregnancy and antenatal care at all levels of prevention with the active participation of the individual in appropriate self-care behaviors including smoking and alcohol abstention, appropriate exercise and nutrition as well as multivitamin supplements, up-to-date immunization, and secondary and tertiary care. Prepregnancy care includes daily folic acid intake. Antenatal care includes regular check-ups, multivitamin supplements, healthy diet, smoking and alcohol cessation, prevention of infectious diseases, as well as good nutrition and exercise. Newborn screening and prevention (early case-finding) of birth defects and their management is crucial to optimal care of the newborn.

Community-wide prevention has seen some highly effective measures introduced including iodine fortification of salt to prevent iodine deficiency brain damage, folic acid fortification of flour to prevent NTDs, and rubella immunization and eradication to prevent CRS. Screening and follow-up for STDs in the community to prevent infecting the fetus and the newborn with congenital syphilis, gonococcal and cytomegaloviruses (CMV), hepatitis B and C, HIV infections along with hepatitis B immunization to prevent maternal-fetal transmission facilitate control of these infections. Community organization for education, premarital screening for common genetic disorders with genetic counseling, has been shown to be effective in reducing thalassemia and Tay Sachs disease and can be applied to other genetic disorders (see Chapter 18).

Environmental prevention is the safe management of environmental pollutants that can lead to neurodevelopmental defects and diseases. Perera et al. reported that environmental pollutants are important in the causation of birth defects. Vector control is important in reducing environment-associated risks such as Zika. This virus spread in mosquito friendly environments constitutes a major threat for spread in tropical and semitropical areas including in the United States, the Caribbean, and potentially in Africa and other countries. Schizophrenia and coronary heart disease have been associated with early fetal exposure to famine. Other dangerous pollutants include asbestos, chemicals used in agriculture, and radiation including disasters such as nuclear explosions at Hiroshima and Nagasaki (1945) and the nuclear reactor accidents in Three Mile Island accident (1979) in the US, Chernobyl (1986) in the Ukraine and Fukushima (2001) in Japan.

Prepregnancy and Prenatal Prevention

Preparation for pregnancy and prenatal care, before and throughout pregnancy, should include screening for risk factors, education, medical care, and counseling. Cessation of smoking, alcohol, and drug intake are essential as is good nutrition and physical fitness. Prepregnancy and pregnancy nutrition counseling is important to promote optimal fetal development. This should include family history, genetic screening and counseling for parents at risk. Education should include avoidance of nonessential medication, and smoking, drug, and alcohol cessation, stressing regular supplements of iron, folic acid, preferably as multivitamins supplements. Immunization during pregnancy for influenza, pneumococcal pneumonia, pertussis, diphtheria and tetanus are recommended to protect the newborn from serious infections before their own immunization comes into play. Exposure to teratogenic agents before and during pregnancy should be avoided such as anesthetic agents, pesticides, lead and mercury, and to mosquitoes in Zika-infected areas.

Results of risk assessment may require referral to a high-risk clinic. Prenatal care protocols should start in the first trimester and include appropriate counseling. Safe delivery in a general hospital is recommended.

Follow-up care includes genetic counseling regarding care of the affected newborn and preparation for future pregnancies (see Table 20.1).

Newborn Screening for Birth Defects and Follow-up Management

In 1952 Dr. Virginia Apgar, an anesthesiologist from a New York hospital, developed a scoring system to evaluate the physical condition of newborns based on appearance, pulse, grimace, activity, and respiration. The APGAR score is used worldwide as an international standard for initial assessment of health of a newborn.

The 1993 US federal State Children's Health Insurance Program (SCHIP) provided health care coverage for up to five million children. It was followed by the 1998 Birth Defect Prevention Act and the Children's Health Act of 2000, establishing a National Center on Birth Defects and Developmental Disabilities, and the Newborn Screening Saves Lives Act. The Food and Drug Administration has undertaken to promote voluntary fortification of corn (masa) flour in addition to wheat flour with folic acid to further reduce the incidence of NTDs.

Newborn screening in the United States for hearing loss increased from 46.5 percent in 1999 to 96.9 percent in 2008. The percentage of infants found with deficient hearing screening diagnosed by an audiologist before age three months as either normal or having permanent hearing loss increased from 51.8 percent in 1999 to 68.1 percent in 2008. Lack of screening for critical congenital heart disease (CCHD) puts newborns at risk of disability or death if their condition is not diagnosed soon after birth. CCHD screening is included in many hospitals but not currently included in all state screening panels. Newborns identified with a CCHD are referred to pediatric cardiologists for assessment and ongoing care to prevent disability and death early in life.

Newborn screening and follow-up are cost-effective preventive measures leading to early diagnosis and treatment of conditions that threaten the well-being and life of the newborn. PKU screening was the first classic screening test, and it led to the prevention of large numbers of children with severe intellectual development disorders ending up in institutionalized settings. Early intervention with strict dietary care provides the opportunity for normality. Similarly early finding of CH allows for prompt treatment to prevent irreversible brain damage.

The development of newborn screening now includes many conditions for which early and long-term care can reduce severity and improve life quality and longevity. Newborn screening has expanded in its scope and effectiveness to many conditions for which genetic and medical sciences are providing effective interventions helping to reduce the prevalence and incidence of under age five years child mortality including congenital anomalies and birth defects. Screening before and during pregnancy in addition to new-born screening, which have long been practiced in high-income countries with success, are indicated.

Since the introduction of the Guthrie test for PKU, screening has been implemented in all State health programs in the United States, with increasing types of tests included. In 2017 all states in the US require newborn screening for at least 29 panel of health conditions including hearing, and heart disorders; some states include many more tests. At least four million babies are screened annually and significant disorders detected in some 5,000 babies.

The US Department of Health and Human Services (DHHS) screening program is not obligatory and each State conducts its own set of tests, but they are all influenced by the DHHS recommended schedule, which includes metabolic disorders (e.g., PKU); endocrine disorders (e.g., CH); hemoglobinopoathies (e.g., thalassemia, sickle-cell disease); and other disorders (e.g., congenital heart disease, hearing loss, and cystic fibrosis.). New York State has implemented the largest number of screened conditions in the United States and considers this to be a high-priority public health program.

The blood sample from a heel prick of the newborn placed on a filter paper is sent to a state central laboratory where the tests are read by an automated machine with the results sent to the referring hospital and listed family physician. Abnormal results are followed up to confirm and the patient is referred to a specialized congenital abnormality unit in a teaching hospital for follow-up. In 2000, 35 percent of US states screened for fewer than five conditions; by 2009, 49 states screened for 21 conditions or more. The CDC Newborn Screening Quality Assurance Program (NSQAP) provides quality assurance services to more than 650 newborn screening laboratories in the United States and for more than 75 countries around the world and has 32 newborn screening test manufacturers.

A 2015 review of the development of newborn screening programs globally indicates that the industrialized countries have implemented increasing numbers of tests with improving laboratory technology. In Europe most countries have newborn screening generally more limited than that in North America with great variation and no general EU guidelines. More mid-level income countries in the Americas and Asia are joining this trend but many low-income countries are not yet. China has recently successfully implemented a national program, but India has not yet done so (Therrell et al., 2015).

CURRENT RELEVANCE

Birth defects are an important population health issue because of the burden of diseases, disability, and death associated with multiple causes. With growing scientific advances in genetics, more conditions have been identified as being of genetic and environmental origin, some with appropriate clinical intervention. Prevention has been demonstrably effective in reducing or eradicating measles or congenital rubella syndrome (CRS) by widespread use of an effective vaccine to eradicate the virus. Screening has been shown to be effective in managing newborns with PKU, CH, and Rh incompatibility over many decades. Screening and genetic counseling have helped to eliminate thalassemia major as a public health problem in many countries. Credé in the mid-19th century applied silver nitrate to the eyes of all newborns in a Vienna obstetric hospital leading to elimination of gonoccocal ophthalmia neonatorum as a widespread cause of blindness. This practice is considered vital newborn care and continues to be essential in the 21st century as STDs (e.g., gonorrhea) have again become common in high-, middle-, and low-income countries (see chapters 3, 4, 5, and 12). Silver nitrate solution or anti-biotic ointments are used for this purpose. Screening, treatment, and immuni-zation are important for prevention of birth transmission of important infectious diseases to newborns including maternal syphilis and other STDs such as HIV, hepatitis B, hepatitis C, and CMV.

In 2016 Zika virus syndrome emerged to become a public health emer-gency of international concern (PHEIC) declared by WHO with many coun-tries now coping with the disease in travelers returning home from visiting infected countries. Infected travelers can transmit the disease via local Aedes mosquitoes as well as through sexual transmission. Zika causes a major birth defect of microcephaly and severe damage to fetal brain development during the first, second, or third trimester of pregnancy of Zika-infected mothers and even in the infant following birth. Initially reported in Brazil, the virus has migrated with travelers, transmitted sexually and from affected persons to local mosquitos who then spread the disease to wider populations in South America, the Caribbean, and parts of the United States. Rapid transmission and local endemicity in the United States and other countries have increased alarm levels about the importance of vector control, delay in pregnancy, avoidance of visits to infected areas or countries, and protection against mos-quitoes (i.e., *Aedes aegypti*). Development of vaccines to prevent this horrific disease causing birth defects is in fast track development but will not be available for field use during the next several years.

Vitamin K by injection adopted as a mandatory practice in New York State, and subsequently in all US states, has eliminated vitamin K bleeding disorders in the country. Vitamin K is not used universally by injection but given orally in some countries, which is less effective especially against late onset VKDB up to age six months, requires multiple doses, and com-promises compliance. Parental refusal of injections and failures of oral vita-min K result in cases of late VKDB usually within six weeks of birth. Schulte et al. reported seven cases of VKDB in Tennessee in 2013 resulting from parental refusal of vitamin K including three with brain damage due to intraventricular bleeding with serious long-term consequences and others requiring intestinal surgery to stop life-threatening bleeding. Parental refusal of vitamin K injection is related to refusals of other preventive care including immunizations to protect the individual child and the community.

Structural birth defects such as congenital heart defects, congenital cataracts, cleft lip/palate, and clubfoot can be corrected with strategies for care by appropriate surgery. Children with diseases such as thalassemia, sickle cell disorders, and CH can benefit from appropriate treatment. Prevention is even more successful with global efforts to fortify salt with iodine and thus a major reduction in iodine deficiency disorders.

An estimated 7.9 million children are born annually with a serious birth defect of genetic or partially genetic origin (March of Dimes). La Franchi reported that only 30 percent of newborns of the world population were screened for CH with 82−84 percent in Europe and Americas, but only 38 percent in Oceania and Africa and 24 percent in Asia. As a result, approximately 30,000 babies are born worldwide with CH not diagnosed or treated early in life and are at risk for mental retardation. CH is not clinically obvious at birth but unless detected early and treated with thyroid hormone results in serious and irreversible brain damage and severe learning disability. CH cases detected at birth and treated have major improvements in neurodevelopmental outcomes. Screening costs are just over US $15,000 per case identified whereas lifetime costs of care of untreated children in developed countries are reported as US $1.3 million.

Countless other children are at risk of intellectual (IQ) deprivation due to maternal iodine deficiency levels that, despite a century of iodine supplements and fortification, are still inadequately managed even in high-income countries of Western Europe as reported by Andersson et al. Even where iodization of salt has been implemented for many decades, a re-evaluation of maternal supplements of iodine and monitoring of pregnant women and schoolchildren are essential to protecting newborns from subclinical iodine deficiency brain damage (see Chapter 10).

Folic acid supplementation prepregnancy and flour fortification are still underimplemented even though more than 80 countries have adopted mandatory flour fortification. In the United States, Grosse et al. report that fortification of the grain food supply with folic acid reduced NTDs by one third annually, with cost savings estimated at over US $600 million annually. In Europe, a study by Khoshnood et al. reported that mandatory folic acid fortification of flour has not been adopted. The study was a population-based observational study of data from 28 EUROCAT (European Surveillance of Congenital Anomalies) registries. Of 12.5 million births in 19 countries between 1991 and 2011, there were 11,353 cases of NTD, including 4,162 cases of anencephaly and 5,776 cases of spina bifida. The main outcome measures were total and live birth prevalence of NTDs. The trend patterns for anencephaly and spina bifida were similar, but neither anomaly decreased substantially over time. Atta et al. published an extensive literature review showing that national mandatory folic acid fortification resulted in lower prevalence of spina bifida regardless of the type of birth cohort. In contrast, spina bifida is significantly more common in world regions without government legislation mandating folic acid fortification of the food supply, with Asian and European countries lagging. Some African nations are beginning to adopt folic acid legislation. Failure to implement preventive measures for micronutrient deficiency for much of the world's population leaves NTDs as a major global health problem.

ETHICAL ISSUES

The UN Declaration of the Rights of Disabled Persons (1975) and the UN Declaration of the Rights of the Child (1990) spell out the obligations of member states of the United Nations to protect children and support the rights of disabled persons including those with birth defects. The aim of the Millennium Development Goals (MDGs) for 2000–15 was to mobilize nations to reduce child and maternal mortality including birth defects and the associated multiple risk factors such as socioeconomic conditions of the population. The follow-up Sustainable Development Goals (SDGs) for 2016–30 with impressive international consensus will continue and expand the range of global efforts to improve life, well-being, and survivability. The ethical commitment to global health is supported by most nations and many international agencies and donors. In part these goals are based on the ethical commitments of the UN declarations of the rights of the child and disabled persons.

Controversies arose in the UK and Ireland over retaining the PKU heel blood test filter papers with identification on the grounds that they could be used for other testing including DNA for genetic disorders, but this seems to have dissipated. In the early years of the Guthrie test concern arose over potential for damage done by false positives tests, but this has also disappeared as an issue since the accuracy of more recently developed tests based on the heel prick test has reduced false positives, and no significant harm was done to children with false positive tests subsequently shown not to indicate they suffered from PKU.

Ethical debates center on the fact that many of the new diseases being tested for are rare and have no current known treatment. Other diseases need not be treated until later in life. More concern is raised that there may be no available treatment for the disease making the test superfluous or even harmful (Goldenberg and Sharp, 2012). These issues are in part answered by the dynamic evolution of improved prevention and management of more of the disorders discovered with improved survival and quality of life for affected children. The US Recommended Uniform Screening Panel (RUSP) has increased the recommended panel of screening tests to 32 core conditions and 26 secondary targets after thorough reviews of risks and benefits, public health impact, consequences, and available treatment. The potential for genetic treatment methods is also promising for future interventions.

Developing screening programs for newborns in low income countries should be added to the priorities of national and international agencies. Sickle cell anemia and thalassemia with high prevalence rates have been recently reported in Tanzania, so that routine screening in low-, middle-income countries (LMICs) can offer affected children hope for preventive care to help their survival and relatively good health.

Vitamin K at birth is sometimes met with parental refusal and inconsistent recommendations for oral vitamin K (which is less effective) versus injected vitamin K have led to a mandatory requirement in many countries. But parental refusal is becoming more common and cases of VKDB are reported, as in Tennessee in 2013 when a cluster of five infants presented with VKDB in Nashville. Similarly, screening for birth defects is standard practice or mandatory in many countries and contributes to protection of the child from failure to treat manageable congenital disorders that threaten the well-being and survival of many children from conditions that cannot be readily detected by routine medical care.

Ethical issues are raised regarding potential genetic modification techniques might be applied to "designer babies" and selection bias as in countries where termination of female fetuses took place in male preference societies such as occurred on a mass scale in China. The unintended consequences of such selection is a generation of young men with few opportunities to find a female partner. On the other side of the scale is the clear advantage given to the screening at birth to protect against serious development and health consequences by timely preventive care. Non attention to proven cost effective measures to prevent birth defects such as NTDs by fortifying a basic food with folic acid, as is the case in Europe, would seem to be unethical policy and public health malpractice comparable to failure to ensure up to date immunization content and coverage.

Slow adoption of neonatal screening in many high-, medium- and low-income countries is a factor in continued high rates of neonatal mortality as well as morbidity and thus requires increased awareness among policymakers for inclusion in development of child health services. This topic has not been emphasized as a high priority among low-income countries where the birth defects are the most common nor by the nations themselves, by international donors and organizations, although birth defects are major contributors to neonatal/child mortality and disability.

Refusal of vaccination by newly pregnant women or refusal to take essential supplements such as multivitamins or individual supplements of iron, folic acid, and vitamin D create a burden for healthy survival of the newborn infant, as does smoking and alcohol consumption. These could be seen as neglect or even abuse of a child just as nonplacement of a young child in a safe seat in a motor vehicle.

ECONOMIC ISSUES

Prevention of birth anomalies/defects is a cost-effective population-based approach. Prenatal and neonatal screening saves lives and provides the opportunity for provision of appropriate preventive care and treatment of affected individuals. Primary prevention, screening and effective care can prevent further damage to newborns which would otherwise require costly health care, while improving quality and length of life. These all have economic implications.

Model et al. report that inherited hemoglobin disorders (sickle cell disorders and thalassemias) with defective hemoglobin and red blood cells, which die much earlier than the normal red blood cell span of 120 days, were in the past characteristic of tropical and subtropical regions, but are now common worldwide due to migration. Hemoglobin disorder endemicity has risen from 60 percent to 71 percent in 229 countries. Prevention is making, only a small impression: affected birth prevalence is estimated at 2.6/1,000 live births. In high-income countries, affected children survive with quality care until the age of 40 years or more. Affected children in low-income settings do not receive the quality of care needed and mostly die before the age of five years. Hemoglobin disorders cause 3.4 percent of mortality in children up to five years of age worldwide and 6.4 percent in Africa. Annually there are over 332,000 births globally with hemoglobin disorders including 275,000 with sickle cell disorder, which can greatly benefit from early diagnosis and long-term prophylactic medical care. Some 56,000 cases of beta thalassemia major are born annually, with over 30,000 needing regular transfusions and iron-reducing chelating therapy to reduce iron overload in key organs in the body to enable the patient to survive and live. Prevention of hemoglobinopathies has shown remarkable success in Cyprus and other Mediterranean countries in preventing new cases by community education, premarital genetic screening and careful monitoring of pregnancies at risk (see Chapter 18).

Prevention of neural tube defects (NTDs) has become highly effective since the 1990s. The cost of preventing NTDs is far outweighed by the cost of care of affected children. Folic acid supplements taken in the 3 months before pregnancy prevent some 70 percent of NTDs, but compliance has been less than 40 percent of women and about half of pregnancies are unplanned. The option of folic acid fortification of basic foods has been adopted since 1998 in over 80 countries, but astonishingly no countries in Western Europe.

Arth et al. at the CDC reported that birth defect-associated hospitalizations account for 3.0 percent of all hospitalizations and 5.2 percent of total hospital costs, with an estimated annual cost in the United States in 2013 of $23 billion. This includes hospital costs for people with a congenital heart defect of about $6 billion in 2013. Spina bifida costs based on a

2012 study from Florida showed hospital costs for a typical baby born with spina bifida were about $21,900 (but ranging up to $1,350,700), and for a baby with Down syndrome medical costs were 12−13 times higher than a child without Down syndrome and much more if the child also had a heart defect. These do not include emotional, societal, and family expenses.

Stephenson et al. report that the risk of death for cystic fibrosis is 34 percent lower and longevity 10 years longer in Canada than in the United States, attributed to the differences in health care delivery systems, especially for the disadvantaged. Grosse et al. reported on US cost savings of prevention of NTDs by folic acid fortification and supplementation with an estimated reduction in spina bifida cases of between 614 and 767 cases per year since the fortification mandate was implemented in 1998. CDC data for 2003 on costs of NTD disabilities includes average costs of lifetime care for intellectual disability of over $1 million USD, cerebral palsy of US $920,000, hearing loss over US $400,000, and over US $566,000 for vision impairment (see Table 20.2). For spina bifida the total cost of care per infant affected is estimated at US $577,000. Savings from prevention of 600−700 NTDs for each birth year cohort in the United States is estimated to save over US $600 million; more than the cost of flour fortification (CDC 2017).

A CDC analysis of 2013 data found an annual cost of US $22.9 billion for hospitalizations due to birth defects in that calendar year. Although birth defects accounted for only three percent of the hospitalizations, the cost represented 5.2 percent of total costs, indicating the high cost of treating patients with birth defects. The share of costs was even sharper in the case

TABLE 20.2 Estimated Lifetime Costs of Selected Developmental Disabilities in the United States

Developmental Disabilities	Total Cost (US$ millions)	Average Cost Per Person (US$)
Intellectual disability	$51.2	$1,014,000
Cerebral palsy	11.5	921,000
Hearing loss	1.9	383,000
Vision impairment	2.6	601,000

Note: Present value estimates, in 2003 dollars, of lifetime costs for persons born in 2000, based on a 3% discount rate.
Source: Honeycutt A, Dunlap L, Chen H, al Homsi G, Grosse S, Schende D. National Center on Birth Defects and Developmental Disabilities, CDC. Economic costs associated with mental retardation, cerebral palsy, hearing loss, and vision impairment—United States, 2003. Morb Mort Wkly Rep MMWR. 2004;53(03):57−59 https://www.cdc.gov/mmwr/preview/mmwrhtml/mm5303a4.htm; Errata: vol. 53, no. 3: Morb Mort Wkly Rep MMWR. 2006;55(32):881 Available at: https://www.cdc.gov/mmwr/preview/mmwrhtml/mm5532a5.htm (accessed 17 February 2018).

of infants with birth defects at 35.0 percent of all hospitalization costs for patients under one year of age. The analysis found that cardiovascular defects (8,1000 live births) accounted for the highest portion of the costs (US $6.1 billion), followed by central nervous system defects (US $1.7 billion), eye defects (US $44,441), and ear defects (US $11,349).

GENOMICS/GENETICS

The development of the PKU Guthrie test opened the field of newborn screening for genetic conditions and genomic sciences. Genetics focuses its study on a single gene while the focus of genomics is on the interrelationship and combined effect on growth and development of all genes on the organism. The National Human Genome Research Institute supports research in many of the areas including the function of genes; the interrelationship of DNA, proteins, and the environment; and strategies for diagnosis and management of diseases, including the study of ethical, legal and social issues related to genomics and genetics. The rapid development of the fields of genetics and genomes has important implications for health policy and health insurance coverage policies.

The Institute of Clinical and Economic Review reported in March 2017 that gene therapy is a new approach to treat, cure, or ultimately prevent disease by changing the genetic makeup of affected persons. Gene therapies can potentially repair, deactivate, or replace dysfunctional genes that cause disease, with the aim of reestablishing normal function. Around 4,000 diseases have been linked to gene disorders, and thus gene therapy could, in principle, positively affect millions of lives. Two gene therapies have been approved in the European Union, but none have yet been approved by the USFDA due to concerns that premature promotion of insufficiently proven therapies may be exploited for commercial purposes. One application is being submitted to the US Food and Drug Administration (USFDA) for a gene therapy for retinal dystrophy, an inherited form of blindness. Some 12−14 gene therapies for additional ultra-rare conditions and some for more common conditions, such as hemophilia and sickle cell disease, are under developmental and expected to reach regulatory approval by 2020.

Prevention of birth defects should be viewed in the context of prevention of late-term abortions, stillbirths, and low birth weight newborns. This requires upgrading the skills of community care providers with access to health systems for referrals, resuscitation training, and case reviews by community and district public health managers. The AAP recommends that management of low- and very low birth weight (i.e., between 500 and 1,500 grams birth weight) newborns should be provided in regional centers with high levels of expertise and facilities.

CONCLUSION

Newborn screening pioneered by Robert Guthrie has become a standard method of improving newborn care. Screening is valuable because it identifies diseases and disorders before symptoms appear making an enormous contribution to the quality of life and survivability of the child affected. Many of the diseases tested today are not currently curable, but identifying them can enable supportive care to help normalize the child's life. The prevention of neural tube defects as established by Nicholas Wald opened a major new parameter of population health by the fortification of basic foods with folic acid. Advances in vaccinology, nutritional, and genetic sciences will bring many more advances in this field.

Widespread adoption of Guthrie's PKU test from 1962 onward has steadily enriched newborn screening by technological advances with a host of new tests being developed in the following years. This included newborn screening for congenital hypothyroidism (CH) the commonest cause of treatable mental retardation first pioneered in 1972 in Quebec, Canada by Dussault.

New technology provided testing for many inborn errors of metabolism, hemoglobinopathies (thalassemia and sickle cell anemia) followed rapidly expanding the capacity of newborn screening to become an essential part of quality maternal/ infant clinical care and public health. The application of these advances was characterized by elimination of virtually all cases of beta thalassemia major in Cyprus and other Mediterranean countries in the 1970s. In 1969, an enzyme test to show carrier status for a horrific genetic disease called Tay-Sachs in which children afflicted wasted away and died by age five years was developed. A community based education, screening and genetic counseling program was implemented and the disease was practically eradicated since the mid-1980s in New York and California orthodox Ashkenazi Jewish populations.

The topic of newborn screening has medical, moral and economic justifications but also bears with it controversial ethical and moral aspects for diseases without current effective treatment. Many benefits of the screening/ diagnostic tests have led to effective preventive care (PKU, CH, thalassemia, Tay Sachs, sickle cell anemia and others). For others there is no current effective curative treatment but screening allows for genetic counseling to provide carrier couples the option to terminate an affected fetus while the next pregnancy could be disease free. But there are also concerns arising from deep seated anxieties that birth defect screening can lead to branding a child for life with potential for harmful measures such as promoted by the eugenics movement and tragically implemented in the first half of the twentieth century (see Chapter 13). Nevertheless the practical application of newborn screening has enabled saving of lives and health of large numbers of children whose fate otherwise was pain, suffering and early death. The pioneering phase quickly moved into the real world of public health and fetal/

newborn screening will undoubtedly benefit from the rapidly growing potential of genetics for alteration of disease causing genetic abnormalities of children, and also for adults bearing cancer-causing genetic variants.

Prevention of birth defects should be a central issue in public health practice and development. Routine preventive practices have shown remarkable success through fetal screening, immunizations, nutritional support by multivitamin supplements, and fortification of basic foods. These measures have saved untold numbers of newborns from the range of serious birth defects such as NTDs and other less obvious delays in brain development and delay in overall growth due to micronutrient deficiencies. Early intervention and treatment can save the child from serious developmental harm. Vector control is important in reducing environment-associated risks. Public health challenges in reducing birth anomalies and defects are many and are vital to population health and protection.

Education of the public and policymakers of the multiple levels and methods of prevention is needed to reduce congenital anomalies and birth defects as an important component of the maternal and child health strategy and initiatives. This is a shared responsibility of clinical caregivers, parents, and most definitely the public health community and governments. Reminders of immunization and antenatal care requirements are becoming available on personal communication devices. Standards of preventive care continue to evolve and require clinical and community support to be most effective.

In 2010, the World Health Assembly (WHA) adopted a resolution on birth defects calling all member countries to promote primary prevention and improve the health of children with congenital anomalies by:

- developing and strengthening registration and surveillance systems;
- developing expertise and building capacity;
- strengthening research and studies on etiology, diagnosis, and prevention; and
- promoting international cooperation.

Robert Guthrie founded newborn screening for PKU in the early 1960s and this has developed over the years into an import public health endeavor to discover birth defects as early as possible to prevent serious consequences for the child and the family and society. Nicholas Wald established the effect of pre-pregnancy folic acid to prevent neural tube defects. Together these measures have added important prevention measures to protect the health of newborns along with measures such as vitamin K and eye care as standard care for all newborns. New knowledge of genetic diseases and hopefully improved methods of treating them perhaps with stem cells will add greatly to public health effectiveness in the coming decades.

RECOMMENDATIONS

1. All international health agencies, donors, and countries should develop fetal and neonatal screening as part of essential public health programs.
2. Routine screening at birth and at-risk populations for important birth defects should be promoted by international agencies, professional associations, national governments, and donors as part of a standardized, recommended and funded priority program in fetal and neonatal health.
3. All newborns should receive antibiotic eye care to prevent eye infection that can lead to blindness and vitamin K by injection within six hours of birth to prevent vitamin K bleeding disorders.
4. All countries should develop routine newborn screening, preferably as a mandatory free service to protect the fetus and newborns from otherwise preventable congenital anomalies and birth defect conditions. These should include at least: PKU, CH, thalassemia, sickle cell disease, CF, and some inborn errors of metabolism.
5. Infrastructure development for birth defect detection requires regional public service laboratories and trained staff with capacities for standardized screening and confirmation services available to analyze blood by standardized methods to carry out the screening tests.
6. Staff development of laboratory personnel as well as personnel for follow-up procedures and expert clinical services should include validation of positive screening tests and clinical care for the affected child, including provision of essential foods (e.g., phenylalanine diet; CH, thyroid replacement therapy, and monitoring).
7. Education for infectious disease prevention and treatment in pregnant women is crucial to prevent congenital defects such as CRS, microcephaly, and those caused by STDs.
8. Education for prevention of micronutrient deficiency conditions among women, pre-pregnancy and during pregnancy, which cause damage to the fetus.
9. Mandatory fortification of basic foods, such as flour with folic acid, vitamin B complex, iron, and vitamins D and B12; iodine in salt; and vitamins A and D in milk products including milk substitutes should be advocated and promoted by international aid agencies and donors and by national governments.
10. Renewed education for avoiding alcohol, smoking, and illicit and other drugs or medications before and during pregnancy and lactation.
11. Education and promotion of awareness of infection control of STDs, including syphilis, gonorrhea, HIV, and others, which can affect the fetus during pregnancy, and immunization and HIV and hepatitis B treatment before or during pregnancy to protect the fetus and newborn infant.
12. Promotion of delivery in sanitary, professionally supervised facilities; avoidance of home delivery as an unnecessary risk for newborn and mother.

13. Promotion of breastfeeding for a minimum of six months, with multivitamin supplements for lactating mothers. Breast fed infants require similar supplements and introduction of solid foods at age-appropriate timing.

14. Promotion of research on causes of major congenital anomalies and birth defects as a major challenge in reaching MDGs/ SDGs child health goals.

15. Global efforts should be included in SDGs to develop newborn screening and preventive measures as key efforts to reduce neonatal and child mortality and to save children from lifelong serious disability.

RECOMMENDED READINGS

1. American Academy of Pediatrics. Policy statement: committee on fetus and newborn: controversies concerning vitamin K and the newborn. Pediatrics. 2003;112(1):191−192. Available at: http://pediatrics.aappublications.org/content/pediatrics/112/1/191.full.pdf (accessed 16 March 2017).

2. American Academy of Pediatrics. Policy statement: committee on fetus and newborn policy: levels of neonatal care. Pediatrics. 2012;130(3):587−597. Available at: http://pediatrics.aappublications.org/content/pediatrics/130/3/587.full.pdf (accessed 16 March 2017).

3. Andermann A, Blancquaert I, Beauchamp S, Costea I. Guiding policy decisions for genetic screening: developing a systematic and transparent approach. Public Health Genomics. 2011;14(1):9−16. Abstract available at: https://www.karger.com/Article/Abstract/272898 (accessed 16 March 2017).

4. Andersson M, Karumbunathan V, Zimmermann MB. Global iodine status in 2011 and trends over the past decade. J Nutr. 2012;142(4):744−750. Available at: http://jn.nutrition.org/content/142/4/744.long (accessed 16 March 2017).

5. Arth AC, Tinker SC, Simeone RM, Ailes EC, Cragan JD, Grosse SD. Inpatient hospitalization costs associated with birth defects among persons of all ages—United States, 2013. Morb Mortal Wkly Rep. 2017;66(2):41−46. Available at: https://www.cdc.gov/mmwr/volumes/66/wr/mm6602a1.htm (accessed 16 March 2017).

6. Atta CA, Fiest KM, Frolkis AD, Jette N, Pringsheim St T, Germaine-Smith C, et al. A global birth prevalence of spina bifida by folic acid fortification status: a systematic review and meta-analysis. Am J Public Health. 2016;106(1):e24−e34. Available at: https://www.ncbi.nlm.nih.gov/pubmed/26562127 (accessed 16 March 2017).

7. Baraona F, Gurvitz M, Landzberg MJ, Opotowsky JR. Hospitalizations and mortality in the United States for adults with Down syndrome and congenital heart disease. Am J Cardiol. 2013;111(7):1046−1051. Available at: https://www.ncbi.nlm.nih.gov/pubmed/23332593 (accessed 16 March 2017).

8. Berry RJ, Bailey L, Mulinare J, Bower C. Folic acid working group. Fortification of flour with folic acid. Food Nutr Bull. 2010;31(1 Suppl):S22−S35. Abstract available at: https://www.ncbi.nlm.nih.gov/pubmed/20629350 (accessed 16 March 2017).

9. Bestwick JP, Huttly WJ, Morris JK, Wald NJ. Prevention of neural tube defects: a cross-sectional study of the uptake of folic acid supplementation in nearly half a million women. PLoS One. 2014;9(2):e89354. Available at: http://www.ncbi.nlm.nih.gov/pmc/articles/PMC3929694/ (accessed 16 March 2017).

10. Bhutta ZA, Darmstadt GL, Haws RA, Yakoob MY, Lawn JE. Delivering interventions to reduce the global burden of stillbirths: improving service supply and community demand.

BMC Pregnancy Childbirth. 2009;9(Suppl 1):S7. Available at: https://www.ncbi.nlm.nih.gov/pmc/articles/PMC2679413/ (accessed 16 March 2017).

11. Behrman RE, Butle AS, editors. Institute of Medicine, Committee on Understanding Premature Birth and Ensuring Healthy Outcomes. Preterm birth: causes, consequences, and prevention. Washington, DC: National Academies Press, 2007. Available at: https://www.ncbi.nlm.nih.gov/books/NBK11362/ (accessed 16 March 2017).

12. Black MM, Walker SP, Fernald LCH, et al. Early childhood development coming of age: science through the life course. Lancet. 2017;389(10064):77–90. Available at: https://www.ncbi.nlm.nih.gov/pubmed/27717614 (accessed 16 March 2017).

13. Blencowe H, Cousens S, Oestergaard MZ, Chou D, Moller A-B, et al. National, regional, and worldwide estimates of preterm birth rates in the year 2010 with time trends since 1990 for selected countries: a systematic analysis and implications. Lancet. 2012;379:2162–2172. Available at: http://www.thelancet.com/pdfs/journals/lancet/PIIS0140-6736(12)60820-4.pdf (accessed 9 July 2017).

14. Board of Global Health, Committee on Improving Birth Outcomes. Improving birth outcomes: meeting the challenge in the developing world. Washington, DC: National Academies Press, 2003. Available at: https://www.nap.edu/read/10841/chapter/1#ii (accessed 16 March 2017).

15. Boyle C. Birth defects and developmental disabilities: CDC activities. National Center on Birth Defects and Developmental Disabilities, Centers for Disease Control and Prevention. Available at: http://www.ncsl.org/print/health/CBoyle807.pdf (accessed 16 March 2017).

16. Britto PR, Lye SJ, Proulx K, Yousatzai AK, Matthews SG, Vaivada T, et al. Nurturing care: promoting early childhood development. Lancet. 2017;389(10064):91–102. Available at: http://www.thelancet.com/journals/lancet/article/PIIS0140-6736(16)31390-3/abstract (accessed 16 March 2017).

17. Burgard P, Cornel M, Di Filippo F, Haege G, Hoffmann GF, Lindner M, et al. Short executive summary of the report on the practices of newborn screening for rare disorders implemented in member states of the European Union, candidate, potential candidate and EFTA countries, 18 October 2011. Available at: http://ec.europa.eu/chafea/documents/news/Summary_20120110.pdf (accessed 9 July 2017).

18. Centers for Disease Control and Prevention. Achievements in public health, 1900–1999: healthier mothers and babies. Morb Mort Wkly Rep. 1999;48(38):849–858. Available at: https://www.cdc.gov/mmwr/preview/mmwrhtml/mm4838a2.htm (accessed 16 March 2017).

19. Centers for Disease Control and Prevention. Alcohol use among pregnant and nonpregnant women of childbearing age—United States, 1991–2005. Morbid Mortal Wkly Rep. 2009;58(19):529–532. Available at: https://www.cdc.gov/mmwr/preview/mmwrhtml/mm5819a4.htm (accessed 16 March 2017).

20. Centers for Disease Control and Prevention. Birth defects are costly, January 20, 2014. Available at: https://www.cdc.gov/features/birthdefectscostly/ (accessed 16 March 2017).

21. Centers for Disease Control and Prevention. Spina bifida basics, October 17, 2016. Available at: https://www.cdc.gov/ncbddd/spinabifida/facts.html (accessed 19 March 2016).

22. Centers for Disease Control and Prevention. Facts about microcephaly, December 7, 2016. Available at: https://www.cdc.gov/ncbddd/birthdefects/microcephaly.html (accessed 19 March 2016).

23. Centers for Disease Control and Prevention. Birth defects, last updated June 26, 2017. Available at: https://www.cdc.gov/ncbddd/birthdefects/index.html (accessed 16 March 2017).

24. Centers for Disease Control and Prevention. Cytomegalovirus MV and congenital CMV infection. Available at: https://www.cdc.gov/cmv/congenital-infection.html (accessed 16 March 2017).

25. Centers for Disease Control and Prevention. Fetal alcohol spectrum disorder, June 6, 2017. Available at: http://www.cdc.gov/ncbddd/fasd/data.html (accessed 16 March 2017).

26. Centers for Disease Control and Prevention. Folic Acid: birth defects COUNT. Neural tube defects, last updated 20 May 2016. Available at: https://www.cdc.gov/ncbddd/birthdefects-count/basics.html (accessed 9 July 2017).

27. Centers for Disease Control and Prevention. Laboratory and quality assurance and standardization programs: about the program, updated July 6, 2017. Available at: http://www.cdc.gov/labstandards/nsqap_about.html (accessed 16 March 2017).

28. Centers for Disease Control and Prevention. Newborn screening portal. Available at: https://www.cdc.gov/newbornscreening/ (accessed 16 March 2017).

29. Centers for Disease Control and Prevention. Ten great public health achievements—United States, 2001−2010. Morb Mortal Wkly Rep. 2011;60(19):619−623. Available at: https://www.cdc.gov/mmwr/preview/mmwrhtml/mm6019a5.htm (accessed 16 March 2017).

30. Centers for Disease Control and Prevention. Trends in wheat-flour fortification with folic acid and iron—worldwide, 2004 and 2007. Morb Mortal Wkly Rep. 2008;57(01):8−10. Available at: https://www.cdc.gov/mmwr/preview/mmwrhtml/mm5701a4.htm (accessed 16 March 2017).

31. Centers for Disease Control and Prevention. Grand Rounds: Additional opportunities to prevent neural tube defects with folic acid fortification. Morb Mortal Wkly Rep. 2010;59 (31):980−984. Available at: https://www.cdc.gov/mmwr/preview/mmwrhtml/mm5931a2. htm#fig1 (accessed 21 June 2017).

32. Centers for Disease Control and Prevention. Use of supplements containing folic acid among women of childbearing age—United States, 2007. Morb Mortal Wkly Rep. 2008;57:5−8. Available at: https://www.cdc.gov/mmwr/preview/mmwrhtml/mm5701a3. htm (accessed 16 March 2017).

33. Centers for Disease Control and Prevention. Zika virus, Updated 2 February 2018. Available at: https://www.cdc.gov/zika/ (accessed 5 February 2018).

34. Christianson A, Howson CP, Modell B. March of dimes: global report on birth defects; the hidden toll of dying and disabled children. White Plains, NY: March of Dimes Birth Defects Foundation, 2006. Available at: http://www.marchofdimes.org/materials/ global-report-on-birth-defects-the-hidden-toll-of-dying-and-disabled-children-full-report. pdf (accessed 16 March 2017).

35. Cornel M, Rigter T, Weinreich S, et al. Newborn screening in Europe: expert opinion document. 2011. http://www.iss.it/cnmr/index.php?lang = 1&id = 1621&tipo = 72 (accessed 9 July 2017).

36. Cornel M, Rigter T, Weinreich S, Burgard P, Hoffmann GF, Lindner M, et al. Newborn screening in Europe: expert opinion document. Brussels: European Union, 2012. Available at: http://ec.europa.eu/chafea/documents/news/Expert_opinion_document_on_NBS_20120108_ FINAL.pdf (accessed 16 March 2017).

37. Cystic Fibrosis Foundation. Newborn screening for CF. Available at: https://www.cff.org/ What-is-CF/Testing/Newborn-Screening-for-CF/ (accessed 23 August 2017).

38. Czeizel AE, Dudas I. Prevention of the first occurrence of neural-tube defects by periconceptional vitamin supplementation. N Engl J Med. 1992;327:1832−1835. Available at: http://www.nejm.org/doi/full/10.1056/NEJM199212243272602 (accessed 16 March 2017).

39. Czeizel A. Periconceptional care: an experiment in community genetics. Commun Genet. 2000;3:119−123. Abstract available at: https://www.karger.com/Article/Pdf/51120 (accessed 16 March 2017).

40. Darmstadt GL, Howson CP, Walraven G, Armstrong RW, Blencowe HK, Christianson AL, et al. Prevention of congenital disorders and care of affected children: a consensus

statement. JAMA Pediatr. 2016;170(8):790−793. Available at: http://jamanetwork.com/journals/jamapediatrics/article-abstract/2529986 (accessed 9 July 2017).

41. Dupuis A, Hamilton D, Cole DE, Corey M. Cystic fibrosis birth rates in Canada: a decreasing trend since the onset of genetic testing. J Pediatr. 2005;147(3):312−315. Abstract avalble at: https://www.ncbi.nlm.nih.gov/pubmed/16182667/ (accessed 16 March 2017).

42. Farrell PM. The prevalence of cystic fibrosis in the European Union. J Cystic Fibrosis. 2008;7(5):450−453. Available at: http://www.sciencedirect.com/science/article/pii/S1569199308000349 (accessed 16 March 2017).

43. Fintel B, Samaras AT, Carias E. The thalidomide tragedy: lessons for drug safety and regulation. Helix: Science in Society, Northwestern University, 2009. Available at: https://helix.northwestern.edu/article/thalidomide-tragedy-lessons-drug-safety-and-regulation (accessed 16 March 2017).

44. Fisher DA, Dussault JH, Foley TP, Klein AH, LaFranchi S, Larsen PR, et al. Screening for congenital hypothyroidism: Results of screening one million North American infants. J Pediatrics. 1979;94(5):700−705. Abstract available at: http://www.jpeds.com/article/S0022-3476(79)80133-X/pdf (accessed 21 August 2017).

45. Fitzgerald B, Boyle C, Honein MA. Birth defects potentially related to Zika virus infection during pregnancy in the United States. JAMA. Published online January 25, 2018. Available at: https://doi.org/10.1001/jama.2018.0126. Available at: https://jamanetwork.com/journals/jama/fullarticle/2671017 (accessed 30 January 2018).

46. Friberg AK, Jorgensen FS. Few Danish pregnant women follow guidelines on periconceptional use of folic acid. Dan Med J. 2015;62(3):A5019. Available at: http://www.ncbi.nlm.nih.gov/pubmed/25748861 (accessed 16 March 2017).

47. Ginsberg G, Tulchinsky TH, Filon D, Goldfarb A, Abramov L, Rachmilevitz EA. Cost-benefit analysis of a national thalassemia prevention programme in Israel. J Med Screen. 1998;5(3):120−126. Available at: http://msc.sagepub.com/content/5/3/120.full.pdf (accessed 16 March 2017).

48. Goldenberg AJ, Sharp RR. The ethical hazards and programmatic challenges of genomic newborn screening. JAMA. 2012;307(5). Available at: https://doi.org/10.1001/jama.2012.68. Available at: https://www.ncbi.nlm.nih.gov/pmc/articles/PMC3868436/pdf/nihms513756.pdf (accessed 12 September 2017).

49. Gomes S, Lopes C, Pinto E. Folate and folic acid in the periconceptional period: recommendations from official health organizations in thirty-six countries worldwide and WHO. Public Health Nutr. 2016;19(1):176−189. Available at: https://www.ncbi.nlm.nih.gov/pubmed/25877429 (accessed 16 March 2017).

50. Gonzalez J, Willis MS. Ivar Asbjörn Følling: discovered Phenylketonuria (PKU). Lab Med. 2010;41(2):118−119. Available at: https://doi.org/10.1309/LM62LVV5OSLUJOQF (accessed 3 October 2017).

51. Graves JC, Miller KE. Maternal serum triple analyte screening in pregnancy. Am Fam Physician. 2002;65(5):915−921. Available at: http://www.aafp.org/afp/2002/0301/p915.html (accessed 16 March 2017).

52. Grosse SD, Berry RJ, Tilford JM, Kucik JE, Waitzman NJ. Retrospective assessment of cost savings from prevention: folic acid fortification and spina bifida in the US. Am J Prev Med. 2016;50(5):S74−S80. Available at: http://www.sciencedirect.com/science/article/pii/S0749379715006893 (accessed 16 March 2017).

53. Grover JK, Vats V, Gopalakrishna R, Ramam M. Thalidomide: a re-look. Natl Med J India. 2000;13(3):132−141. Available at: https://www.ncbi.nlm.nih.gov/pubmed/11558112 (accessed 16 March 2017).

54. Guthrie P. Life happens, science follows. The Robert Guthrie Legacy Project. Available at: http://www.robertguthriepku.org/newborn-screening/ (accessed 5 February 2018).

55. Hamburg M. 50 years after thalidomide: why regulation matters, posted on February 7, 2012 by US FDAVoice. Available at: http://blogs.fda.gov/fdavoice/index.php/2012/02/50-years-after-thalidomide-why-regulation-matters/ (accessed 16 March 2017).

56. Honein MA, Paulozzi LJ, Mathews TJ, Erickson JD, Wong LY, et al. Impact of folic acid fortification of the US food supply on the occurrence of neural tube defects. JAMA. 2001;285(23):2981−2986. Abstract available at: https://www.ncbi.nlm.nih.gov/pubmed/11410096 (accessed 11 June 2017).

57. Howson CP, Kinney MV, Lawn JE. Born too soon: the global action report on preterm birth. The March of Dimes Foundation, PMNCH, Save the Children, World Health Organization, 2012. Available at: http://www.who.int/pmnch/media/news/2012/preterm_birth_report/en/ (accessed 9 Mar 2017).

58. Institute of Clinical and Economic Review. Gene therapy: understanding the science, assessing the evidence, and paying for value: a report from the 2016 ICER membership policy summit, March 2017. Available at: https://icer-review.org/material/white-paper-gene-therapy/ (accessed 11 June 2017).

59. Jägerstad M. Folic acid fortification prevents neural tube defects and may also reduce cancer risks. Acta Paediatr. 2012;101(10):1007−1012. Available at: http://onlinelibrary.wiley.com/doi/10.1111/j.1651-2227.2012.02781.x/epdf (accessed 16 March 2017).

60. Kaye CI; Committee on Genetics, Accurso F, La Franchi S, Lane PA, Northrup H, Pang S, Schaefer GB. Introduction to the newborn screening fact sheets. Pediatrics. 2006;118 (3):1304−1312. Abstract available at: https://www.ncbi.nlm.nih.gov/pubmed/16960984 (accessed 9 July 2017).

61. Kirby RS. Population surveillance for microcephaly. BMJ 2016;354:i4815. Available at: http://www.bmj.com/content/354/bmj.i4815 (accessed 14 July 2017).

62. Khoshnood B, Loane M, de Walle H, Arriola L, Addor MC, Barisic I, et al. Long term trends in prevalence of neural tube defects in Europe: population based study. BMJ. 2015;351:h5949. Available at: https://www.ncbi.nlm.nih.gov/pmc/articles/PMC4658393/ (accessed 16 March 2017).

63. LaFranchi SH. Worldwide coverage of newborn screening for congenital hypothyroidism: a public health challenge. US Endocrinol. 2014;10(2):115−116. Available at: https://www.touchendocrinology.com/wp-content/uploads/sites/5/2015/07/StephenHLaFranchi_0.pdf (accessed 16 March 2017).

64. Lawn JE, Cousens S, Zupan J. Lancet neonatal survival steering team. 4 million neonatal deaths: when? where? why? neonatal survival series #1. Lancet. 2005;365(9462):891−900. Abstract available at: https://www.ncbi.nlm.nih.gov/pubmed/15752534 (accessed 16 March 2017).

65. Leger J, Olivieri A, Donaldson M, Torresani T, Krude H, van Vliet G, et al. European Society for Paediatric Endocrinology consensus guidelines on screening, diagnosis, and management of congenital hypothyroidism. J Clin Endocrinol Metab. 2014;99(2):363−384. Available at: https://www.ncbi.nlm.nih.gov/pmc/articles/PMC4207909/ (accessed 16 March 2017).

66. Li X, Dumolard L, Patel M, Gacic-Dobo M, Hennessey K. Implementation of hepatitis B birth dose vaccination − worldwide, 2016. Wkly Epid Rec WER. 2018;93:61−72. Available at: http://apps.who.int/iris/bitstream/10665/260207/1/WER9307.pdf (accessed 16 February 2018).

67. Lloyd-Puryear MA, Tonniges T, van Dyck PC, Mann MY, Brin A, Johnson K, et al. American Academy of Pediatrics Newborn Screening Task Force recommendations:

how far have we come? Pediatrics. 2006;117(5 Pt 2):S194–S211. Available at: http://pedi-atrics.aappublications.org/content/117/Supplement_3/S194.long (accessed 16 March 2017).

68. Loane M, Morris JK, Addor M-C3, Arriola L, Budd J, Doray B, et al. Twenty-year trends in the prevalence of Down syndrome and other trisomies in Europe: impact of maternal age and prenatal screening. Eur J Human Genetics. 2013;21:27–33. doi:10.1038/ejhg.2012.94; Available at: https://www.ncbi.nlm.nih.gov/pmc/articles/PMC3522199/pdf/ejhg201294a.pdf (accessed 14 July 2017).

69. Loeber JG, Burgard P, Cornel MC, Rigter T, Weinreich SS, Rupp K, et al. Newborn screen-ing programmes in Europe; arguments and efforts regarding harmonization. Part 1-from blood spot to screening result. J Inherited Metab Dis. 2012;35(4):603–611. Abstract avail-able at: https://www.ncbi.nlm.nih.gov/pubmed/22552820 (accessed 9 July 2017).

70. Lopez-Camelo JS, Orioli IM, da Graca Dutra M, Nazer-Herrera J, Rivera N, Ojeda ME, et al. Reduction of birth prevalence rates of neural tube defects after folic acid fortification in Chile. Am J Med Genet A. 2005;135(2):120–125. Abstract available at: https://www.ncbi.nlm.nih.gov/pubmed/15846825 (accessed 16 March 2017).

71. Lupton C, Burd L, Harwood R. Cost of fetal alcohol spectrum disorders. Am J Med Genet C Semin Med Genet. 2004;127C(1):42–50. Abstract available at: https://www.ncbi.nlm.nih.gov/pubmed/15095471 (accessed 16 March 2017).

72. Mai CT, Kucik JE, Isenburg J, Feldkamp ML, Mareng LK, Bugenske EM, et al. Selected birth defects data from population-based birth defects surveillance programs in the United States, 2006 to 2010: featuring trisomy conditions. Birth Defects Res A Clin Mol Teratol. 2013;97(11):709–725. Available at: https://www.ncbi.nlm.nih.gov/pmc/articles/PMC4636004/pdf/nihms702834.pdf (accessed 21 August 2017).

73. March of Dimes. Website 2017. Available at: http://www.marchofdimes.org/ (accessed 16 March 2017).

74. Mathews TJ. Trends in spina bifida and anencephalus in the United States, 1991–2006. National Center for Health Statistics, April 2009. Available at: http://www.cdc.gov/nchs/data/hestat/spine_anen/spine_anen.pdf (accessed 16 March 2017).

75. May PA, Chambers CD, Kalberg WO, Zellner J, Feldman H, Buckley D, et al. Prevalence of fetal alcohol spectrum disorders in 4 US communities. JAMA. 2018;319(5):474–482. Available at: https://doi.org/10.1001/jama.2017.21896. Abstract available at: https://jamanetwork.com/journals/jama/article-abstract/2671465?utm_source = silverchair&utm_medium = email&utm_campaign = article_alert-jama&utm_content = etoc&utm_term = 020618&redirect = true (accessed 7 February 2018).

76. McNulty B, Pentieva K, Marshall B, Ward M, Molloy AM, Scott JM, McNulty H. Women's compliance with current folic acid recommendations and achievement of optimal vitamin sta-tus for preventing neural tube defects. Hum Reprod. 2011;(6), 1530–1536. Available at: https://www.ncbi.nlm.nih.gov/pubmed/21441543 (accessed 14 March 2017).

77. MedlinePlus. G-6-phosphate dehydrogenase test, 2017. Available at: https://medlineplus.gov/ency/article/003671.htm (accessed 16 March 2017).

78. Modell B, Darilson M. Global epidemiology of haemoglobin disorders and derived service indicators. Bull World Health Organ. 2008;86(6):480–487. Available at: http://www.who.int/bulletin/volumes/86/6/06-036673/en/ (accessed 16 March 2017).

79. MRC Vitamin Study Research Group. Prevention of neural tube defects: results of the Medical Research Council Vitamin Study. Lancet. 1991;338:131–137. Abstract available at: https://www.ncbi.nlm.nih.gov/pubmed/1677062 (accessed 3 February 2018).

80. National Center on Birth Defects and Developmental Disabilities. Strategic plan 2011–2015. Atlanta, GA: Centers for Disease Control and Prevention, February 2011.

Available at: http://www.cdc.gov/NCBDDD/AboutUs/documents/NCBDDD_StrategicPlan_ 2-10-11.pdf (accessed 16 March 2017).

81. National Institute of Health, MedlinePlus. Gaucher disease, updated March 9, 2017. Available at: https://medlineplus.gov/ency/article/000564.htm (accessed 16 March 2017).

82. Oakley GP, Tulchinsky TH. Folic acid and vitamin B12 fortification of flour: a global basic food security requirement. Public Health Reviews. 2010;32(1):284−295. Available at: https://www.biomedcentral.com/track/pdf/10.1007/BF03391603?site=publichealthre-views.biomedcentral.com (accessed 5 February 2018).

83. Parker SE, Mai CT, Canfield MA, et al. Updated national birth prevalence estimates for selected birth defects in the United States, 2004−2006. Birth Defects Res A Clin Mol Teratol. 2010;88:1008−1016. Available at: http://onlinelibrary.wiley.com/doi/10.1002/ bdra.20735/abstract (accessed 14 July 2017).

84. Perera F, Herbstman J. Prenatal environmental exposures, epigenetics, and disease. Reprod Toxicol. 2011;31(3):363−373. Available at: https://www.ncbi.nlm.nih.gov/pmc/articles/ PMC3171169/ (accessed 16 March 2017).

85. PKU Test in History. Everything about Phenylketonuria, 9 March 2011. Available at: http://www.pkutest.com/2011/03/09/what-is-pku-test/ (accessed 12 September 2017).

86. Pyeritz RE, Tumpson JE, Bernhardt BA. The economics of clinical genetics services. I. Preview. Summary. Am J Hum Genet. 1987;41:549−558. Available at: https://www. ncbi.nlm.nih.gov/pmc/articles/PMC1684311/pdf/ajhg00133-0037.pdf (accessed 16 March 2017).

87. Rajaratnam JK, Marcus JR, Flaxman AD, Wang H, Levin-Rector A, Dwyer L, et al. Neonatal, postneonatal, childhood, and under-5 mortality for 187 countries, 1970−2010: a systematic analysis of progress towards Millennium Development Goal 4. Lancet. 2010;375(9730):1988−2008. Abstract available at: https://www.ncbi.nlm.nih.gov/pubmed/ 20546887 (accessed 16 March 2017).

88. Rasmussen SA, Jamieson DJ, Honein MA, Peterson LR. Zika virus and birth defects— reviewing the evidence for causality. N Engl J Med. 2016;374:1981−1987. Available at: http://www.nejm.org/doi/full/10.1056/NEJMsr1604338 (accessed 16 March 2017).

89. Rodwell C, Aymé S (editors). 2014 report on the state of the art of rare disease activities in Europe, July 2014. Available at: http://www.eucerd.eu/upload/file/Reports/ 2014ReportStateofArtRDActivitiesV.pdf (accessed 14 July 2017).

90. Rose SR, Brown RS, Wilkins L, (American Academy of Pediatrics, American Thyroid Association, Pediatric Endocrine Society). Update of newborn screening and therapy for congenital hypothyroidism. Pediatrics 2006;117(6):2290-2303. doi:10.1542/peds.2006-0915. Abstract available at: http://pediatrics.aappublications.org/content/117/6/2290.short (accessed 21 August 2017).

91. Ryan-Harshman M, Aldoori W. Folic acid and prevention of neural tube defects. Can Fam Physician. 2008;54(1):36−38. Available at: https://www.ncbi.nlm.nih.gov/pmc/articles/ PMC2329900/ (accessed 16 March 2017).

92. Save Babies Through Screening Foundation. Newborn screening. Available at: http://save-babies.org/video.html (accessed 16 March 2017).

93. Schalock RL, Borthwick-Duffy S, Bradley VJ, et al. Intellectual disability: definition, classi-fication, and systems of supports. 11th edition. Washington, DC: American Association on Intellectual and Developmental Disabilities, 2010. Available at: https://aaidd.org/publications/ bookstore-home/product-listing/intellectual-disability-definition-classification-and-systems-of-supports-(11th-edition)#.WXDQQYTys4g (accessed 20 July 2017).

94. Schulte R, Jordan LC, Morad A, Naftel RP, Wellons JC, Sidonio R. Rise in late onset vita-min K deviancy bleeding in young infants because of omission or refusal of prophylaxis at

birth. Pediatr Neurol. 2014;50(6):264–568. Abstract available at: http://www.pedneur.com/article/S0887-8994(14)00141-6/pdf (accessed 16 March 2017).

95. Scotet V, Duguépéroux I, Saliou P, Rault G, Roussey M, Audrézet MP, et al. Evidence for decline in the incidence of cystic fibrosis: a 35-year observational study in Brittany, France. Orphanet J Rare Dis. 2012;7:14. doi:10.1186/1750-1172-7-14. Available at: https://www.ncbi.nlm.nih.gov/pmc/articles/PMC3310838/ (accessed 16 March 2017).

96. Simeone RM, Oster ME, Cassell CH, Armour BS, Gray DT, Honein MA. Pediatric inpatient resource use for congenital heart defects. Birth Defects Res A Clin Mol Teratol. 2014;100(12):934–943. Available at: https://www.ncbi.nlm.nih.gov/pmc/articles/PMC4422978/ (accessed 5 February 2018).

97. Simopoulos AP. Genetic screening: programs, principles, and research – thirty years later: reviewing the recommendations of the committee for the study of inborn errors of metabolism (SIEM). Public Health Genomics. 2009;12(2):105–111. Available at: https://www.karger.com/Article/Pdf/156114 (accessed 16 March 2017).

98. Sly PD, Brennan S, Gangell C, de Klerk N, Murray C, Mott L, et al. Lung disease at diagnosis in infants with cystic fibrosis detected by newborn screening. Am J Respir Crit Care Med. 2009;180(2):146–152. Available at: http://www.atsjournals.org/doi/abs/10.1164/rccm.200901-0069OC#readcube-epdf (accessed 16 March 2017).

99. Snodgrass SD, Poissant TM, Thomas AR. Notes from the field: underreporting of maternal hepatitis C virus infection status and the need for infant testing—Oregon, 2015. MMWR Morb Mortal Wkly Rep. 2018;67:201–202. Available at: https://doi.org/10.15585/mmwr.mm6706a6. Available at: https://www.cdc.gov/mmwr/volumes/67/wr/mm6706a6.htm?s_cid=mm6706a6_e (accessed 16 February 2018).

100. So SA, Urbano RC, Hodapp RM. Hospitalizations of infants and young children with Down syndrome: evidence from inpatient person-records from a statewide administrative database. J Intellect Disabil Res. 2007;51(Pt 12):1030–1038. Available at: https://www.ncbi.nlm.nih.gov/pubmed/17991010 (accessed 18 March 2017).

101. Steinburg SJ, Moser AB, Raymond GV. X-linked adrenoleukodystrophy (X-ALD). Gene Rev (Internet), update April 9, 2015. Available at: https://www.ncbi.nlm.nih.gov/books/NBK1315/ (accessed 16 March 2017).

102. Stephenson A, Sykes J, Stanojevic S, Quon BS, Marshall BC, Petren K, et al. Survival comparison of patients with cystic fibrosis in Canada and the United States: a population-based cohort study. Ann Intern Med. 2017;166(8):537–546. doi:10.7326/M16-0858. Abstract available at: http://annals.org/aim/article/2609289/survival-comparison-patients-cystic-fibrosis-canada-united-states-population-based (accessed 16 March 2017).

103. Sustainable Development Goals. The global strategy for women's, children's and adolescents' health: survive, thrive, transform (2016–2030). New York: United Nations, 2015. Available at: http://globalstrategy.everywomaneverychild.org/ (accessed 16 March 2017).

104. Tan CH, Denny CH, Cheal NE, Sniezek GE, Kanny D. Alcohol use and binge drinking among women of childbearing age—United States, 2011–2013. MMWR Morb Mortal Wkly Rep. 2015;64(37):1042–1046. Available at: https://www.cdc.gov/mmwr/preview/mmwrhtml/mm6437a3.htm (accessed 16 March 2017).

105. Tong VT, Farr SL, Bombard JD, D'Angelo D, Ko JY, England LJ. Smoking before and during pregnancy among women reporting depression or anxiety. Obstet Gynecol. 2016;128(3):562–570. Available at: https://www.ncbi.nlm.nih.gov/pmc/articles/PMC5013536/ (accessed 5 February 2018).

106. Tulchinsky TH, Patton MM, Randolph LA, Myer MR, Linden JV. Mandating vitamin K prophylaxis for newborns in New York State. Am J Public Health. 1993;83 (8):1166–1168. Available at: https://www.ncbi.nlm.nih.gov/pmc/articles/PMC1695173/ pdf/amjph00532-0096.pdf (accessed 16 March 2017).

107. UNICEF. State of the world's children 2016: a fair chance for every child. New York: United Nations Children's Fund, 2016. Available at: http://www.unicef.org/sowc2016/ (accessed 16 March 2017).

108. United Nations. Convention on the rights of persons with disabilities. Available at: http:// www.ohchr.org/EN/HRBodies/CRPD/Pages/ConventionRightsPersonsWithDisabilities.aspx (accessed 16 March 2017).

109. United Nations Human Rights. Convention on the rights of the child, 1990. Available at: http://www.ohchr.org/EN/ProfessionalInterest/Pages/CRC.aspx (accessed 16 March 2017).

110. US Department of Health and Human Services. Advisory Committee on Heritable Disorders in Newborns and Children. Recommended uniform screening panel, November 2016. Available at: https://www.hrsa.gov/advisorycommittees/mchbadvisory/ heritabledisorders/recommendedpanel/ (accessed 16 March 2017).

111. US Department Health and Human Services. Human Genome Research Institute. What are the next steps in genomic research? March 14, 2017. Available at: https://ghr.nlm.nih. gov/primer/genomicresearch/nextsteps (accessed 18 March 2017).

112. US National Library of Medicine. Genetic Home Reference. Glucose-6-dphosphate dehydrogenase deficiency, March 14, 2017. Available at: https://ghr.nlm.nih.gov/condition/ glucose-6-phosphate-dehydrogenase-deficiency (accessed 16 March 2017).

113. US National Library of Medicine. Genetic Home Reference. Down syndrome, July 17, 2017. Available at: https://ghr.nlm.nih.gov/condition/down-syndrome (accessed 16 March 2017).

114. US National Library of Medicine. Gaucher disease, updated July 5, 2017. Available at: https://medlineplus.gov/ency/article/000564.htm (accessed 16 March 2017).

115. Vanderbilt AA, Wright MS. Infant mortality: a call to action overcoming health disparities in the United States. Med Educ Online. 2013;18:22503. doi:10.3402/meo. v18i0.22503. Available at: https://www.ncbi.nlm.nih.gov/pmc/articles/PMC3772318/pdf/ MEO-18-22503.pdf (accessed 5 February 2018).

116. Walani SR, Biermann J. March of Dimes Foundation: leading the way to birth defects prevention. Public Health Rev. 2017;38:12. Available at: https://publichealthreviews.bio-medcentral.com/articles/10.1186/s40985-017-0058-3 (accessed 9 July 2017).

117. Wald N, Leck I (editors). Antenatal and neonatal screening, second edition. Oxford University Press 2000, pp. 573. ISBN: 019-262826-7.

118. Wald NJ, the Vitamin Study Research Group Medical Research Council (MRC). Prevention of neural tube defects: results of the Medical Research Council vitamin study. Lancet. 1991;338(8760):131–137. Abstract available at: http://www.thelancet.com/journals/ lancet/article/PII0140-6736(91)90133-A/fulltext (accessed 5 February 2018).

119. Wald NJ. Folic acid and the prevention of neural-tube defects. N Engl J Med. 2004;350 (2):101–103. Available at: http://www.nejm.org/doi/full/10.1056/NEJMp038186 (accessed 5 February 2018).

120. Wald NJ. The cause of neural tube defects—a journey of discovery and the challenge of prevention. Hamdan Med J. 2012;5:285–292. Available at: http://hamdanjournal.org/journal/ index.php?journal=HAMDAN&page=article&op=view&path%5B%5D=211&path% 5B%5D=pdf (accessed 16 March 2017).

121. Wald NJ, Morris JK, Blakemore C. Public health failure in the prevention of neural tube defects: time to abandon the tolerable upper intake level of folate. Public Health Reviews.

2018;39(2). Available at: https://doi.org/10.1186/s40985-018-0079-6. Available at: https://publichealthreviews.biomedcentral.com/articles/10.1186/s40985-018-0079-6 (accessed 31 January 2018).

122. Wappner R, Cho S, Kronmal RA, Schuett V, Seashore MR. Management of phenylketonuria for optimal outcome: a review of guidelines for phenylketonuria management and a report of surveys of parents, patients, and clinic directors. Pediatrics. 1999;104(6):e68. Available at: http://pediatrics.aappublications.org/content/pediatrics/104/6/e68.full.pdf (accessed 16 March 2017).

123. Wang H, Bhutta Z, Coates MM, Coggeshall M, Dandona L, Diallo K, et al. GBD 2015 Child Mortality Collaborators. Global, regional, national, and selected subnational levels of stillbirths, neonatal, infant, and under-5 mortality, 1980–2015: a systematic analysis for the Global Burden of Disease Study 2015. Lancet. 2016;388(10053):1725–1774. Available at: http://www.thelancet.com/journals/lancet/article/PIIS0140-6736(16)31575-6/fulltext (accessed 5 February 2018).

124. Watson MS, Mann MY, Lloyd-Puryear MA, Rinaldo P, Howell RR, editors. American College of Medical Genetics Newborn Screening Expert Group. Newborn screening: toward a uniform screening panel and system–executive summary. Pediatrics 2006;117(5):S296–S307. Available at: http://pediatrics.aappublications.org/content/117/Supplement_3/S296.long (accessed 16 December 2017).

125. WHO/CDC/ICBDSR. Birth defects surveillance: atlas of selected congenital anomalies. Geneva, Switzerland: WHO, 2014. Available at: http://apps.who.int/iris/handle/10665/127941 and available at: http://apps.who.int/iris/bitstream/10665/127941/1/9789241564762_eng.pdf?ua=1 (accessed 16 March 2017).

126. Williams J, Mai CT, Mulinare J, Isenburg J, Flood TJ, Ethen M, et al. Updated estimates of neural tube defects prevented by mandatory folic acid fortification—United States, 1995–2011. Centers for Disease Control and Prevention. MMWR Morb Mort Wkly Rev. 2015;64(01):1–5. Available at: https://www.cdc.gov/mmwr/preview/mmwrhtml/mm6401a2.htm (accessed 9 July 2017).

127. Wilson, JMG, Jungner G. The principles and practice of screening for disease. Public Health Papers no. 34. Geneva: World Health Organization Geneva, 1968. (p. 26). Available at: http://apps.who.int/iris/bitstream/10665/37650/17/WHO_PHP_34.pdf (accessed 14 July 2017).

128. World Health Organization 63rd Assembly, Agenda Item 11.7. Birth defects, 21 May 2010. Available at: http://apps.who.int/gb/ebwha/pdf_files/WHA63/A63_R17-en.pdf (accessed 3 June 2017).

129. World Health Organization. WHO statement on the first meeting of the International Health Regulations (2005) (IHR 2005) Emergency Committee on Zika virus and observed increase in neurological disorders and neonatal malformations. WHO statement, February 1, 2016. Available at: http://www.who.int/mediacentre/news/statements/2016/1st-emergency-committee-zika/en/ (accessed 18 March 2017).

130. World Health Organization. Congenital anomalies: fact sheet, updated September 2016. Available at: http://www.who.int/mediacentre/factsheets/fs370/en/ (accessed 16 March 2017).

131. World Health Organization. Preterm birth fact sheet, updated November 2017. Available at: http://www.who.int/mediacentre/factsheets/fs363/en/ (accessed 12 February 2018).

132. World Health Organization. Human genomics in global health. WHO definitions of genetics and genomics, 2017. Available at: http://www.who.int/genomics/geneticsVSgenomics/en/ (accessed 18 March 2017).

133. World Heath Organization. Birth defects around the world. Page last updated 12 April 2017. Available at: https://www.cdc.gov/features/birth-defects-day/index.html (accessed 8 December 2017).

134. World Health Organization. WHO guidelines: maternal, reproductive and women's health. Geneva, Switzerland: WHO, 2013. Available at: http://www.who.int/publications/ guidelines/reproductive_health/en/ (accessed 16 March 2017).

135. World Health Organization. Maternal, newborn, child and adolescent health, 2017. Available at: http://www.who.int/maternal_child_adolescent/en/ (accessed 16 March 2017).

136. Yi Y, Lindemann M, Colligs A, Snowball C. Economic burden of neural tube defects and impact of prevention with folic acid: a literature review. Eur J Pediatr. 2011;170 (11):1391–1400. Available at: https://www.ncbi.nlm.nih.gov/pmc/articles/PMC3197907/ (accessed 5 February 2018).

137. Zaganjor I, Sekkarie A, Tsang BL, Williams J, Razzaghi H, Mulinare J, et al. Describing the prevalence of neural tube defects worldwide: a systematic literature review. PLoS One. 2016;11(4):e0151586. doi:10.1371/journal.pone.0151586. Available at: http://journals.plos. org/plosone/article?id = 10.1371%2Fjournal.pone.0151586 (accessed 31 July 2017).

138. Zipursky A. Prevention of vitamin K deficiency bleeding in newborns. Br J Haematol. 1999;1064:430–437. Available at: http://onlinelibrary.wiley.com/doi/10.1046/j.1365-2141.1999.01104.x/epdf (accessed 16 March 2017).

Chapter 21

Marc Lalonde, the Health Field Concept and Health Promotion

ABSTRACT

During the 20th century, public health evolved with increasing capacity for disease prevention as scientific breakthroughs occurred in microbiology, immunology, nutrition, and other sciences. Disease-control advanced and new epidemiologic evidence identified risk factors for the growing burden of noncommunicable diseases such as the cardiovascular diseases, cancer, and others. Medical care also improved and became more accessible through health insurance systems both in the private and governmental sector. Health systems became more combined public–private endeavors, with health insurance for medical- and hospital-care taking center stage.

Epidemiology blossomed as a science following World War II, producing vital insights and evidence of contributory factors to noncommunicable diseases. In the 1960s the cumulative evidence of smoking as a direct cause of lung cancer and heart disease was identified as a major public health challenge. These relationships became clear and increasingly accepted after the US Surgeon General's Report in 1964.

In 1974, Hon. Marc Lalonde, Canada's Minister of National Health and Welfare issued the book A New Perspective on the Health of Canadians, which identified genetic, environmental, personal lifestyle, and medical care as equally important issues in personal and population health.

New Perspectives led to the "Ottawa Charter" in 1986 which defined health promotion and has become a vital issue in public health. The health promotion movement immediately found a crucial role in smoking reduction and diet change to deal with the pandemics of lung cancer and heart disease. In the 1980s health promotion found itself at the frontline dealing with the HIV pandemic when there were no biomedical means to stem the pandemic of death from AIDS. Public health had to find new and effective instruments for disease control. A renewed emphasis on social inequalities in health in the 21st century exemplified in the Millennium Development Goals (MDGs) addressed vulnerable populations with linked targets of reducing poverty, promoting education and gender equality, safer environment, and biomedical disease-control measures as global health policy. This more holistic approach to population health has become a leading element in modern public health largely based on the intellectual contribution of Marc Lalonde.

Case Studies in Public Health. DOI: http://dx.doi.org/10.1016/B978-0-12-804571-8.00028-7

523

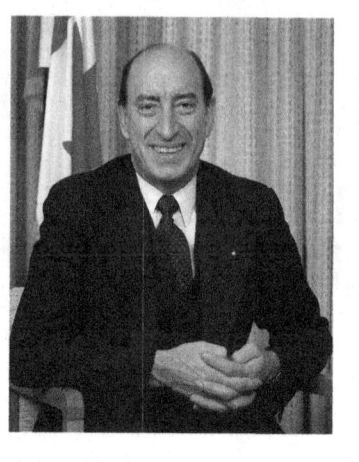

Honorable Marc Lalonde, PC, OC, QC, LLL, MA, Minister of National Health and Welfare, Canada, 1972–77. He was responsible for *A New Perspective on the Health of Canadians* in 1974. Photo provided by Mr LaLonde with personal permission, 2017.

BACKGROUND

Marc Lalonde was born in 1929 at Île Perrot, Quebec, and obtained a Master of Law degree from the Université de Montréal, a master's degree from Oxford University, and a further diploma from the University of Ottawa. He served in 1959 as special advisor to the federal Justice Minister of Canada and then moved to practice law in Montreal returning to Ottawa in 1967 as an advisor in the Prime Minister's Office under Liberal Prime Minister Lester B. Pearson. He remained when Pierre Trudeau became Prime Minister of Canada in 1968, serving as Principal Secretary. Lalonde entered federal politics in 1972, was elected as a Liberal Member of Parliament for Quebec, and joined the Cabinet as Minister of National Health and Welfare. During 1972–77 he served as Minister of National Health and Welfare and in 1974 published a landmark document *A New Perspective on the Health of Canadians* that brought him international renown. This document was the cornerstone for the reconceptualization of public health policy, as it has evolved since its publication.

After serving in various other ministerial positions, Lalonde retired as a Cabinet minister in 1984 and currently practices law in Montreal. In 1989, he was made an Officer of the Order of Canada and in 2004 he was inducted into the Canadian Medical Hall of Fame. In 1988, he received the World Health Organization Medal for *"exceptional contribution to health policy"* and in 2002 he was honored by the Pan American Health Organization (PAHO). As part of its 100th anniversary celebration, Lalonde was named by PAHO as one of 12 *"Public Health Heroes of the Americas, in recognition of their noteworthy contributions to public health in the Region of the Americas."*

A New Perspective on the Health of Canadians is widely regarded as a ground-breaking document issued by a government recognizing that other strategies beyond biomedical methods are needed to improve the health of a population. The *New Perspective* document introduced what was called the Health Field Concept that health is a result of four major elements: human biology, health care systems, environment, and lifestyle. In Canada, and many other countries, the focus of health policies in those days was on health insurance for hospital and medical care. Public health was marginal in priority, but awareness was growing from research on smoking and other cardiovascular disease risk factors, such as emerged from research in Britain on smoking, lung cancer, and the many other studies of risk factors for cardiovascular diseases (see Chapter 14). The landmark publication of the US Surgeon General's Report on Smoking in 1964, the Framingham study in Massachusetts, and others indicated that many of the key risk factors for disease were due to lifestyle issues, i.e. personal habits influenced by societal factors including diet, smoking, and exercise as well as access to medical care. New Perspectives proved to be a major contribution to public health policy generally providing the basis for the health promotion movement which became a fundamental element of current public health globally.

The traditional approach to health as generally accepted in the 1960–70s focused on advancement in the science and practice of medicine as the major tools for improvements in health. National health insurance enables people to access medical care and hospital care, along with the biomedical instruments of public health such as sanitation and immunization. The level of a population's health was, justifiably, seen as dependent on access to and the quality of medical care. However, as a consequence, health policy was directed toward acute care hospital and physician-centered expenditures. Emphasis in Canada was on provincial Medicare plans of universal coverage hospital and medical insurance plans, and their financing with federal standards and cost sharing. Health promotion and disease prevention were of lower priority in Canada at that time, lacking schools of public health and a federal equivalent of the US Centers for Disease Control, with lack of political, media and public attention and public financing for public health (see Chapters 8 and 15).

Following a period of doubts and debate, Canada adopted the New Perspectives approach to become one of the leading countries in health promotion. The public dialogue that had been previously been dominated by concerns about universal health insurance, the costs and delivery of health care services, began to direct attention to other health issues, especially those relating to personal behaviors such as smoking, diet and physical activity as well as inequalities in universal health systems.

The World Health Organization (WHO) sponsored the famous 1978 Alma Ata Conference articulating a policy of "Health for All" with a focus on primary health care. The Alma Ata Declaration promoted global recognition of health needs and national orientation that health depends on more than medical care.

The First International Conference on Health Promotion, organized by WHO and held in Ottawa, Canada, in November 1986 largely stimulated by the Health Field Concept, produced a formal definition of health promotion which was to become a conceptual stimulus to development of a new discipline and major factor in public health policy. The Ottawa Charter adopted the basic Lalonde concepts, defining health promotion as: "*the process of enabling people to increase control over, and to improve, their health. To reach a state of complete physical, mental and social well-being, an individual or group must be able to identify and to realize aspirations, to satisfy needs, and to change or cope with the environment. Therefore, health promotion is not just the responsibility of the health sector, but goes beyond healthy lifestyles to well-being.*"

The Lalonde concept linked medical care, genetics, environment, and self-care, including the biomedical Germ, the environmental Miasma and the political Social Medicine theories of the 19th century. This promoted innovations in national and global health leading to major health achievements in all countries in the late 20th century and early 21st century. The concepts of New Perspectives were articulated operationally by global consensus in the Millennium Development Goals (MDGs, 2000−15), and the follow-up Sustainable Development Goals (SDGs, 2016−30). Both had specific health targets (reduced child and maternal mortality and addressing HIV, tuberculosis and other global disease issues), but in the context of poverty reduction, improved nutrition, education and environmental conditions, rights of women and social and economic advances.

In 1979 the United States issued health promotion guidelines with stated health targets. "Healthy People" was a landmark in the history of US public health, characterized as a document "*to encourage a second public health revolution.*" It reflected an emerging consensus among the health community that the nation's health strategy should emphasize the prevention of disease. This document has been periodically updated since then through a broad consultative process providing guidelines for preventive approaches to clinicians as well as public health organizations including state and local authorities. US national policy articulated health objectives for the nation with specific targets related to preventable conditions, and has sustained this approach with renewal of targets each decade since.

Concurrently, findings of research in epidemiology, health policy, and health economics, made it convincingly clear that investment in the promotion of health and prevention is cost-effective and more beneficial to improving quality of life than solely focusing health expenditures on medical care. It became increasingly accepted that the state has responsibility for the health of its citizens, and to allocate resources to carry out that responsibility. But Health Promotion also emphasizes the responsibility of the individual and the community, as well as medical care providers, to prevent adverse health conditions and events. The concept and challenge of individual behavior measures as an important part of the health field requires training, legislative, policy and fiscal support as a domain where health policy can act successfully to promote health and prevent avoidable disease.

New Perspectives demonstrated the limitations of predominant reliance on medical and hospital care for addressing the main causes of morbidity and mortality. The wider view of health, frankly addressed the importance of self-imposed and socio-economic and environmental risks as major factors in population health. The data clearly showed the main causes for morbidity and mortality related to preventable conditions. Considering that the Canadian health system was already one of the most advanced and accessible health systems at the time, Lalonde called for a wider holistic view of health with a focus on moderating self-imposed health risks, improving the environment and considering human genetics, as well as classical health care systems. In an acceptance speech to the PAHO meeting in 2002 on the 28th anniversary of the publication of *New Perspectives* awarding him the honor "Public Health Hero of the Americas," Lalonde put the issue this way:

> *"It is important to reassert the fundamental validity of the Health Field Concept and the interrelationship between its four components: human biology, environment, lifestyle, and health care organization. Although conceived in the context of an economically advanced country, the strength and the appeal of the Health Field Concept are its universal application. The specific plans of action would obviously need to reflect local conditions, but the general strategies are capable of application in developing as well as developed countries. New Perspective cannot be dismissed as a document of interest only to rich countries. If we really want to improve the health of our citizens, we cannot concentrate only on the health care organization."*

The Health Field Concept (HFC) brought a new emphasis to health thinking which had previously primarily focused on medical and hospital care with insurance to cover payment for those services as a national responsibility. The HFC articulated what was recognizable as a more holistic approach including the role of genetics, self-care, lifestyle habits and the environment, as well as medical care. The timing was important: it came a decade after the famous 1964 US Surgeon General's Report on Smoking which had a strong effect on public and legislator opinion with a growing public call for public law to control promotion and advertising of cigarette consumption, placing the powerful cigarette industry in a defensive mode which continued to deny the health threat.

The immediate Canadian response to *New Perspectives* was mixed, including apathy, charges of "blaming the victim," excuses for reducing federal financial support for costs of provincial health insurance plans, and various conspiracy theories. The "Lalonde doctrine" was criticized as deficient in unequivocal scientific evidence which would justify taking action against potentially harmful factors. The main challenge came from the health sector complaining of unsatisfactory evidence in certain issues. But at the same time, a growing flood of epidemiologic evidence identified risk factors and successful methods of intervention to prevent disease or consequences of disease such as smoking reduction, control of hypertension, poor diet, lack of exercise and others (see Chapter 14). New Perspectives was also criticized as overemphasizing lifestyle with little attention to environment including poverty, education, housing and other social inequalities. Moreover, health in Canada is a provincial responsibility, while the federal level had no clear public health structures to implement the recommendations of the report. Lessons learned later in Canada from the 2003 severe acute respiratory syndrome (SARS) epidemic led to development of the federal Public Health Agency of Canada, created in 2004 to develop capacity to anticipate and respond effectively to public health threats and to promote disease prevention. Similarly, in the same time period many regional laboratories and schools of public health sprang up across the country with a new public health orientation.

New Perspectives was received positively outside of Canada and to this day is recognized in Europe especially, as a game-changer for health policy, generating similar reports in Britain, Finland, Sweden, and the United States. The report remains a landmark contribution to the transformation in thinking about health that has occurred with the emergence of the health promotion movement.

Following publication of *New Perspectives*, Canada has continued taking an important international role in the discussion of health determinants as exemplified in the first International Conference on Health Promotion in Ottawa, Canada in 1986 and the Ottawa Charter. The Ottawa Charter defines prerequisites for health as the fundamental conditions and resources resulting from the social and physical environments. The means of action toward health promotion, as defined in the Charter, includes the creation of supportive environments and development of personal skills, hence enabling people to exercise more control over their own health context as well as make their personal and family lifestyle choices more conductive to health. This also requires reorientation of health services toward prevention and health promotion.

The Ottawa Charter called for a new direction for public health, with a pledge to health promotion:

- *"to move into the arena of healthy public policy, and to advocate a clear political commitment to health and equity in all sectors.*
- *to counteract the pressures toward harmful products, resource depletion, unhealthy living conditions and environments, and unhealthy nutrition; and to focus attention on public health issues such as pollution, occupational hazards, housing, and settlements.*
- *to respond to the health gap within and between societies, and to tackle the inequities in health produced by the rules and practices of these societies.*

- *to acknowledge people as the main health resource; to support and enable them to keep themselves, their families and friends healthy through financial and other means, and to accept the community as the essential voice in matters of its health, living conditions, and well-being.*
- *to reorient health services and their resources toward the promotion of health and primary prevention; and to share power with other sectors, other disciplines and, most importantly, with people themselves.*
- *to recognize health and its maintenance as a major social investment and challenge; and to address the overall ecological issue of our ways of living"* (Ottawa Charter for Health Promotion, 1986).

During the 1980s, new disease challenges were appearing with no bio-medical means of care let alone cure. HIV/AIDS was the classic case, but this was followed by hepatitis C and other conditions for which care was essentially palliative. In the early years of the AIDS pandemic, preventive care depended on health promotion initiatives to change unsafe sexual behavior and illicit drug practices to reduce transmission and stem the spread of the pandemic, with education, condom and needle distribution. This was the case while millions died of HIV/AIDS until the late 1990s when effective biomedical measures became available using powerful new classes of antiretroviral life saving drugs for treatment and prevention of transmission. Health promotion measures were the only real option in the form of partnership with the most vulnerable gay community in dealing with the growing pandemic of HIV and illicit drug use. Even in the second decade of the 21st century, health promotion is vital in AIDS control to promote preventive treatment for HIV-positive pregnant women and to reduce backsliding on safe sex practices among treated AIDS patients to reduce reappearance of other sexually transmitted diseases thought to have been controlled.

CURRENT RELEVANCE

The Health Field Concept marked an important leap forward from the traditional perception of health focused and funded mostly in terms of medical and hospital care toward a more inclusive approach. However, the *New Perspectives* definition of four health fields, by its very nature and as acknowledged in the report, is also limiting. The health field terminology has evolved to incorporating the term "holistic" health.

In order to give the proper attention required to health issues, a broad perspective is needed for recognition by national and international policy makers as reflected in policies and resource allocation. Planning for health has had many definitions incorporating the fundamentals of *New Perspectives*. The US Department of Health and Human Services, *Healthy People 2020* defines determinants of health as the social environment,

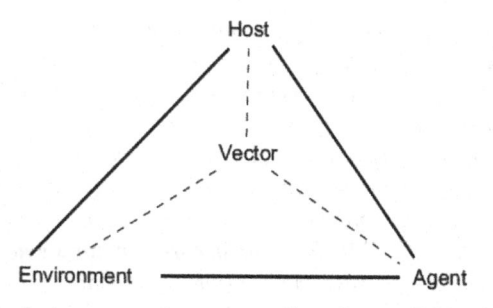

FIGURE 21.1   The host–agent–environment paradigm. Source: *Tulchinsky TH, Varavikova EA. The new public health. 3rd edition. San Diego, CA: Academic Press/Elsevier, 2014, p. 49.*

physical environment, genetic endowment, health care, and individual biological and behavioral factors. It distinguishes outcomes of disease, well-being, and prosperity and suggests a causal pathway linking determinants and outcomes. The Health in All Policies for state and local health departments in the United States focuses on:

- Promotion of health, equity, and sustainability;
- Support for intersectoral collaboration;
- Benefits from multiple partners;
- Engagement of stakeholders; and
- Creation of structural or procedural change, institutionalizing change in existing or new structures.

The classical epidemiologic triangle of host-agent-environment causation of disease based on the Germ Theory has proven to be dramatically successful in approaching and in many cases diminishing or even eradicating important infectious diseases such as smallpox, poliomyelitis, measles, and rubella. It has drastically reduced others such as HIV, malaria, and tuberculosis and even neglected tropical diseases (NTDs) such as onchocerciasis (river blindness), dracunculiasis (guinea worm disease), leprosy, and others. Since the period following World War II, evidence of new methods of interventions to reduce the heavy burden of cardiovascular disease and cancer by lifestyle and nutritional measures, and improved medical care, have shown remarkable success in reducing stroke, coronary heart disease mortality, and mortality from cancer of the lung, cervix, liver, stomach, and colon-rectum. The classical Germ Theory is represented in the epidemiologic triangle in Figure 21.1. Figure 21.2 represents the transition of single causation of disease to a multifactorial paradigm including genetics, personal life habits, and a broad range of other societal factors including socio-economic and physical environmental conditions. This might be seen as a transition from a purely biomedical model to a "renewed miasma theory," including sanitation, and an entire range of new health policy and Social Medicine as pioneered in the

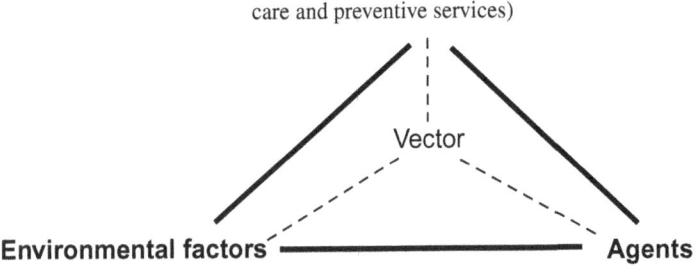

Host factors
(age, gender, genetics, nutrition, mental health, education, occupation, employment, family situation, socioeconomic status, residence, access to medical care and preventive services)

Vector

Environmental factors

(pollution of air, water, exposure to toxic, microbiological and vector growth factors, radiologic chemical exposure factors, socioeconomic and security environment, residence, employment, housing, poverty, inequality, lack of education.

Agents

(microbiological, chemical, physical, radiologic agents, employment risks, food safety and nutritional insecurity, war and insecurity factors.

FIGURE 21.2 The expanded host−agent−environment holistic paradigm. Source: *Tulchinsky TH, Varavikova EA. The new public health. 3rd edition. San Diego, CA: Academic Press/Elsevier, 2014, p.49.*

19th century by Rudolph Virchow in Germany. Finding common ground in a much broader holistic range of risk factors for the host-agent-environment paradigm has emerged with this transition stimulated by the Health Field Concept supported by great progress in evidence from epidemiology, medical sciences, and public health experience of success. The two figures represent the epidemiologic transition, which is often focused on evolution of predominance of infectious diseases to overwhelming dominance of noninfectious diseases over the past century.

Health in All Policies are being adopted and implemented in many jurisdictions in Europe and in the United States. The California-based Public Health Institute, as an example, conducts an extensive program of advocacy, research and consultation in developing climate control measures, healthy urban environments and many other aspects of healthy public policy. It has influenced state policies on many issues including vehicle emission standards, urban planning and others. The US Preventive Services Task Force (USPSTF) created in 1984 is an independent, volunteer panel of national experts in prevention- and evidence-based medicine. The Preventive Services Task Force works with wide consultative approaches to improve the health of all Americans by making evidence-based recommendations about clinical preventive services such as screening, counseling, and preventive medications, such as low dose aspirin, statins, and antihypertensive medications to people with risk factors for cardiovascular diseases, and vaccinations for pneumonia and influenza for the chronically ill, the elderly, pregnant women and many others. All recommendations are published online and/or in peer-reviewed journals. Similar organizations have been created in Britain, Sweden, and other countries to continuously update guidelines for preventive services with best available evidence. The United Kingdom NICE (National Institute for Health and Care Excellence) for clinical and policy guideline in the National Health Service, is followed by other countries as well.

ETHICAL ISSUES

Another downstream effect from *New Perspectives* is a return to the issue of inequalities in health including in countries with highly developed health insurance for national health services. Sir Michael Marmot, Research Professor of Epidemiology and Public Health, University College, London, famously led a research group on health inequalities for some 30 years. The Whitehall studies of British civil servants showed a striking inverse social gradient in morbidity and mortality providing evidence for the importance of reducing social inequalities in health. Marmot, who was knighted in 2000 for his outstanding epidemiological leadership, was the Chair of the Commission on Social Determinants of Health set up by the World Health Organization in 2005. This document's theme returned to earlier versions of Social Medicine seeing health as a political issue as promoted by Rudolph Virchow (1821–1902) a preeminent German medical scientist of the mid-19th century and pioneer developer of cellular pathology.

Virchow, who opposed the Germ Theory, Darwin's theory of evolution and the hand washing practices of Semmelweis, was a strong advocate of the idea that if living conditions could be improved, there would be fewer epidemics. Epidemics, he said, were best treated politically rather than medically and fostered the concept of Social Medicine that improving people's living conditions, hygiene, and diet would be highly beneficial to their general health and well-being. He considered health as a universal human aspiration and a basic human need. Marmot and The Commission on Social Determinants of Health renewed focus on the "causes of the causes" of health inequality as socially determined conditions in which people grow, live, work, and grow old. Ethical and economic issues together influenced the international consensus on the Millennium Development Goals and the Sustainable Development Goals.

Health promotion became a transformational element of public health generating strong advocacy and growing signs of success in anti-tobacco campaigns, and in addressing cancer and cardiovascular diseases with anti-smoking education and associated legal limitations on advertising, tobacco sales to minor children, smoking in public places and an higher cost of cigarettes by taxation, along with dietary change, exercise and biomedical care.

Health promotion became the only feasible public health activity when the HIV/AIDS epidemic storm arrived in the 1980s when there were no effective biomedical measures available. Health promotion provided some useful measures such as education, condom and syringe distribution, in high-risk groups to reduce the spread of the disease, until effective antiretroviral drugs came available in the late 1990s.

There is also a growing use of expanded data sets in health to show regional and individual health care process and outcome measures of morbidity and mortality. This provides a growing base for quality control and financial incentives for improvement as well as sanctions for poorer performance and outcome measures. Regional, social class status, and ethnic disparities in health have increasingly come to light even where universal access systems have been in place for many years such as in the United Kingdom, but also in the costliest health system in the world in the United States. These inequalities have important social, political and ethical implications for health policy.

ECONOMIC ISSUES

The World Bank since 1993 has promoted the economic value of improving equity in health in developing countries. The European Union has articulated a similar position for high-income countries that health investment improves economic growth (Suhrke and McKee 2006). This concept influenced the global consensus on the Millennium Development Goals and the follow-up Sustainable Development Goals. The burden of illness and its cost are high whether the payment is private, or by health insurance through place of work, or by governmental insurance or service systems (see Chapters 8 and 15). Many diseases once thought to be treatable but not preventable are now avoidable by self care, community action or by medical care whether immunizations or treatment of hypertension. The economic gains of preventing disease or the complications of disease are enormous. Investment in prevention thus gains economic rationale. This applies in countries at all economic levels. A payment system that covers medical care but excludes preventive services or public health promotion is behaving irrationally from an economic viewpoint. Thus health insurance systems adopt new methods of screening for cervical or colo-rectal cancer as part of their benefit system.

The World Health Organization (WHO) actively promotes Health in All Policies to address inequalities and society-based issues causing ill health including nutrition and food fortification. This includes many activities of State and local authorities, such as reducing air pollution, using sustainable clean fuels, home use of fuels, compact and efficient urban planning, construction standards for safe housing, low emission public transport, recreation and shopping facilities in urban neighborhoods. It also includes general sanitation, safe water and waste management including reduction in plastics use, and recycling/reuse. These activities require political leadership of state and local authorities with incentives to reduce poverty, unemployment, drug abuse, and pollution, and to improve urban planning, transportation, access to quality foods and other efforts to reduce inequality in health. Education and support systems to help people make healthy lifestyle choices are the crucial elements of modern public health.

The UN sponsored Millennium Development Goals (MDGs) developed by consensus of almost all nations in large part as a derivative of the *New Perspective's* holistic approach to health improvement globally in the context of social and environmental changes. Three of the eight goals established by consensus of 190 countries are specifically on health topics: reducing child mortality; reducing maternal mortality; and, combating HIV/AIDS, malaria, and other diseases. The other goals are reducing poverty; achieving universal primary education; reducing gender inequality and empowerment of women; ensure environmental sustainability; and, development of a global development partnership. The MDG achievements between 2000 and 2015 were remarkable, particularly in reducing poverty, child mortality, maternal mortality, increasing education accessibility especially for girls, access to safe water, management of HIV, malaria, tuberculosis, and others. This was achieved by the consensus of nations on the issues and building public–private cooperation between nations and donors, international aid and recognition that education, the social and physical environments, and public health are the crucial issues. The initiative was followed by Sustainable Development Goals (SDGs, 2015–30) which are even broader in scope, but recognizing that health is part of, and dependent on, many factors including access to medical care, again widely credited internationally in large part due the intellectual legacy of Marc Lalonde and the Health Field Concept of the *New Perspective*. The economic rationale for investment in prevention of chronic diseases is that there is proven track record of reducing cardiovascular and cancer deaths by relatively inexpensive intervention including those of health promotion, such as smoking and alcohol reduction, and those of biomedical intervention, such as low-dose aspirin, blood pressure control, immunizations, and nutritional fortification of basic foods. Cost utility studies for individual preventive interventions have become a necessary analysis for policy determination of priorities. WHO estimated in 2005 that an additional 2% reduction in chronic disease death rates worldwide, per year, over the next 10 years would prevent 36 million premature deaths by 2015, stating that the scientific knowledge to achieve this goal already exists (WHO, 2005). Global burden of disease studies indicate that behavioral, environmental and occupational, and metabolic risks can explain half of the global mortality providing many opportunities for prevention (Global Burden of Disease, 2015).

CONCLUSION

The Health Field Concept in the *New Perspective* in 1974 opened a new paradigm of public health thinking and policy that health is a benefit and resultant of a broad range of causes and responses to address those causes. The Health Field Concept was an articulation based on decades of research and controversy, with continuing expanding of biomedical capacity of medical care and vaccines, and with research defining risk factors for the major disease groups. Together these strongly influenced a true renaissance of public health, or what has been called The New Public Health.

The Health Field Concept articulated in *A New Perspective on the Health of Canadians* (1974) was one of the most influential health policy documents of the 20th century. It was a working paper addressing the concepts of health and the basic principles as a basis for health policy, but it indicated and led to a wider approach to public health policy. It marked a change in the way to perceive and promote a holistic approach to health, moving from a predominantly biomedical focus in the mid-twentieth century toward a wider view, including the examination of determinants in each of four health fields: human biology, lifestyle, health care organization, and the environment.

Lalonde's *New Perspective* challenged traditional views of health urging new health policies and priorities. It placed the individual as a key factor in his/her own health status, applying to the community level as well. It emphasized advocacy or health promotion and the development of prevention-oriented national health strategies involving personal and community health behavior including many aspects of the community physical and social environment. In modern terms, it is a 21st century balanced cohesion between the Germ and the Miasma theories or more broadly the biomedical and the sanitation and social hygiene movements of the 19th century.

The Health Field Concept was a major contributor to development of a new paradigm for public health. In this new articulation of health promotion, health protection, disease prevention including universal access to medical care, and long-term community care, are all of importance for population and individual health. There was also attention to the concept of vulnerable populations, based not only on individual behavioral, but also societal factors. This has implications for resource allocation and recognition of demographic and epidemiologic changes as well as important additions to public health capabilities with new vaccines to prevent infectious diseases and cancers, for example. The once-dominant position of hospitals and medical care in health spending has changed, with increased emphasis on community care, prevention and health promotion.

The global impact of a holistic concept of health was important in formulation of global health policy in the Millennium Development Goals and their achievements up to 2015, for the follow-up Sustainable Development

Goals for the years 2015—30, and new initiatives to reduce inequalities in health. The impact of New Perspectives also contributed to the movement led by Sir Michael Marmot to focus on reducing national and global inequalities in health. Lalonde's contribution to this process was of great significance to national and global health progress in stimulating a renaissance of the public health community and indeed population health, that is a work still in process.

Even the purest biomedical aspect of public health has implications for health promotion including different aspects, including legal, ethical, economic and public education, whether a topic is environmental impact on health, nutrition, prevention of cancer and cardiovascular diseases, vaccination policies or legal requirements for public health as is pasteurization of milk, or mandatory use of car seats for children. The principle issues outlined in the Health Field Concept and the 1986 Ottawa Charter on health promotion are essential to carry public health forward in the 21st century. This requires continuing advocacy of translation of public health policies into programs essential for protecting and improving population health for high-, medium- and low-income countries.

RECOMMENDATIONS

1. National and international leaders of government and organizations should apply the broadened Health Field Concept for adaptation and implementation for low, middle and high income countries especially for vulnerable population groups.
2. Decision makers and policy analysts should stress the elements of health promotion as defined in the Ottawa Charter including:
   - Building public health policy, including biomedical, epidemiological, ethical, legal and economic aspects;
   - Creating supportive environments by promoting public awareness and political support;
   - Strengthen community actions by working with local, regional, state and national authorities as well as voluntary organizations, and the private sector for promoting health on the public agenda;
   - Developing personal responsibility, skills and commitment to explain and advocate policies for promoting a health agenda;
3. Reorient health service priorities with continuous evaluation by studying quantitative and qualitative values of disease prevention and health promotion.
4. The fundamentals of the Health Field Concept should be incorporated in all basic training in public health and in ongoing in-service training, so that future managers and workers in all sectors of public health incorporate this orientation in planning and providing for current and future public health challenges.

5. Funding to academic institutions for implementing training programs, and transitional funding to health authorities to adapt these principles into re-orientation of health systems should be provided by national, state/provincial/regional and local government authorities.

6. Case studies of issues dealt with in public health primarily by health promotion approaches should be incorporated in study programs including continuing education.

7. Professional journals should be encouraged to require authors of scientific papers relevant to population health submitted for publication to include observations of potential translational aspects of the work in discussions of findings addressing the actual or potential relevance of the work to population health.

STUDENT REVIEW QUESTIONS

1. How does the gap between a biomedical model and health promotion aspects of the new public health reflect the 19th century conflict between the Germ, Miasma and Social Medicine theories?

2. How has each contributed to advancing population health over the past century and relevance in coming decades?

3. How was defining human behavior as a key factor in individual and population health a step forward in public health policy?

4. Give examples of important disease groups where individual behavior is a major contributory or causative factor.

5. How does health promotion fit with traditional topics of public health to create a "New Public Health"?

6. How does health promotion fit with climate change initiatives?

7. How does health promotion fit with traditional biomedical aspects of public health such as immunization and nutritional issues of micronutrient deficiencies?

8. What intervention principles are needed to mitigate health inequalities/disparities in countries with advanced universal healthcare systems with interventions based on population-health approaches?

RECOMMENDED READINGS

1. Axworthy L, Spiegel J. Retaining Canada's health care system as a global public good. CMAJ. 2002;167(4):365−366. Available at: http://www.cmaj.ca/content/167/4/365.full (accessed 28 January 2017).

2. Canadian Medical Hall of Fame. Hon Marc Lalonde, 2008. Available at: http://cdnmedhall. org/inductees/marclalonde (accessed 9 February 2018).

3. Catford J. The Bangkok Conference: steering countries to build national capacity for health promotion. Health Promot Int. 2005;20(1):1−6. Available at: https://academic.oup. com/heapro/article/20/1/1/797609 (accessed 9 February 2018).

4. Centers for Disease Control and Prevention. Health objectives for the nation. MMWR Morb Mort Wkly Rep. 1989;38(37);629–633. Available at: https://www.cdc.gov/mmwR/preview/mmwrhtml/00001462.htm (accessed 9 June 2017). 27

5. de Leeuw E, Tang KC, Beaglehole R. Ottawa to Bangkok—Health promotion's journey from principles to "glocal" implementation. Health Promotion Int. 2007;21(Suppl 1). http://doi.org/10.1093/heapro/dal057. Available at: https://pdfs.semanticscholar.org/ef45/6c2dc6214b84ef80af386887f971cf83abed.pdf (accessed 11 May 2017).

6. European Observatory. Health in all policies: seizing opportunities, implementing policies. Leppo K, Ollila E, Peña S, Wismar M, Cook S., editors. Geneva, Available at: http://www.euro.who.int/__data/assets/pdf_file/0007/188809/Health-in-All-Policies-final.pdf (accessed 28 January 2017).

7. Famous Scientists. Rudolf Virchow. Available at: www.famousscientists.org/rudolf-virchow/ (accessed 14 May 2017).

8. Friedman DJ, Starfield B. Models of population health: their value for US public health practice, policy, and research. Am J Public Health. 2003;93(3):366–369. Available at: https://www.ncbi.nlm.nih.gov/pmc/articles/PMC1447744/pdf/0930366.pdf (accessed 11 May 2017).

9. Frohlich KL, Potvin L. The inequality paradox: the population approach and vulnerable populations. Am J Public Health. 2008;98(2):216–221. Available at: http://health-equity.lib.umd.edu/935/1/Trancending_the_Known_in_Public_Health.pdf (accessed 6 May 2017).

10. Global Burden of Disease. Risk Factors Collaborators. Global, regional, and national comparative risk assessment of 79 behavioural, environmental and occupational, and metabolic risks or clusters of risks in 188 countries, 1990–2013: a systematic analysis for the Global Burden of Disease Study 2013. Lancet. 2015 December 5. 2013;386(10010):2287–2323. https://doi.org/10.1016/S0140-6736(15)00128-2. Available at: http://europepmc.org/articles/pmc4685753 (accessed 20 February 2018).

11. Glouberman S, Millar J. Evolution of the determinants of health, health policy, and health information systems in Canada. Am J Public Health. 2003;93(3):388–392. Available at: https://www.ncbi.nlm.nih.gov/pmc/articles/PMC1447749/ (accessed 11 May 2017).

12. Government of Canada. Public Health Agency of Canada. Modified 1 February 2018. Available at: https://www.canada.ca/en/public-health.html (accessed 20February 2018).

13. Groff P, Goldberg S. The health field concept then and now: snapshots of Canada, a Document of the Health Network. Canadian Policy Research Networks, 2000. Available at: http://studylib.net/doc/8129911/towards-a-new-perspective-on-health-policy-background-paper (accessed 28 January 2017).

14. Hancock T. Lalonde and beyond: looking back at "A New Perspective on the Health of Canadians." Health Promot Int. 1986;1(1):93–100. Abstract available at: https://www.ncbi.nlm.nih.gov/pubmed/10286856 (accessed 6 May 2017).

15. Institute of Medicine (US). Committee on the National Quality Report on health care delivery. In: Hurtado MP, Swift EK, Corrigan JM, editors. Envisioning the national health care quality report. Washington (DC): National Academies Press (US), 2001. Available at: https://www.ncbi.nlm.nih.gov/books/NBK223318/ (accessed 7 May 2017).

16. Kindig D, Stoddart GL. What is population health? Am J Public Health. 2003;93:380–383. Available at: https://www.ncbi.nlm.nih.gov/pmc/articles/PMC1447747/ (accessed 8 February 2018).

17. Kickbusch RE. The contribution of the World Health Organization to a new public health. Am J Public Health. 2003;93:383–388. Available at: https://www.ncbi.nlm.nih.gov/pmc/articles/PMC1447748/ (accessed 8 February 2018).

18. Lalonde M. A new perspective on the health of Canadians: a working document. Ottawa: Department of National Health and Welfare, 1974, 1981. Available at: http://www.phac-aspc.gc.ca/ph-sp/pdf/perspect-eng.pdf (accessed 6 May 2017).

19. Lalonde M. A new perspective on the health of Canadians 28 years later. Pan Am J Public Health. 2002;12(3). Available at: http://www.scielosp.org/pdf/rpsp/v12n3/12867.pdf (accessed 7 May 2017).

20. MacDougall H. Reinventing public health: a new perspective on the health of Canadians and its international impact. J Epidemiol Commun Health. 2007;61(11):955−959. http://dx.doi.org/10.1136/jech.2006.046912. Available at: https://www.ncbi.nlm.nih.gov/pmc/articles/PMC2465617/ (accessed 6 May 2017).

21. Marmot M. Economic and social determinants of disease. Public Health Classics. Bull World Health Organ. 2001;79(10):988−989. Available at: http://www.who.int/bulletin/archives/79(10)988.pdf (accessed 8 February 2018).

22. Marmot MG, Bosma H, Heminway H, Brunner E, Stansfeld S. Contribution of job control and other risk factors to social variations in coronary heart disease incidence. Lancet. 1997;350:235−239. Abstract available at: https://www.ncbi.nlm.nih.gov/pubmed/9242799 (accessed 9 June 2017).

23. Marmot MM. Commission on social determinants of health. Achieving health equity: from root causes to fair outcomes. Lancet. 2007;370(9593):1153−1163. Abstract available at: http://www.thelancet.com/pdfs/journals/lancet/PIIS0140-6736(07)61385-3.pdf (accessed 28 January 2017).

24. McLeroy KR, Bibeau D, Steckler A, Glanz K. An ecological perspective on health promotion programmes. Health Educ Q. 1988;15(4):351−377. Available at: https://www.ncbi.nlm.nih.gov/pubmed/3068205 (accessed 7 May 2017).

25. NICE. Improving health and social care through evidence-based guidance. Available at: https://www.nice.org.uk/ (accessed 7 May 2017).

26. Office of Health Promotion and Disease Prevention. Healthy People 2020 topics and objectives. objectives A−Z. Site last updated 8 June 2017. Available at: https://www.healthypeople.gov/2020/topics-objectives (accessed 9 June 2017).

27. Ottawa Charter for Health Promotion. First international conference on health promotion, Ottawa, 21 November 1986. Available at: http://www.who.int/healthpromotion/conferences/previous/ottawa/en/ (accessed 27 January 2017).

28. Overview 7th Global Conference on Health Promotion, Nairobi 2009. The urgency of health promotion. Available at: http://www.who.int/healthpromotion/conferences/7gchp/overview/en/ (accessed 11 May 2017).

29. Rose G. Sick individuals and sick populations. Public Health Classics Available at .Bull World Health Organ. 2001;79(10):990−996. Available at: http://apps.who.int/iris/bitstream/10665/70950/1/bu1409.pdf (accessed 8 February 2018).

30. Rudolph L, Caplan J, Ben-Moshe K, Dillon L. Health in all policies: a guide for state and local governments. Washington, DC and Oakland, CA: American Public Health Association and Public Health Institute, 2013. Available at: http://www.phi.org/uploads/files/Health_in_All_Policies-A_Guide_for_State_and_Local_Governments.pdf (accessed 28 January 2017).

31. Sachs JD. Commission on macroeconomics and health. Macroeconomics and health: investing in health for economic development. Geneva: World Health Organization, 2001. Available at: http://apps.who.int/iris/bitstream/10665/42435/1/924154550X.pdf (accessed 28 January 2017).

32. Suhrcke M, McKee M, Stuckler D, Sauto Arce R, Tsolova S, Mortensen J. The contribution of health to the economy in the European Union. Public Health. 2006;120

(11):994−1001. Available at: https://ec.europa.eu/health/archive/ph_overview/documents/health_economy_en.pdf (accessed 28 January 2017).

33. Szreter S. The population health approach in historical perspective. Am J Public Health. 2003;93:421−431. Available at: https://www.ncbi.nlm.nih.gov/pmc/articles/PMC1449802/ (accessed 12 May 2017).

34. Tang K-C, Beaglehole R, O'Byrne D. MenuPolicy and partnership for health promotion—addressing the determinants of health. Bull World Health Org. 2005;83(12):881−968. http://www.who.int/bulletin/volumes/83/12/editorial31205html/en/ (accessed 28 January 2017).

35. The Fifth Global Conference on Health Promotion. Geneva: World Health Organization, 2000. The Fifth Global Conference on Health Promotion (5GCHP)−Health Promotion: Bridging the Equity Gap−was held 5−9th June, 2000 in Mexico City. Available at: http://www.who.int/healthpromotion/conferences/previous/mexico/en/hpr_mexico_report_en.pdf (accessed 12 May 2017).

36. The 6th Global Conference on Health Promotion, Bangkok, August 2005. Policy and partnership for action: addressing the determinants of health. Available at: http://www.who.int/healthpromotion/conferences/6gchp/en/ and http://www.who.int/healthpromotion/conferences/hpr_special%20issue.pdf?ua=1 (accessed 11 May 2017).

37. The 8th Global Conference on Health Promotion; Helsinki. Health in all policies. 2013. Available at: http://www.who.int/healthpromotion/conferences/8gchp/outcomes/en/ (accessed 11 May 2017).

38. Tulchinsky TH, Varavikova EA. What is the "New Public Health"? Public Health Reviews. 2010;32:25−53. Available at: https://publichealthreviews.biomedcentral.com/articles/10.1007/BF03391592 (accessed 8 February 2018).

39. United Nations. Millennium development goals report 2015. Available at: http://www.un.org/millenniumgoals/2015_MDG_Report/pdf/MDG%202015%20rev%20(July%201).pdf (accessed 8 February 2018).

40. United Nations. Sustainable development goals. Available at: http://www.un.org/sustainabledevelopment/sustainable-development-goals/ (accessed 8 February 2018).

41. US National Library of Medicine. Reports of the surgeon general: the 1964 report on smoking and health. Available at: https://profiles.nlm.nih.gov/ps/retrieve/Narrative/NN/p-nid/60 (accessed 7 May 2017).

42. US Preventive Services Task Force. About the USPTF, December 2016. Available at: https://www.uspreventiveservicestaskforce.org/Page/Name/about-the-uspstf (accessed 7 May 2017).

43. US Public Health Service. Healthy People: The Surgeon General's Report on Health Promotion and Disease Prevention. Washington, DC: US Department of Health, Education, and Welfare, Public Health Service, 1979. DHEW publication no. (PHS)79-55071. Available at: https://profiles.nlm.nih.gov/ps/access/NNBBGK.pdf (accessed 9 June 2017).

44. World Bank. 1993. World Development Report 1993: Investing in Health. New York: Oxford University Press. © World Bank. Available at: https://openknowledge.worldbank.org/handle/10986/5976 License: CC BY 3.0 IGO (accessed 10 June 2017).

45. World Health Organization. The Ottawa Charter for Health Promotion: first international conference on health promotion, Ottawa, 21 November 1986. Available at: http://www.who.int/healthpromotion/conferences/previous/ottawa/en/ (accessed 3 September 2017).

46. World Health Organization. The Bangkok Charter for Health Promotion in a globalized world. Geneva; 2005. Available at: http://www.who.int/healthpromotion/conferences/6gchp/bangkok_charter/en/index.html (accessed 20 February 2018).

47. World Health Organization. Neglected tropical diseases. Available at: http://www.who.int/neglected_diseases/diseases/en/ (accessed 10 June 2017).

48. WHO Global health promotion conferences. Available at: http://www.who.int/healthpromotion/ conferences/en/(accessed 9 June 2017).

49. World Health Organization. Declaration of Alma-Ata international conference on primary health care, Alma-Ata, USSR, 6–12 September 1978. Available at: http://www.who.int/ publications/almaata_declaration_en.pdf (accessed 6 May 2017).

50. World Health Organization. International Conference Dedicated to the 30th Anniversary of the Alma-Ata Declaration on Primary Health Care. 15–16 October 2008. Available at: http://www.who.int/whr/2008/en/ (accessed 20 February 2018).

51. World Health Organization. The world health report 2008—primary health care (now more than ever). http://www.who.int/whr/2008/en/.

52. World Health Organization. World health report 2002–Reducing risks, promoting healthy life. Geneva: World Health Organization, 2002. Available at: http://www.who.int/whr/ 2002/en/ (accessed 9 May 2017).

53. World Health Organization. Ministry of Social Affairs and Health, Finland. Health in all policies: Helsinki statement: framework for country action. 2014. Available at: http:// apps.who.int/iris/bitstream/10665/112636/1/9789241506908_eng.pdf?ua=1 (accessed 6 May 2017).

54. World Health Organization. Public health, environmental and social determinants of health (PHE): health in all policies-progressing the sustainable development goals, 30–31 March 2017. International Conference, Adelaide, South Australia. Available at: http://www.who. int/phe/events/HiAP-conference-March2017/en/ (accessed 6 May 2017).

55. World Health Organization. Health in all policies training manual. Geneva, Switzerland: World Health Organization, 2015. Available at: http://apps.who.int/iris/bitstream/10665/ 151788/1/9789241507981_eng.pdf (accessed 27 January 2017).

56. World Health Organization. Social determinants of health: Sir Michael Marmot, Chair of the Commission on Social Determinants of Health. Available at: http://www.who.int/ social_determinants/thecommission/marmot/en/ (accessed 14 May 2017).

Chapter 22

Warren, Marshall, *Helicobacter Pylori*, Peptic Ulcers and Gastric Cancer

ABSTRACT

Chronic peptic ulcer disease (CPUD) was a disease group with severe complications requiring long-term medical care, surgery in many cases, and death from perforation or hemorrhage, known as a major medical problem from antiquity until the late 20th century. In the 1970s, the discovery of histamine receptor (H$_2$ receptor) was a breakthrough, identifying a principal factor in gastric acid secretion, which responded to treatment with H$_2$ antagonists. This proved to be a safe and effective therapy for CPUD. However, in 1982, a new medical discovery of the cause of the condition was made by Drs. Robin Warren and Barry Marshall at the Royal Perth Hospital in Perth, Western Australia, offering the answer to the cause of CPUD and providing a simple and inexpensive antibiotic therapy cure and, jointly winning them the Nobel Prize in 2005. CPUD became curable, and emptied medical and surgical departments of CPUD patients for gastrectomies, vagotomies, and other procedures that previously filled these departments, as well as reducing death from severe complications of peptic ulcers including hemorrhage and perforation, and the incidence of cancer of the stomach. The causative relationship of treatable H pylori to CPUD, one of the commonest medical problems, and to gastric cancer and its prominence as the third leading cancer cause of death globally makes control and ultimate eradication of this infection a major public health challenge for the coming decades. This was one of the great breakthroughs in medicine and public health of the 20th century.

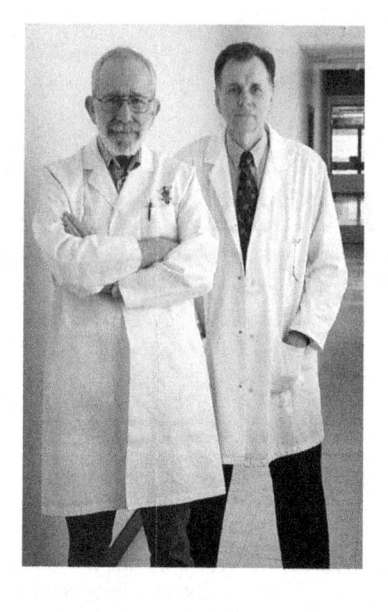

J. Robin Warren and Barry J. Marshall, co winners of the Nobel Prize in Medicine in 2005 for their joint work in discovery of Helicobacter pylori as the cause of peptic ulcer disease and curative treatment for it. *Photo courtesy of Drs Warren and Marshall, University of Western Australia, Adelaide, Australia*

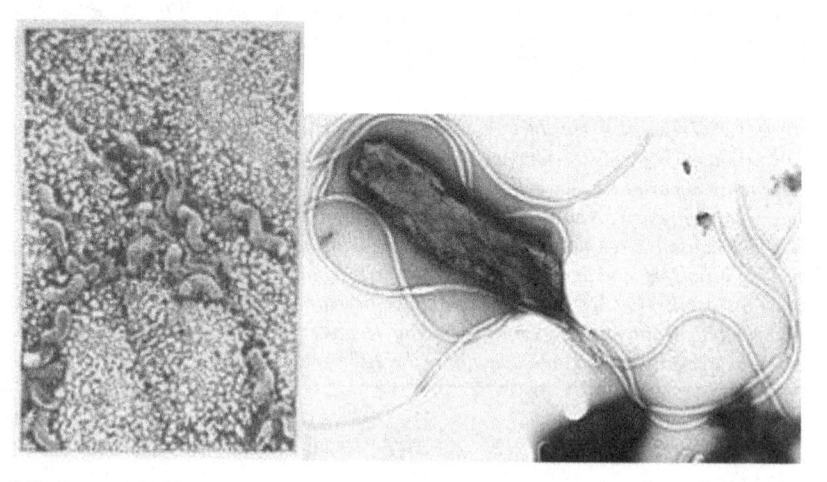

Helicobacter pylori is a bacterium protected against stomach acidity by producing the chemical urease and burrowing in crypts in the lining of the stomach causing peptic ulcer disease. H. pylori is estimated to exist in over 50% of the world's population but the rates are declining where hygiene and socio economic conditions improve. *Source: National Institute of Health Consensus Statement 1994;12(1)1−23. Available at: https://consensus.nih.gov/1994/ 1994HelicobacterPyloriUlcer094html.htm (accessed 8 February 2018) and Helicobacter pylori. Available at: https://upload.wikimedia.org/wikipedia/commons/thumb/d/d6/EMpylori.jpg/220px-EMpylori.jpg (accessed 23 February 2018).*

BACKGROUND

A peptic ulcer is a sore or hole in the lining of the stomach or duodenum (the first part of the small intestine) resulting from acidic juices. The most common ulcer symptom is gnawing or burning pain in the upper abdomen. The pain often occurs when the stomach is empty, between meals, and in the early morning hours, but it can occur at any other time. It may last from minutes to hours and may be relieved by eating food or taking antacids. Less common symptoms include nausea, vomiting, or loss of appetite. Ulcers may present with chronic bleeding causing anemia, weakness, and fatigue, or heavy chronic bleeding, which may appear in vomitus or stools or as an acute life-threatening hemorrhage or perforation. Hospital medical and surgical wards were heavily populated by acute and chronic peptic ulcer disease patients with large numbers of surgical operations in most of the 20th century.

In 1982 J. Robin Warren and Barry J. Marshall, pathologist and gastroen-terology resident respectively, in Perth, Australia, discovered and grew the bacteria *Helicobacter pylori* (H. pylori) and established its role as the cause of chronic peptic ulcer disease. They were awarded the Nobel Prize for Medicine in 2005 for *"their discovery of the bacterium Helicobacter pylori and its role in gastritis and peptic ulcer disease" (Nobel Prize Award 2005)*, one of the great scientific breakthroughs directly applicable in clinical medicine and pub-lic health in recent decades.

This discovery strengthened evidence of the potential of infectious organ-isms to cause chronic diseases. This specific case led to a simple, inexpen-sive cure for one of the important groups of chronic diseases. *Helicobacter pylori* is associated with not only chronic peptic ulcers, but also life-threatening perforations, bleeding and gastric cancer. Establishing H. pylori as the curable cause of peptic ulcer diseases also raised hopes that clinical peptic ulcers can be eliminated, along with reduction of gastric cancer and the ultimate hope of eradicating this group of diseases.

Chronic bacterial infections of the stomach with *H. pylori* mainly begin dur-ing childhood. If persistent, these may cause chronic gastritis often leading to peptic ulcer disease (PUD) later on in life. It is estimated that more than half of the world's population harbor *H. pylori*, in particular in low-income populations and countries. *Helicobacter pylori* lodges in crypts in the stomach lining and produces urease, a chemical that reduces the acidity of the surroundings allow-ing the bacteria to survive and multiply (See Figures 22.1 and 22.2).

Since antiquity and throughout most of the 20th century, peptic ulcers were thought by the medical community to be the result of stress and dietary factors. Treatment included special diets as well as rest and hospitalization for complications of chronic peptic ulcer disease (CPUD). Later treatments focused on the reduction of acidity in the digestive tract, using antacids and special diets until proton pump blockers became available. However, despite these treatments relieving the symptoms of ulcer, high recurrence and severe complications including bleeding and even death remained major problems.

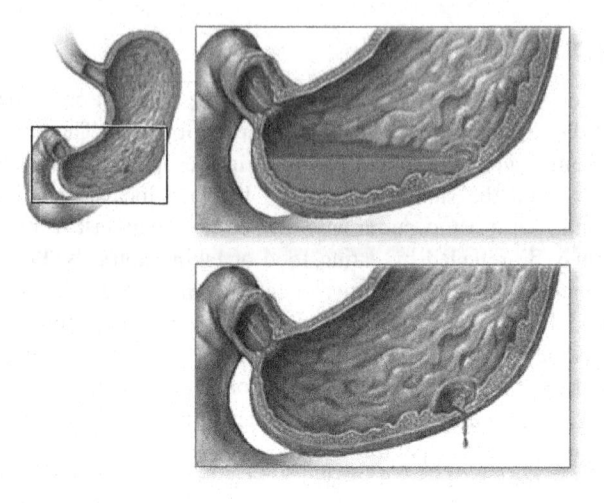

FIGURE 22.1 Peptic ulcers bleeding and perforation in the stomach. *Source: Reproduced from U.S. National Library of Medicine. Available at: https://medlineplus.gov/ency/article/000206.htm (accessed 8 February 2018).*

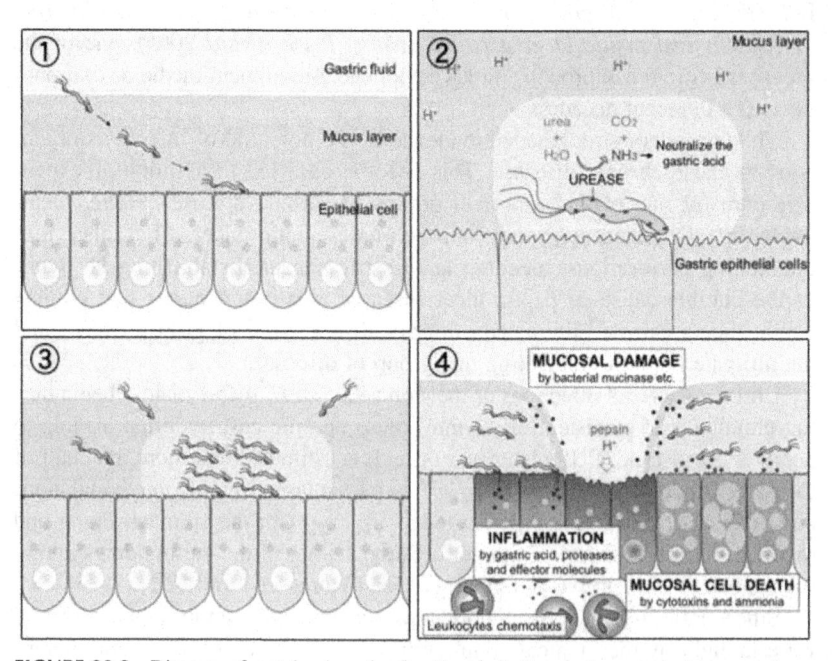

FIGURE 22.2 Diagram of gastric ulceration by *H. pylori*. *H. pylori* penetrate the mucus layer of host stomach and adhere to the surface of gastric mucosal epithelial cells; produce ammonia from urea by urease. The ammonia neutralizes gastric acid to prevent elimination of the bacteria which proliferate and migrate from the infectious site. The gastric ulcer develops by destruction of mucosa, inflammation and mucosal cell death. *Source: Ytambe. GNU Free Documentation License, 6 January 2006. Available at: https://commons.wikimedia.org/wiki/File:H_pylori_ ulcer_diagram_en.png (accessed 8 February 2018).*

Physicians and scientists around the world preceded the Warren and Marshall work with the discovery of *H. pylori*, a spiral rod shaped bacteria initially called campylobacter, but none successfully demonstrated a causal relationship with peptic ulcers. The first recorded work on *Helicobacter* was described by the Italian pathologist Giulio Bizzozero in 1892. Others followed and added more knowledge and understanding about *Helicobacter* mostly concentrating on classification, in vitro culture, and histopathology, but none made the actual discovery until Warren and Marshall followed through with demonstration and proof of causation.

Medical dogma taught that bacteria could not survive in the acidic environment of the stomach and all medical therapy was concentrated on reducing the acidity by diet and other measures. During the 1970s a histamine receptor (H_2 receptor) in the lining of the stomach and duodenum was demonstrated to control gastric acid secretion. Antagonists of this receptor were developed and found to be safe and effective therapy for PUD. Later, inhibitors of the proton pump ($H+,K+$-ATPase) in gastric lining cells to reduce acidity also proved to be rapidly effective and potent antiulcer drugs to treat the symptoms but not to cure the disease.

J. Robin Warren was born in 1937 in North Adelaide Australia, to a middle class family of fifth generation Australians. His father was a winemaker expert in viniculture. Robin grew up during World War II and developed grand mal epilepsy in his teens. Not good at sports, he excelled in school studies and entered University of Adelaide Medical Faculty in 1955. After graduation, he went on to specialize (Royal Melbourne Hospital) in clinical pathology, and during the 1970s focused on gastric biopsies for peptic ulcers.

In his work as a senior pathologist at the Royal Perth Hospital, Robin Warren in 1979, at age 42, made the key observation in pathological specimens of gastric ulcers or gastritis of helical bacteria-like bodies located in the crypts of the gastric lining near ulcers, raising the hypothesis that these bacteria could be causing the ulcers. His research work on the digestive tract and his first major related finding was that the presence of spiral-shaped bacteria correlated with infiltration of leukocytes. This led to Warren's hypothesis that the stomach was not bacteria-free as previously believed by generations of physicians.

Barry J. Marshall was born in Kalgoolie, a gold rush town in Western Australia. His father was an apprentice fitter and turner, who found work in a whaling town, and his mother a nurse, later moving to Perth for educational opportunities for their children. Barry was an adventurous child but a good scholar and entered medical school at the University of Western Australia in 1975. He married and the couple had four children. In 1981 he began training in the field of gastroenterology and met Robin Warren with the two agreeing to work together continuing Warren's work on Helicobacter. In literature reviews, Marshall found many reports of gastric bacteria and hypothesis that they were linked with gastritis. He engaged in the Helicobacter project on a full time basis with moral and financial support from his wife Adrienne. In 1982, the initial report of their work was published. It was much criticized as premature in its conclusions, but their follow-up publications in 1983 and 1984 were more convincing.

Together they demonstrated the link between the presence of a bacterium, identified as *H. pylori*, and peptic ulcers. They grew a pure culture of a gram-negative, spiral urease-producing organism on their 35th attempt where the culture was left for 5 days over a holiday weekend rather than the usual 3 days of incubation. In 1985, Marshall subsequently ingested a broth culture of the bacteria and developed severe symptoms of acute gastritis which were relieved by antibiotic and bismuth treatment. They clearly established the causative role *H. pylori* plays in gastritis and peptic ulcers rather than just the correlation based on their cumulative work and thus fulfilled the classical 19th century "Koch postulates" proving causative relationship of an organism to a specific disease (see Chapter 7). The medical community focused on the new antacid therapies remained highly skeptical and rejected this work delaying acceptance and adoption of Warren and Marshall's conclusions.

This work was enhanced by the development of the flexible endoscopy instrument for easier sampling of urease for diagnosis and treatment using antibiotics for the treatment of a bacterial infection, which gradually won general acceptance bringing relief to millions of people suffering from peptic ulcers. The urease was protective of the organism against stomach acidity. A non invasive diagnostic breath test for urea produced by urease was developed by Marshall and colleagues which indicated the presence of H pylori. This innovation made the condition readily identifiable with very high accuracy for diagnosis of the presence of gastric H pylori. Gastroscopy remains important to rule out gastric cancer in a symptomatic person. The adoption of treatment protocols with antibiotics and antacid treatment proved to be curative for those countless patients worldwide suffering from gastritis and CUPD.

Helicobacter pylori is the causative agent of a number of important medical conditions including chronic gastritis, gastritis and CPUD with its many complications, with the increasingly strong evidence linking it to gastric cancer as well as esophageal cancer, is recognized as carcinogenic. The evidence of a link between the bacterium and gastric cancer was convincingly demonstrated in four case control studies which quantified and confirmed that *H. pylori* is associated with stomach cancer. A strong correlation was also shown via the demonstration of antibodies and growth of the organism before and after diagnosis of cancer, and in one of the studies, a dose response was found showing a relation between severity of infection and risk of stomach cancer. Gastric cancer has been declining steadily in industrialized countries for many decades as public sanitation, food safety and widespread use of antibiotics for other reasons reduced *H. pylori* prevalence. Nevertheless, gastric cancer remains the fifth most common cause of cancer death worldwide.

In 1993 a US National Institutes of Health (NIH) Consensus Conference concluded that there is a strong association between *H. pylori* and peptic ulcer as well as with gastric cancer and recommended that patients with

H. pylori infection be treated with antibiotics both for cure of symptoms and as a preventive measure for gastric and esophageal cancer. In 1994, WHO and the International Agency for Research in Cancer (IARC) declared infection with H. pylori to be a class 1 carcinogen and a definite cause of gastric adenocarcinoma in humans.

Parkin in 2006 estimated total infection-attributable cancers in 2002 numbered 1.9 million cases, or 17.8 percent of the global cancer burden. The principal microorganisms causing cancer were *Helicobacter pylori* (5.5% of all cancer), the human papilloma viruses (HPV 5.2%), the hepatitis B and C viruses (4.9%), Epstein-Barr virus (1%), and HIV (0.9%).

In 2012, WHO estimated 952,000 new cases of stomach cancer in the world; this was 6.8 percent of all cancers or the fifth most common malignancy globally after lung, breast, colorectal, and prostate. The incidence of gastric carcinoma in the United States and Western Europe has declined dramatically over the past century but in much of Latin America and Asia the incidence remains high but declining in some previously high-prevalence countries. Improved social and environmental conditions are associated with reduction in incidence of *Helicobacter* infection; high-income populations have lower prevalence than low-income groups in countries of varying socioeconomic development. Some 70 percent of gastric cancers are located mainly in East Asian countries: China, Japan, and Korea account for 60 percent of total cases, primarily in men. The lowest rates are reported in the United States, in Africa and the Eastern Mediterranean region.

Japan experienced a reduction of 60 percent in gastric cancer between 1965 to 1995. A literature review of case findings among asymptomatic Asian individuals with *H. pylori* showed a marked reduction in incidence of gastric cancer in healthy asymptomatic infected persons as compared to nontreated control groups with moderate evidence of reduction. A 2016 review of survey of *H. pylori* and gastric cancer showed prevalence is higher in less affluent regions of Europe, although *H. pylori* prevalence and gastric cancer incidence declined throughout Europe with annual reduction of just over two percent from 1993 to 2007 (Roberts et al., 2016).

Despite major therapeutic advances, as of 1995, 75 percent of peptic ulcer patients in the United States were still primarily treated with medications to reduce acid secretion and only five percent received antibiotics. Medical practice was slow to adopt and implement the new therapeutic method of antibiotics and patients' awareness of the bacterial cause of their medical condition was low (about 10%); most people continued to attribute CPUD to anxiety and diet.

After antibiotic treatment of ulcer was first approved in 1996, a multisectoral project involving the US Centers for Disease Control (CDC), government agencies, academic institutions, and industry representatives focused on educating the public about peptic ulcer being a curable infection. The project also stressed that health can be greatly improved and economic burden of the disease can be relieved by disseminating information about *H. pylori* and its simple inexpensive and non-invasive diagnosis and cure.

CURRENT RELEVANCE

Helicobacter pylori is estimated to be present in over half of the world's population primarily in low-income countries due to poverty, poor sanitation of food and environmental conditions allowing widespread transmission of the organism. In western countries, estimates indicate that 20 percent of all adults have persistent or recurrent upper-abdominal symptoms including pain, heartburn, bloating, and nausea. Currently, some 25 million Americans are estimated to suffer from PUD, with one out of 10 Americans suffering from this condition during their lifetime.

Peptic ulcer disease is primarily caused by *H. pylori*, so testing ulcer patients for *H. pylori* infections and providing antibiotic treatment should be a high priority for patient care. Improvement of health and reduced suffering are dramatic in patients who suffer from chronic PUD, and the diagnosis and cure of the infection with antibiotics also has an important economic impact on care costs. Antibiotics shorten ulcer healing time and significantly reduce the ulcer recurrence rate compared with traditional ulcer therapies such as acid-reducing medications. *Helicobacter pylori* infection can usually be cured with a two-week regimen of antibiotics. In more than 80 percent of patients, the ulcer is cured but antibiotic resistance is increasing.

With *H. pylori* responsible for 75–80 percent of gastric cancer, hundreds of studies are published every year comparing the efficacy of treatments (as well as diagnostic tools), constantly aiming to improve the medical solution offered for this widespread clinical condition. Recommendations change rapidly and a variety of treatments are available. In addition, recent genetic mapping of *H. pylori* has allowed better understanding of pathogenicity, virulence factors, and host-pathogen interactions of this highly variable organism. Another recent issue is the finding of *H. pylori* in surface water, suggesting the existence of an important environmental reservoir that could probably be eliminated via proper treatment of drinking water.

Gastric cancer remains an important public health problem in Asia as the third most common cancer after breast and lung cancer even as incidence and mortality rates are slowly declining, presumably with reduction in *H. pylori* prevalence. Incidence and mortality rates vary within the Region closely related to the prevalence of *H. pylori* and its molecular virulent characteristics. Gastric cancer mortality rates per 100,000 population reported in 2014 vary widely by region: world 14.0; 18.5 in Asia; 10.3 in Europe; 4.2 in North America; and 4.0 in Africa (Rahman et al., 2014). WHO reported that cancer accounted for 8.8 million deaths in 2015. The commonest causes of cancer death globally were: lung (1.69 million deaths); liver (788,000); colorectal (774,000); stomach (754,000); and breast (571,000) (WHO 2018).

Gradually improving socioeconomic conditions are associated with lower *H. pylori* seroprevalence rates and reduced gastric cancer incidence. Studies from developing countries have shown high rates of *H. pylori* prevalence, such as 22.6 percent in Vietnamese children aged <3 years, 46.7 percent in Mexican children <5 years, 33 percent in Egyptian children <6 years, 80 percent in Bangladeshi children <5 years, 57 percent in Indian children <5 years, 40 percent in Brazilian children <6 years, 32.4 percent in Saudi children <10 years, and 41 percent in Turkish children <6 years. Studies in Portugal, Spain, and the Netherlands show trends toward reduced prevalence of *H. pylori* and a decline in gastric cancer, which nevertheless remains a serious public health challenge. It may be that increased use of antibiotics and sanitation since World War II have been a factor in reducing *H. pylori* and gastric cancer prevalence but would not explain the still high prevalence in Japan, for example.

H. pylori is spread by oral-fecal contamination via direct contact, as well as from contaminated food and water. It is more prevalent in poorer countries or poor populations in wealthy countries. Discussions of eradication based on clinical screening for case finding and cure is one current method of reducing the burden of disease including gastric cancer. Screening is not yet widely adopted as a standard procedure. Improving social and economic conditions are important and community water treatment is a basic necessity. A vaccine is being sought as the infection affects a large global population and antibiotic resistance is becoming commoner.

ETHICAL ISSUES

Successful treatment and cure of CPUD has radically transformed surgical wards in hospitals in the industrialized countries by curing CPUD patients medically, but providing care for sufferers of PUD in low-income countries is not available due to lack of access to health care and the costs of diagnosis and treatment. Ultimately treatment for ulcer disease and gastritis demands the eradication of a bacterium, so that potential antibiotic resistance has to be taken into account with permanent alertness to changes in efficacy of treatments. As a result, physicians face an important challenge, requiring their awareness of scientific up-to-date advances in this domain.

Eradication of a bacterial infection in individual patients involves 7–14 days of treatment with proton pump inhibitors (PPI) plus two antibiotics and bismuth to remove *H. pylori* infection. For an infection that affects half the world population treatment is discussed as a method of prevention of gastric cancer. Searching for and eradicating *H. pylori* in healthy asymptomatic persons would entail an enormous use of resources and will not be feasible until vaccines are developed supplemented by environmental measures. Recognition of the importance of this issue has not yet reached the level of priority needed for a policy commitment.

Research for *H. pylori* vaccines is not listed among the high priorities of WHO, but there is some activity. Some recent partial success indicates that this may be feasible, but is not yet ready for public immunization programs. Findings showed the benefit resulting from mucosal routes of vaccination, leading to the reduction of *H. pylori* density in the human gastric mucosa, but the advance is only partial, as no serologic response has been produced so far.

Helicobacter is also an environmental issue due to its presence in contaminated water. Thus environment management and general living conditions including housing, food quality, and water treatment by filtration, coagulation, and chlorination are important in reducing CUPD and cancer of the stomach. Poverty, crowding and poor sanitation are the key factors in the widespread contamination of children with H pylori which may also cause anemia as well as chronic gastritis and PUD.

ECONOMIC ISSUES

Prior to the Warren and Marshall identification of *H. pylori* as the cause of chronic peptic ulcer diseases, hospitals were largely occupied by CPUD patients for medical treatment and surgical wards for the commonly used gastrectomies and vagotomies. Following general adoption of antibiotic treatment these conditions have largely disappeared in the high-income countries. Hospitalizations for which the diagnosis was *H. pylori* infection were also drastically reduced. The age-adjusted hospitalization rate in the US for PUD decreased by 21%; from 71.1/100,000 population in 1998 to 56.5/100,000 in 2005. Rates were highest for adults >65 years of age, and higher for men than for women (Feinstein et al., 2010). The US Centers for Disease Control reports that millions of Americans suffer from peptic ulcer disease during their lifetime. Ulcers cause an estimated 1 million hospitalizations and 6,500 deaths per year. In the United States, annual health care costs of PUD have been estimated at nearly $6 billion: $3 billion in hospitalization costs, $2 billion in physician office visits, and $1 billion in decreased productivity and days lost from work for health care. The annual cost of treating gastric cancer in the US, a low-risk country, is estimated at approximately $2 billion (Herrero, 2014).

In the 1980s, pharmaceutical manufacturers were making a billion dollars per year from the current Tagamet. Zantac, the second drug to reduce acid production, sold more at rates of over $3 billion USD per year for most of the 1980's. The only other way that ulcers could be controlled medically was with chalky antacid in large amounts over four weeks. Cure of PUD often required removal of the lower third of the stomach by surgery (Marshall, 2008).

Eradication of *H. pylori* infection is a controversial issue in the gastrointestinal medical world due to concern that it may increase incidence of esophageal cancer. Studies in China, a country with high gastric cancer rates, suggest there is a real benefit for case-finding and treatment approaches. In Japan where gastric cancer rates are also high, search and treat strategies to eradicate the bacterium through the country's universal insurance system are being implemented. Case finding and treatment are important, but long term benefit in CUPD and gastric cancer control will depend on improved hygiene, food and water safety, improved socioeconomic conditions for deprived populations, with many benefits in prevention of CUPD and many other diseases.

CONCLUSION

Successful treatment with antibiotics to eliminate *H. pylori* cures PUD and is an enormous achievement of medical science and practice. As the initial infection with this bacterium mainly occurs during infancy, childhood and old age. Environmental improvements in water quality and sanitation will gradually reduce the prevalence of *H. pylori* infection. Diagnosis and adequate antibiotic treatment permanently cures CPUD and prevents gastric cancer. Curing peptic ulcers and preventing their possible recurrence relieves suffering, greatly improves the quality of life and also diminishes the economic burden caused by surgery and hospitalization (which previously was common), as well as doctor visits, medications, and sick leave from school or work.

Despite major advancement in the understanding and treatment of PUD (gastritis, ulcers) and the bacterial cause, continuous research is still needed and is needed in many research centers. However, there is an additional aspect to treatment of gastric ulcers: health care provider and patient awareness of the cause and most efficient treatment of this medical condition. Until recently PUD was a lifelong disease with only symptomatic relief available, but today it is a curable condition when appropriate treatment is chosen. This has changed the lives of countless people who suffered from this burdensome condition and associated risk of stomach cancer.

Current estimates suggest that more than half the world's population is affected by *H. pylori*. Clinical screening and treatment is possible in high-income countries but not accessible to the majority in low-income countries with high rates of prevalence of *Helicobacter* infection, so that clinical approaches are much less feasible than in industrialized countries. An effective and safe vaccine is elusive but vital for a population-based approach. Vaccine research is under way, but thus far none of several *H. pylori* vaccine candidates have proven effective in humans. Increasing antibiotic resistance leads to trial and error in therapeutic combinations. The search for an effective vaccine is essential for control of PUD and its costly and severe consequences to half the world's population.

The future for PUD and gastric cancer seems hopeful. Surgical wards have reported few such cases in recent years in the industrialized countries. High prevalence of *H. pylori* in high-, medium-, and especially low-income populations and developing countries, such as in India. First Nation Canadians are at high risk of PUD and gastric cancer.

In a 2014 viewpoint in the Journal of the American Medical Association (JAMA). Hererro and colleagues state: "*it is estimated that more than*

700,000 people will die of gastric cancer, making this disease the third most common cause of cancer death globally. Although gastric cancer rates have been declining by approximately 2 percent per year, the numbers of cases and deaths are expected to increase in coming years, reflecting increasing numbers of older (and thus, higher-risk) individuals in the world. Despite its importance, gastric cancer receives little attention from research funding agencies or public health organizations."

Warren and Marshall opened the door to great new possibilities to relieve widespread suffering from PUD and to prevent gastric cancer deaths. Their breakthrough was rapidly accepted by sufferers from CPUD whose family physicians responded, and despite initial rejection by the gastroenterology community the translation of science to practice was relatively rapid over the decade following the discovery. At the same time, elimination of *H. pylori* caused diseases requires long term improvement in hygiene, food and water quality, and the development of a safe, effective and low cost vaccine. This will require recognition of CPUD and gastric cancer as high priority in global health with mobilization of international agencies, and donors, as well as national public health systems and the medical community.

CPUD should be included in disease risks in natural disaster and mass refugee situations when sanitation is poor, water and food safety inadequate in crowded the conditions are breeding grounds for gastrointestinal, nutritional and other diseases. CPUD is still not high on the public health agenda globally nor even in high-income countries. Even beyond the specific diseases caused by *H. pylori* is the growing list of cancers proven to be caused by microorganisms alongside *H. pylori*, HIV, hepatitis B and C, *Schistosoma haematobium*, and Human papilloma virus (HPV), and there will be others.

The challenges for medical sciences, clinical medicine, and for public health in the coming decades are daunting, but there is potential to prevent chronic diseases as common and clinically important as CPUD including cancer. With improved screening and treatment, CPUD and gastric cancer can be greatly reduced even in low- and medium-income countries. Improving sanitation and developing a hoped for vaccine will provide the opportunity to reduce and possibly eliminate this group of diseases as important public health problems globally. The Warren and Marshall brilliant demonstration of *H. pylori* as the cause of CPUD, and later demonstrated by others to be the cause of most gastric cancer added a major new challenge for clinical medicine and in the larger context for public health. It was a great gift to humanity.

RECOMMENDATIONS

1. Helicobacter pylori infection is global in spread in high but varying percentages of populations, depending on levels of public and private sanitation and hygiene; continued and expanded efforts in these public health

fields are additional reasons for their high priority in development plans for reducing the continuing widespread infection with *Helicobacter*.

2. The search for a safe, effective and inexpensive vaccine for the fight against *Helicobacter pylori* should be among the high priority targets of funders and researchers in vaccinology.

3. Clinical care providers should be highly alert to the possible presence of *Helicobacter pylori* as a causative organism of related abdominal symptoms which is easily detected and inexpensively and effectively eradicated preventing potentially dangerous consequences.

4. Planning for eradication of *Helicobacter pylori* may require screening of age categories most likely to be infected e.g., those over 45 years of age, or all ages of populations in areas where poor standards of hygiene, water safety and food hygiene may be common.

5. In the coming decades reduction in case load, transmission and environmental contamination will provide for evidence-based public health measures.

STUDENT REVIEW QUESTIONS

1. Why was the idea of infection as the cause of peptic ulcers rejected by medical doctors until the 1990s when repeated studies had shown there was a strong case for a change in the preconception that bacteria could not survive in the high acidity level in stomachs?

2. What was the discovery by Warren and Marshall in 1982 that proved that bacteria were the cause of chronic peptic ulcer disease?

3. Why was there skepticism and opposition among medical bodies to the Warren and Marshall theory?

4. What convinced the medical community that the Warren and Marshall theory was correct?

5. What is the estimated prevalence of Helicobacter globally? In developing countries?

6. What was the economic impact of the adoption of antibiotic therapy and improved case finding diagnostics of CUPD on hospital surgical patient case load?

7. What is the evidence that *H. pylori* is the major cause of gastric cancer?

8. What are possible and hoped for public health responses to this worldwide phenomenon?

RECOMMENDED READINGS

1. American Cancer Society. Can stomach cancer be prevented? Revised March 16, 2015. Available at: http://www.cancer.org/cancer/stomachcancer/detailedguide/stomach-cancer-prevention (accessed 18 July, 2017).

2. Beaulieu N, Bloom R, Stein R. Breakway: the global burden of cancer—challenges and opportunities. The Economist Intelligence Chart, 2009. Available at: http://graphics.eiu.com/upload/eb/EIU_LIVESTRONG_Global_Cancer_Burden.pdf (accessed 3 September 2017).

3. Blaser MJ. Hypotheses on the pathogenesis and natural history of Helicobacter pylori-induced inflammation. Gastroenterology. 1992;102:720−727. Available at: http://www.gastrojournal.org/article/0016-5085(92)90126-J/pdf (accessed 8 February 2018).

4. Brown LM. *Helicobacter pylori*: epidemiology and routes of transmission. Epidemiol Reviews. 2000;22:283−297. Available at: https://pdfs.semanticscholar.org/7c90/c587293e2c016b0fd9fe880f423ae3736308.pdf (accessed 3 September 2017).

5. Carcas LP. Gastric cancer review. J Carcinog. 2014;13:14. Available from: http://doi.org/10.4103/1477-3163.146506. Available at: http://www.ncbi.nlm.nih.gov/pmc/articles/PMC4278094/ (accessed 31 July 2017).

6. Centers for Disease Control and Prevention Division of Bacterial Diseases (DBD). Economics of peptic ulcer disease and *H. pylori* infection, October 1998. Available at: http://www.cdc.gov/ulcer/economic.htm (accessed 3 September 2017).

7. Centers for Disease Control and Prevention. Knowledge about causes of peptic ulcer disease—United States, March-April 1997. MMWR Morb Mortal Wkly Rep. 1997;46 (42):985−987. Available at: http://www.cdc.gov/mmwr/PDF/wk/mm4642.pdf (accessed 3 September 2017).

8. Centers for Disease Control and Prevention. Helicobacter pylori: fact sheet for health care providers updated: July 1998. Available at: https://www.cdc.gov/ulcer/files/hpfacts.pdf (accessed 23 September 2017).

9. Danesh J, Punder RE. Commentary: eradication of *Helicobacter pylori* and non-ulcer dyspepsia. Lancet. 2000;355(9206):766−767. Abstract available at: http://www.thelancet.com/pdfs/journals/lancet/PIIS0140-6736(00)90005-9.pdf (accessed 3 September 2017).

10. Dalton-Griffin L, Kellam P. Infectious causes of cancer and their detection. J Biol. 2009;8 (7):67. Available from: http://doi.org/10.1186/jbiol168. Available at: http://www.jbiol.com/content/8/7/67 (accessed 27 July 2017).

11. Dominici P, Bellentani S, DiBiase AR, Saccoccio G, Le Rose A, Massutiti F, et al. Familial clustering of *Helicobacter pylori* infection: population based study. BMJ. 1999;319:537. Available at: http://www.bmj.com/content/319/7209/537 (accessed 3 September, 2017).

12. Dubois A. Spiral bacteria in the human stomach: the gastric Helicobacters. Emerg Infect Dis. 1995;1(3):79−85. https://doi.org/10.3201/eid0103.950302. Available at: https://wwwnc.cdc.gov/eid/article/1/3/pdfs/95-0302.pdf (accessed 8 February 2018).

13. Fashner J, Gitu AC. Diagnosis and treatment of peptic ulcer disease and *H. pylori* infection. Am Fam Physician. 2015;91(4):236−242. Available at: http://www.aafp.org/afp/2015/0215/p236.pdf (accessed 27 July 2017).

14. Feinstein LB, Holman RC, Yorita Christensen KL, Steiner CA, Swerdlow DL. Trends in hospitalizations for peptic ulcer disease, United States, 1998−2005. Emerg Infect Dis. 2010;16(9):1410−1418. Available at: http://wwwnc.cdc.gov/eid/article/16/9/09-1126 (accessed 27 July 2017).

15. Flahault A, Tulchinsky TH. From science to public health: the *Helicobacter pylori* case. Public Health Reviews. 2010;32:7−9. Available at: http://www.publichealthreviews.eu/show/a/20 (accessed 3 Sept 2015).

16. Fock KM, Ang TL. Epidemiology of *Helicobacter pylori* infection and gastric cancer in Asia. J Gastroenterol Hepatol. 2010;25:479−486. Available at: http://onlinelibrary.wiley.com/doi/10.1111/j.1440-1746.2009.06188.x/pdf (accessed 3 September 2017).

17. Ford AC, Forman D, Hunt R, Yuan Y, Moayyedi P. Helicobacter pylori eradication for the prevention of gastric neoplasia. Coch. Database Syst. Rev. 2015;7. Art. No.: CD005583. doi:10.1002/14651858.CD005583.pub2. Available at: http://onlinelibrary.wiley.com/doi/10.1002/14651858.CD005583.pub2/pdf (accessed 23 September 2017).

18. Ford AC, Forman D, Hunt RH, Yuan Y, Moayyedi P. *Helicobacter pylori* eradication therapy to prevent gastric cancer in healthy, asymptomatic infected individuals: systematic review and meta-analysis of randomized controlled trials. BMJ. 2014;348:g3174. Available at: http://www.bmj.com/content/348/bmj.g3174.long (accessed 3 September 2017).

19. Forman D, Newell D, Fullerton F, Yarnell J, Stacey A, Wald N, et al. Association between infection with *Helicobacter pylori* and risk of gastric cancer: evidence from a prospective investigation. BMJ. 1991;302:1302−1305. Available at: http://www.bmj.com/content/302/6788/1302.full.pdf + html (accessed 3 September 2017).

20. Fuccio L, Zagari RM, Eusebi LH, et al. Meta-analysis: can *Helicobacter pylori* eradication treatment reduce the risk for gastric cancer? Ann Intern Med. 2009;151:121−128. Available at: http://www.ncbi.nlm.nih.gov/pubmed/19620164 (accessed 3 September 2017).

21. Grad YH, Lipsitch M, Aiello AE. Secular trends in *Helicobacter pylori* seroprevalence in adults in the United States: evidence for sustained race/ethnic disparities. Am J Epidemiol. 2012;1:54−59. Available at: http://aje.oxfordjournals.org/content/early/2011/11/14/aje.kwr288.full (accessed 3 September 2017).

22. Graham DY. History of Helicobacter pylori, duodenal ulcer, gastric ulcer and gastric cancer. World J. Gastroenterol. 2014;20(18):5191−5204. Available at: https://www.ncbi.nlm.nih.gov/pmc/articles/PMC4017034/pdf/WJG-20-5191.pdf (accessed 10 February 2018).

23. Herrero R, Parsonnet J, Greenberg ER. Viewpoint: prevention of gastric cancer. JAMA. 2014;312(12):1197−1198. Available from: http://doi.org/10.1001/jama.2014.10498. Abstract available at: http://jama.jamanetwork.com/article.aspx?articleid=1906623 (accessed 31 July 2017).

24. Jamal A, Bray F, Center MM, Ferlay J, Wrad E, Forman D. Global cancer statistics. CA Cancer J Clin. 2011;61:69−90. Available at: http://onlinelibrary.wiley.com/doi/10.3322/caac.20107/full (accessed 3 September 2017).

25. Jenks S. Renewed focus on preventing gastric cancer. J Natl Cancer Inst. 2015;107(1):dju501. Available from: http://doi.org/10.1093/jnci/dju501. Available at: http://jnci.oxfordjournals.org/content/107/1/dju501.full (accessed 3 September 2017).

26. Jones NL, Chiba N, Fallone C, Thomson A, Hunt R, Jacobson K, et al. *Helicobacter pylori* in First Nations and recent immigrant populations in Canada. Can J Gastroenterol. 2012;26(2):97−103. Available at: http://canhelpworkinggroup.ca/downloads/publications_83_3828538179.pdf (accessed 3 September 2007).

27. Marshall BJ, Goodwin CS, Warren JR, Murray R, Blincow ED, Blackbourn SJ, et al. Prospective double blind trial of duodenal ulcer relapse after eradication of Campylobacter pylori. Lancet. 1988;ii:1437−1442. Abstract available at: https://www.ncbi.nlm.nih.gov/pubmed/2904568 (accessed 8 February 2018).

28. Marshall BJ. Virulence and pathogenicity of *Helicobacter pylori*. J Gastroenterol Hepatol. 1996;(2), 121−124. Abstract available at: https://www.ncbi.nlm.nih.gov/pubmed/1912416 (accessed 8 February 2018).

29. Marshall BJ, Plankey MW, Hoffman SR, Boyd CL, Dye KR, Frierson Jr HF, et al. A 20-minute breath test for helicobacter pylori. Am J Gastroenterol. 1991;86(4):438−445. Abstract available at: https://www.ncbi.nlm.nih.gov/pubmed/2012046 (accessed 8 February 2018).

30. Marshall BJ. Banquet Speech. Nobelprize.org. Nobel Media AB 2014. Available at: http://www.nobelprize.org/nobel_prizes/medicine/laureates/2005/marshall-speech.html (accessed 2 October 2017).

31. Marshall B, Adams PC. Helicobacter pylori: a Nobel pursuit? Can J Gastro. 2008;22(11):895−896. Available at: https://www.ncbi.nlm.nih.gov/pmc/articles/PMC2661189/ (accessed 10 October 2017).

32. de Martel C, Ferlay J, Franceshi S, et al. Global burden of cancers attributable to infections in 2008: a review and synthetic analysis. Lancet Oncol. 2012;13:607−615. Abstract available at: http://www.thelancet.com/journals/lanonc/article/PIIS1470-2045(12)70137-7/abstract (accessed 3 September 2015).

33. Marshall BJ, Warren RJ. Unidentified curved bacilli in the stomach of patients with gastritis and peptic ulceration. Lancet. 1984;323(8390):1311−1315. Abstract available at: http://www.thelancet.com/journals/lancet/article/PIIS0140-6736(84)91816-6/abstract (accessed 20 September 2017).

34. Morais S, Ferro A, Bastos A, Castro C, Lunet N, Peleteiro B. Trends in gastric cancer mortality and in the prevalence of *Helicobacter pylori* infection in Portugal. Eur J Cancer Prev. 2015;25(4):275−281. Abstract available at: http://www.ncbi.nlm.nih.gov/pubmed/26186469 (accessed 31 July 2017).

35. Moayyedi P, Soo S, Deeks J, Delaney B, Harris A, Innes M, et al. Eradication of Helicobacter pylori for non-ulcer dyspepsia. Cochrane Database Syst Rev 2006;(2). http://doi.org/10.1002/14651858. CD002096.pub4. Art. No.: CD002096. Available at: https://pdfs.semanticscholar.org/5217/33e786baba62f87c9ca413587fc879d59178.pdf (accessed 20 September 2017).

36. National Cancer Institute. *H. pylori* and cancer: fact sheet, 5 September 2013. Available at: http://www.cancer.gov/about-cancer/causes-prevention/risk/infectious-agents/h-pylori-fact-sheet (accessed 3 September 2017).

37. Nobel Prize in Physiology and Medicine 2005. Barry J. Marshall and J. Robin Warren for their discovery of the bacterium *Helicobacter pylori* and its role in gastritis and peptic ulcer disease. Available at: http://www.nobelprize.org/nobel_prizes/medicine/laureates/2005/ (accessed 25 July 2017).

38. Normark S. Presentation speech of the Nobel Prize for Physiology or Medicine, 2005. On behalf of the Nobel Foundation, Karolinska Institute, December 10, 2005. Available at: http://nobelprize.org/nobel_prizes/medicine/laureates/2005/presentation-speech.html (accessed 25 July 2017).

39. Parkin DM. The global health burden of infection: associated cancers in the year 2002. Int J Cancer. 2006;18:3030−3034. Available at: http://onlinelibrary.wiley.com/doi/10.1002/ijc.21731/full (accessed 30 September 2017).

40. Parsonnet J. *Helicobacter pylori* in the stomach—a paradox unmasked. N Engl J Med. 1996;335:278−280. Abstract available at: http://www.nejm.org/doi/full/10.1056/NEJM199607253350411 (accessed 31 2017).

41. Parsonnet J, Friedman GD, Vandersteen DP, Chang Y, Vogelman JH, Orentreich N, et al. *Helicobacter pylori* infection and the risk of gastric carcinoma. N Engl J Med. 1991;325 (16):1127−1131. Available at: http://www.nejm.org/doi/full/10.1056/NEJM199110173251 603#t = articleTop (accessed 25 September 2017).

42. Peek RM, Blaser MJ. Reviews: *Helicobacter pylori* and gastrointestinal cancer tract adenocarcinomas. Nat Rev Cancer. 2002;2(1):28−37. Abstract available at: http://www.ncbi.nlm.nih.gov/pubmed/11902583 (accessed 25 September 2017).

43. Peleteiro B, Bastos A, Ferro A, Lunet N. Prevalence of *Helicobacter pylori* infection worldwide: a systematic review of studies with national coverage. Dig Dis Sci. 2014; 59(8):1698−1709. Abstract available at: http://www.ncbi.nlm.nih.gov/pubmed/24563236 (accessed 5 September 2017).

44. Poddar U, Yachha SK. *Helicobacter pylori* in children: an Indian perspective. Indian Pediatr. 2007;44:761−770. Available at: http://www.ncbi.nlm.nih.gov/pubmed/17998576 (accessed 3 September 2017).

45. Rahman R, Asombang AW, Ibdah JA. Characteristics of gastric cancer in Asia. World J Gastroenterol. 2014;20(16):4483−4490. Available at: http://www.ncbi.nlm.nih.gov/pmc/ articles/PMC4000485/ (accessed 19 September 2017).

46. Roberts SE, Morrison-Rees S, Samuel DG, Thorne K, Akbari A, Williams JG. Review article: the prevalence of *Helicobacter pylori* and the incidence of gastric cancer across Europe. Aliment Pharmacol Ther. 2016;43(3):334−345. https://doi.org/10.1111/apt.13474. Available at: http://onlinelibrary.wiley.com/doi/10.1111/apt.13474/full (accessed 8 February 2018).

47. Ruggiero P, Censini S. *Helicobacter pylori*: a brief history. Diseases. 2014;2:187−208. Available at: http://www.mdpi.com/2079-9721/2/2/187/htm (accessed 3 September 2017).

48. Salih BA. *Helicobacter pylori* infection in developing countries: the burden for how long. Saudi J Gastroenterol. 2009;15(3):201−207. Available at: http://www.ncbi.nlm.nih.gov/ pmc/articles/PMC2841423/ (accessed 3 September 2017).

49. Santiago P, Moreno Y, Ferrús MA. Identification of viable *Helicobacter pylori* in drinking water supplies by cultural and molecular techniques. Helicobacter. 2015;20(4):252−259. Abstract available at: https://www.ncbi.nlm.nih.gov/pubmed/25655472 (accessed 25 July 2017).

50. Sonnenberg A. Time trends of ulcer mortality in Europe. Gastroenterology. 2007; 132(7):2320−2327. Available at: http://www.gastrojournal.org/article/S0016-5085(07) 00634-8/pdf (accessed 8 February 2018).

51. Thomson M. Familial clustering of *Helicobacter pylori* infection: population based study: Commentary: *Helicobacter pylori*-the story so far. BMJ. 1999;319:537. Abstract available at: http://www.bmj.com/content/319/7209/537 (accessed 25 July 2017).

52. van Blankenstein M, van Vuuren AJ, Ouwendijk M, Kuipers EJ. The prevalence of *Helicobacter pylori* infection in the Netherlands. Scand J Gastroenterol. 2013; 48(7):794−800. Abstract available at: http://www.ncbi.nlm.nih.gov/pubmed/23795659 (accessed 3 September 2017).

53. Wang C, Weber A, Graham DY. Age, period, and cohort effects on gastric cancers in Asia. Dig Dis Sci. 2015;60(2):514−523. Abstract available at: http://www.ncbi.nlm.nih.gov/ pubmed/25274157 (accessed 31 July 2017).

54. Wang AY, Peura DA. The prevalence and incidence of *Helicobacter pylori*−associated peptic ulcer disease and upper gastrointestinal bleeding throughout the world. Gastrointest Endosc Clin N Am. 2011;21(4):613−635. Abstract available at: https://www.ncbi.nlm.nih. gov/pubmed/21944414 (accessed 25 July 2017).

55. Warren JR, Marshall B. Unidentified curved bacilli on gastric epithelium in active chronic gastritis. Lancet. 1983;1(8336):1273−1275. Available at: https://www.ncbi.nlm.nih.gov/ pubmed/6134060 (accessed 10 September 2017).

56. Warren RJ. Reminiscences on *Helicobacter pylori*. Public Health Reviews. 2010;32:10−14. Available at: https://link.springer.com/content/pdf/10.1007/BF03391589. pdf (accessed 27 September 2017).

57. Warren JR. Nobel Lecture: Helicobacter − the ease and difficulty of a new discovery. Nobelprize.org. Nobel Media AB 2014. Available at: http://www.nobelprize.org/nobel_ prizes/medicine/laureates/2005/warren-lecture.html (accessed 2 October 2017).

58. World Health Organization. Initiative for vaccine research: state of the art of new vaccine research and development (*Helicobacter pylori*). Geneva, Switzerland: WHO, 2006. Available at: http://apps.who.int/iris/bitstream/10665/69348/1/WHO_IVB_06.01_eng.pdf; http://www.who.int/vaccine_research/documents/Helicobacter_pylori/en/index.html (accessed 1 September 2017).

59. World Health Organization. Media Centre. Cancer Fact Sheet, February 2018. Available at: http://www.who.int/mediacentre/factsheets/fs297/en/ (accessed 23 February 2018).

60. Zeng M, Mao X-H, Li J-X, Tong W-D, Wang B, Zhang Y-J, et al. Efficacy, safety, and immunogenicity of an oral recombinant *Helicobacter pylori* vaccine in China: a randomised, double-blind, placebo-controlled, phase 3 trial. Lancet. 2015;386 (10002):1457−1464. http://doi.org/10.1016/S0140-6736(15)60310-5. Abstract available at: http://www.ncbi.nlm.nih.gov/pubmed/26142048 (accessed 5 September 2017).

Index

Note: Page numbers followed by "*f*," "*t*," and "*b*" refer to figures, tables, and boxes.

A

Accountable Care Organizations (ACO), 153, 361–362, 377
ACE inhibitors, for cardiovascular diseases, 337–338
Acute flaccid paralysis (AFP), 385–386, 390–391, 393–395, 398, 400
Acute gastroenteritis (AGE), 458–460
Advisory Committee on Immunization Practices (ACIP), 39
Advocacy, 7, 46, 90, 135, 204, 213–214, 218, 266, 290, 432–433, 436, 531–532, 535
Aedes aegypti, and birth defects, 496–497, 501
Affordable Care Act of 2010 (ACA), 152, 154–155, 159, 161, 169–170, 262, 360–362, 365, 377–378
AIDS. *See* HIV/AIDS
Air, Water and Places, Hippocrates, 105–106
Alcohol consumption, and birth defects, 481, 489
Allocation of resources, 134, 162, 166–167, 282, 300, 303, 376
Alpha fetoproteins (AFP), 482–483
Alpha-thalassemia, 425
American Academy of Family Physicians, 340–341
American Academy of Pediatrics (AAP), 158, 238, 456
  delayed intellectual development, 488–489
  genetic disorders, 507
  measles, 39
  vitamin K deficiency bleeding, 408, 413
American Cancer Society, 322
American Civil War, 58–59, 191
American College of Medical Genetics (ACMG), 430–431, 477
American College of Obstetricians and Gynecologists (ACOG), 158
  vitamin K deficiency bleeding, 408, 413
American College of Physicians, 340–341
American Heart Association (AHA)
  cardiovascular diseases, 322, 330, 332–333, 340–341, 343, 346
American Medical Association (AMA), 204
  Council of Food and Nutrition, 188

American Public Health Association (APHA), 204, 322, 358–359
  principles of ethical public health practice, 302–303, 304*b*
American Thyroid Association, 208
Anemia, Cooley's. *See* Beta thalassemia major (BTM)
Anson, Commodore George, 2
Anthrax, 85, 119, 121–123, 306
  vaccines, 103–104, 107–109, 113
Anthrax bacillus, 121
Antibiotics, for peptic ulcer disease, 551, 553
Antimicrobial resistance, 126–127
Antioxidants, 7
Antisepsis, 60–63, 71
Antiseptic techniques, 61–63
Apgar, Virginia, APGAR score, 499
Army Service Medical Corps, 183–184
Arthralgia, 258–259
Ascorbic acid, 7
Aseptic meningitis, 385–386
Asian flu vaccine, 445
Atherosclerosis, 329–330
Attenuation of organisms, 104, 106–107, 112
Attlee, Clement, 143–144
Auto-immune diseases, 450
Avian influenza, 307

B

Bacillus anthracis, 109
Barré-Sinoussi, Françoise, 111
Basket of services, 137, 142
Beneficence, 281
Beriberi, 230
Beta blockers, for cardiovascular diseases, 337–338
Beta thalassemia major (BTM), 423, 427*f*, 493–494
  current relevance, 428–432
  economic issues, 433–434
  ethical issues, 432
  prevalence, 425, 429
  prevention, 429–430, 435
  recommendations for prevention, 435–436
  screening, 427–428, 430–431
Beveridge, Sir William, 132*f*

Beveridge, Sir William (*Continued*)
  Beveridge model National Health Service, 133, 142−144, 361
  Beveridge Report, 143
Bill and Melinda Gates Foundation, 306, 457−458. *See also* Global Alliance for Vaccination Initiatives (GAVI)
  polio eradication, 391−392, 394, 399
  rubella vaccine, 268
  smallpox eradication, 25
  vitamin K deficiency bleeding, 414
Biomedical model
  of causation of disease, 117−130
  in public health, 286−287
Birth defects/disorders, 266
  background, 473−500
  beta thalassemia major, 424, 427*f*
  causes, 479*t*
  current relevance, 500−503
  defined, 473
  economic issues, 505−507, 506*t*
  ethical issues, 503−504
  genomics/genetics and, 507
  hematologic disorders, 493−495
  infectious diseases, 495−497
  management, 497−498
  newborn screening for congenital disorders and follow-up management, 499−500
  nutritional deficiencies and, 474−481
  prenatal prevention, 498−499
  recommendations for prevention, 510−511
  screening and prevention, 471−522
  types, 482−484
Bismarck, Otto von, 132*f*, 141, 169−170
  Bismarckian health system, 141−142, 361
Bizzozero, Giulio, 547
Blane, Gilbert, 3
Bleeding. *See also* Hemorrhage
  vitamin K deficiency and, 407
Blumberg, Baruch, 448−449
Board of Health, 107
Body mass index (BMI), 236, 239
Bordet, Jules, 110
Boston University
  Framingham Heart Study, 320, 322−324, 323*t*
Boussingault, Jean-Baptiste, 2
Bovet, Daniel, 111
Bovine spongiform encephalopathy (BSE), 85
Brazil, Russian Federation, India, China, and South Africa (BRICS)
  vaccine coverage in, 458, 459*t*

British Medical Council (BMC), 230
Breath test for Helicobacter, 123, 548
Broad Street pump
  background, 79−83
  contaminated water, 80, 83, 87−88, 93−94
  current relevance, 84−88
  economic burden and prevention, 91−93
  epidemics, 79−85, 82*t*, 87, 90−91
  ethical issues, 88−91
  Snow, John, cholera epidemic, London, 80−83
  waterborne and infectious diseases and outbreaks, 85−86
  waterborne disease in London's water distribution systems (1854), 82*t*, 83, 84*f*
Brucellosis, 108
Budd, William, typhoid fever, 106

C

Calcium channel blockers, for cardiovascular diseases, 337−338
Campylobacter, 86
Canada Health Act 1984, 146
Canadian Broadcasting Corporation (CBC)
  "The Greatest Canadian", 148−149
Canadian health system, provincial responsibility, 144−149
Cancer
  cervix, 156, 298−299, 446, 450−452, 533
  gastric, 548
  infectious causes, 113
  liver, 448−452, 458
  stomach, 530−531, 548−549, 552−553
Capitation payment system, 141−143, 153, 373*t*
Carbolic acid (phenol), 61−62
Cardiopulmonary resuscitation (CPR), 341
Cardiovascular diseases (CVD)
  background, 318−333
  current relevance, 333−341
  economic issues, 343−345
  epidemiology, 317−356
  ethical issues, 341−343
  morbidity, 329−330
  mortality rate, 327*t*, 328*f*, 331*f*, 332*f*, 333*f*
  prevalence, 337*f*
  and public health importance, 329−330
  risk factors, 319−320, 322−330, 326*t*, 333−340, 337*f*, 342−348
Carter Foundation, 306
Causation of disease

biomedical model, 117–130
  environmental, 123
  genetic, 124–125
  lifestyle, 120, 124–125
  socioeconomic factors, 126
Centers for Disease Control and Prevention
    (CDC), 149–151
  anthrax, 109
  beta thalassemia major, 430–431
  birth defects, 473, 478–481, 505–507
  cardiovascular diseases, 322, 332–333
  cholera, 84, 86
  fetal alcohol syndrome disorder, 489
  healthcare-acquired infections, 70
  HPV vaccine, 298–299
  Legionella, 91
  measles, 38–39
  Morbidity and Mortality Weekly Report
    (MMWR), 157
  *National and State Healthcare-Associated
    Infections Progress Report*, 70
  National Center for Public Health
    Informatics, 157–158
  National Nosocomial Infection
    Surveillance, 65
  Newborn Screening Quality Assurance
    Program, 500
  pellagra, 186–189
  polio, 389–390, 399
  public health ethics, 280
  rickets, 232
  rubella, 262–263, 265–268
  severe acute respiratory syndrome, 148
  smallpox, 21, 23
  syphilis, 124
  vaccines, 457–458
  vitamin K deficiency bleeding, 408–409,
    412
  Zika virus infection, 497
Cerebral palsy (CP), 487–488
Certificate of Need (CON), 358–359,
    367–368
Chicken cholera, vaccines for, 103, 106
Chickenpox vaccine (varicella), 452–453
Childbed (puerperal) fever, Semmelweis,
    60–61
Child health
  birth defects, 473–476, 478–481,
    488–492, 499–506
  immunization, 259–260
  low birth weight, 473–474, 478–481,
    487–490, 507

measles, 41
  nutrition, 38
Chlorination in community water, waterborne
    disease prevention, mortality rates for,
    84*f*
Cholera, 119–123
  background, 79–83
  Broad Street pump, 79–94, 82*t*
  contaminated water and, 80, 83, 87–88,
    93–94
  current relevance, 84–88
  economic burden, 91–93
  epidemics, 79–85, 82*t*, 87, 90–91
  ethical issues, 88–91
  in London's water distribution systems
    (1854), 82*t*, 83, 84*f*
  outbreaks, 86
  prevention, 91–93
  Snow, John, 77–100
  waterborne diseases, 82*t*, 83, 84*f*, 85–86
Chorionic villus testing, 429
Chronic peptic ulcer disease (CPUD), 543
  background, 545–549
  bleeding and perforation, 546*f*
  current relevance, 550–551
  economic issues, 552–553
  ethical issues, 551–552
  H. pylori and, 545, 547–555
  recommendations for prevention, 554–555
  treatment for, 551–553
Churchill, Winston, 143
CINDI (Countrywide Integrated
    Noncommunicable Disease
    Intervention), 329, 335–336, 345
Circulating vaccine-derived poliovirus
    (cVDPV), 392–395
Cleanliness, 60
  in surgery, 62–63
Clinton, Bill, 154, 293–294
Cod liver oil
  antirachitic properties, 231
  Mellanby, Sir Edward, 231
  for rickets/osteoporosis prevention,
    227–256
Committee on Economic, Social, and Cultural
    Rights of the UN Economic and Social
    Council, 92–93
Committee on the Costs of Medical Care, 150
Commonwealth Fund, 163
Commonwealth of Independent States (CIS),
    162
Community rights, 283–286, 284*t*

Community health workers, 22, 49–50, 335, 342–343, 347
Congenital disorders of hemoglobin, 426
Congenital hypothyroidism (CH), 424, 431, 478, 490, 499, 502
Congenital rubella syndrome (CRS), 257–276, 461*b*, 476, 496, 501. *See also* Measles; Rubella
and congenital cataract, 258, 258*f*
current relevance, 261–265
economic issues, 266–268
eradication, 260
recommendations for, 270–271
vaccine, 259–260, 261*f*
Contaminated water, and cholera, 80, 83, 87–88, 93–94
Continuum of health services, 365, 365*f*, 374
Convention on the Rights of the Child, 92–93
Cook, n James, 3
Cooley, Thomas Benton, 423*f*, 425
Cooley's anemia. *See* Beta thalassemia major (BTM)
Cooley's Anemia Foundation, 429–430
Cooperative Commonwealth Federation (CCF), 144–146
Copenhagen Conference, 216
Corn theory, pellagra, 183
Coronary heart disease (CHD), 319, 330
Cost and benefits, 281
Cost constraints, 152, 168
Council of Food and Nutrition (American Medical Association), 188
Cowie, David, 202*f*
iodization of salt, 204
Credé, Carl Franz, 58*f*
opthalmia neonatorum, 59, 63, 66, 69–71
Cretinism, 205–210
Crimean War, 58–59, 63–64
Congenital heart disease (CCHD), 499
Cryptosporidium, 91
Cyprus
Cyprus National Programme for Management of Hepatitis B and AIDS, 426
Cyprus Paediatric Society, 426
Cystic fibrosis (CF), 430, 476, 478, 491–492
Cystic Fibrosis Foundation, 492
Cytomegalovirus (CMV), 496

D

Dam, Henrik, 408*f*
Vitamin K, 408

Dawber, Thomas, Framingham Study, 318*f*
De Contagione (Fracastoro Girolamo), 106
Deafness. *See* Hearing loss
Defibrillation, 341
Delayed intellectual development, 488–489
Dementia, and pellagra, 182, 191
Department of Agriculture US
National School Lunch Program, 150–151, 156
Women, Infant and Children (WIC) program, 156, 159–160
Department of Health and Human Services (US DHHS), 156, 529–530
congenital disorders in newborn, 500
Healthy People 2010, 156
Healthy People 2020, 157–159
Healthy People 2030, 330, 342–343
Office of Minority Health, 157
Depression, and pellagra, 182, 191
Dermatitis, and pellagra, 182, 191
Desalination of seawater, 213
Developmental disabilities, estimated lifetime costs of, 506*t*
Diagnosis-related group (DRG) payment system, 141–142, 153–154, 363–364, 368–369, 372–374
Diagnostic Related Group (DRG) creep, 363
Diarrhea, and pellagra, 182, 191
Diphtheria, 108
Directly Observed Therapy (DOT), 370–371
Disability Adjusted Life Years (DALYs), 167
Disadvantaged, 24–25, 267, 342–343, 506
Disaster planning, 194–195, 308
Disparities in health, 144, 306, 532–533
Disseminated intravascular coagulation in newborn (DIC)
vitamin K deficiency and, 408–411
Doisy, Edward, 408*f*
Vitanin K, 408
Doll, Sir Richard, 319, 482
"Do not resuscitate", 302
Douglas, Honorable Thomas C ("Tommy"), 132*f*, 144–146, 148–149
Down syndrome, 473, 491
DPT (Diphtheria, pertussis, tetanus), 452–453
Drug addiction, and birth defects, 481
"Dying with dignity", 301–302
Dysentery, 87

E

Ebola virus, 85, 306–308, 358, 449, 456–457
Economic issues

of beta thalassemia major, 433−434
of birth defects/disorders, 505−507, 506*t*
of cardiovascular diseases, 343−345
of chronic peptic ulcer disease, 552−553
of congenital rubella syndrome, 266−268
of controlling hospital infections, 70−71
of infectious diseases, 112
of iodine deficiency disorders, 216
of pellagra, 192
of poliomyelitis, 398−399
of rickets, 240−241
of scurvy, 9−10
of smallpox eradication, 24−25
of universal health coverage, 166−168
of vitamin K deficiency bleeding, 414
Economics of health, 357−382
    background, 358−374
    health policy, 375−376
    market forces
        classical, 371−374, 372*b*
        modified, 371−372, 373*t*
        regulatory, 374*b*
    recommendations for, 377−378
Edmonston-Enders strain, 448−449
Edmonston strain, 448−449
Ehrlich, Paul, 117*f*, 119, 121−125
Emergency Medical Service, US, 143
Enders, John, 384*f*, 386−387, 448−449
Enhanced strength inactivated (Salk) vaccine
    (eIPV), 388−389, 392
Environment, 524−528, 535
    physical, 528, 534−535
    social, 528−530, 534−535
Epidemiologic studies, 106, 189−190,
    319−322, 324
Epidemiologic transition, 162, 170, 318−319,
    530−531
Elimination of diseases, 17−21, 39, 41*f*,
    43−46, 48−51, 61, 89, 102−103,
    124−125, 154−157, 184, 201,
    260−265, 268−270, 287−288, 306,
    341, 343−344, 389−390, 392,
    394−399, 423, 450−451, 455,
    458−462, 464, 476, 493, 501−502,
    508, 545, 550, 553−554
Equity, 281
Eradication of diseases, 124−125, 193, 234,
    238−239, 345, 435, 451, 456,
    458−460, 462, 464, 493, 533−534,
    551−553
    of iodine deficiency disorders, 206,
        213−214, 217

of measles, 35, 262−263, 501
of poliomyelitis, 105, 383
of rubella, 260−271, 497−498, 501
of smallpox, 17−34
Erythroblastic anemia. *See* Beta thalassemia
    major (BTM)
Escherichia coli (*E. coli*), 103, 105, 108
    and gastroenteritis, 85−86
Ethical issues
    of beta thalassemia major, 432
    of birth defects/disorders, 503−504
    of cardiovascular diseases, 341−343
    of chronic peptic ulcer disease, 551−552
    of congenital rubella syndrome, 265−266
    of controlling hospital infections, 67−70
    of hospital bed supply/economics of health,
        374−375
    of infectious diseases, 111−112
    of iodine deficiency disorders, 214−215
    of pellagra, 191−192
    of poliomyelitis, 396−398
    of public health, 277−316
    of medical research, 292*t*
    of rickets, 237−240
    of scurvy, 6−8, 8*f*
    of smallpox eradication, 23−24
    of universal health coverage, 164−166
    of vaccines, 454−457
    of vitamin K deficiency
        bleeding, 413−414
Ethical Review Boards (ERBs), 291−293
Ethics, 279−280
    confidentiality, 279
    human rights, 280
    informed consent, 279
    scientific integrity, 280
Eugenics, 286−288, 290*b*
Europe, measles in, 43*b*
European Centers for Disease Prevention and
    Control (ECDC), 453−455
    measles, 44
    healthcare-acquired infections, 65
    rubella, 260
European Society for Pediatric Endocrinology
    (ESPE)
    Consensus Group, 238
European Thyroid Association, 210−212
Euthanasia, 282, 287−288, 290
    versus Sanctity of Life, 301−302
Exercise, 10, 295, 302, 320, 333−334, 339,
    344−346, 528
Evans, Sir Richard, 287

F

Fabrication, 299
Falsification, 299
Familial Mediterranean fever, 489
Federal–Provincial Committee on the Costs
    of Health Services, 147–148
Fee-for-service payment system, 152, 363
Fetal alcohol syndrome disorder (FASD), 481,
    489
Fetal hypothyroidism, 205
Finland, 8, 208, 320, 325–327, 329–330,
    335–336
Fleming, Sir Alexander, 123–124
Foege, William, 22
Folic acid, 282–283, 473–474, 482–483,
    485, 488, 509
    deficiency, 478–482
    fortification, 485–487, 486f, 487f,
        497–498, 502–503, 505–506, 508
    supplementation, 485, 502–503
Food and Agricultural Organization (FAO)
    iodine deficiency disorders, 206–207,
        210–212
    scurvy, 11
    vitamin D deficiency, 237
Food and Drug Administration (US FDA),
    149–150, 157, 185–186
    anthrax, 109
    cardiovascular diseases, 344
    genetic disorders, 507
    neural tube defects, 282–283, 483
    public health ethics, 305
    rubella vaccine, 259–260
    smallpox eradication, 21, 23
    vaccines, 448
Fortification
    folic acid, 270, 297, 302–303, 485–487,
        486f, 487f, 497–498, 502–503,
        505–506, 508
    of foods, 4–5, 7, 9–10, 150, 183,
        185–188, 191–192, 194–195, 214,
        218, 282–283, 305–306, 435, 510
    iodine, 190–192, 204–208, 210, 213–218
    iron, 478–481, 510
    vitamin A, 231, 478–481, 510
    vitamin B complex, 510
    vitamin B12, 510
    vitamin D, 192, 231–232, 236–240,
        242–243, 510
Food and Drug Control Act of 1906 (US)
Fracastoro, Girolamo. *See De contagione*
    (Fracastoro Girolamo)

France, 42, 102–105, 112, 262–263,
    369–370, 425
Framingham Heart Study, 320, 322–324,
    323t, 345, 347
Friendly Societies, 142–143
Funding models for hospitals, 362–364
    DRG payment system, 363–364, 368–369,
        372–374
    fee-for-service method, 363
    historical method, 362–363
    normative method, 364
    per diem payment, 362
Funk, Casimir, vital amines, 2, 183–184,
    193–195, 230

G

Galactosemia, 474–475
Galen, 58–59, 230
Game Theory identification, 376
Gastric cancer, 545, 548–554
Gastroenteritis, 85–86
Gatekeeper function of care givers, 374
Gaucher's disease, 489–490
GAVI, the Vaccine Alliance. *See* Global
    Alliance for Vaccine Initiative (GAVI)
General Motors, 151–152
Genetic diseases, and birth defects, 478, 479t,
    502, 507
Genetic diseases, dominant and
    recessive, 478
Genocide, 288–291, 290b
George, David Lloyd, 142–143
German measles. *See also* Rubella
Germ theory, 36–38, 59–63, 71, 80, 102,
    105–106, 108, 113, 120, 125–126,
    286, 530–531, 535
Giardia, 86
Giardia lamblia, 91
Glisson, Francis, 230
Global Alliance for Vaccine Initiative
    (GAVI), 25, 48–49, 295–296, 306,
    458
    polio eradication, 391–392, 394, 399
    smallpox eradication, 25
    rubella vaccine, 268
Global Burden of Disease study 2017, 167
Global health, 137
Global Measles and Rubella Strategic Plan:
    2012–2020, 458–460, 460b
Global Polio Eradication Initiative (GPEI),
    390–391, 398–399
Global public health ethics, 306–308

Global Working Group of the European Society of Pediatric Endocrinology, 234

Glucose-6-phosphate dehydrogenase deficiency (G6PD), 495

Goiter
endemic, 201
goiter belt, 203

Goldberger, Joseph, 181−186, 181*f*, 187*b*, 188, 193

"Greatest Canadian, The" Tommy Douglas, 148−149

Gregg, Norman McAlister, 257−276, 257*f*

Gross domestic product (GDP), 133, 139, 140*f*, 141−142, 149, 162, 167−168, 368−370

Gross national product (GNP), 147−148

Guthrie, Robert, 472*f*, 474−477, 508−509

Guthrie test, for phenylketonuria, 474−477, 490, 500, 507

H

Hadjiminas, Minas, Cyprus Thalassemia Project, 426

Harmonization of vaccine policy, 457−460, 464

Hand hygiene, 65−67

Haworth, Norman, 4

Hayflick, Leonard, 446
human cell line WI-38 strain, 446−448

Hayflick Limit, in cellular ageing, 446−448

Healthcare-acquired infections (HAI), 64−68, 70−71

Health Care and Education Reconciliation Act of 2010. *See* Affordable Care Act of 2010 (ACA)

Health Care Financing Administration (HCFA), 157, 363

Health care organization, 535

Health expenditures, 140*f*

Health Field, 148

Health Field Concept (HFC), Marc Lalonde, Health Promotion, 524−527, 529−531, 534−535

"Health for All," Alma Ata, 526

Health in All Policies, 529−534

Health indicators, 147*b*, 149*b*

Health information, 157−158

Health insurance, 301

Health Insurance Plan of Greater New York, 152−153

Health insurance population coverage, 155*b*

Health Maintenance Organizations (HMOs), 152−154, 361−362, 365, 377

Health policy, economics and, 375−376

Health Promotion, 133, 135−136, 138, 146−148, 158−161, 166−169, 524−526, 528−529, 532−533, 535
defined, 526

Health Resources and Services Administration US, 477

Health system, defined, 134

Health targets, 158−159

Healthy People 2000, 158−159

Healthy People 2010, 156

Healthy People 2020, 157−159, 334−335, 529−530

Hearing loss, 424
rubella and, 258−259

HeLa cells, 446−448

Helicobacter pylori (*H. pylori*), 123
gastric cancer, 85−86, 545, 548−554
gastritis, 545, 548
peptic ulcer disease, 85−86, 545, 547−555

Helsinki Declaration, 288, 291−293, 310

Helsinki Research Ethics Committees.
See Institutional Review Committees

Hematologic disorders, 493−495

Hemolytic disease of the newborn (HDN), 494

Hemophilus influenza type b (Hib) vaccine, 452−453

Hemorrhage. *See also* Bleeding
intracerebral, 410−411

Hemorrhagic disease of the newborn (HDN), 408−411

Henderson, Donald, 18*f*, 22

Henle, Jacob, 119−120

Henry J. Kaiser Industries, 152−153

Hepatitis A, 85−87

Hepatitis B, 69
immunization, 451−452
vaccine, 454, 458

Hepatitis B surface antigen (HBsAg), 448−449

Hepatitis C, 529
vaccine, 454, 458

Hepatitis E, 85−87

Herd immunity, 126, 450−451

Hetzel, Basil Stuart, 202*f*
iodization of salt, 205−206

High-risk groups, 7, 135−136, 230, 238, 242, 298, 335, 349, 377, 410−411

Hill, Austin Bradford, criteria of causation, 319

Hill Burton Act of 1946, 150–151, 361, 364, 367

Hilleman, Maurice Ralph, 443, 443*f*
Haemophilus influenzae bacteria, 459*t*
hepatitis A, 446–448, 458
hepatitis B, 448–452, 454, 458–460, 464
measles, 448–460, 460*b*
meningitis, 456
MMR, 259–260, 448, 452–456, 458–460
mumps, 448, 450–451
pneumonia, 448, 450, 452–453
rubella, 259–260, 446–448, 450–451, 457–460, 461*b*
vaccines, 38, 443
Hippocrates, 58–59
Historical method of funding to hospitals, 362–363
HIV/AIDS, 85, 124, 137, 298, 495–496, 529, 534
Holmes, Oliver Wendell, 59
Holocaust, 286–291, 301
Home care, 147–148
Hospital bed supply
background, 358–374
costs, 368–371
economics, 368–371
ethical issues, 374–375
management, 364–365, 370*b*
recommendations, 377–378
Roemer's Law, 358–360, 364–365, 367–369, 371–372, 375–378
utilization, 357–382, 369*t*, 370*f*
Hospital infections, controlling, 57–76
background, 58–64
current relevance, 64–67
economic issues, 70–71
ethical issues, 67–70
recommendations for prevention, 71–72
Hospital Insurance and Diagnostic Services Act (Saskatchewan 1946), 145–146
Hospital Trusts UK, 143–144
Host–agent–environment paradigm, 530–531, 530*f*, 531*f*
Human biology, 524–525, 535
Human Development Index (HDI), 139
Human experimentation, 291–294, 292*t*
Human Genome Project, 431–432
Human papillomavirus (HPV) vaccine, 298–299, 451–452
Hurricane Matthew, 84
Hygiene, 63–64, 66–68, 71

Hypertension, and cardiovascular diseases, 342–344
Hyperthyroidism, 258
Hypothyroidism, fetal, 205
Hypovitaminosis D, 240

I

Illinois Pellagra Commission, 189–190
Immunization
for influenza, 67, 69, 156, 169
for measles, 45, 47
parental refusal, 45, 126, 262, 266–267, 269, 298–299, 397, 413, 455–456
routine child immunization, 263, 267
for rubella, 259–260
Immunosuppressive agents, 66–67
Inactivated (Salk) vaccine (IPV), 386–387, 389–390, 392–393, 395–398, 400, 452–453
enhanced strength, 388–389, 392
Inborn errors of metabolism, 431–432, 477, 508
Independent Practice Associations (IPAs), 153–154
Indian Health Service US, 151–152
Individual human rights, 281
Individual rights, 283–286, 284*t*
Inequalities, 144, 159, 165–166, 168–169
Infantile paralysis, poliomyelitis, 385–386
Infections, and birth defects, 479*t*
Infectious diseases, 105–108, 113
current relevance, 109–111
during pregnancy, 495–497
economic issues, 112
ethical issues, 111–112
Influenza, 67, 69, 85, 156, 169, 307–308, 386–387, 445, 448, 452, 457
Informed consent, 279
Inoculation (variolation), for smallpox, 19
Institute of Clinical and Economic Review (US ICER), 507
Institute of Medicine (US IOM), 236
cardiovascular diseases, 344
public health ethics, 305
Institutional Review Boards (IRBs), 288, 291–293
Institutional Review Committees (IRCs), 288, 300
Integration of health services, 365, 366*f*
lateral, 371, 377
vertical, 365, 366*f*, 377

Intellectual (IQ) deprivation, maternal iodine deficiency and, 502
Intellectual impairment, 207, 488–491
International Agency for Research in Cancer (IARC)
  chronic peptic ulcer disease, 548–549
International Bill of Human Rights, 92–93
International Classification of Disease (ICD 9, ICD10), 409
International Conference on Health Promotion, 528
International Council for Control of Iodine Deficiency Disorders, 205, 210–212
International Health Regulations, 306
International Monetary Fund (IMF), 376
International Thalassemia Federation (ITF), 429
Intracerebral hemorrhage (ICH), vitamin K deficiency and, 410–411
Iodine
  endemic goiter and elimination, 201
    economic issues, 216
    ethical issues, 214–215
    historical milestones, 211*b*
    recommendations for, 218
  fortification, 204–208, 210, 213–218
  and intellectual deprivation, 502
  levels, monitoring, 218
  public health severity, assessment criteria for, 207*t*
  recommended dietary allowances for, 213*t*
  spectrum, 209*t*
  supplemention, 218
    during pregnancy, 484
Iodine Global Network, 213–214, 218
Iodization of salt, 204–206, 210–214, 216
  universal, 209–210, 214–215, 218
Iodized salt
  access to, in low -and lower-middle-income countries, 205–214
  Cowie, David, 204
  Hetzel, Basil, 205–206
  Marine, David, 203–204
Iron supplementation, during pregnancy, 485
Israel
  Central Virus Laboratory, 396
  hospital bed supply, 369–370
  polio eradication, 396

J
Jacob, François, 111
Jenner, Edward, 17–34, 18*f*

Jeryl Lynn, mumps virus, 444*f*, 448
Johnson, President Lyndon B, 132*f*, 151, 169–170, 361

K
Kaiser Permanente system, 152–153, 365, 377
Kannel, William, Framingham Study, 318*f*
Karrer, Paul, 4
Katz, Samuel L., 448–449
Kennedy, John F., 322
Keys, Ancell, 319–320
Kiwanis International, 210–212
Koch, Robert, 59, 83, 103–104, 107, 112, 117*f*, 119–122, 124–125
Koch–Henle postulates, 59, 120, 122–123, 548
Koop, Everett, 204–205

L
Lalonde, Hon. Marc, 524, 524*f*, 526–528, 530–531, 534–536
Laudable pus, 58–59, 61
Laveran, Charles Louis, 110
Legionella, 91
Length-of-stay (LOS), 365
  average, 368
Levin, Simon, 203
Life expectancy, 139*t*
  at birth, 163*f*
Life of Louis Pasteur, The, 108
Lifestyle, 524–525, 527–528, 530–531, 535
Lind, James, 1*f*, 105
  clinical epidemiologic experiment, 3–4
  HMS Salisbury, 2
  Royal Navy, 2–3
  scurvy, 1–16
Lions Club International
  rubella vaccine, 268
Lister, Lord Joseph, 58*f*, 59–63, 69–71, 108–110
Listeria, 103, 105
Live attenuated vaccines, 105
London's water distribution systems (1854), waterborne diseases in, 82*t*, 84*f*
Long-term care (LTC), 65, 69, 240, 329, 332–333, 361, 364, 370–371, 376, 499–500
Low -and middle-income countries (LMICs)
  vaccine coverage in, 457–458
Low-density lipoprotein (LDL), 7

Lwoff, André, 111
Lynn, Jeryl
  mumps virus, 448
Lyophilization, 22

M

Magic Bullets, 121–122, 124–126
Magna Carta, 279
Mahler, Halfdan, 20–21
Mal de rosa, pellagra, 182
Managed care, 153–154
Mandatory
  driving regulations, 282
  helmet, 51
  immunizations, 282
  seat belts, 215, 283–286, 334–335
Mandatory health insurance (MHI), 162
Maple syrup urine disease (MSUD), 474–475
March of Dimes (MOD), 430–431
  birth defects, 502
  low birth weight, 268
Marine, David, 202*f*, 203–204
Market forces in health
  classical, 371–374, 372*b*
  modified, 371–372, 373*t*
  regulatory, 374*b*
Marmot, Sir Michael, 319, 532
Marshall, Barry J., 544*f*, 545, 547–548, 554
Maternal and Child Health Bureau US, 477
Maternal infections, and birth defects, 478
Maternal mortality, 60–61, 67–68, 71
  rates, 68
Maternal smoking, and birth defects, 481
McCollum, Elmer, 227–256, 228*f*
Measles, 35, 125
  background, 36–39
  current relevance, 39–47
  economic issues, 48–49
  eradication, 50
  ethical issues, 47–48
  in Europe, 43*b*
  German. *See* Rubella
  immunization, 45
  recommendations for prevention, 51
  transmission, 66, 69–70
  vaccination, 38, 38*f*, 40*f*, 41, 41*f*, 45,
    47–48, 448, 453–454, 458–460,
    460*b*
Measles-containing vaccine (MCV), 38*f*, 40,
  44–45
Medécins sans Frontiére (MSF), 306
Media coverage of health-related topics, 158

Medicaid, 151, 154–157, 159, 359–361, 378
Medical research, ethical issues of, 292*t*
Medicare, 146, 148–149, 151, 154–155, 159,
  165, 365, 367, 378
Mediterranean anemia, 425, 493
Medium- and low-income countries
  universal health coverage, 133, 135, 137,
    149, 163–164, 167–168, 170
Melanpus, 2
Mellanby, Edward, 227–256, 228*f*
Meningitis, 456
Mental defects, Iodine deficiency and, 207
Men who have sex with men (MSM), 298
Merck & Company, 445, 448
Metabolic syndrome, 336
Metchnikoff, Ilya, 110
Methicillin-resistant *Staphylococcus aureus*
  (MRSA), 65, 69
Meyer, Harry, 259–260
Miasma theory, 36–38, 58–60, 63–64, 80,
  106, 120, 286, 535
Microcephaly, 488
Micronutrient deficiencies (MNDs), 4, 6–7, 10
  iodine deficiency disorders, 218
  pellagra, 191–192, 194–195
Micronutrient Initiatives (MIs), 213
Migrant health, 432–433, 493
Military health coverage, 151–152
Millennium Development Goals (MDGs),
  165, 169–170, 526, 532, 534–536
  birth defects, 474
  child mortality rates, 67–68, 473–474, 534
  cholera, 90, 94–95
  congenital rubella syndrome, 266
  maternal mortality rates, 68
  MDG 4, 412–413
  public health ethics, 306
  rickets, 233–234
  waterborne diseases, 93
Minority rights, 156–157, 284*t*
Mixed public–private health insurance
  systems, 149–161
MMR (Measles, Mumps, Rubella) vaccine,
  38, 45, 48, 50, 259–263, 265,
  267–269, 297, 448, 452–456,
  458–460
Modell, Bernadette
  thalassaemia epidemiology, 426
MONICA (Multinational MONItoring of
  trends and determinants in
  CArdiovascular disease), 320, 329,
  335, 345

Monod, Jacques, 111
Montagnier, Luc, 111
Montagu, Lady Mary, 19
Moraten strain of measles virus, 38
Morbidity and Mortality Weekly Report
    (MMWR), 157
Morris, Jeremy, 319
MPOWER program, WHO Framework
    Convention on Tobacco Control, 334
Muni, Paul, 105, 108

N

National Academy of Science, Institute of
    Medicine, 158
National Center for Health Statistics (US
    NCHS), 156–157
National Center for Public Health Informatics
    (US NCPHI), 157–158
National Health and Nutrition Examination
    Survey (US NHANES), 8, 208, 295
National health expenditures, 360t
National health insurance, 133, 135, 141–143,
    145–152, 154, 159, 169–170
National Health Insurance Act, 142–143
National Health Service (NHS, Britain), 65,
    133, 142–144, 159–160, 169–170,
    299, 375, 533–534
National health systems, 137–140, 163,
    165–168, 170
  elements of, 136b
  rationale for, 138b
National Heart, Lung, and Blood Institute (US
    NHLBI), 322–323
  cardiovascular diseases, 322–323
  coronary heart disease, 338
  Framingham Heart Study, 320, 322–324,
    323t
National Human Genome Research Institute
    (US NCHGR), 507
National Immunization Days (NIDs),
    389–392, 394
National Institute for Health and Care
    Excellence (UK NICE), 533–534
National Institutes of Health (US NIH),
    149–151, 157, 320, 361
  Framingham Heart Study, 320, 322–324,
    323t
  Office of Dietary Supplements, 234–235,
    234t
  scurvy, 7
National Insurance Act of 1946 (UK),
    143–144

National Nosocomial Infection Surveillance
    (CDC NNIS), 65
National Nutrition Conference for Defense
    (US 1941), President Franklin D.
    Roosevelt, 186–187
National Nutrition Survey, US
    NHANES–National Health and
    Nutrition Examination Survey, 148
National School Lunch Program, US
    Department of Agriculture, 150–151
National Tuberculosis Association, 322
Neonatal mortality, 68, 473–474, 494–495,
    504
Neosalvarsan, syphilis, 122
Neural tube defects (NTDs), 282–283, 473,
    477, 482–487, 487f, 508–509
  prevalence, 486f
  prevention, 497–498, 502–503, 505–506,
    509
Newborns
  for congenital disorders and follow-up
    management, 499–500
  Newborn screening (NBS), 474–478, 492,
    497, 507–508
  for phenylketonuria, 477, 499, 509
  Vitamin K deficiency bleeding prevention
    in, 407
Newborn Screening Quality Assurance
    Program (US NSQAP), 500
Newborn Screening Saves Lives, US Act of
    2007, 430–431
Newborn Screening Saves Lives US Act of
    2008, 477
New Deal, President Franklin D Roosevelt, 150
New Perspective on Health of Canadians,
    Marc Lalonde, 148, 524–525,
    527–530, 532, 534–535
New Public Health, The, 308, 376, 535
New York State Department of Health, 409
New York State Public Health Council, 411
Nicolle, Charles Jules Henri, 111
Nightingale, Florence, 58f, 59, 63–64, 69–71
Nobel Prize for Medicine and Physiology
  Dam, Henrik, 408, 408f
  Doisy, Edward, 408, 408f
  Ehrlich, Paul, 117f
  Enders, John Franklin, 38, 384f
  Koch, Robert, 83, 117f, 119–122
  Marshall, J. Barry, 544f, 545
  Warren, Robin J., 544f, 545
Noncommunicable diseases (NCDs),
    320–321, 325, 327, 333–335, 348

Nongovernmental organizations (NGOs), 157
Noninvasive infection-resistant methods, 65–66
Nonmalfeasance, 281
Nontariff barriers to health, 165–166, 169
Normative method of funding to hospitals, 364
North Karelia Project, 320, 325–327, 326*t*,
　　327*t*, 328*f*, 329, 335–336, 345,
　　347–348
Nosocomial infections, 65, 70–71
Nuremberg trials, 288, 291, 292*t*, 310
Nutritional deficiencies, and birth defects,
　　474–481, 479*t*
Nutritional epidemiology, 2–3, 7, 181

O

Obama, President Barack, 132*f*, 152,
　　154–155, 159, 169–170
Obamacare. *See* Affordable Care Act of 2010
　　(ACA)
Ocular prophylaxis, 66
Office of Minority Health (US OMH), 157
Ophthalmic infection of newborns, *opthalmia
　　beonatorum*, 63
Oral live (Sabin) attenuated vaccine (OPV,
　　oral polio vaccine), 387–398, 400
Oral rehydration therapy (ORT), for diarrheal
　　diseases, 91–92
Organization for Economic Cooperation and
　　Development (OECD), 139, 146,
　　160–161, 166, 170, 336, 346, 368
Osteomalacia, 229, 232, 234, 237–243
Osteoporosis, vitamin D deficiency and,
　　229–230, 234–237, 239–243
Ottawa Charter, 124–125, 148, 526, 528–529
Out-of-pocket spending, 163–164

P

Palestinian Ministry of Health
　polio eradication, 396
Pan American Health Organization (PAHO),
　　46, 87, 263–264, 524, 527
Panum, Peter Ludwig, 37–38, 38*f*, 47,
　　50–51, 106
　measles epidemiology, Faroe Island, 36–37
Paramyxovirus, 36
Parkman, Paul, 259–260
Pasteur, Louis, 59–63, 101, 101*f*, 119
　discoveries, 110*b*
Pasteur, Sanofi, 449
Pasteur Institute (*Institut Pasteur*), 102,
　　104–105, 110–111, 113

Patient care ethics, 300–301
Patient-Centered Medical Home (US PCMH),
　　153
Patient Protection and Affordable Care Act,
　　US. *See* Affordable Care Act of 2010
　　(ACA)
Patients' rights, 300–301
Pauling, Linus, 7
Pasterization, 103, 105, 108, 112
Pay for Performance systems, 372–374
Peebles, Samuel, 38
Pellagra, Goldberger, Joseph, 181
　background, 182–190
　current relevance, 190–191
　deaths by sex, 185*f*
　economic issues, 192
　ethical issues, 191–192
　outbreaks in emergency-affected
　　populations, 190*t*
　recommendations for, 195–196
Peptic ulcer disease, chronic. *See* Chronic
　　peptic ulcer disease (CPUD)
Per diem payment, 153, 362
Personal belief exemption (PBE), 47–48
Personal responsibility, 284*t*
Phenylketonuria (PKU), 424, 431, 477–478,
　　490, 500–501
　blood screening test for, 474–475
　Guthrie test for, 474–477, 490, 500, 507
　newborn screening for, 477, 499, 509
Physician-aided suicide, 301
Plagiarism, 300
Plotkin, Stanley, 259–260
　rubella virus, 259–260
Pneumococcal vaccine, 448, 452, 453*f*
Polio eradication, 125, 383, 386*f*
Poliomyelitis, 383
　background, 385–392
　current relevance, 392–396
　economic issues, 398–399
　ethical issues, 396–398
　recommendations eradication, 399–400
　vaccines. *See* Inactivated (Salk) vaccine
　　(IPV); Oral live (Sabin) attenuated
　　vaccine (OPV, oral polio vaccine)
Polysaccharide vaccine, 448
Population health, 7–8, 10, 50, 112, 133, 137,
　　146–147, 149–150, 159, 165,
　　167–169, 283, 286, 294–295, 300,
　　302, 307, 318–319, 334–335,
　　339–340, 368–370, 374, 508, 527,
　　535–536

Population Health Management System
    (PHMS), 153
Postsurgery infections, 61
Poverty, and cardiovascular diseases, 330
Precautionary Principle, 281
Preferred Provider Organizations (US PPOs),
    153−154
Pregnancy, and rubella, congenital rubella
    syndrome, 258−259, 261−262,
    264−265, 270
Premature births, cytomegalovirus and, 496
Prenatal prevention, of birth defects/disorders,
    498−499
Prepaid group practice (US PGP), 152−153
Preventive Services Task Force, US, 156
Private health insurance (PHI), 141−142
Proportionality, 281
Proton pump inhibitors (PPI), for chronic
    peptic ulcer disease, 551
Public health, 182−186, 188−189, 191−195
    ethics. *See* Public health ethics
    importance, 329−330
    scurvy, 2, 4, 6−7, 9−10
Public health emergency of international
    concern (PHEIC), 501
Public health ethics, 277−316, 281*b*
    eugenics, 290*b*
    global, 306−308
    human experimentation, 291−294, 292*t*
    imperative to act or not act, 302−306
    individual and community rights, 283−286,
        284*t*
    patient care, 300−301
    principles, 281*b*, 304*b*
    in recent decades, 296−306
    recommendations for, 308−309
    research misconduct, definition of, 299−300
    research, 294−296
    successes and failures, 286−291
    teaching, 307−308
Pucini, Filipo, 83
Puerperal fever, 59−60
Puska, Pukka, North Karelia Project, 318*f*,
    325, 327

Q

Quality Adjusted Life Years (QALYs), 167

R

Rabies, 102, 112−113
    vaccine, 102, 104−105, 107−109

Racial and Ethnic Adult Disparities in
    Immunization Initiative, 156
Randomized control trial (RCT), 3−4
Rationing, 374−375
Reasonableness, 281
Recessive diseases, 478
Reciprocity, 281
Recommended dietary allowances (RDAs), for
    iodine, 213*t*
Red Cross, International, 90−91
Reform, 65, 70, 107, 142−145, 147−149,
    154−155, 170, 303, 333−334,
    361−362, 364
Regional Health Authorities, 143−144
Report of the Committee on Scientific
    Inquiries in Relation to the Cholera
    Epidemic of 1854, 80
Research misconduct, definition of, 299−300
Resources, 9−10, 48, 50, 64−65, 90, 134,
    144, 162−168, 240, 267, 282,
    299−300, 302−303, 308−309,
    338−339, 362−364, 367−370, 376,
    378, 399−400, 526−528, 551
Respiratory distress syndrome (RDS), vitamin
    K deficiency and, 410−411
Responsibility to act, 281
Responsive to needs, 281
Rickets, 227−256
    current situation, 232−237
    economic issues, 240−241
    ethical issues, 237−240
    history, 230−231
Risk factors, Framingham study, 323−324,
    345, 348, 524−525
Rockefeller Foundation, 185−186
Roemer, Milton, 358−359, 358*f*, 361−362
Roemer's Law, 358−360, 364−365,
    367−369, 371−372, 375−378
Roosevelt, Eleanor, 279*f*
Roosevelt, Franklin D., 150, 186−187, 204
Rotary Club International, 25, 306
    polio eradication, 391, 394, 399
Rotavirus, 86
    and gastroenteritis, 85−86, 88
    vaccines, 88−89
Royal Commission on Health Services (Canada
    "Hall Commission"), 145−146
Royal Navy, 2−3
Rubella, 259*f*, 461*b*. *See also* Congenital
    rubella syndrome (CRS); Measles
    during pregnancy, 258, 261−262
    vaccine, 259−262, 261*f*

Rubella-containing vaccine (RCV), 263–264, 269
Rubin, Benjamin, Rubin needle, 22
Russian health system, 161–163

S

Sabin, Albert Bruce, 384f, 386–388, 449
Sabin live attenuated polio vaccine (OPV), 387–398, 400
Salisbury HMS, 2
Salk, Jonas, 384f, 386–387, 449
Salk inactivated (killed) polio vaccine IPV, 446
Salvarsan, 122–124
Sambon, Louis W., 183
Sanctity of Human Life (*Pikuah Nefesh*), 280–281
    versus euthanasia, 301–302
Sanitary Movement, 105–106, 120
Saskatchewan Hospital and Diagnostic Services Act, 1946, 145–146
School lunch programs, 156
Scurvy, 230
    background, 2–4
    clinical epidemiologic experiment, 3–4
    current relevance, 4–6
    dietary deficiency, 8, 10
    economic issues, 9–10
    ethical issues, 6–8, 8f
    investigation, 2–3
    Lind, James, 1–16
    recommendations for prevention, 11–12
    Royal Navy (British), 2–3
Self-esteem, and cardiovascular diseases, 330
Semashko, Nikolai, 132f, 161–163
Semmelweis, Ignaz, 58f, 62–63, 108
Sepsis, vitamin K deficiency and, 410–411
Seven Countries Study, 319–320
Severe acute respiratory syndrome (SARS), 85, 145, 148, 306, 527–528
Sexually transmitted diseases (STDs), 495–496
Sheppard-Towner Act of 1921, 150
Shigella, and gastroenteritis, 85–86
Sick Funds (*Krankenkassen*), 141–142, 169–170, 361
Sickle cell disease (SCD), 424, 426, 430–431, 435, 476, 478, 494
Sleeping sickness, 183
"Slippery Slope", the, 277–316
Smallpox, Edward Jenner, 125
    vaccination, 17–34

    economic issues, 24–25
    ethical issues, 23–24
    inoculation (variolation) for, 19
Snow, John, 78f, 80, 106, 119
    Broad Street pump, 79–94, 82t
    cholera epidemic, 77–100
    waterborne diseases, 82t, 83, 84f, 85–86
Social hygiene movement, 286
Social inequities, 155–157, 161
Social Insurance and Health Services, 143
Social Security Act of 1935 (SSA), 150, 169–170, 361
    Title XVII, 151
    Title XIX, 151
Socioeconomic status (SES), and cardiovascular diseases, 330
Solidarity principle, 281
Soranus, 230
Soviet health system, 299, 364
Spanish flu pandemic 1918, 445
Spontaneous generation, 102, 106
Stanford Community Study, 320, 327–328
Stanford School of Medicine, 325–326
State Children's Health Insurance Program (SCHIP), 151
Statutory Health Insurance (SHI), 141–142
Stereochemistry, 102
Sterile techniques, 63
Sterilization, 61–63, 65–66, 286–288, 290
Stewardship, 281
Stillbirths, 474
    iodine deficiency and, 207
Streptococcal infection, in childbirth, 60–61
Stroke, cerebrovascular disease, 321, 330, 338–340, 343
"Stroke Belt" USA, The, 330–331
Structural birth defects, 502
Stunted growth, iodine deficiency and, 207
Subacute Sclerosing Pan Encepahalitis (SSPE), measles, 38–39
Supplementary/special immunization activities (SIAs), 390–396, 398–399
Surgery
    cleanliness in, 62–63
    postsurgery infections, 61
Surgical site infections (SSI), 70
Sustainable Development Goals (SDGs), 133, 165, 169, 194, 415, 526, 532, 534–536
    birth defects, 474
    cholera, 94–95
    of congenital rubella syndrome, 266

measles, 45, 49−51
  public health ethics, 306
  waterborne diseases, 93
Syphilis, 59, 121−126
Szent-Györgyi, Albert, 4
Szmuness, Wolf, 448−449

T

Tay−Sachs disease, 431, 491
Terry, Luther, Surgeon General, 322
Thalassemia, 423, 478. *See also* Alpha-
  thalassemia; Beta thalassemia major
  (BTM)
Thalidomide, 481
That Mothers Might Live, 108
Thompson−McFadden Pellagra Commission,
  183−184, 189−191
Thyroid deficiency, 207
Thyroid stimulating hormone (TSH),
  206−207
Tobacco Framework Convention on Tobacco
  Control, 341−342
Townsend, CW, 408
Toxoplasmosis, 496
Transfats, 333−334, 341, 344
Transparency, 281
Treponema pallidum, 121
Triple oral polio vaccine (TOPV), 388−389,
  395−396
Trotter, Thomas, 3
Truman, President Harry S., 150−151, 361
Trump, President Donald, 159
Trust, 281
Trypanosomiasis, 183
Tryptophan deficiency, 182
Tuberculosis (TB), 103, 105, 108, 120−124,
  127
Tuskegee experiment, 293−294, 294*b*, 310
Tuskegee experiment, syphilis, ethics,
  293−294, 294*b*
Typhoid fever, 87
  mortality rates for, 84*f*

U

UK General Medical Council
  polio eradication, 397
UK National Screening Committee
  beta thalassemia major, 431
UN Convention on Prevention and
    Punishment of the Crime of Genocide
    (UNPPCG), 289

UN Declaration of the Rights of Disabled
    Persons, 503
UN Declaration of the Rights of the Child,
    503
UN Economic and Social Council
  Committee on Economic, Social, and
    Cultural Rights, 92−93
UNICEF, 306
  genocide, 289
  Global Vaccine Alliance, 458
  iodine deficiency disorders, 207, 210−212,
    214, 218
  polio eradication, 391−392, 394
  rubella vaccine, 268
  vitamin D deficiency, 237
  vitamin K deficiency bleeding, 412, 414
Uninsured, 152, 154−157, 159−160, 296
United Kingdom Childhood Cancer Study,
    411
United Nations, 92*b*
  cholera, 85
  human rights to water and sanitation, 92*b*
  Millennium Development Goals, 67−68,
    90, 93−95, 165, 169−170, 233−234,
    266, 306, 412−413, 473−474, 526,
    532, 534−536
  Sustainable Development Goals, 45,
    49−51, 93−95, 133, 165, 169, 194,
    266, 306, 415, 474, 526, 532,
    534−536
Universal access, 133−135, 149, 155−156,
    159−163, 165, 167−168, 170−171
Universal Declaration of Human Rights, 164,
    279, 281, 292*t*, 310
  Article 25, 164
Universal health coverage (UHC), 131−180
  background, 133−163
  Beveridge system, 133, 142−144
  Bismarckian system, 141−142
  building blocks for, 134*b*
  Canadian system, 144−149
  changing US health care environment,
    151−155
  current relevance, 163−164
  defined, 138
  economic issues, 166−168
  ethical issues, 164−166
  management, 166−168
  Medicaid, 151
  Medicare, 151
  national health systems, 138−140
  reform pressures and initiatives, 147−149

Universal health coverage (UHC) (*Continued*)
  Russian system, 161–163
  US mixed public–private health insurance
    systems, 149–161
Universal health insurance (UHI), 166–167
Universal salt iodization (USI), 209–210,
    214–215, 218
US AID, 214
US Department of Health and Human
    Services, 156, 529–530
  congenital disorders in newborn, 500
  Healthy People 2010, 156
  Healthy People 2020, 157–159
  Healthy People 2030, 330, 342–343
  Office of Minority Health, 157
US health care system
  challenges and strengths, 160*b*
  environment, changing, 151–155
  health information, 157–158
  health targets, 158–159
  social inequities, 155–157
US pellagra epidemic, 181
US Preventive Services Task Force
    (USPSTF), 158, 531–532
  cardiovascular diseases, 335, 338
US Public Health Service (USPHS),
    156–158, 184, 262, 293–296, 361
US Public Health Service Commissioned
    Corps (USPHS), 149–150
US STOP program, 392
US Surgeon General, 149–150, 157
  Healthy People, 158–159
  Report on Smoking, 524–525, 527

V

Vaccination Assistance Act of 1962, 259–260
Vaccination refusals, problem of, 303
Vaccine-associated paralytic poliomyelitis
    (VAPP), 389–390, 390*f*, 392–396
Vaccine-derived poliomyelitis, (VDPV),
    389–390, 397
  circulating, 392–395
Vaccine-preventable diseases (VPDs), 67,
    261–262, 267, 270
Vaccines, 443
  anthrax, 103–104, 107–109, 113
  Asian flu, 445
  background, 444–449
  chicken cholera, 103, 106
  current relevance, 449–454
  economic implications, 457–461, 459*t*,
    460*b*, 461*b*
  ethical issues, 454–457

  measles, 38, 38*f*, 45, 448
  MMR, 38, 45, 48, 50, 259–263, 265,
    267–269, 297
  pneumococcal pneumonia, 448
  polysaccharide, 448
  rabies, 102, 104–105, 107–109
  rotavirus, 88–89
  rubella-containing, 263–264, 269
  timeline of development or licensure, 447*t*
  varicella, 452–453
  using WI-38 cells, 446–448
Vaccinology, 105, 112, 448–449, 454, 464
van Leeuwenhoek, Anton, microscope, 106
Varicella vaccine, 452–453
Veterans Administration (VA), 150–152
Veterans Affairs Department, 149–150
Vibrato cholera (*V. cholera*), 79, 83, 87, 92
Vibrio, 85
Vibrio cholerae, 120
Vibrio cholera pucini, 83
Vienna Lying-in Hospital, 59–60
Virchow, Rudolf, 60, 106, 120, 532
Vital amines, 2, 4, 183, 194–195, 230
Vitamin B3 (niacin) deficiency, 182, 188
Vitamin C, 4–5
  deficiency, 5–7, 10
  supplementation, during pregnancy, 485
Vitamin D, 4
  deficiency, and rickets/osteoporosis
    prevention, 227–256
  recommended daily intake, 234–235, 234*t*
  supplementation, during pregnancy,
    484–485
Vitamin K
  intramuscular (IM) administration, 411
  prophylaxis, 408, 411–415
Vitamin K deficiency bleeding (VKBD),
    494–495, 501–502, 504
  current relevance, 411–413
  economic issues, 414
  ethical issues, 413–414
  prevention, in newborns, 407
  stages, 409
von Liebig, Justus, 230

W

Wagner-Murray-Dingell Bill (US 1946),
    150–151
Wakefield, Andrew
  Wakefield Effect, 42–44, 296, 297*b*
Wald, Sir Nicholas, 472*f*, 482–483, 508–509
Walsh, Barry, 123
War Order Number One, 186–187, 204

Warren, J. Robin, 123, 544*f*, 545, 547−548, 554
Waterborne diseases, 77−100
cholera, 85−86
Helicobacter pylori, 85−86
London, 82*t*, 84*f*
rotavirus, 85−86
Weapons of mass destruction (WMD), 22−23
Welfare state, 133
West Bank, polio eradication, 395−396
WI-38 cells, 446−448
Wild poliovirus (WPV), 388−398, 400
types, 395−396
Wistar Institute, 446−448
Women, Infants and Children (USDA WIC) program, 156, 159−160
Woodall, John, 2
World Bank, 166, 306
Global Vaccine Alliance, 458
health expenditure, 376
iodine deficiency disorders, 209−212, 214, 216−218
smallpox eradication, 25
vaccines, 457−458
vitamin K deficiency bleeding, 414
World Health Assembly (WHA), 206
antimicrobial resistance, 126−127
beta thalassemia major, 426
birth defects, 509
of congenital rubella syndrome, 266
measles, 39−40
polio eradication, 393
smallpox eradication, 21−23
Tobacco Framework Convention on Tobacco Control, 341−342
World Health Organization (WHO), 164, 166, 533−534
beta thalassemia major, 426−428, 434−435, 493
birth defects, 473−474, 478−481
cardiovascular diseases, 333−334, 336, 341−343
cholera, 84, 90−91, 93−94
chronic peptic ulcer disease, 548−549, 551−552

CINDI, 329, 335−336, 345
Framework Convention on Tobacco Control (FCTC), 344−345
Global Measles and Rubella Strategic Plan: 2012−2020, 49−50, 458−460, 460*b*
Global Task Force on Cholera Control, 90, 93−94
healthcare-acquired infections, 64−65
"Health for All", 526
health system, defined, 134
iodine deficiency disorders, 205−207, 210−214
measles, 36, 39−40, 44−45
MONICA, 320, 329, 335, 345
MPOWER program, 334
pellagra, 190−191
polio eradication, 389−392, 394−400
rotavirus vaccines, 88
rubella vaccine, 262−269
scurvy, 7, 11
smallpox eradication, 21−23, 25−26
Strategic Advisory Group of Experts on Immunization, 49−50, 399−400
2016 Midterm Review of the Global Vaccine Action Plan, 265
vaccines, 449, 456−457
vitamin D deficiency, 237
vitamin K deficiency bleeding, 412−413
World Health Report, 134
Zika virus infection, 497, 501
World Health Organization European Region, Health for All Database, 8*f*, 163*f*, 331*f*, 332*f*, 370*f*
World Health Report, 134
World Heart Federation, 340
World Medical Association, 288
World Summit for Children (1990), 206, 210−212
Wound healing, 58−59

Z
Zidovudine (AZT), 295−296
Zika virus, 85, 270, 306, 358, 449, 456−457, 496−497, 501

Printed in the United States
By Bookmasters